Ex Libris

SHERWYN M. WOODS
M.D.

OXFORD MEDICAL PUBLICATIONS

HENDERSON AND GILLESPIE'S
TEXTBOOK
OF PSYCHIATRY

HENDERSON AND GILLESPIE'S

TEXTBOOK

OF PSYCHIATRY

FOR
STUDENTS AND PRACTITIONERS

NINTH EDITION

Revised by

SIR DAVID HENDERSON
M.D., D.Sc., LL.D., F.R.C.P., F.R.F.P.S.G.
Professor Emeritus of Psychiatry, University of Edinburgh

AND

IVOR R. C. BATCHELOR
M.B., Ch.B., F.R.C.P.E., D.P.M., F.R.S.E.
Physician Superintendent, Dundee Royal Mental Hospital;
Lecturer and Head of Department of Psychiatry,
University of St. Andrews

LONDON
OXFORD UNIVERSITY PRESS
NEW YORK   TORONTO
1962

Oxford University Press, Amen House, London E.C.4

GLASGOW NEW YORK TORONTO MELBOURNE WELLINGTON
BOMBAY CALCUTTA MADRAS KARACHI LAHORE DACCA
CAPE TOWN SALISBURY NAIROBI IBADAN ACCRA
KUALA LUMPUR HONG KONG

First Edition 1927
Ninth Edition 1962

Printed in Great Britain

In respectful and affectionate remembrance
of
ADOLF MEYER (1866–1950), M.D., LL.D.
Professor of Psychiatry and Director of the
Henry Phipps Psychiatric Clinic
Johns Hopkins Hospital, Baltimore

*

His imaginative leadership instituted a new era
in psychiatric thought and practice

CONTENTS

PREFACE TO THE NINTH EDITION

Since the previous edition of this textbook was published the progress of psychiatry has undergone many changes which have altered or modified its genetic, social, clinical, pharmacological, psychological and legal aspects. We have endeavoured to keep abreast of the new developments and have selected for incorporation in this edition whatever has seemed to us to be sufficiently well validated. Our main object is to provide our readers with a reliable guide so that they may pursue their psychiatric studies and practice not only with interest and enthusiasm, but with a critical outlook as well. That is why we continue to emphasize the paramount importance of the psychological factor, however it may have been determined, in influencing every type of illness, bodily or mental. The one reverberates on the other and it is the knowledge of that fact which means so much not only in the treatment of the specific disorder, but in coming to an understanding of the total personality. Psychiatry is not a narrow specialty but forms such an essential component part of general medicine that its principles should permeate and be taught throughout the entire medical curriculum. In our attempt to implement that viewpoint we have throughout this edition stressed the immense medico-social problems with which psychiatry has to deal, and the need for much more intensive teaching and research. This has led to the introduction of a new chapter dealing with the interrelationship of psychiatry and general medicine, and to the rewriting of those sections dealing with history, classification, aetiology, neuroses, sexual anomalies, schizophrenia, certain organic affections of the nervous system, and mental subnormality.

The new Mental Health Acts (1959–1960) applicable to the United Kingdom are now in operation. They mark a further advance in the understanding of mental illness which should lead to many beneficial changes in hospital administration and in the treatment of patients; the chapter dealing with Psychiatry and the Law has been brought into conformity therewith.

So far as methods of treatment are concerned we continue to maintain an eclectic attitude, and advise the use of whatever methods seem to be best suited to the individual circumstances. We cannot stress too strongly the necessity of taking sufficient time to establish a reasonably accurate diagnosis before any form of treatment is prescribed; time is sometimes sacrificed on the basis of expediency, a custom which is to be deprecated. An accurate clinical and statistical analysis of the after-results of treatment should always be determined.

Finally we report that we have discarded, with much reluctance, a number of case records which had been used in previous editions to illustrate our clinical material. It has been like bidding good-bye to old friends to whom one has been deeply attached. But in the passage of time many of the vivid clinical pictures of former days have become dimmed, have taken on a new look, one not nearly so terrifying as formerly.

We wish to thank the Oxford University Press who for so many years have sponsored our efforts, and spurred us on to new ones. We trust that the Ninth Edition may continue to merit the generous approval accorded to previous ones.

D. K. H.

I. R. C. B.

Edinburgh
July 1961

PREFACE TO THE FIRST EDITION

Our aim in this book has been to present psychiatry as a living subject, with important relations not only to general medicine, but to the social problems of everyday life. Recent work in psychopathology has given to the study of mental disorders a human and a scientific interest which was too often lacking before. Most of all, the biological viewpoint of Adolf Meyer and his followers of the American school has seemed to us to shed fresh light on the nature of mental illness, and to offer new hope in its prevention and treatment. This biological hypothesis regards mental illness as the cumulative result of unhealthy reactions of the individual mind to its environment, and seeks to trace in a given case all the factors that go to the production of these reactions. We hope to have shown to some extent in the following pages how much of understanding and interest these and other recent researches have added to psychiatry.

Nomenclature we have sought to make as simple as possible, as we believe that the facts are best expressed in ordinary language, and that the use of technical terms should be restricted to occasions where brevity and convenience demand them. One thing will be apparent to the reader; namely, how much regarding the nature of mental disorder remains unknown. We have presented the facts and the chief interpretations of them, indicating what among the latter seems most likely to be verified. We believe the time has come when mental illness need no longer be regarded as the mysterious preserve of a few specialists now that a working knowledge of psychiatry is within easy reach of the general practitioner, with all that that implies in the way of early recognition, prevention and treatment.

We have made a point of quoting at length clinical records of cases in our own practice, so far as space permits; and this for several reasons. Mental illness is an individual affair. Its symptoms have little meaning apart from the setting in which they occur. This setting includes not only the general mental and physical condition at the time, but the individual's personality, circumstances and history from his earliest days. Hence general descriptions of clinical syndromes, while interesting, are not of the first importance. What is wanted always is an understanding of the patient as a human being, and of the problems which he is meeting in a morbid way with his 'symptoms'. It is in accordance with these principles, and with what is called the 'dynamic' view, that we have utilized clinical records so extensively.

The clinical material upon which the book is largely based was observed at the Glasgow Royal Mental Hospital; the Henry Phipps Psychiatric Clinic of the Johns Hopkins Hospital, Baltimore; the Psychiatric Institute of the New York State Hospital, Ward's Island, New York; the Cassel Hospital, Penshurst, Kent; and Guy's Hospital.

We have appended only a brief bibliography. To have furnished a comprehensive list of references would have meant much additional space. We must therefore content ourselves with acknowledging our indebtedness to many of the standard textbooks and to monographs dealing with special topics. Throughout the text we refer to a number of these, but where we have failed to make acknowledgement we now do so.

D. K. H.
R. D. G.

May 1927

HISTORICAL REVIEW OF THE CARE
AND TREATMENT OF MENTAL ILLNESS

Mental disorder, in one form or another, has been recognized from time im-
memorial, but it is only in comparatively recent years that serious attempts have
been made to study and understand it. Progress in this branch of medicine has
been slow, but the difficulties to be contended with—professional apathy, public
prejudice and the inherent complexity of the subject—have been very great, and
the advance which has actually taken place has not been sufficiently recognized.
To give perspective to modern psychiatric problems, therefore, we have thought it
wise to mention some of the more important landmarks in the social history of
psychiatry.

Writers on the history of psychiatry have habitually referred to records, in
Greek poetry and mythology, of episodes of frenzy affecting the Heroes, but it
is quite impossible at this date to form a definite opinion of the relationship of
these states to mental disorder as it is understood to-day. Early Egyptian papyri
contain references to mental disturbances. Thus, about 1500 B.C., it was written
of senility that 'The heart grows heavy, and remembers not yesterday.' This
statement may have had a basis, even at that time, in anatomical as well as in
psychological observations; Elliot Smith has demonstrated arteriosclerosis in his
dissections of mummies. The first authentic cases of mental disorder are recorded
in the Books of the Old Testament, where Saul, David and Nebuchadnezzar are
famous examples. Epilepsy was the type of mental illness with which the ancients
were specially familiar. It was long known to them as the 'sacred disease', but
Hippocrates, with his customary insight, stated that 'The sacred disease (epilepsy)
appears to me to be nowise more divine nor more sacred than other diseases, but
has a natural cause from which it originates like other affections. Men regard its
nature and cause as divine from ignorance, and wonder because it is not like
other diseases.' Cambyses, the King of Persia, is a much-quoted example.

An early reference, perhaps the first, to the treatment of the insane is contained in Plato's *Republic* (Bk. xi. c. 13). 'If anyone is insane let him not be seen
openly in the city, but let the relatives of such a person watch over him at home
in the best manner they know of, and if they are negligent let them pay a fine.'
In the time of Hippocrates, it was the custom for the mentally afflicted to visit
the temple of Aesculapius, where sacrifices and prayer were offered. Incantations
and purifications seem to have been specially recommended for epilepsy. Hippocrates himself, however, believed that the brain was the organ of mind, and he
denied that there was anything occult or mysterious about the occurrence of a
mental disorder. Democritus, in his correspondence with Hippocrates, made the
curious statement that 'Hellebore when given to the sane pours darkness over
the mind, but to the insane is very profitable'! Haemorrhoids and varicose veins

were alleged to relieve a disturbed mind. The treatment attributed traditionally to Asclepiades (who flourished in the first century B.C.) was later described in the Christian era by Celsus, who advocated two widely divergent methods. On the one hand, he had a use for such methods as starving, chains and flogging; because under such treatment, it was said, those who had refused food started to eat, and in certain cases the memory was refreshed. On the other hand, he deprecated venesection and the use of fomentations of poppy and hyoscyamus, maintaining that everything possible should be done to divert the melancholic, and commenting favourably on sports, music, reading aloud, rocking in a hammock and the sound of a waterfall as methods of treatment. Themison, another disciple of Asclepiades, recommended a liberal diet, baths and fomentations. Titus has the invidious distinction of recommending stripes. Caelius Aurelianus is worthy of much praise, for he placed his patients under the best conditions of light, temperature and quiet, and recommended that everything of an exciting character should be excluded. Of particular interest are his references to tactfulness in attendants for the avoidance of antagonism, and to the limited and cautious use of physical restraint. The physician, he said, should not see the patient too frequently, lest his authority be undermined. Theatrical entertainments, riding, walking and work were all recommended, particularly during the period of convalescence. Topics of conversation were to be such as would suit the patient's condition. Later, excursions by land and water, and various other distractions, were to be used. He denounced semi-starvation, bleeding, chains and excessive drug therapy. Galen, basing his treatment on humoral pathology, recommended a just balance between 'moisture' and 'dryness'. Aretaeus, probably a contemporary of Galen, advised bleeding to relieve the liver in melancholy, purging by means of aloes, and baths; and, in convalescence, natural hot baths for their sulphur and bitumen.

Mediaeval Europe left the treatment of mental illness to priests, and superstitious beliefs in witchcraft and the like flourished. Special reference may be made to contemporary customs in the British Isles. Treatment by herbs, and binding in chains and fetters, are mentioned in old Saxon chronicles. Certain wells were considered to have special virtue. Of these, the most famous were St. Fillans, St. Ronans, Struthill, and a well on a small island on Loch Maree, in Scotland; St. Winifred's Well in Wales; and some in England, particularly in Cornwall. The Valley of Glen-na-Galt in Ireland had more than a local reputation.

Lunacy legislation in England dates from 1320 when it was enacted during the reign of Edward II that the property of lunatics should be vested in the Crown. Bethlem, which had been founded in London in 1247 as a priory of the Order of the Star of Bethlem, was the first hospital in the British Isles to care for the insane. It is recorded that in 1403 six lunatics were confined there. In 1546 Henry VIII granted St. Bartholomew's Hospital and Bethlem to the laity; in 1618 Dr. Helkiah Crooke was appointed Keeper and Physician to Bethlem.

In the seventeenth century the great Sydenham prescribed for 'mania' after long agues a cordial, generous indeed, consisting of Venice treacle (which contained the flesh and blood of vipers, and sixty-one more ingredients), canary wine and honey. This was given three times a day, with rest in bed; even pregnancy was no contra-indication. In addition Sydenham strongly recommended bleeding in the treatment of 'mania', saying, 'Young subjects, if of a sanguine habit, are to be bled to the extent of nine ounces on two or three occasions, with three days between each bleeding.' A caution was given not to exceed this amount of bleeding, 'otherwise idiocy and not recovery will result'. The bleeding was followed by a course of purgative pills. In place of venesection, Denis, of Paris, in 1667, introduced the transfusion of blood. This he employed in the case of a love-sick youth, with fatal results, and an ensuing action for damages.

In the next century the treatment of King George III, who suffered from recurrent attacks of maniacal excitement, served to arouse much public interest and controversy. His physician was a Dr. Willis, who had acquired a high reputation for his skill in dealing with such cases through his experience derived from the management of a private mental home in Lincolnshire which provided accommodation for twenty patients. Willis allowed his maniacal patients much freedom. If they escaped, the wages of the delinquent attendant were withheld until the patient returned. The Royal patient was treated with singularly little respect. No hesitation was evinced in knocking him down, and one attendant was even heard to boast that he had knocked him 'as flat as a flounder'. Willis ascribed great value in the King's case to the use of Peruvian bark, but other physicians who were consulted did not agree with him. In consequence of the rivalry, jealousy and differences of opinion which were revealed, the House of Lords decided to appoint a Committee to institute a detailed inquiry. This served a most useful purpose not only by directing greater attention to the King's treatment, but also to the medical and nursing care of all mentally afflicted throughout the whole country.

The modern era of the treatment of mental illness dates from the end of the eighteenth century, and may be divided into four periods:
1. The period of humane reform with which are associated the names of Pinel, Esquirol and Daquin in France; Tuke in England; Fricke in Germany; Morgagni and Chiarugi in Italy; Andrew Duncan in Scotland.
2. The introduction of non-restraint by Gardiner Hill, Charlesworth and Conolly in England, and by Bond, Kirkbride and Rush in the United States of America.
3. The hospital period.
4. The social and community period.

These periods will be discussed separately even although there is considerable overlapping.

HUMANE REFORM

It was in 1794 that Philippe Pinel was appointed to the medical staff of the Bicêtre Hospital, Paris. For several years he had shown great interest in the care and treatment of those who were mentally ill, and wrote a number of papers in which he discussed 'moral' treatment; one of his papers was entitled 'The most efficacious means of treating Mental Diseases occurring before Old Age'. It has been said that Thouret, an influential member of the Assembly, was impressed by Pinel's dissertation, and supported his candidature for the vacant post at Bicêtre Hospital. Pinel was a shy, timid, self-conscious man, but like many other sensitive people he had great tenacity of purpose, and it was not long before he was able to institute the beneficent and humanitarian reforms which were so close to his heart, and which have become so indissolubly associated with his name. At that time Bicêtre housed upwards of 200 male patients who were regarded not only as incurable but also as extremely dangerous. Some had been chained and fettered and confined in dungeons for many years, and yet Pinel was convinced that they were only unmanageable because they had been robbed of air and liberty, and freedom of action. His highest hopes were amply justified; the happy results proved the correctness of his opinions. Instead of blows and chains he introduced light and fresh air, cleanliness, workshops and promenades, but above all kindliness and understanding. The reforms which had proved so successful at Bicêtre were duplicated at the Salpêtrière, a mental hospital for women, where at a later date Esquirol became the physician in charge. A great epoch in the treatment of the mentally ill had been ushered in, which was acclaimed and had its reverberations in every country where psychiatry was practised.

Pinel was much more than a mental hospital administrator and physician. He set a high standard of medical care and practice, insisted on good case-taking, and made outstanding contributions to psychiatric literature. He taught by his writing and character more than by word of mouth.

Jean Étienne Dominique Esquirol, who may be described as Pinel's most distinguished pupil and interpreter, was appointed in 1812 to the medical staff of the Salpêtrière. He also managed a small private mental hospital at 23 Rue de Buffon, Paris, and in 1825 was appointed Chief Physician of the Charenton Mental Hospital. He became recognized as an authority on mental hospital construction—he founded no less than ten—but he was especially famous for instituting the first clinical lecture course on psychological medicine. He became known as a great teacher, and attracted students and doctors from all over the world. For instance, Sir Alexander Morison's lectures on psychiatry, and his textbook on mental diseases, were based on Esquirol's teaching; Dr. Andrew Combe and Sir Robert Christison were other distinguished Edinburgh physicians who attended Esquirol's lectures. Esquirol may be regarded as one of the first, if not the first, to establish a school of psychiatry.

After Esquirol came Ferrus, who received the new title, 'Inspecteur-Général du Service des Aliénés'. He had the distinction of starting a farm worked by patients who were being cared for at Bicêtre hospital. From his advocacy resulted the law of 1838 for the establishment of new mental hospitals in every department of France, and the improvement of the existing ones.

Almost simultaneously with these epoch-making reforms in France, the humanitarian efforts of William Tuke and Lindley Murray resulted in the opening in 1796 of the York Retreat in England. In Scotland, in 1792, Dr.

Andrew Duncan, who was Professor of Medicine, Edinburgh University, and President of the Royal College of Physicians, Edinburgh, sponsored an appeal for funds to establish the Royal Edinburgh Mental Hospital, which was opened in 1813.

In Germany the modern era began with Fricke, who in Brunswick in 1793 applied humane medical treatment and greatly reduced mechanical restraint. In 1803 Reil published a volume entitled *Rhapsodies on the Use of Psychic Treatment in Mental Disorder*, and in 1805 the first journal devoted to the study of mental disorders—the *Magazin für Nervenheilkunde*—was edited by Reil and Kayssler.

The reforms begun in England by Tuke, which resulted in the establishment of the York Retreat, were followed by the introduction of a Bill into Parliament for the better treatment of the insane. This became known as 'Wynn's Act', and was introduced in 1808 with the purpose of providing 'better care and maintenance of lunatics being paupers or criminals in England'. Amending Acts were introduced in 1811, 1815, 1819 and 1824 which laid the basis for the ensuing lunacy administration of this country. The Lunacy Commission, which was established in 1845, became reorganized in 1913 as the Board of Control, England, which now in terms of the 1959 Mental Health Act has been merged in the Ministry of Health.

In 1815 a Committee was appointed to investigate the conditions in 'madhouses' in England. The Report stated that keepers of houses for the insane admitted a greater number of persons than they were calculated for, there was an insufficient staff, too much restraint was used, the certificates on which the patients were received were often faulty and the visitation and inspection of private madhouses was inefficient. The Report drew attention to the flagrant abuses which existed, but no immediate action was taken. For instance, at the York Lunatic Asylum it was found that there had been great neglect and cruelty. Of 365 patients who had died, the deaths of only 221 had been reported; a patient had been killed and his body disposed of so as to avoid an inquest; and two sets of books had been kept. When Dr. Munro, the Superintendent of Bethlem, was questioned about the treatment of his patients, he said: 'Patients are ordered to be bled about the latter end of May, according to the weather. After they have been bled they take vomits once a week for a certain number of weeks. After that we purge the patients. That has been the practice for years, long before my time.' It is true there were no strait-jackets—irons were held in more esteem! Patients were chained in a state of nudity to tables. A female patient in a hospital at Bethnal Green was confined in a quondam pigsty. Male attendants not infrequently had charge of female wards (the practice appears to be returning) and the immorality and depravity which existed beggar description. In 1828 an Act (9 Geo. IV, c. 40) was passed appointing fifteen Metropolitan Commissioners to visit Homes in which the insane were detained.

It is obvious from what has been said that there was urgent need for the introduction of courses of instruction in psychiatry. In 1753 Dr. William Battie

B

attained the distinction of being the first psychiatrist in the British Isles to give clinical instruction at St. Luke's Hospital, London; 'young physicians well-recommended' visited the hospital with Dr. Battie, and were able to observe the treatment of the patients. Robertson (1928) states that Battie 'gave occasional clinical lectures to a few pupils'. In 1823 in Edinburgh, Sir Alexander Morison, who, as stated previously, had been a pupil of Esquirol, instituted a course of nine systematic lectures in psychiatry; in 1826 these lectures were duplicated in London, and this dual arrangement was maintained until 1852—a truly remarkable and unique performance. It can be claimed, therefore, with considerable justification, that Morison was the first teacher of systematic psychiatry in this country.

In the United States of America, Bond, Kirkbride and Rush were all responsible for instituting reforms which were very much in line with what was happening in France and Great Britain. The otherwise enlightened Rush (he was a graduate of Edinburgh University) published *Observations on the Human Mind*, in which he advocated copious bleeding, low diet, purges, calomel and opium. These methods came to be discarded by his successors, who were more in favour of 'supporting treatment'.

While the above changes, indicative of a more humanitarian outlook in regard to the treatment of the mentally disordered, were being engendered and spread over the civilized world, it is of interest to recall that even in 1731 Jonathan Swift, the famous Dean of St. Patrick's, Dublin, had foreshadowed the changes which might occur. It was in that year that he wrote his ode entitled *Verses on the Death of Dr. Swift*, the concluding lines of which consisted of the well-known quip or jest:

> He gave the little wealth he had
> To build a house for fools and mad;
> And show'd, by one satiric touch,
> No nation wanted it so much.

In 1745, at the time of his death, it was found that he had bequeathed a sum of between ten and eleven thousand pounds to found a hospital for the treatment of the insane. St. Patrick's Hospital was the first to be established in Ireland. The charter for erecting and endowing it was obtained in 1746, and in 1757 the first patients were admitted. It continues to maintain the great tradition of its past.

ABOLITION OF RESTRAINT

This period was initiated in 1837 by Gardiner Hill and Charlesworth at the Lincoln Asylum. In 1827, in the asylum, there were 72 patients. Of these, 39 were constantly in restraint and the total number of hours of restraint per annum amounted to 20,424. Under the regime of Hill and Charlesworth a revolution was effected; out of 130 patients only two were under restraint for a total period of 28 hours per annum. Subsequently mechanical restraint was entirely abolished. The patients showed a great improvement in their physical and mental health, their conduct was more controlled and the numbers of accidents and suicides was greatly decreased. Conolly in 1838 at Hanwell Asylum became an enthusiastic advocate of non-restraint, and in one of his reports he wrote: 'There is no asylum in the world in which all mechanical restraints may not be abolished, not only with perfect safety, but with incalculable advantage.' In 1856 he embodied his wide experience and his wisdom in a book entitled *The Treatment of the Insane without Mechanical Restraint.* The *Edinburgh Review* in 1870, commenting on Conolly's remarkable achievement, wrote as follows: 'To Conolly belongs a still higher crown, not merely for his courage in carrying out a beneficent conception on a large scale and in a conspicuous theatre, but for his genius in extending it. To him, hobbles and chains, handcuffs and muffs, were but material impediments that merely confined the limbs; to get rid of these he spent the best years of his life; but beyond these mechanical fetters he saw there were a hundred fetters to the spirit which human sympathy, courage and time only could remove.'

One of the most outstanding and courageous personalities among the early pioneers was the American school teacher Dorothea Lynde Dix. This remarkable woman, handicapped as she was by her upbringing and poor physical health, showed a spirit and an enterprise in relation to the welfare of the mentally disordered which has reverberated throughout the world. In America she was not only responsible for effecting great improvements but also founded approximately thirty-two institutions. 'Could all the prisons on new and better plans she carried Bills for, and all the almshouses she caused to be thoroughly reconstructed be added to these, and then all brought vividly before the mind's eye, the impressions would be amazing indeed.' Here in Scotland we are under a particular debt of gratitude to her. She had come to Great Britain to recuperate from a serious physical illness. She came to Edinburgh and visited a number of houses and hospitals where mentally ill patients were being cared for. Some were reasonably well-conducted but in others she discovered the most serious abuses. She tried to interest the local authorities, lawyers and doctors in what she felt was wrong but her protestations were received with coldness and contempt. She was dubbed 'the American invader', an interfering busybody. She was, however, a woman of great determination, and irrespective of all obstacles and local antagonism she journeyed to London, and was successful in obtaining an interview with the Home Secretary. The evidence which she presented so impressed him that in a few weeks a Royal Commission was appointed to inquire into the condition of lunatic asylums in Scotland, and the existing state of the law of that country in reference to lunatics and lunatic asylums. The Commission was appointed on April 3, 1855, and it was largely as a result of its findings that public mental hospitals were established throughout Scotland. She had accomplished in a few months what others during many years had striven to do.

It was due to the lack of suitable hospital organizations for the care and treatment of mental patients that a system of colony care arose which met with gratifying success. The colonies of Gheel and Lierneux in Belgium, of Clairmont (Oise) near Paris, and of those in Hanover and Moravia deserve special mention.

The one at Gheel is the best known. Its fame as a place of cure for the mentally ill arose from the legend of Dymphna, the beautiful daughter of an Irish king, who had made incestuous proposals to her. She refused, fled in a state of alarm to Belgium, but was followed, captured and beheaded by her father. Among those who witnessed this dreadful crime were some mentally afflicted persons who were stated to have, immediately, recovered their sanity. The scene of the crime became hallowed ground, pilgrimages were organized for the mentally sick and many remained to live among the inhabitants, so forming the first 'colony'. As organized at present it consists of a central psychiatric hospital of 200 beds, and in addition more than 2000 patients live, under supervision, in private homes and are employed, principally, in agricultural work. The patient lives as one of the family, and has no restrictions placed upon his freedom, except that he must be home by eight o'clock in the summer and by four o'clock in the winter. He is not allowed to enter an inn, or be served with alcohol, without special permission. On admission to the colony the patient is placed in an observation hospital and after his mental state has been carefully determined he is transferred to a family residence where he is likely to be suitably cared for. This system ensures a good degree of personal liberty, it is economical and promotes recovery through individualization and association with other persons who are able to behave and think in a normal manner.

Boarding Out. This is the term used in Scotland to describe the system of care and treatment whereby certain easily managed, long-continued-treatment cases can be maintained under guardianship in private homes. The patients are not segregated in one colony, as at Gheel, but are placed in those parts of the country where the most suitable guardians and houses are available. Minute inquiries are made beforehand as to the domestic arrangements, the amount of accommodation available, the facilities for occupation, recreation, social activities and, most important of all, the experience of the guardians. The possible exploitation of the patients requires to be safeguarded. Some patients may be 'boarded out' direct from their own homes, but the majority are transferred from a mental hospital or colony for the subnormal where they have been under treatment. The sanction of the Mental Welfare Commission must be obtained in all cases. If, for any reason, the arrangements do not prove satisfactory the patient may be re-transferred to the mental organization from which he was 'boarded out'. During the period he is under private care his welfare is safeguarded by visits of inspection, four times a year by the district medical officer, twice a year by a public assistance employee, and once a year by a deputy medical commissioner or Commissioner of the Mental Welfare Commission. A record of visits requires to be kept. Patients under private care are either placed singly or in numbers not exceeding four of the same sex in any one house; the more usual arrangement is for one patient only. The above system has been in operation since the middle of the last century, and has much to commend it. It provides, under sheltered conditions, an approximation to home life which is not only beneficent and humanitarian but also much more economic than continued residence in a mental hospital organization. The statistics published in 1957 show that in Scotland there were 2551 boarded out subnormal and 307 boarded out mental patients. In Scandinavia, Canada and the United States, similar schemes are being put into operation.

THE HOSPITAL PERIOD

Since the beginning of the century the modernization and up-grading of mental hospitals has been a continuing process which has resulted in numerous beneficial changes. Their administration, medical and nursing staffing, the employment of psychiatric social workers, occupational therapists, psychologists, chiropodists and hairdressers, have raised the standard of care and treatment to a level of which we can be proud. The introduction of the National Health Service Act (1948) acted as a spur to our efforts and government funds became available whereby old hospitals could be renovated, and extensive reconstruction programmes could be undertaken. Our object is to develop the preventive and curative side of mental hospital work, and, *pari passu*, to educate our professional brethren and the public so that they may regard the mental hospital as an asset to the medical service of the community. The new Mental Health Acts (1959 and 1960) whereby patients can be admitted to such hospitals 'informally' just as to general hospitals, will do much to facilitate the disappearance of the shades of the prison-house.

In order to gain a proper perspective it is of interest and value to recapitulate, summarily, some of the more important changes which have been effected.

After the period of 'non-restraint' had run its course, a system of 'seclusion' for dangerous impulsive patients who could not be trusted was introduced. This consisted of the use of single rooms—sometimes referred to as strong rooms—and of padded rooms which were locked, and in which patients might be confined both during the day and at night. Those in favour of the above system argued that it prevented struggling with the patient, it obviated serious accidents and there was much less necessity to use powerful sedatives. Furthermore it eased the burden and responsibility of a small, often sorely-tried medical and nursing staff. As the medical and nursing staffs became increased, both in quantity and quality, it soon became evident that the vast majority—if not all—of the so-called single room cases responded more co-operatively when cared for and nursed in open wards where they could be adequately supervised. The single rooms and padded rooms of the past have now been converted into comfortable bed-sitting rooms which are appreciated by those who are accustomed to privacy. We believe that the above-mentioned changes received a considerable impetus when as long ago as 1841 Dr. Samuel Hitch, who founded the Royal Medico-Psychological Association, suggested that much benefit might result from the employment of female nurses in the male wards of mental hospitals. At the Gloucester General Lunatic Asylum (as it was then called) he employed the wives of his married male nurses, to assist their husbands. In 1854 Dr. Browne, the Medical Superintendent of the Crichton Royal, Dumfries, instituted classes for the training of nurses, and in 1877 a similar systematic course of instruction was put into effect at the McLean Hospital, Boston, Massachusetts. In 1880 Dr. Campbell Clark conceived the idea that the standard of mental hospital nursing could be advanced to a higher level by the appointment of a general hospital trained nurse as matron of the Lanarkshire Mental Hospital at Bothwell; he was also responsible for the publication of a *Handbook for Attendants on the Insane* which has been greatly extended and brought up to date. It is still in use by mental hospital nurses who are preparing for the examinations conducted by the General Nursing Council and Royal Medico-Psychological Association.

Clouston, Turnbull and Robertson were a few of the distinguished Scottish psychiatrists who were ardent protagonists of the introduction of general hospital nurses to positions of high responsibility, *e.g.* matrons, and assistant matrons, and of female nurses in the male wards. It has been our experience that male patients respond more naturally and politely to female nurses. But at the same time we appreciate that well-trained male nurses (many of whom now combine general and mental hospital training) are an indispensable and essential part of any mental hospital organization. Indeed the pendulum has been swinging in the contrary direction, and in some mental hospitals and psychiatric units male nurses are being appointed to senior posts on the female wards. We deprecate such an arrangement but have felt that it was incumbent to mention it.

The care of patients in mental hospitals has been made easier by the establishment of smaller ward units, and by making special arrangements for attractive admission wards, hospital units for those requiring special nursing, *e.g.* acute mental states, convalescent cases, and those requiring more prolonged care. A special department for geriatric patients is to be desired.

The medical staffs of mental hospitals have been greatly increased. The post of Medical Superintendent has lost its administrative and clinical importance; the duties formerly undertaken by one person are now shared by lay administrators, by medical committees, and by consultant psychiatrists (whole and part-time) who assume clinical responsibility for departments or wards under their particular direction. Whether or not these are steps in the right direction remains to be seen. There are some of us who believe that a mental hospital with all its special activities which require co-ordination should be under unitary control, and that the splitting of authority is apt to lead to discordance not only in the care and treatment of the patients—which is the main issue—but also in the control of the nursing, domestic and artisan staff.

However that may be, the fact remains that the mental hospital to-day has established outside contacts and interests which, previously, did not exist. The medical staff are not only engaged in indoor duties, but their experience and training has been broadened by their participation in out-patient clinics, child-guidance clinics, domiciliary consultations, medico-legal work and university departments of psychiatry. The scope and training of the young psychiatrist have been developed so much that he has every opportunity to become familiar with preventive medico-social aspects of psychiatry which were not in the purview of his predecessors. Instead of locked doors and high walls we are developing anew the open door system where the wards are unlocked, and where the patients are given the freedom of the grounds and of the adjoining city or countryside. Following the lead of Professor Ewen Cameron, McGill University, Montreal, we have established Day and Night hospitals which can be of enormous advantage in the convalescence and rehabilitation of those patients who may require additional help before they are fully able to resume their previous positions either at home or at work. In addition, in a large number of areas in Great Britain, Holland, Canada and the United States, determined attempts are being made to treat larger numbers of patients in their own homes. This is made possible through the co-operation of Public Health officials, out-patient departments, family practice units, psychiatrists, psychiatric social workers and health visitors. Our aim is to diminish our mental hospital admission rates and to maintain patients at work so long as it is compatible with their well-being.

We should stress particularly the advantages to be gained by establishing closer liaison with general practitioners, and with medical, surgical and other specialists. Such teamwork is not only of enormous benefit to the psychiatrist but serves the dual purpose of familiarizing the other members of our profession with the significance of the psychological factors in all forms of illness. It is by such co-ordinated methods that the prejudice and stigma so traditionally associated with mental illness will be eliminated.

A prerequisite for the extension of psychiatric work and service revolves round a comprehensive development of undergraduate and postgraduate psychiatric education. Psychiatry has earned a more prominent place in the medical curriculum. We advocate the establishment of chairs of psychiatry in every medical school, and the incorporation of a professional examination in psychiatry in the final medical examination. A medical student should be as adequately trained in psychological as in physiological principles, and we believe that this can be effected by blending these disciplines throughout his undergraduate career. There is still a place for systematic lectures as well as for seminars, and from the angle of clinical instruction there is no better training ground than the psychiatric out-patient department of a large general hospital. We meet there a good cross-section of the medico-social problems which occur in general practice; we can demonstrate methods of examination; we can emphasize the salient features which will require further investigation under more private conditions. Our experience has convinced us that patients who are tactfully dealt with become most co-operative, and gain a sense of pride and prestige from the interest, understanding and sympathy which is shown them; and successful treatment can be more readily accomplished.

From the postgraduate angle much has been done to extend the training and experience of the psychiatric specialist. The University of Edinburgh in 1912 set up regulations governing examination for the Diploma of Psychiatry. In the examination for Membership of the Royal College of Physicians of Edinburgh the candidate, in addition to his examination in general medicine, is allowed to choose a selected subject of which psychiatry is one. This scheme ensures that the successful candidate not only has to reach a very high standard in general medicine, but also a more than usually good knowledge of psychiatry.

While therefore we must continue to increase the efficiency of the medical, nursing, research and administrative aspects of every mental hospital, yet our ability to keep people out of mental hospitals, and to build up the preventive and curative side of our work, will be the ultimate tokens of our success. We recommend the even more widespread establishment of psychiatric clinics as an integral part of every teaching general hospital. The necessary out-patient departments, social service and other ancillaries such as research laboratories would be indispensable adjuncts. Where it may not be possible to establish a separate unit it is quite feasible to reserve certain wards in the general hospital for psychiatric cases. In our opinion every large general hospital would benefit by providing 5–10 per cent. of its beds for that purpose. Modern methods of treatment by means of drugs, electricity, leucotomy and appropriate psychotherapy have made it possible to treat a wide variety of nervous and mental illness without disturbing the amenity of the general hospital. Psychiatry will thus assume an equal status with general medicine to the advantage of both.

To ensure the success of our preventive work we must constantly remind ourselves that the seeds of many nervous and mental disorders are sown in childhood. For this reason we advocate that departments of child psychiatry should be integrated with paediatric hospitals. This has been done in many places and countries, in the United States, Canada, Scandinavia, Great Britain and Germany. Such departments widen the scope of Child Guidance Clinics, where the resources of psychiatrist, psychologist, educationist and social worker can be utilized as a team. Childhood constitutes the golden period for the inculcation of mental hygiene; it is the plastic period of development, the time when prophylactic work should have its greatest reward. A modification of environment and social circumstances can work wonders, and the vast majority of personal emotional difficulties can be dealt with at an objective level; relatively few—but they can be important and difficult—may require prolonged investigation at a subjective and subconscious level. Again we require to have the complete co-operation of parents, schoolmasters, the law courts, employers of labour, and social organizations concerned with the problems of children. Emotional and social security is the greatest safeguard against all subsequent disorder of life and conduct (Henderson, 1955).

While we note the changes which have occurred in psychiatric work and practice we would remind the psychiatrists of to-day that it has been an evolutionary process rather than a revolutionary one. It is salutory to remember the work of our predecessors, and to disabuse our minds of the idea that the real study of psychiatry stemmed from Kraepelin, Freud, the World Wars or the introduction of physical methods of treatment. For instance, in the middle of the nineteenth century Thomas Laycock held the joint appointment of Professor of Medicine of Edinburgh University and Lecturer in Medical Psychology and Mental Diseases. In 1840 he published a book entitled *Nervous Diseases of*

Women to be followed in 1860 by *Mind and Brain*. As an example of his imaginative foresight he stressed the reciprocal action of body and mind and stated that 'a practical knowledge of mental science is essential to parents, jurists and legislators, governors of jails, schoolmasters, and teachers, ministers (gospel), naval and military officers, and employers of labour'. In Laycock's estimation psychiatry was not a narrow specialty but a discipline for general application in studying the conduct of man. Laycock combined his lecture course with clinical demonstrations by Skae at the Royal Edinburgh Hospital for Mental Disorders. In 1879 Clouston was appointed to the Lectureship of Mental Diseases in Edinburgh University.

As regards research it was in 1866 that the West Riding Mental Hospital Reports (Crichton Browne) were published. They incorporated the work of Ferrier on the *Localisation of Brain Function* and inspired much of the subsequent work of the British school of neurology.

In 1895–96 Pathological Laboratories for the development of research were inaugurated almost contemporaneously in Edinburgh (by Clouston), in London (Mott) and in New York (van Giesen). Observation wards for the study and treatment of acute psychiatric disorders were under the charge of Greisinger in 1865 at the Royal Charité (general hospital), Berlin. Similar wards were in 1889 inaugurated by Dr. John Carswell in Barnhill Parochial Hospital, Glasgow. Such pioneer efforts were the forerunners of the psychiatric clinics and out-patient departments which are so indispensable.

COMMUNITY PERIOD

The establishment of Departments or Institutes of Social Medicine in every university illustrates the changed outlook on the prevention of illness in preference to its cure. In the past Public Health Departments had an objective, mechanistic approach, confined for the most part to the betterment of physical and environmental conditions, to vital statistics, sanitary problems, the purity of water and milk supplies, the control of infectious diseases and epidemics. Now we seek to promote measures which will protect the individual and the community so that man's mental and physical capacity can be maintained at its peak. For this purpose investigations into the social, genetic, environmental and domestic factors are being undertaken in the hope that we may acquire greater knowledge in relation to the epidemiology of human disease, and of those more subtle influences which produce nervous and mental instability. The whole personality of man has to be studied in relation to his social setting. Psychiatrists were doing just that, applying the psychobiological principles formulated by Adolf Meyer, long before Institutes of Social Medicine had been inaugurated, but that is not gainsaying the most valuable contributions which they are making. The fact that of every 100 children born 8 will have a nervous breakdown and 3 will spend some part of their lives in a mental hospital is alarming enough, but it completely fails to express the anxiety, distress and unhappiness of sorrowing relatives. The fact, too, that the combined number of mentally ill and defective is closely approximate to all those under treatment in general hospitals is indicative of the social and economic burdens for which the healthier members of the community have to assume responsibility. A more concrete example has been reported by Canby Robinson (1942), who in a study of 174 patients admitted to the medical wards of Johns Hopkins Hospital, Baltimore, found that no less than 66 per cent. presented social problems that were related to their illness, and in 36 per cent. social and emotional factors were the chief precipitating cause of illness. More specifically still Aubrey Lewis (1951) writes as follows: 'Of all the studies in this field, I think those called "ecological" have been the most promising and informative. . . . The chief of them was carried out by E. L. Faris and Warren Dunham. They examined the origin of nearly 35,000 patients admitted to Chicago mental hospitals between 1932 and 1934, and they found that those areas which had the highest rate of incidence of mental disorder had the highest indices of social disorganization: suicide, venereal disease, family disruption, juvenile and adult crime, high mobility in the population, poverty, demoralization, cultural heterogeneity were also at a high level in these areas.' At another point he comments: 'And in his daily work the psychiatrist, even more than other physicians, is incessantly forced to consider the social relations of his patients.'

It is evident from what has been said that further important developments in the medico-social field lie ahead of us. But while we look forward, a glance to the past will help us to keep our ideas in reasonable perspective. No history of psychiatry would be complete without reference to that remarkable American humanitarian Clifford W. Beers, who in 1907 wrote an autobiographical study entitled *A Mind That Found Itself.* Therein he described his experiences while he had been a patient in mental hospitals, and made constructive suggestions as to the improvements which might be effected. In furtherance of his ideas, in 1908 he founded the Connecticut Society for Mental Hygiene, and soon every state in the Union had its own Mental Hygiene Society. Other civilized countries soon followed the example which had been set, and in 1930 the First International Congress of Mental Hygiene was held in Washington: representatives attended from all over the world. The International Association of Mental Hygiene has now been superseded by the World Federation of Mental Health. In addition, the World Health Organization with its headquarters in Geneva has a highly efficient psychiatric department. The expressed objects of these organizations are to enlist the co-operation of the public in developing those preventive measures which may lead to greater social solidarity and individual well-being. If we are successful in our efforts we may be able to effect a substantial reduction in those seeking admission to psychiatric clinics and mental hospitals, and with the aid of civic organizations, education authorities, trained social workers and general practitioners, build up an effective community health service. Querido in Amsterdam has established a Psychiatric Consultative Bureau where psychiatrists and social workers maintain a 24-hour service. The Bureau assists the family doctor in the treatment of the patient in his own home, or may arrange for his admission to a psychiatric clinic or mental hospital, depending on the particular nature and acuteness of the illness. In addition the Bureau works in close association with the public assistance department and the labour exchange, and may take an active part in rehabilitation. Such a type of organization serves the dual purpose of preventing the admission of patients to hospital and of facilitating their discharge by means of a well-organized after-care service.

REFERENCES AND FURTHER READING

Beers, C. W. (1908) *A Mind That Found Itself*, New York.
Bucknill, J. C., and Tuke, D. H. (1858) *Psychological Medicine*, Philadelphia.
Ciba Symposium (1950) *French Psychiatry*.
Conolly, John (1849) *On Some Forms of Insanity*. Reprinted by St. Bernard's Hospital Management Committee, July 1960.
Deutsch, Albert (1937) *The Mentally Ill in America*, New York.
Guthrie, D. (1957) *Med. Hist.*, **1**, 307.
Harms, E. (1960) *Amer. J. Psychiat.*, **116**, 1037.
Henderson, D. (1955) *Brit. med. J.*, **2**, 519.
Janet, P. (1925) *Psychological Healing*, London.
Jones, E. (1953–55) *Sigmund Freud; Life and Work*, London.
Lewis, A. (1951) *Edinb. med. J.*, **58**, 214, 231.
Robertson, G. M. (1928) *Edinb. med. J.*, **35**, 192.
Robinson, G. C. (1942) *Clinics*, **1**, 842.
Tiffany, F. (1890) *Dorothea Lynde Dix*, Boston.
Tuke, T. H. (1882) *History of the Insane*, London.
Tuke, T. H. (1892) *Dictionary of Psychological Medicine*, London.
Whitwell, J. R. (1943) *Historical Notes on Psychiatry*, 2nd ed., London.
Zilboorg, G., and Henry, G. W. (1941) *A History of Medical Psychology*, New York.

2

PSYCHIATRY AND GENERAL MEDICINE

It is not so long ago since a wide gap separated psychiatry from general medicine. It was not until the twentieth century that psychiatry became a compulsory subject in the medical curriculum, and even then the amount of teaching was meagre, and was confined almost entirely to the psychoses, so that the young graduate entered into the practice of his profession with a very limited knowledge and understanding of the implications of psychiatric work. Psychiatry was a minor specialty practised almost entirely in mental hospitals; the neuroses—when recognized as such—were the particular province of the neurologists—and were treated by galvanism, faradism, hypnotism and a Weir-Mitchell regime.

As time has gone on great changes have been effected—professorial chairs of psychiatry have been established in some of our medical schools; a professional examination in psychiatry forms part of the final examination in medicine; the teaching of psychiatry has come to occupy an increasing part of the medical curriculum; the extramural, social and community aspects of psychiatry have been enormously increased; the crippling legal enactments which differentiated mental illness from physical illness have been abolished. The gap, therefore, between psychiatry and general medicine is being bridged, and it may be hoped that, in the not too distant future, psychiatry in its preventive aspects will become a part of general medical practice. It has, of course, its important specialist aspects but our aim is to train the general practitioners of the future so that they may become as interested in and as able to treat their psychiatric patients as those who are physically involved; the psychic and somatic constantly react on one another and cannot be completely separated. That is why we stress the treatment of the whole man, and not merely the particular disease from which he may be suffering. To do so effectively we must know his background, his personality structure plus his environmental situation, and the biological manner in which he has been able to adapt to the various exigencies of a physical or psychological nature which he has been called upon to meet. The general practitioner, therefore, must be as expert in conducting a psychological examination of his patient as a physical one, and in the long run he can rest assured that he will save much more time than he wastes. He will acquire a more comprehensive viewpoint, he will inspire greater confidence, he will be able to exercise a stronger influence, he will be able to go to the core of the situation. Among other things he will find that many of the bodily states which have not responded to surgery or pharmacology will disappear, miraculously, once the underlying psychological factors have been disclosed. It is for such reasons that we believe that all medical students at the beginning of their training should be informed that there is a mind as well as a body, that the two work in harmony, are delicately balanced and must be handled with the greatest care; the one is complementary to the other. All good doctors in general practice recognize those things, their success in practice depends on them, but there are others who say that they are too busy to listen to the complaints of their nervous patients, who dismiss them summarily, tell them 'there is nothing wrong', 'forget it', 'it is all imagination', 'take a long sea trip to Africa', etc., but our view is that it is implicit in the doctor's calling and his obligation to relieve distress wherever he finds it irrespective of its psychological or physical nature; and it is his failure to do so which renders so many patients disappointed with orthodox medicine so that they turn, in despair, to the arts of the unqualified. There may have been an excuse in the past, but now that the Faculties of Medicine of our great universities are becoming better orientated towards the teaching of psychiatry and the part it should occupy in the medical curriculum, it should not be long before all practitioners of medicine will deal more expertly with the preventive and curative sides of nervous and mental illness. We may need more psychiatric specialists, but our particular and most urgent need is an increase of general practitioners with psychological insight. They will acquire the confidence to treat more patients in their own homes, to keep them at work while treating them as outpatients, and to diminish the admission rate to mental hospitals and to psychiatric clinics. All such things have become more possible due to our greater knowledge of psychotherapy, and potent pharmacological and physical remedies; but for these agents to act to the best advantage it is essential that a good rapport, an empathy, should have been established between doctor and patient. A good doctor will not be hasty and impatient in his judgement; he will take time, he will not dismiss the subjective complaints of his patients as sheer nonsense but will consider them worthy of investigation. If his careful physical examination has failed to disclose an objective organic cause, he will at once extend his inquiries into the possibility of constitutional anomalies and emotional problems as being the causative agents.

What are the particular nervous and mental states which the general practitioner is most commonly called upon to deal with? We would suggest the following which have been more fully discussed under the general heading of the neuroses and psychosomatic states, e.g. anxiety states with a fear of impending death (angor animi); conversion hysterical symptoms (which are much less common than they used to be); obsessive thinking with compulsive tendencies; the asthmatic, duodenal ulcer, and dermatological conditions which so often reflect emotional immaturity; depressive states with suicidal impulses; and certain cases of sexual anomaly.

While the above states can be discriminated by the different forms they assume the root factor which is common to all is fear. Most of us at one time or another have experienced a quick beating of the heart, a cold sweat, hurried breathing, dryness of the mouth, a tendency to yawn, a catch in the throat, fluttering in the abdomen, which are the accompaniments of fear. Montaigne exclaimed: 'The thing in the world I am most afraid of is fear; that passion in the trouble of it exceeding all other accidents.' The physiologists in their investigation of such distressing and painful bodily phenomena have correlated them with an oversensitization of the autonomic nervous system, which may be sparked off by causes which seem trivial and insignificant, so that Ernest Jones came to define morbid fear as 'a disproportion between the intensity of the emotion and the occasion of its occurrence'. He regarded fear as the most frequent single symptom in psychopathology and perhaps in all medicine. 'It is', he said, 'the Alpha and Omega of practical psychiatry.' (Jones, 1911.) In his elaboration of the above opinion Jones accepted the Freudian hypotheses that morbid fears of external objects or situations are projections of internal mental processes; that every fear is the obverse of a wish, that fear and desire are intimately associated; and that fears have their origin on a sexual basis. According to that theory there is a never-ending struggle between Eros and Death with fear as a fundamental component.

We believe that a much broader interpretation is more satisfying and agree with Suttie's criticism of the Freudian doctrine when he lays the emphasis on love as a protective mechanism, giving rise to a sense of security. According to Suttie, the source of love is dependent on the mechanism of self-preservation, on the need of food, and not sexual desires and sensations; the original object of love is the mother, and it is the innate need for companionship which is the infant's only way for self-preservation. The infant's mind, from the beginning, is dominated by the need to retain the mother, a need which, if not satisfied, may produce intense emotional distress such as anger, rage, terror, as the loss of the mother may symbolize death itself (Henderson, 1939). Emancipation, therefore, may prove to be a highly traumatic event not only at birth, but later in life as well. Anxious fears, indecision, a lack of emotional maturity may come to dominate the person's life, and it is because of those facts that all doctors and intelligent parents should study the psychic needs of the developing child as much as its physical hygiene, and should minimize their impact as much as possible. We have seen how the wrong choice of a school, of a career, of a wife or a husband may produce the most disastrous results, and we believe that the family doctor with his intimate knowledge of family resources and potentialities could be an infinitely better guide if he took time to consider that he would be doing valuable preventive work in dealing with the difficulties and disharmonies of everyday life. That point of view was envisaged at the time when the National Health Act was introduced and sentiments were expressed then which even yet contain an important message. For instance, it was stated: 'Health is a way of living, it is not a negative state, it involves more than the mere absence of disease'; and, 'the medical practitioner and the medical services should view the individual as a living organism in relation to his whole environment'; and again: 'In the future the doctor's work will be more and more educational and less and less curative. He will deal more with physiology and psychology and less with pathology. This re-orientation of his education and his work is overdue.'

We have stressed the above points because we believe that they form the background of most of the cases of nervous illness with which the family doctor should be familiar. If he does not have them in mind, and does not realize how much they mean to his patient, he is likely to fail in coping with the presenting symptoms which are merely the symbols of strong underlying conflicts and resentments. And it is important to deal with the symptoms in the first place, even although a much longer time may be required to straighten out the personality disturbance. Like the surgeon we require to let the acute inflammatory symptoms subside before a radical operation is undertaken. The fact that painful, crippling symptoms have been cured helps to establish a good jumping-off ground for more detailed investigations. The change may be brought about simply enough. It may be a change in the environment, an easement of tension, better sleep at night-time, a readjustment of habits, rather than the employment of any highly specialized technique, which will make the position more acceptable. Kindness, consideration, encouragement, a transitory rest in hospital or nursing home, a careful case-history, taking into consideration the adequacy or failure of biological adjustment, can work wonders. Medical students in their training appreciate that point of view, it interests them, they want much more of it, it gives them something to work with in the treatment of their patients, which is far more important than coming to a formal diagnosis. They are warned that they are not likely to see or effect the quick results which occur in other branches of medical work, but if they have patience they may experience the great satisfaction of contributing to the art of living, to harmonious relationships, to the prevention of illness rather than to the mere dispensing of medicine for intractable complaints which have never been traced to their source. That is why we maintain that psychiatry is hardly a 'specialty' at all—it is not like brain surgery, ophthalmology, otology—but it may be part and parcel of all forms of medical work. That is the reason why we will welcome the day when all teachers of medicine, surgery and the special subjects will regard it as imperative to draw attention to the personality of the patient, to his environment, and to the influence of the psychological factors. Such advice coming from the physician, the surgeon, the gynaecologist will be more impressive and carry more weight than if uttered by the psychiatrist; the psychiatrist, however, can supply the ammunition. The whole theme and endeavour of this book has been to broaden the education of the medical student so that he may become a better informed medical practitioner equally conversant with the management of physiological and psychological anomalies. Whitehorn expressed the same idea in this way: 'to prepare the medical student to deal intelligently and skilfully with patients as persons, and to provide him with the basic knowledge of psychological and social problems and resources in relation to health and disease'. The idea inherent in such attempts at definition is surely to widen our horizons and to recognize that medicine (all forms of medicine) is concerned not only with the treatment of the ill but with the wider task of the welfare of society.

From a more detailed and practical angle the new Mental Health Acts which have been introduced into England and Scotland are likely to make it much easier for general practitioners to make arrangements for the treatment of acute psychiatric emergencies. It is now possible for any patient in need of treatment for mental disorder to be admitted to any hospital or nursing home and receive treatment there without any legal formalities, and in the same informal way as patients suffering from physical conditions. No doubt there will always be a certain number of patients who are so unco-operative that compulsory measures may be required, but the majority will be glad to avail themselves of the informal provisions. This should result in earlier treatment and in better prospects of recovery, and the doctor will be relieved of legal responsibilities which often appeared to be formidable.

Acute psychiatric cases, however, have never assumed a large proportion of the general practitioner's work, and when they have occurred they have usually necessitated treatment and care in clinic or hospital. But even a considerable number of these cases may be successfully treated in their own homes by their own doctors with the specialist assistance provided by domiciliary consultations, psychiatric social workers and health visitors. The build-up of a community health service has much to be said for it, both in regard to the treatment of the patient and the education of the medical profession.

The real problem of general practice centres round the treatment of the large numbers of neurotic and psychosomatic patients who congregate in the out-patient departments of every large general hospital, who are regular visitors to health centres and private consulting rooms. Many of them must consume a fortune in the form of sedatives, tranquillizers and tonics, and their numbers seem to increase, rather than to lessen. What is responsible for this? Are we becoming too health-conscious? What has been the effect of documentary and commercial television with its seductive advertising? Is it just sheer bad doctoring due to our one-sided training and inability to understand the whole-man aspect? Is it the discontent which seems to permeate all ranks of society leading to futile, silly strikes or threats of strikes on the basis of larger pay claims and shorter hours of work? Whatever it may be, the result is tending towards a selfish, individualistic society without much thought of family, business, profession or patriotic obligations. It breeds unhappiness and inefficiency and domestic disharmony, and it is these medico-social phenomena which require to be put right if we are to make much progress in dealing with the many neurotic, dissatisfied persons we have to treat. Psychotherapy in its various forms can accomplish much—but the real secret is for a better mental hygiene of childhood, better homes to live in and a more contented, philosophical outlook on life's problems.

Sleeplessness, carrying in its train a variety of other symptoms, is the most frequent premonitory indication of a nervous system which is becoming over-strained. Sometimes it may be helped by simple measures such as a frank discussion of possible causes, a readjustment of the environment, e.g. home, work, etc., an appropriate sedative. If, however, the sleeplessness becomes more intractable, fails to respond adequately to sedatives and is accompanied by anxiety, fear, fatigue, hypochondriasis, a decision may require to be taken as to whether it would be advisable to 'down tools' completely, and seek treatment in hospital or nursing home. It is not an easy decision to make—it is not wise to be arbitrary —and the sensitivity and reactions of the person should always be taken into careful consideration. Some people do not like hospitals or nursing homes, they are afraid of them, they feel they may be influenced by the condition of others, they miss the privacy of their own homes, and not infrequently a patient's condition may be aggravated rather than helped. Sometimes, although a risk is being taken, it is wiser to treat the patient as an out-patient, to keep him at work even although he may require the aid of drugs, because work is often a good remedy and allows the patient to retain his prestige. We have known many patients whom we have been able to assist by keeping in touch with them, advising and encouraging them, and using sedatives and hypnotics as stabilizers. It is impossible to state what the best drugs are, they vary according to the person, and can be changed as the occasion may arise. There are a considerable number of patients who are ambivalent in regard to sleep. They may long for it but are afraid of it, afraid of sinking into unconsciousness, of the unknown, of death. Such patients fight against sedatives, they are not willing to be dominated, they waken with a start if they should fall asleep, and more and more sedatives confuse and befuddle them rather than produce the desired effect. Sleep, it should be understood, is a symbol of death. W. H. Hudson records (*Far Away and Long Ago*) his feelings when he was present at the burial of a favourite dog. It was Mr. Trigg, the schoolmaster, who made the grave-side address: 'That's the end. Every dog has its day and so has every man; and the end is the same for both. We die like old Caesar, and are put into the ground, and have the earth shovelled over us.' Hudson, when he heard those words, recalls: 'Now these simple, common words affected me more than any other words I have heard in my life. They pierced me to the heart. I had heard something terrible— too terrible to think of, incredible, and yet if it was not so why had he said it.' It was only when Hudson realized that the part 'that really mattered, the myself, the I am I, which knew and considered things would never perish', that sudden immense relief was obtained. That short extract exemplifies the intensity of the fear reaction and illustrates how relief can come, almost miraculously, once faith and confidence and insight are attained. Sensitive people cannot be bludgeoned out of their fears and forebodings, they require more delicate measures, especially the so-called vasovagal victims suffering from the tormenting distressing feeling that they 'will fall down dead'.

We would like to emphasize once more that the general practitioner should bring the same interested attitude to bear whether he is dealing with bodily or psychological symptoms. He should have patience to investigate, the ability to see the position as it appears to the patient, to establish confidence so that time will be available in which to come to a true estimate of the symptoms. This approach may be sufficient to instil a feeling of reassurance, optimism and security. It puts the patient at his ease, allows him to talk naturally, so that the physician becomes a sort of father-confessor. In that rôle he is able to gather together the besetting problems of a personal, domestic or business nature which have influenced his patient's life, and may be able to direct them into healthier channels. The ability to keep in touch with the patient, even although the practitioner may feel that he is not contributing anything, may accomplish far more than he thinks. It is by working together, by co-operation and mutual trust that the patient may be led gradually to acquire that greater insight and

c

self-knowledge whereby he gains confidence and independence. And that is the very best type of psychotherapy which can be utilized. It is not abstruse, mystical nor concerned with symbolic interpretation (which can be dangerous), but deals with the patient's reactions, of a bodily or psychological nature, from the point of view of a dynamic psychobiology. If by any chance the general practitioner should feel out of his depth, or if the patient himself is dissatisfied with his progress, then there should be no delay in referring the patient to a suitable consultant, or to a specialized hospital where more expert and prolonged treatment is available. Under the National Health Service there is no one in Great Britain who cannot have the benefit of the best advice available whenever or wherever it may be desired.

REFERENCES

Henderson, D. K. (1939) *Psychopathic States*, London.
Jones, E. (1911) *J. abnorm. soc. Psychol.*, 6, 81.
Suttie, I. D. (1935) *Origins of Love and Hate*, London.

3

CLASSIFICATION

In the time of Hippocrates a few comprehensive types of mental disorder were recognized, so-called 'mania', 'melancholia' and 'dementia', but their significance was ill-defined, and for two thousand years little advance was made. It could hardly be otherwise, so long as supernatural agency was invoked to account for mental disorder, and so long as physiologists believed in humours, spirits and bizarre localization of function, and had no constant recognition of the interrelation of mind and brain.

With the beginning of pathological investigation and its correlation with clinical symptoms by Willis in the seventeenth century, by Haslam towards the end of the eighteenth, and by Bayle in his classical description of general paralysis which appeared in 1820, the foundations were laid for a more fruitful psychiatric classification.

The principles adopted for subdivision have been symptomatological, aetiological, psychological and physiological. Often two or more of these have been simultaneously used in the same classification.

PSYCHOLOGICAL CLASSIFICATIONS

In this method, *a priori* formulations have been made usually from current academic psychology, and an attempt made to fit all cases into the rack thus constructed. Linnaeus (1763) was early in this field, and divided his cases into Ideales, Imaginarii and Pathetici. Arnold (1782) had two main divisions, Ideal and Notional, or as we should say, disorders of perception and imagination, and conceptual disorders. Crichton (1798) described insanity under the headings of Faculties (including attention, etc.), Principles (including volition and consciousness) and Passions. Pritchard's two divisions (1822) were Moral Insanity and Intellectual Insanity. His 'moral insanity' was corrupted into 'moral imbecility' or 'moral defectiveness' and now is recognized by the term 'psychopathic state'; it will be considered separately and in detail in another chapter. Heinroth's analysis was more searching, and included disorders of the understanding, disorders of the will or propensities, and mixtures of these. Bucknill and Tuke, following the Scots metaphysicians, had two main divisions, Intellectual and Affective, the latter being subdivided into the moral sentiments and the animal propensities. Ziehen classified mental disorders into those without and those with intellectual defect, and the former into affective and intellectual forms, while the latter are subdivided into congenital and acquired.

The disadvantages of psychological classifications have been chiefly these: they have been derived from speculation remote from the field of psychopathology;

disorders have been forced into one psychological category, when they may more correctly belong to several; and they bring together in one group psychoses essentially different (Kraepelin).

PHYSIOLOGICAL CLASSIFICATIONS

The primary and damning disadvantage of this method is that so little is known of the physiology of normal mental processes, and still less of abnormal ones. Further, the method often involves ill-established hypotheses of localization. Conolly's is an early example. 'All forms of mental disorder are dependent on one of three states of the nervous system: a state of increased or diminished or unequal excitement.' Laycock made much use of a hypothetical localization, *e.g.* he wrote of 'disorders of encephalic centres subservient to emotions and sentiments'—'the ideogenic or sensorial substances' of the cerebellum and hemispheres, but he stressed especially the reciprocal influence of body and mind. Tuke (1892) based his classification on the divisions of sensory, motor and ideational centres, with their corresponding disordered manifestations of hallucinations, paralysis and dementia. Meynert's scheme (1884) was partly dependent on physiological assumptions. His groups were: 1. clinical forms arising from anatomical changes; 2. disorders of nutrition involving (*a*) cortical excitement, mania and melancholia, (*b*) subcortical irritation or feebleness (*e.g.* delusions and hallucinations), and (*c*) disorders of subcortical vascular centres (*e.g.* epilepsy); and 3. intoxications. Wernicke made several sweeping psychophysiological assumptions which were fundamental for his grouping. Making use of the doctrine of specific nerve-energies, he first of all assumed that every content of consciousness was dependent on a definite set of nervous elements. Further, he took his aphasic scheme as the paradigm for mental processes in general, which consisted for him in a chain containing a psychosensory, an intrapsychic and a psychomotor element. In mental disorders interruption might occur at any point ('sejunction'), and the function of any element might be either increased or diminished. Accordingly he arranged the disorders of the associative chain as follows:

PSYCHOSENSORY SPHERE	INTRAPSYCHIC SPHERE	PSYCHOMOTOR SPHERE
Anaesthesia	Afunction	Akinesis
Hyperaesthesia	Hyperfunction	Hyperkinesis
Paraesthesia	Parafunction	Parakinesis

Wernicke believed in the localization of memories, and that hallucinations were caused by irritation of the memory-image centres and irradiation thence to perception-cells. His classification depended equally on the above assumptions and on his division of concepts into those of the outside world, of the personality, and of the body—'allopsychic', 'autopsychic' and 'somatopsychic'. Neither his rigid application of the doctrine of specific nerve-energies nor his theories of localization and sejunction were valid.

AETIOLOGICAL CLASSIFICATIONS

Classification according to cause has obvious disadvantages—the multiplicity of causes and imperfect knowledge of most of them, and the fact that one cause may produce vastly different clinical pictures in different persons, and, conversely, that very various clinical pictures may arise from the same apparent cause. Jacobi was a pioneer in this method, and, in 1830, boldly declared that insanity existed solely as the result of disease in the bodily system.

Morel (1860) described hereditary, toxic, idiopathic and sympathetic insanity, and insanity 'from transformation of other diseases'. Skae went much further, and his classification had a type of mental disturbance for almost every common physical disorder—gout, phthisis, uterine, ovarian, etc.

Clouston followed Skae's example, and had a number of 'more or less important clinical varieties'—anaemic, diabetic, metastatic and a dozen others.

Tuke made classification easy by enumerating, like Skae, all disorders associated with known organic conditions, and by throwing all the rest into a group covered by 'disease of the generative system'—a sweeping aetiological theory which had no more than a coincidental foundation at that time.

SYMPTOMATOLOGICAL CLASSIFICATIONS

Kraepelin has been the outstanding exponent of this method, and he obtained his most valuable inductions from it. Yet even his method involves much aetiology as well. The symptomatological method is essentially the method of clinical psychiatry, and if only for that reason is to be commended; for it stimulates observation, and, if broadly used, has valuable consequences. It includes the principles of other methods without falling into their errors and becoming involved in their unnecessary assumptions. It is true, of course, that in this method, as in Nature generally, there are no hard and fast boundaries, and that a given symptom will appear in several symptom groups; but 'the agreement of a great number of cases in certain signs', as Griesinger puts it, is the justification for the construction of an empirical division. If further, not simply a 'cross-section' of each case is taken, but a 'longitudinal section' also, so that the evolution of the psychosis is taken into account in the symptomatology, a more comprehensive foundation is obtained for classification.

A distinction, first made by Kahlbaum, arises here—that between the fundamental underlying disease and the temporary symptom-complex which it displays. The method of observation which has just been commended enables this distinction to be made, and allows us to speak of episodes arising in the course of a disorder, such as hysterical symptoms in a schizophrenic psychosis, and depressive periods in the course of general paralysis. This distinction of Kahlbaum's was carried further, so that the mental disorder itself was regarded as the expression of a fundamental innate disposition (*e.g.* Bleuler's 'schizoid' disposition).

It was Kraepelin who first furnished a systematic symptomatological grouping with special attention to the course and outcome of the various types of disorder. This he accomplished by following them over a long period of years.

ADOLF MEYER'S CLASSIFICATION

Meyer constructed a classification round the root word 'ergasia', meaning function, or the total behaviour of the individual. The appropriate descriptive prefix is added, *e.g.* merergasia—the usual neurotic reactions.

Thymergasia—the primary affective disorders, divided into hyperergastic or other active manic states and hypoergastic or depressive retarded states.

Parergasia—the fantastic, incongruous schizophrenic states.

Dysergasia—the toxic delirious states.

Anergasia—with defect traits characteristic of the organic group.

Oligergasia—the group of constitutionally defective states.

The truth is that no attempt at psychiatric classification is entirely satisfactory, and consequently that 'diagnosis', or the placing of the patient in the appropriate class, is on an unstable foundation. But, fortunately, it is not diagnosis only that matters, but the understanding of the disorder, and of the patient who suffers from it—under what circumstances it arose, how it is related to the patient's normal condition, what the disorder means, what light is shed on his problems, and what can be done to help towards a favourable outcome. In Adolf Meyer's words, it is not the patients we are to sort out, but the facts; and while in the following pages the case records will be arranged in groups for the sake of more or less systematic description, the disorders exhibited will be considered as the individual reactions of a specifically endowed, and often constitutionally loaded, organism to the environment.

Nevertheless, classification is useful and necessary; first, for the student, that he may more readily grasp and arrange his cases; and second, for the compilation of a uniform set of statistics by institutions and administrative authorities, in order to make comparison possible, both within and between countries. Epidemiological research depends upon classification.

Following Meyer, in this book, we speak of different types of mental disorder as different types of reaction. We use the term 'reaction-types' instead of referring to mental diseases, as expressing the point of view which concentrates upon the study of the individual as a psychobiological organism perpetually called upon to adapt to a social environment. We recognize that in many instances the constitutional element is the important factor, that the environmental influences in a number of cases are of relatively minor importance and that there are all degrees of relative participation of these two factors. But we also recognize that there is an internal environment and that what is regarded as a 'constitutional' type of mental disorder may often be the reaction of the mind to inner stimuli to which it finds difficulty in maintaining a healthy adjustment.

CURRENT CLASSIFICATIONS

The two classifications at present most widely used are, in this country, that of the *International Classification of Diseases, 1955*, published by the World Health Organization; and, in the U.S.A., the American Psychiatric Association's *Standard Classification, 1952*.

Section V of the *International Classification of Diseases* comprises 'Mental, Psychoneurotic and Personality Disorders'. The classification is as follows (the detailed subheadings are not given):

PSYCHOSES

> Schizophrenic disorders
> Manic-depressive reaction
> Involutional melancholia
> Paranoia and paranoid states
> Senile psychosis
> Presenile psychosis
> Psychosis with cerebral arteriosclerosis
> Alcoholic psychosis
> Psychosis of other demonstrable aetiology
> Other and unspecified psychoses

PSYCHONEUROTIC DISORDERS

> Anxiety reaction without mention of somatic symptoms
> Hysterical reaction without mention of anxiety reaction
> Phobic reaction
> Obsessive-compulsive reaction
> Neurotic-depressive reaction
> Psychoneurosis with somatic symptoms (somatization reaction) affecting circulatory system
> Psychoneurosis with somatic symptoms (somatization reaction) affecting digestive system
> Psychoneurosis with somatic symptoms (somatization reaction) affecting other systems
> Psychoneurotic disorders, other, mixed, and unspecified types

DISORDERS OF CHARACTER, BEHAVIOUR AND INTELLIGENCE

> Pathological personality
> Immature personality
> Alcoholism
> Other drug addiction
> Primary childhood behaviour disorders
> Mental deficiency
> Other and unspecified character, behaviour and intelligence disorders

This classification has been used since 1948 in the National Health Service in this country, but has been accepted only by a very few other countries. It has been criticized for failing to include all psychiatric disorders: transient deliria are specifically excluded; G.P.I. is classified under the Infective and Parasitic Diseases (Syphilis and its sequelae); and, to give a further example, Puerperal Psychosis comes under Complications of the Puerperium. More serious criticisms can be made of the category of Disorders of Character, Behaviour and Intelligence; here the section on Mental Deficiency is seriously out of date, and the section on Childhood Behaviour Disorders scanty, including only jealousy, masturbation, tantrum and juvenile delinquency. Psychopathic Personality is included under the heading Antisocial Personality: and more strangely, Inadequate Personality is included under the Pathological Personalities although there is a separate category of Immature Personality. Other complaints which have been made have been more matters of opinion: for example, that a neurotic-depressive reaction is acknowledged, and that a phobic reaction is distinguished both from anxiety and obsessive-compulsive reactions. There is no glossary of definitions.

The I.C.D. classification has had few champions. It has also had less than just treatment from many of its users, who are too often bored by problems of classification and deviate sometimes wilfully and unnecessarily from its categories.

The American Psychiatric Association's *Standard Classification* is as follows (the detailed subheadings are not given):

Disorders Caused by or Associated with Impairment of Brain Tissue Functions

ACUTE BRAIN DISORDERS

Disorders due to or associated with infection
Disorders due to or associated with intoxication
Disorders due to or associated with trauma
Disorders due to or associated with circulatory disturbance
Disorders due to or associated with disturbance of innervation or of psychic control
Disorders due to or associated with disturbance of metabolism, growth or nutrition
Disorders due to or associated with new growth
Disorders due to unknown or uncertain cause
Disorders due to unknown or uncertain cause with the functional reaction alone manifest

CHRONIC BRAIN DISORDERS

Disorders due to parental (constitutional) influence
Disorders due to or associated with infection
Disorders associated with intoxication
Disorders associated with trauma
Disorders associated with circulatory disturbances
Disorders associated with disturbances of innervation or of psychic control
Disorders associated with disturbance of metabolism, growth or nutrition

Disorders associated with new growth

Disorders associated with unknown or uncertain cause

Disorders due to unknown or uncertain cause with the functional reaction alone manifest

MENTAL DEFICIENCY

Disorders due to unknown or uncertain cause with the functional reaction alone manifest; hereditary and familial diseases of this nature

DISORDERS OF PSYCHOGENIC ORIGIN OR WITHOUT CLEARLY DEFINED PHYSICAL CAUSE OR STRUCTURAL CHANGE IN THE BRAIN

PSYCHOTIC DISORDERS

Disorders due to disturbance of metabolism, growth, nutrition or endocrine function

Disorders of psychogenic origin or without clearly defined tangible cause or structural change

Affective reactions

Schizophrenic reactions

Paranoid reactions

Psychotic reaction without clearly defined structural change, other than above

PSYCHOPHYSIOLOGIC AUTONOMIC AND VISCERAL DISORDERS

Disorders due to disturbance of innervation or of psychic control

PSYCHONEUROTIC DISORDERS

Disorders of psychogenic origin or without clearly defined tangible cause or structural change

PERSONALITY DISORDERS

Disorders of psychogenic origin or without clearly defined tangible cause or structural change

Personality pattern disturbance

Personality trait disturbance

Sociopathic personality disturbance

Special symptom reactions

TRANSIENT SITUATIONAL PERSONALITY DISORDERS

This classification is based on aetiological groupings, so far as the data seem to allow. The basic division is into 'mental disorders associated with organic brain disturbance, and those occurring without such primary disturbance of brain function, and NOT into psychoses, psychoneuroses and personality disorders'. Psychosomatic syndromes are classified under the heading 'Psychophysiologic Autonomic and Visceral Disorders'. Hysteria is not classified as such, but can be placed under the heads of 'Dissociative Reaction' or 'Conversion Reaction'.

There are perhaps two main areas of this classification which are open to criticism. Subnormality (Mental Deficiency) comes rather awkwardly under two heads—'Chronic Brain Disorders' and 'Mental Deficiency' itself: the subnormal (feeble-minded) will mostly come into the latter category. (The terms idiot, imbecile and moron have been abandoned.) The groupings suggested for the Personality Disorders also seem rather arbitrary and uncertain. While Schizoid Personality is classified under the 'Personality Pattern Disturbances', Compulsive Personality is classified as a 'Personality Trait Disturbance'. The term Sociopathic Personality is preferred to Psychopathic Personality, and the category includes both sexual deviation and addiction. Speech disturbances and enuresis are classified under Personality Disorders, though the latter certainly would seem to come more readily under the Psychophysiologic Autonomic and Visceral Disorders. Somnambulism is also listed under the Personality Disorders.

The A.P.A. classification is backed by a most useful *Diagnostic and Statistical Manual*, which defines terms and gives guidance about the recording of psychiatric conditions.

The A.P.A. classification gives corresponding code equivalents in the I.C.D. However, when Brooke (1960) coded 200 diagnoses both by the I.C.D. and by the A.P.A., and then used the A.P.A. categories to translate back to the I.C.D., she found she obtained agreement not in 100 per cent. of cases but only in 40 per cent. The two systems of classification are therefore far from being interchangeable in their present forms.

In general, psychiatrists agree fairly well in their diagnoses of the major psychoses, except for argument about the independence of the syndromes of Involutional Melancholia and Paranoid Psychosis. It is in the field of the Neuroses and Psychopathic States that diagnoses are so frequently discordant that statisticians have been inclined to think them haphazard.

FUTURE DEVELOPMENTS

It seems most probable that the classification of the future, as it moves towards a more comprehensive aetiological basis, will include conceptions derived from the same sources as the classifications hitherto existing.

The types of reaction classified as neurotic, for example, will probably continue to include all those syndromes in which the pathology is essentially the pathology of personal relationships—in that they result either from a maladaptation to contemporary circumstances or a perpetuation of faulty mental attitudes acquired in early life.

Another large group will consist of the mental disorders in which a definite brain pathology has been revealed. Recent advances in genetics, which have highlighted the importance of constitutional factors, and the success of physical methods of treatment, have raised hopes that pathological physiology may be shown to underlie certain 'functional' conditions, such as manic-depressive, involutional and schizophrenic psychoses which, although they may be precipitated by personal factors or accidental physical stresses, are apt to run a self-limiting or self-perpetuating course.

While we need to classify the phenomena of mental illness for purposes of research and communication, we must accept that we are likely to remain dissatisfied with our classifications because they will always clearly reflect the patchiness of our clinical knowledge. But undoubtedly we can improve upon the classifications currently used. The World Health Organization is currently giving a lead by reviewing the problem. On its behalf Stengel (1959) has made an extensive critical survey of existing classifications and has discussed the principles of psychiatric classification. The problem having been focussed, one of the main preconditions for progress has been fulfilled. Nothing, however, is to be gained from trying to tidy clinical data prematurely into the neat pigeonholes of a consistent classification. What was written in another connection is perhaps relevant here: 'in the present state of our faculties, any system which is without its paradoxes, is by the same token as suspicious as an exact correspondence of several witnesses in a trial at the Old Bailey'.

REFERENCES

Brooke, E. (1960) *Proc. roy. Soc. Med.*, **53**, 128.
Stengel, E. (1959) *Bull. Wld Hlth Org.*, **21**, 601.

4

AETIOLOGY

The relative importance of the various causative factors of nervous and mental illness is most difficult to evaluate. Our inability to do so constitutes one of the fundamental problems of psychiatry. There is no specific relationship between cause and effect such as exists in physical illness, but rather are we called upon to deal with a constellation of causes of an hereditary, constitutional or personality nature plus an almost bewildering variety of environmental stresses. That is why in the organization of preventive and remedial psychiatry it is always so necessary, in every case, to consider the man in the setting of his environment, and not as a mere disease entity.

The economic burden involved in providing care and treatment for those who are incapacitated by some form of nervous or mental disease is enormous, but the accompanying individual, family and social problems are even more distressing and alarming. New laws, new drugs, other new methods of treatment, and greatly improved hospital conditions are all having a beneficial impact, but the statistics which we are about to quote indicate the urgent need for more intensive efforts entailing greater research.

The Secretary of the General Board of Control for Scotland has provided us with the most recent statistics. In Scotland, a country with a population of approximately 5,000,000 persons, there were as at December 31, 1960, a total of 20,044 mental patients. In addition there were 8480 mental defectives of whom 6090 were in institutions, and 2430 were under guardianship. Since the introduction of the Mental Health Act (1960) the number of mental defectives, on an informal basis, amounts to 520. Apart from those who are being cared for in hospitals or under guardianship it has been estimated that 10 per cent. of the total population of school age are so dull and backward that special schools, special classes, occupation centres, and sheltered workshops are required for their training and happiness. The mere ascertainment of the numbers involved is, in itself, a formidable task.

In England and Wales at March 31, 1959, the total number of patients in mental hospitals amounted to 136,176. During that year there were 95,350 admissions to designated mental hospitals compared with 91,558 in 1958, and 55,856 in 1950. Admissions to all institutions and to private single care numbered 98,243 in 1959, an increase of 2275 over the previous year. In addition the total number of mentally defective or subnormal persons in hospitals or under guardianship amounted to 63,893. Furthermore, 60,522 subnormal persons were living in the community under statutory supervision, and 19,338 under voluntary supervision.

Both in Scotland and in England and Wales there has been a gratifying increase of the number of patients who seek treatment on a voluntary or informal
basis; the number of certified patients has been showing a steady decrease. In
Scotland, in 1959, 80 per cent. of the total admissions were voluntary patients;
in England and Wales, in 1959, voluntary and informal admissions amounted
to 88 per cent. of the total of 98,243, while the number of certified patients fell
by 2196 to 10,672 (10·9 per cent.).

The high admission rate of so many voluntary and informal patients has been
accompanied by a considerably increased discharge rate, due to early and
improved methods of treatment, but it is disquieting to find that there is a comparatively high readmission level. It is a reminder that therapeutic successes may
be more apparent than real, and might benefit by even greater refinement. For
instance, in Scotland in 1959 out of a total of 12,428 admissions to mental hospitals 4480 (36 per cent.) had been previously admitted. Of that number, 1139
(9 per cent. of the total) were readmitted within 3 months of discharge; 886 (7
per cent.) between 3–6 months after discharge; 624 (5 per cent.) between 6–9
months after discharge; 365 (3 per cent.) between 9–12 months after discharge,
and 1466 (12 per cent.) were readmitted more than a year after discharge.

For England and Wales the Registrar General has calculated the incidence of
readmissions of mental patients on a percentage base as follows:

1949		1953		1954		1955		1956	
M.	F.	M.	F.	M.	F.	M.	F.	M.	F.
32	32	36	37	38	41	40	43	42	45

While these are the latest figures available yet we may suspect that the readmission rate has not shown any decline.

Current population trends also heighten the seriousness of the problem with
which we have to deal. On June 30, 1960, the estimated population of the
United Kingdom was 52,383,000, an increase of slightly over 10,000,000 from
the 1911 census.

The 1960 estimate of the population aged 0–14 years was 12,214,000 compared
with the 1911 census of 12,969,000. The 1960 estimate of the population aged
60 years and over was 8,865,000 compared with the 1911 census of 3,434,000.
It is, of course, well known that with the increase of the life span there is a greater
liability to bodily and mental incapacity.

In 1960 the estimated population of pensionable age amounted to 7,663,000
(males aged 65 years and over 2,377,000, and females aged 60 years and over
5,286,000).

The economic and social burden made evident by the above statistics is something to be reckoned with as the number of persons of pensionable age constitute
one in seven of the population compared with one in seventeen at the beginning
of the century.

In all other countries it may be taken for granted that an almost similar
state of affairs exists. Everywhere mental hospitals are crowded with patients,

and the numbers of mental defectives and epileptics, for whom hospital accommodation is an urgent necessity, are steadily increasing. To develop constructive measures whereby this social and economic burden of caring for and rehabilitating the increasing number of the unfit is a pressing challenge of our times. Perhaps we are going about it in the wrong way, and would attain better results if we placed even greater emphasis on the positive aspect of ensuring the birth of healthy children. We will do well to remember the slogan: 'To make the unfit fit is a noble task, but to make the fit fitter is a higher and finer achievement'.

Our story is still incomplete. In addition to those who require hospital and institutional care we must direct attention to: 1. neuroses; and 2. social misfits for whom special arrangements require to be made. In the case of the former, amounting approximately to 10 per thousand of the population, a small number may require indoor treatment preferably in clinics integrated with general hospitals, but the vast majority can be treated, to the best advantage, as outpatients.

The social misfit group comprise the inefficient, shiftless, unemployable, morally twisted, delinquents, criminals and prostitutes. Many of them are the recidivists, the 'ins and outs' of the prison system. When their particular disability is combined with mental illness or defect or stems from such disabilities then arrangements are made for care and treatment in our special State organizations, *e.g.* Broadmoor and Rampton in England, and Carstairs in Scotland.

The relationship between all these conditions was summed up by Barrett when he wrote: 'Insanity and mental defectiveness, dependency and crime, social maladjustments and unhealthy mental attitudes are but expressions of a common group of problems that have as their units personalities that have found it impossible to control their mental attitudes and behaviour by reason of a variety of causes'.

Sufficient has been said to indicate that our task of elucidating the aetiology of disorders of the mind with a view to treatment is one of great magnitude which requires to be tackled with all the measures which modern medical concepts provide. The work may prove most rewarding. Our hospital clinics, examination techniques and treatment facilities require even greater development. At the risk of being redundant the question may be asked again as to whether we are tackling our problem in the right way: is it not steadily growing greater because the proper measures are being taken too late? It would be no small reward for our labours if it could be shown that by beginning further back, by treating the causes of mental disorder and of its companions and consequences, criminality, vice, alcoholism, poverty, unemployment and the like, we could render unnecessary much of the misery, money-spending and machinery which these disasters entail. This desirable goal can only be reached by an intense and systematic study throughout the country in well-conceived schemes, and with all the means at one's command, of the causation of mental disorders. To obtain co-operation between all individuals and authorities interested in human betterment the issues have to be clearly defined so that the public can be fully informed of the principles of mental hygiene.

AETIOLOGICAL INVESTIGATIONS

It is customary to discuss aetiology under a series of headings—as to sex, age, race, climate and what not. This does no harm, so long as it is remembered that such items have no necessarily specific aetiological connection with a given case. A mental disorder is the sum of many conditions, and the end-result of a long chain of processes. The earliest of these may have begun in the unfertilized germ-plasm, another may have operated *in utero*, and the rest may be the reactions of an organism thus handicapped to the aids and obstacles which it subsequently meets in the environment in which it finds itself—the influence of parents and teachers, the difficulties in the path of ambition and the ease as well as the hardness of innumerable situations in life. The first of these factors falls, in the usual scheme, under 'heredity', the second under 'congenital' and the next under the headings of age, sex, family, etc. But it is the ensemble of all such factors that is the 'cause'. An examination of our case-records shows that there is never, in a given case, one single aetiological factor, but always a constellation of them. Moreover, the cause is not a bolt from the blue, nor a mysterious entity destined to implant itself at a certain epoch on unprepared soil; the 'cause' is a process —something that moves and shapes itself in the passage of time.

So long as these conceptions are remembered it does no harm, and it is convenient, to consider separately some of the commoner and more easily categorized factors in the production of mental disorder.

HEREDITY

The rôle of heredity in relation to mental disorders is of fundamental importance and demands the closest study. That we do not know more about this aspect of aetiology is probably due to two main causes: first, psychiatrists have tended in recent years to pay greater attention to environmental than to constitutional factors, since the former are in general more easily modified, and there has been a tendency also to equate hereditary determination of an illness with incurability and even untreatability; and second, the facts about human inheritance are not easily obtained.

Experimental human breeding is impossible, and human families with their long intervals between generations and the small numbers of their members do not lend themselves to studies in heredity. Moreover, the members of a family may become widely scattered, and it is often necessary to collect data about ancestors on a hearsay basis only. People dissemble about themselves and their relatives, and even when information is freely given such descriptive terms as nervousness, irritability and the like, so often used by lay persons, make it of little value. However, as Penrose (1950) has pointed out, the genetical study of human beings has the advantages of being the study of a natural population, and 'there are excellent opportunities for examining gene frequencies, modification of genetical characters by environment, mutation rates, changes due to natural selection and the effects of different mating systems'; while 'the length of human life enables medical science, psychology and social investigation to study both the internal physiology and pathology as well as the external environment to an extent unknown elsewhere in the natural history of the animal kingdom'.

In the case of any single individual there is no point in asking which is the more important—nature or nurture, heredity or environment. Both heredity and environment are essential factors for the development of practically every human character, and both are potent factors in causing human beings to differ. There are in fact only three or four inherited human traits which are known to be uninfluenced by environment. When therefore we raise the question of the relative importance of heredity and environment, we are comparing one individual with another and inquiring what has made them different. From the genetic standpoint, 'the term hereditary applies to any mental disorder that would not originate without the presence of a certain gene combination'.

The Mode of Inheritance

Genetics has now become a complex science, and it is impossible here to give an adequate account of its basic data. These facts should be sought in a textbook such as Fraser Roberts's *An Introduction to Medical Genetics*. The following statements will assume some slight background knowledge, and stress what has clinical applications.

In general it is not completely developed traits or abnormal characters which are inherited, but predispositions to them. The hereditary factor in the genesis of abnormal mental states is not a general predisposition to all or many mental illnesses, but a specific predisposition to one or other or to more than one particular illness. The fact that more than one abnormal predisposition may be inherited by the same individual may account in part for the great variety and admixture of clinical syndromes which are encountered.

Classification of a trait as inherited does not imply that all possessors of the gene or genes responsible for the trait will develop it. The genes have a range of variability in their manifestation which is called their expressivity and which is due to their several effects being subject to the background influences of other genes and modified also usually by the environment. Thus in the psychiatric field it is possible that the possessor of an abnormal gene or genes may be clinically (phenotypically) normal, or show a certain type of personality, or in unfavourable circumstances develop a psychosis, according to how completely his abnormal genotype is expressed. It is probable also that clinically similar or apparently identical illnesses may be due in some cases to the effects of different genes.

There seem to be two main modes of hereditary transmission: *single-factor inheritance*, where the trait or character is more or less completely determined by the presence of one gene; and *multifactor inheritance*, where it is determined by the combined action of many genes. Where they are inherited, most gross abnormalities and defects are due probably to the action of single genes. Dominant, recessive and sex-linked types of inheritance depend upon single factors. Sex-linked inheritance does not appear to be of much present importance in the psychiatric field and we shall therefore omit consideration of it: the characteristics of the other two types of inheritance must be clearly appreciated, and they are here set out briefly.

Dominant Inheritance. The gene produces its effect in single or heterozygous form, and whether it is present upon one or upon both chromosomes of the pair concerned. Clinically, the features of complete dominance are:

1. The affected individual has an affected parent. Inheritance is usually from one parent only.
2. One-half of the children are affected where there is a parent affected.
3. Normals related to affected individuals are wholly normal and will produce, when mated with normals, normal children.
4. A pedigree covering three generations of an affected family is often sufficient to reveal the mode of inheritance. Direct transmission of an abnormal, inherited trait through three generations is almost pathognomonic of dominant inheritance.

The classical example in psychiatry of dominant inheritance is Huntington's chorea [see p. 411]. But such a clear clinical demonstration of this type of inheritance is unusual, since in the majority of cases the expression of dominant genes is irregular and incomplete. Occasionally a dominantly inherited defect appears sporadically, and it is assumed that there has been a mutation.

Recessive Inheritance. The gene produces its effect only in double or homozygous form, and when it is present upon both chromosomes of the pair concerned. Clinically, the features of complete recessivity are:

1. The affected individual has usually outwardly (phenotypically) normal parents, who are heterozygous carriers of the gene.
2. Among the children of such heterozygous parents, the expected proportion of affecteds is one-quarter.
3. The parents are more frequently blood relatives than is the case in the general population, *i.e.* they show a higher incidence of consanguineous matings.
4. The pedigree of one affected family is not sufficient to reveal the mode of inheritance. Pedigrees must be pooled. Though the abnormality is frequently manifested in more than one sibling, the gene responsible may be transmitted undetected through many generations.

Recessive inheritance is the most common type of transmission of human abnormalities: and diseases recessively inherited show usually less variation and are usually more severe than those inherited as dominants. A typical example of recessive inheritance is phenylketonuria [see p. 451].

Multifactor Inheritance. Here many genes are involved: their individual effects are small, non-specific and additive, and are combined to produce at least in part those traits or graded characters which distinguish normal people. These traits do not segregate but display a continuous range of variation. It is believed that the greater part of the variability of stature and intelligence in the normal population is due to multifactor or polygenic inheritance. Qualities of temperament and personality are probably also to a considerable degree multifactorially determined, but our knowledge in this area is very scanty.

D

Multifactor inheritance is detected by biometrical methods of some complexity. Mendelian methods of analysis, concerned with genes of large effect which produce discontinuous variation, cannot be applied.

Methods of Genetical Investigation

It must be emphasized that genetical investigations are pointless unless diagnosis of the trait or character under investigation is precise, and unless it is a biological entity. Much of the psychiatric field is not yet sufficiently clearly delineated for this type of research.

The high familial incidence of a rare character strongly suggests that it is inherited, but the familial occurrence of a disease does not of course prove that the disease is inherited. Members of a family may develop similar illnesses because they have been subject to similar environmental influences. Further research is therefore required to separate genetic and environmental factors, and three main methods are employed—pedigree, twin and statistical studies.

Pedigree Studies. Relatives of the affected individual (the propositus) are studied for the presence of similar traits. All near relatives should if possible be examined personally by the investigator, and a family tree constructed. If the pedigree shows that the distribution of an abnormal trait in a family has a Mendelian pattern, the possibility of a genetic aetiology of the trait is raised and must be further tested in investigations of other families with affected members. Single and small pedigrees are often misleading, variation in the clinical expression of genes may make interpretation difficult, and statistical corrections must be made for bias in sampling. The classical example of this method has been the elucidation of the genetic nature of Huntington's chorea. Pedigree studies will also become of considerable importance in investigations of the genetic linkage of heritable traits, which are becoming possible with the recognition of 'marker' genes (*e.g.* genes for the blood groups) for certain chromosome pairs. These more easily recognizable genes may in the future be used to trace the inheritance of genes responsible for mental illness and thus perhaps to predict the occurrence of breakdown.

Twin Studies. Francis Galton (1883) pioneered this approach, and notable contributions have been made amongst others by Lange and Conrad in Germany, by Rosanoff and Kallmann in U.S.A., by Slater in England, and by Sjögren and fellow Scandinavian workers. The method allows a rough assessment to be made of the relative importance of hereditary and environmental factors in the genesis of specific nervous and mental illnesses. It does not, however, provide a quantitative measurement of the hereditary influences, and it gives no information about the mode of inheritance.

The method depends on the recognition and separation of the two types of human twins, and upon their detailed comparison. Uniovular twins, which constitute about one-quarter of all twin pairs, are thought to develop from a single fertilized ovum: they have the same genetical make-up (genotype), and for this reason are frequently called 'identical'. Binovular or fraternal twins, which develop from two separate fertilized ova, are genetically no more alike than other brothers and sisters of a family. Any difference between uniovular twins must be due to effects of the environment, pre- or post-natal. Comparison between binovular twin pairs and their siblings can give some measure of the minimum effects of the environment. In assessing the extent of the hereditary influence in the genesis of some abnormal condition, the proportion of uniovular twin pairs in which the condition has become manifest in both members of a pair (*i.e.* in which the twins are concordant for the abnormality) is compared with the proportion of binovular pairs concordantly affected. Pairs of like sex must be selected for comparison, if the condition shows any differential sex incidence.

It is obvious that the comparison of uniovular and binovular twin pairs can only be revealing if the ovularity of the twins is correctly diagnosed. Unlike sexed pairs are of course binovular. Like sexed pairs must be scrutinized for similarities in characteristics which are determined genetically and whose expression is known to be little influenced by environment. Close resemblances in general appearance and stature are of importance in this discrimination, as is a history of great similarity of the twins when younger: uniovular twins may be easily mistaken for each other when children. More detailed criteria must also be satisfied before a twin pair is accepted as uniovular: there must be close similarity in colour of eyes, in colour and texture of hair, in structure of the ears, in finger, palm and foot prints, and in the ability or inability to taste phenylthiourea. The blood groups of uniovular twin pairs are identical. The minimal criteria for the diagnosis of uniovularity have not yet been laid down. The greater the number of detailed resemblances, the more certain becomes the diagnosis; and qualitative and quantitative analyses of the finger-prints (dermatoglyphics), together with examination of the various blood group systems, are usually now considered necessary.

Where comparison is being made between uniovular and binovular twin pairs, sufficient numbers of cases must be found to allow statistically valid conclusions to be drawn, and care must be taken to avoid biased sampling of the twin population. Single case reports, though often inconclusive, may give fruitful leads for research into aetiology. The study of discordant uniovular twin pairs should be particularly profitable.

Kallmann has expanded the twin method of research to include detailed study of the full sibs, half sibs and step sibs of the twins, and this extended 'twin family method' is to be preferred, as giving a more adequate picture of family constellations and as revealing the responses of genetically dissimilar individuals to similar environments.

Further details of twin studies may be found in Slater and Shields (1953).

Statistical Investigations. Statistical methods are employed particularly in genetical studies of the general population: for example, in the analysis of multifactor inheritance, of problems of gene frequency and mutation rates, and in investigation of the results in a community of departures from random mating. In-breeding, particularly the marriage of cousins, is of importance in fostering the appearance of rare recessive defects: and assortative mating, which is the tendency of individuals to choose marital partners who are in certain respects similar to themselves, may pose serious social problems when those who marry are mentally backward or delinquent.

The Development of Psychiatric Genetics

It was for long a general belief, fostered especially by Esquirol, Morel, and Lombroso, that all types of mental disorder and defect were but the varying manifestations of a common tendency to degeneracy which tended to the elimination of tainted human stocks. This was the so-called 'polymorphic' theory of inheritance, which survived into the present century. Many of the pioneer studies in psychiatric genetics, those, for example, of Koller and Diem in Germany and Rosanoff in U.S.A., though they demonstrated that insanity tended to run in families and clearly indicated the importance of genetical causation, were vitiated by a similar failure to differentiate, and by the habit of aggregating diverse and unrelated conditions, both mental and physical, in the search for a neuropathic diathesis. Insanity and 'neuropathy' were treated as clinical entities: and striking family histories (notably those of the Kallikaks and Jukes) were obtained in an unsatisfactory way and widely and tendentiously quoted. Progress was also very understandably retarded by the elementary state of genetic knowledge and theory. It was believed that mental illness tended to appear at an earlier age and with greater malignancy in succeeding generations. This 'anticipation' or 'antedating', apparently observed in human though not in animal genetical studies, is now known to be a fallacy, the product of a biased selection of data. The inheritance of acquired characters was also much debated, before the lack of experimental evidence in favour of the theory led to its abandonment.

It was Francis Galton who, in his book *Enquiries into Human Faculty* published in 1883, pioneered the scientific comparative study of the effects of nature and nurture. Galton realized that the effects of nurture begin as soon as the ovum is fertilized *in utero*, and came to the conclusion that 'the interaction of nature and circumstance (nurture) is very close, and it is impossible to separate them with precision'. He did, however, succeed in making a major contribution to the separation of their effects, by introducing the study of twins. The problem he put to himself was twofold: 1. whether similar twins educated together for many years subsequently grew alike, and if so, due to what cause; 2. whether dissimilar twins brought up under similar environmental conditions tended to become more like one another. As a result of an extensive analysis, Galton came to the conclusion that nature was probably stronger than nurture, and advanced as a convincing example of the force of nature the cuckoo which sings the same song in various parts of the world, although its eggs are hatched in many different kinds of nests.

Gradually, as psychiatric classification improved and the knowledge of genetics grew, more satisfactory data became available in the psychiatric field. Kraepelin found in manic-depressive insanity evidence of an inherited trait in 80 per cent. of his Heidelberg material. Rüdin, also working in Germany, made important studies of schizophrenia, and demonstrated that clinically dissimilar mental disorders may occur in the same family. Myerson (1925) in U.S.A.

contributed a detailed study of 97 families. Penrose investigated all known cases of mental illness in which two or more members of a family entered one of the Ontario mental hospitals, and found that schizophrenia, affective psychosis, senile psychosis, Huntington's chorea, and mental defect were significantly true to type in members of the same family; schizophrenia and certain affective states were, however, not easily differentiated. In the field of mental deficiency the Brock Report (1934) showed that of 8841 children of 3733 defective parents, nearly one-quarter had died, while of the remaining children about whom details were available, between 40 and 45 per cent. were definitely subnormal in intelligence (dull or actually defective).

In the field of delinquency, Lange's work (1931) has, we believe, been important. He investigated twin pairs, of which at least one member was a criminal. In the case of 13 uniovular twins, the other member of the pair was also a criminal in ten instances. Amongst the 17 binovular twins, in only two cases was the other twin a criminal. This high concordance rate for crime in uniovular, genetically identical, twin pairs and the fact that not only did uniovular twins tend both to be criminals but even to be similar kinds of criminals, allowed Lange to stress the great significance of hereditary tendencies in the genesis of crime. It is, however, not justifiable on the basis of this evidence to ignore or minimize the environmental factors, and to claim simply that crime is destiny.

Detailed and precise knowledge of aetiology is essential for progress in psychiatry, and it may be said that research in psychiatric genetics has not yet been pursued either as widely or as intensively as its importance merits. There is, however, available now to psychiatrists, summarized in such a book as Kallmann's *Heredity in Health and Mental Disorder*, a body of evidence which cannot fail to impress by its authority and to stimulate by its challenge to further investigation.

The Genetics of Mental Illness and Defect

Here only a brief summary of the present position will be attempted. Further details will be found in later pages where the various reaction-types are discussed.

Nervous and Mental Illness. The most clear-cut example of single-factor inheritance is Huntington's chorea, which is transmitted as a simple dominant. Amongst other conditions in which single-factor dominant inheritance is known or suspected, the most important appears to be manic-depressive psychosis, where the penetrance of the gene is notably incomplete. It is possible also that Pick's pre-senile dementia is inherited as a dominant.

Twin studies have provided evidence of the importance of heredity in schizophrenia, and some authorities (Luxemburger, Kallmann) believe that it is recessively inherited and due to a single gene. A major difficulty in this research has been, of course, the delimitation of schizophrenia. Even when the reaction-type is strictly defined clinically, it may be the product of a number of different genotypes.

Though the evidence is as yet very incomplete, multifactor inheritance is thought to play some rôle in the aetiology of the psychoneuroses. The protagonists of this theory conceive the neurotic to be a normal variant.

There is considerable disagreement about the genetic background of the epilepsies. Recent studies seem to support the distinction between idiopathic and symptomatic epilepsy, and to demonstrate the importance of heredity in cases of *petit mal* (*i.e.* those which show a three per second wave and spike pattern in the E.E.G.).

Other conditions in which the importance of genetic factors has been demonstrated are senescence and overt homosexuality.

Subnormality or Mental Defect. In the field of subnormality a broad distinction may be made between subnormal and severely subnormal cases.

In the aetiology of many cases of subnormality (previously designated feeble-minded), constituting probably at least one-third of the total defective population, multiple genes (polygenes) play an important and perhaps predominant rôle, as they do in the aetiology of normal intelligence. These 'sub-cultural', defective individuals occupy the lower part of the normal frequency distribution curve of intelligence, and subnormality is common amongst their relatives. Polygenes probably also play a part in determining some cases of severe subnormality.

Severe subnormality (which includes cases previously designated idiots and imbeciles) comprises a large number of clinical entities, many still not satisfactorily differentiated, of very various aetiology. Amongst these an as yet undetermined but important number are due mainly or wholly to the effects of single genes. Amongst such conditions believed to be dominantly inherited are tuberous sclerosis (epiloia), neurofibromatosis, naevoid amentia and hypertelorism. Recessively inherited defects tend to be even more sharply demarcated, and include amaurotic family idiocy, phenylketonuria, gargoylism (Hurler's disease), hepato-lenticular degeneration, and some forms of diffuse sclerosis (Schilder's disease).

The recently discovered associations between subnormality and chromosome abnormalities are described on pages 454-6.

EUGENICS

By dictionary definition eugenics is the science of the production of fine offspring. In practice, eugenics has usually a wider connotation, and the humanitarian spirit which has inspired this movement for human betterment is more fitly expressed in Francis Galton's own statement (1908): 'Man is gifted with pity and other kindly feelings; he has also the power of preventing many kinds of suffering. I conceive it to fall well within his province to replace Natural Selection by other processes that are more merciful and not less effective.'

Galton's work on *Hereditary Genius*, his study (along with Schuster) of *Noteworthy Families*, and the book of F. A. Woods on *Mental and Moral Heredity in Royalty* all demonstrate that 'a considerable proportion of the noteworthy members in a population spring from comparatively few families'. Furthermore, Galton's investigations in relation to the kinship of the Fellows of the Royal Society, of English judges, and of groups of illustrious men from every walk of life showed that eminent men tend to have eminent relatives, and that this is not dependent on special environmental advantages. Terman, in U.S.A., found among gifted children with an I.Q. of 130 or better that in 53 per cent. the fathers were of the professional class; 37 per cent. were clerical workers; and 10 per cent. were skilled artisans: that is, while the professional class constituted about 2 per cent. of the whole population of a state, this class produced 50 per cent. of the children of high natural endowment.

In Great Britain in recent years the evidence of differential reproductive rates has caused some alarm that less valuable stocks may be multiplying at the expense of the good (Godfrey Thomson et al., 1947). The most highly endowed individuals, irrespective of social or economic class, have been producing the smallest families: and it has been found that there is a negative association of size of family with intelligence test scores—the individual child's test score tends to go down as the number of his siblings goes up. So one might expect as a result of this population trend that, if tested intelligence is, as it appears to be, largely inherited and if the tests applied have been as valid and reliable as has been thought, the average intelligence of our population will show a rather steep decline. It has been estimated, for example, that in 50 years subnormality might be twice as common. In fact, however, there is as yet no evidence that this expected decline in intelligence is taking place. For example, in Scotland in 1932, 90,000 11-year olds had their intelligence tested, and in 1947 a similar sample of the school population was similarly tested: and in 1947 the mean score of those tested was found to be slightly higher than it was in 1932. Yet, despite these figures, adverse selection may be proceeding unobserved, temporarily masked by favourable environmental factors.

The matter is one of which every responsible person must take cognizance, and the situation must continue to be watched closely. Burt has expressed the problem this way: 'As a nation we should know our resources in mind-power as accurately as we do in man-power, iron and coal'.

Other dysgenic influences can be detected, more or less certainly, in our Western civilization. Its wars have led to the mutilation and death of some of its fittest citizens: the advances of preventive and therapeutic medicine and surgery have mitigated the pressures of natural selection and have preserved the lives of many who are constitutionally frail or damaged: the increasing exposure of the population to radiation may produce harmful mutations.

It is of course to combat prejudicial population trends that eugenic movements and societies have taken the field and call for and merit our support. But it is necessary also that we should be broad-minded and somewhat sceptical in our approach to this subject. Natural selection is infinitely more potent than selection by deliberate human agency is ever likely to be, and the general population is a great reservoir, not only of definite good and bad, but of that variety and potentiality without which the healthy development of a society fails. Eugenics is wholly dependent upon our knowledge of genetics, and genetics is still a young science, operating in an area where a great deal is unknown. Also, before we can select effectively we must know clearly what products we desire. We do know in a very general way the kinds of individual whose birth and growth we wish to encourage, but we cannot yet be categorical: while we have had some success in measuring intelligence, the measurement of personality and temperament and of all the subtler qualities of human beings eludes us. It would be quite arbitrary to proceed to measure human beings in terms of some current standard of behaviour or concepts of mental hygiene, and to ignore the contributions which have been made, and will be made, to any society by many who are technically unstable. Again, an emphasis on eugenics must not lead to any undervaluation of environmental factors or to any *laissez-faire* attitude towards economic and social betterment. Finally, we should remember that the ultimate arbiter of our recommendations will be that public opinion which it is always better to seek to educate than to coerce, and which for long has been firmly convinced, with much justice, that it takes all kinds to make a world.

Negative and Positive Eugenic Programmes

Negative Eugenics. By negative eugenics is meant the method whereby a reduction can be effected in those below average, and the measures advocated may be grouped as follows:

1. Celibacy and sexual abstinence.
2. Marriage regulations.
3. Segregation.
4. Contraception.
5. Sterilization.
6. Abortion.

All reasonable people are coming to appreciate that there are certain persons who as a result of hereditary or environmental factors, or both, are either so subnormal (mentally defective) or so temperamentally unstable that they should be discouraged from parenthood, both for their own sake and that of their progeny. In consequence of this it has been advocated that where the person does not himself realize the significance of his disordered state a law should be introduced forbidding the marriage of those likely to transmit undesirable traits. In practice this would mean the establishment of a bureau with the power to grant or withhold marriage certificates. That would inevitably be a cumbrous and costly procedure, and in our opinion the emphasis should be placed more on health education and propaganda than on legislation.

Segregation. In colonies for the subnormal or in mental hospitals segregation is an accepted and beneficent mode of caring for the majority of those who are so mentally incapacitated as to be unable to fit into the social *milieu*. In many instances, particularly in cases of severe subnormality (mental defect), it means the continuous care of the individual throughout his life, but in others treatment may be of a temporary nature resulting in complete recovery medically and socially. Segregation, however, is considerably limited in its application, and for the most part cannot be utilized for the so-called 'social problem' or psychopathic group—a group which constitutes the greatest danger to society.

Contraception or Birth-control. This is regarded by the unthinking and vulgar-minded as a means of affording unlimited sexual expression without the fear of parenthood, and as pandering to the selfishness of the individual. It has, however, a larger significance. It may be true to say that it has been misused, that it has been adopted selfishly by the intelligent and well-to-do, and that in consequence it has been dysgenic rather than eugenic by restricting the birth of those who are worth while. Whereas the average size of a family in this country at the mid-Victorian period was 5·5 children, for couples married in 1925-29 it was 2·2 children: and this reduction in family size has been due mainly to the widespread use of contraception. Nevertheless the establishment of birth-control clinics is proving one of the most useful of modern health developments. The public are now being informed why, for physiological, psychological and sociological reasons, pregnancy should be avoided, and on the positive side how pregnancies may be spaced so as to ensure adequate health for both mother and child. Its efficiency depends on careful and intelligent application and, unfortunately, those are just the qualities which are lacking in the subnormal, psychopathic and unstable members of the community.

Sterilization. Sterilization laws were promulgated in the United States of America in 1910, and are effective in 27 States of the Union. In 1948, for example, 2322 official sterilizations were performed. Similar laws are in force in Scandinavian countries and in Switzerland. In general it may be said that the provisions are aimed mainly against the propagation of mental disease, subnormality and epilepsy, and that the sterilization is on a voluntary basis.

In Britain a Departmental Committee on Sterilization (Brock Report, 1934) advocated that, subject to certain safeguards, voluntary sterilization should be legalized in the case of:

1. A person who is mentally defective or who has suffered from mental disorder.
2. A person who suffers from or is believed to be a carrier of a grave physical disability which has been shown to be transmissible.
3. A person who is believed to be likely to transmit mental disorder or defect.

These proposals, which have not been embodied in law, were both wide and vague, and reflected a more optimistic view than can now be entertained of the efficacy of sterilization as a eugenic measure. There is no justification whatever for advocating sterilization in a wholesale way as a means of improving the quality of a population: but if the measure is kept on an individual basis, if each case is judged on its merits, particular families may be helped and few people would raise any objection to its application.

Abortion. Abortion, especially in cases of rape and incest, meets with a large measure of public approval. It is also entirely justifiable in those cases where the mother becomes seriously ill mentally during her pregnancy, though with recent advances in treatment it is rarely indicated in cases of affective disorder. In Britain it is customary for the family doctor to call for a psychiatrist's opinion before finally allowing the operation by an obstetrician. He thereby secures both the patient's welfare and his own reputation.

How successful can these negative eugenic measures be, which have been described? Deliberate negative selection against traits determined by many genes is very difficult: for example, in the control of subnormality it would entail prevention of the assortative mating and reproduction of subnormal individuals, most of whom are at liberty and employed in the community. More perhaps can be effected in the case of traits determined by single genes, but here too our powers are very considerably limited, especially where the inheritance is recessive.

Natural selection acts to modify or eliminate dominant defects rather rapidly. If the inherited disability is very severe and is developed early in life, the natural rate of elimination is high. A high mutation rate (*e.g.* in epiloia) may, however, balance this loss of genes by early death. It is the severe dominant defects which are not manifested until later in life that are perpetuated by transmission to offspring, and it is against these that we would seek to employ negative eugenic measures. Huntington's chorea is an example of such a defect, and it may be used to illustrate the eugenic possibilities. If all the children of parents with Huntington's chorea were sterilized or otherwise remained childless, the incidence of the condition would rapidly diminish. Two major difficulties, however, arise; first, one-half of the children of a parent with Huntington's chorea will be un-affected, and childlessness would be for many of them a severe privation; and second, the average age of onset of the illness is around 35 years, and we know no way of identifying, before he develops it, the individual who is going to be its victim, and it is likely that in many cases the affected individual will have repro-duced before his illness displays itself. Progress in eugenic control of this severe disease is likely to be made, therefore, only when we have found a means of recognizing the heterozygote at an early age. Moreover, it must be remembered that the occurrence of new mutations makes the disease ineradicable.

Natural selection acts exceedingly slowly against recessive defects. Single genes which cause rare recessive diseases or defects in humans do not usually give rise to any disability in the carriers (heterozygotes). We can rarely detect these carriers: and most of the parents of those who develop recessive disabilities are clinically normal. Negative selective measures such as sterilization can therefore very rarely be applied. Furthermore, it may be said in general that from the eugenic point of view the sufferer from, or carrier of, a recessive abnormality should not be discouraged from marrying, if he does not wish to marry a blood relative or into a family in which the same abnormality has appeared.

With regard to epilepsy, the genetic background of the symptom is by no means clear, and it seems that there are no good grounds for forbidding most epileptics to marry and to have children.

Positive Eugenics. A positive eugenic policy aims at increasing the numbers of those above average. This may be effected in the following ways:

1. Family allowances.
2. Relief from taxation.
3. Educational opportunities.
4. Contraception.
5. Marriage certificates.

The objectives are to encourage those individuals with noteworthy heritable qualities to produce bigger families, and to ensure an optimum upbringing for these children. Much has been done in this country and elsewhere by means of bursaries and scholarships to increase educational opportunities for children and young people showing exceptional aptitudes. Parents get other social welfare aids; but more might still be done in this direction.

One method of encouraging the growth and development of healthy families is by making 'family allowances' to parents. This has become national policy in Italy, for example, and in France and Great Britain. In the latter, under the Family Allowances and National Insurance Act 1956, an allowance of eight shillings per week is paid for the second child and ten shillings for the third and each subsequent child up to the normal school-leaving age (15), and for any further period before the 18th birthday while he or she is full-time at school or apprenticed. This is a step in the right direction, but a small one. It recognizes the economic burden of parentage, but such a flat-rate relief, subject also to income tax, does very little, if anything, to encourage parentage in the higher social groups. The Royal Commission on Population which reported in 1949 recommended increased children's allowances for those at lower, and a sliding scale of tax relief for those at higher, income levels.

In conclusion, it may be said that in most cases of nervous and mental illness the aetiology is multiple, that genetic and environmental factors interact, and that with our present knowledge we are likely to gain more by seeking to control the environmental factors. Though both negative and positive eugenic measures can rightly be advocated, the latter are more important. Even a slight selective advantage would cause an increase in frequency of the polygenes upon which probably depend to a large extent the socially desirable qualities of high intelligence, good physique and stable temperament.

Marriage and Motherhood

Marriage. An unhappy marriage is one of the most potent factors in the production of mental distress. It may cause suspicion and jealousy which can lead to mental and physical cruelty, to alcoholism, divorce and a broken home.

There are people who do ask for help and genetic advice in regard to marriage, but the advice given is usually acted upon only when it coincides with the applicant's own ideas. In order to give a reasoned opinion, we must ascertain the facts about the family history both of the man and of the woman and obtain as complete a record as possible of the health of their relatives. It is in fact rare to find a family tree devoid of all trace of nervous or mental disease, and a positive family history of mental illness does not necessarily indicate a bad heredity; the very salt of the earth may spring from such a stock. Furthermore a family stock may be improved by mating with a healthier stock. There has been a tendency for enthusiasts for eugenics to be too arbitrary in advising against the marriage of people with a family history of psychiatric disabilities. As regards cousin marriages, if the cousins come from healthy families there is no medical bar against marriage: but it must be remembered that recessive defects may become manifest.

The ages and personal medical histories of those who seek advice about marriage must also be considered. With few important exceptions (for example, Huntington's chorea), the person who has attained the age of twenty-five years with a clean bill of mental health and marries a person equally healthy, is likely to have healthy children.

More specifically, a family history of manic-depressive psychosis cannot be considered a bar to marriage: the manic-depressive genotype is very widely distributed in the community and is very often associated with admirable traits of character and with high intelligence and achievement. A personal history of manic-depressive illness must be assessed according to the facts of each individual case; the age of onset, and the frequency and duration of the attacks.

In schizophrenia the position is rather different. The marriage and fertility rates are low. Nature thus tends to act eugenically by limiting the birth of schizophrenics. Kallmann's investigations have shown that of 1087 probands, 562 had no children: the highest degree of childlessness occurred among male hebephrenics and male and female catatonics. It is only after the most careful consideration that a recovered schizophrenic should be advised to marry, and always with the proviso that parenthood is inadvisable.

In addition to the psychoses which have been mentioned, the possible consequences of hereditary predisposition may seriously perturb members of those families who have suffered from neuroses, psychopathic states, organic brain disease, or criminal conduct. Often it is impossible to give the complete reassurance which is so anxiously sought. But we can make sure that each case is carefully investigated, and that an arbitrary and categorical opinion is not expressed. Much may depend on the opinion given and on how it is given. We must take both heredity and environment into account, and we should not be unduly pessimistic. We should always urge the contracting parties to be frank with each other: want of frankness may lead to much unhappiness later, if one or other partner has a breakdown. Ultimately these are matters which we should leave to the individual conscience, while, as our knowledge of genetics deepens, we attempt to mould public opinion to the appreciation of their vast importance. The public must be enlightened so as to realize for themselves the difficulties, the trials and the sorrow which the birth of mentally handicapped children means both to the parents and to the offspring.

It may appear that we are putting a great deal of emphasis on hereditary predisposition and its possible consequences. We make no excuse for doing so. We believe that a healthy constitution is of paramount importance for the welfare of the individual and the race. The application of genetic knowledge may make a valuable contribution to the health of the nation and should be the subject of intensive study in the medical departments of our universities.

Motherhood. This is a matter which, psychiatrically, has never had the attention it deserves. Motherhood is the time, above all others, when the interrelationship between the physiological and the psychological functions requires earnest and thoughtful consideration; they may reverberate on each other to an extreme degree, and may constitute the best example of the concept of psychosomatic medicine. Needless to say, at such a critical period in a woman's life everything possible must be done to conserve her strength—physical and mental—and to ensure her welfare. While we do so we must likewise safeguard the prospects of the unborn child so that the child may be born healthy, and be brought up in a good environment. That means that the mother throughout her pregnancy should have been under skilled medical guidance, and that all the possible physical and psychological complications which might occur would have had adequate consideration. Some of the more common factors which may be present are the worry, anxiety and fear associated with the possible transmission of deleterious hereditary tendencies, previous attacks of nervous or mental instability, too frequent pregnancies, difficult social and economic conditions. Furthermore, the unwanted child, the illegitimate one, and the broken-home child may give rise to emotional situations which may seriously complicate married life, and may operate with disastrous consequences throughout pregnancy, at the time of childbirth, or subsequently. 'It may be said that any condition which gives rise to a conflict about childbirth resulting in an increase of the mental strain may operate as a precipitating factor and may, provided other predisposing conditions exist, result in psychotic reactions.' Many patients, while conscious of their psychological difficulties may never voice them, and it comes as a great shock and surprise when they become aware of their aversion to marital intercourse let alone childbirth. This aversion may amount to antagonism and hostility, and sometimes may be traced to experiences which have been present in the parental home. When the hostility to the husband is projected on to the child, which is by no means uncommon, serious consequences, *e.g.* infanticide, may result. Fortunately, however, psychotic reactions are comparatively rare. If they do occur they may be in the form of deliria due to a toxic-infective focus. But otherwise an endless variety of neurotic reactions are seen which may prove difficult to treat, but usually respond to psychological interpretation and analysis. The somatic symptoms may be in the ascendant and may present as nausea, persistent vomiting, abortion and stillbirth. Sometimes the above symptoms are the result of physiological dysfunction, but in other instances they appear to symbolize the rejection of the unborn child. Such phenomena are usually indicative of anxiety, or a hysterical conversion state, or depression, or even a feeling of unreality which may raise the possibility of a schizophrenic involvement. Even the entire character of a pregnant woman may change. For the time being she may be unreliable and untrustworthy: thieving, lying, having unfounded likes and dislikes, craving for food and drink to which she has never been accustomed, may all prove difficult to treat. Such disorders of conduct seem to point to deep-seated complex factors, *e.g.* a young married woman, five months pregnant, when shopping returned home with bags of apples which she always placed on the floor under a particular chair. Sometimes an illegitimate pregnancy will be concealed and the woman may continue in her employment up until the moment of her delivery. These cases may have serious repercussions, resulting in dangerous attempts to dispose of the unwanted child; the act is determined by a sense of guilt. The state of conflicting emotions was demonstrated in a woman 42 years old, who, when pregnant, described how, alternately, she was surprised, delighted, and afraid. The conflict would resolve itself into one of: 'I shall have a baby' with the opposing negative: 'I shall have no child—I have no right to one—I shall lose it—I shall pay for it with my death'.

Motherhood, then, may be a very complex and difficult problem, one which requires the greatest care and most considerate management. To effect such a purpose it would seem essential to establish the closest possible working arrangements between obstetrical, psychiatric and paediatric departments.

ALCOHOLISM

Alcoholism is an immense social problem, although matters have improved of recent years as a result of improving social conditions. The question of the rôle of alcohol in the production of mental disorders is a complicated one, and is more specifically this: knowing that certain clinical syndromes are usually, if not exclusively, associated with alcoholism, and knowing that alcoholism is very often a symptom of mental illness, whether and to what extent is alcohol productive of mental disorder *de novo*? It has formerly been considered that the responsibility of alcohol in this direction was great. Forel, for example, writing in 1900 declared that 'Experience shows that in all countries where the alcoholic habit reigns, it accounts for from one-half to three-fourths of the crimes, a great share of suicides, of mental disorders, of deaths, of diseases generally, of poverty, of vulgar depravity, of sexual excesses and venereal diseases and of dissolution of families. In Switzerland careful statistics of the fifteen largest cities show that one-third of the male suicides and one-tenth of the deaths in men above twenty years are wholly or essentially referable to alcohol.' One-third of the male admissions to his mental hospital were diagnosed alcoholics. To-day, Forel's statement of the situation is more quantitatively than qualitatively inaccurate, and it still serves to draw attention to the widespread social incapacity and disaster which may follow addiction to alcohol.

Forel also emphasized the importance of the hereditary aspects. He believed that there are two kinds of alcoholic heredity: the transfer to offspring of a disposition to inebriety and to intolerance for alcohol; and—distinct from this—the production of deformed progeny by the direct action of alcohol on the parental germ plasm (blastophthoria). The former he considered relatively unimportant.

Though subsequent research has not found evidence to support it, the belief of Forel and others in alcoholic blastophthoria cannot be scouted. Penrose (1949) has reviewed the evidence, and has commented: 'In view of the recent discoveries that chemical as well as physical agents can increase mutation rate, the subject cannot be lightly dismissed. However, we must ascertain that the concentration of a noxious substance in contact with the germ cells is high enough to have a reasonable probability of being effective. In the case of alcoholism this likelihood seems remote.'

Neither is there any evidence that alcoholism *per se* is heritable, though some workers believe that the alcoholic suffers from a constitutional metabolic anomaly which makes him abnormally intolerant of the effects of alcohol. Alcoholism is, however, usually if not always a symptom either of instability of personality or of overt nervous or mental illness, and hereditary factors may frequently play a part in determining the individual soil in which the symptom develops. Dipsomania, for example, is probably often the expression of an inherited manic-depressive constitution.

Research into the problems of alcoholism has been hindered not only by a frequent lack of precision in medical studies in the use of such terms as 'abnormal drinkers', 'alcoholic addicts', and 'chronic alcoholics' (Jellinek, 1942), but also by difficulties which arise in estimating the extent of the problem. We agree with Lemert (1951) that 'there is no one index which can serve as a measure of the total number of intemperate users of alcohol. The methods which have been employed to throw light upon the quantitative aspect of the alcoholic "problems" include surveys of insurance policy holders, absenteeism records in factories, arrests for drunkenness, death rates caused by alcoholism and admissions to mental hospitals of alcoholics with or without psychosis. All these methods individually suffer from one defect or another so that they cannot be relied upon alone as measures of alcoholism.'

The Influence of Alcohol on the Normal Man. It is generally agreed that alcohol is a depressant and not a stimulant, from the very beginning of its direct action on the central nervous system; and that it reduces both mental and muscular efficiency. The deceptive early appearance of stimulation, and the euphoria which misleads the subject into a too favourable view of his performance after he has taken alcohol, arise from the release of the lower nervous centres from control by the higher, by depression of the functions of the latter. In a dose such as is contained in 2–3 ounces of whisky (alcohol 40 per cent. of volume), alcohol causes a disorder of attention, concentration, memory and powers of reasoning; sensory acuity in all fields and the sense of time are impaired; and sensory-motor co-ordination is disturbed. His inhibitions lowered, his self-criticism blurred, his sense of well-being and confidence usually enhanced, the individual is obviously less able to assess risks and to deal with any situation calling for judgement and discriminating response. There is wide variation in the susceptibility and reactions of different individuals to the same amount of alcohol, so that a quantitative estimate of the amount of alcohol in the individual's body cannot give an accurate measure of the degree of disorder in his behaviour. It has been stated that if the percentage of alcohol in the blood is under 0·1 per cent. the individual's faculties are unlikely to be impaired, while if the percentage rises to 0·15 or over he cannot drive a car without risk to the public. In larger doses, alcohol produces all the well-known symptoms of intoxication. A tolerance for alcohol may be acquired by regular drinking. A heavy drinker may have to drink more than twice as much to produce a given degree of intoxication as an abstainer.

Alcohol then is not only a beverage but a narcotic drug, whose toxic effects lead to clumsy, inappropriate and finally completely disordered responses to the environment. It has, of course, also positive and helpful effects. Alcohol facilitates social contacts and warms festive occasions; it can promote generosity and courage. 'It brings its votary from the chill periphery of things to the radiant core', reducing feelings of shyness and loneliness, and is highly effective (if only transiently so) in relieving tensions and easing guilt, drowning the nagging voices of duty and conscience: so that it is not surprising that so many abuse it.

Alcohol, supplying calories, ranks as a food but cannot of course provide an adequate diet. The more that alcohol displaces other foods in the individual's daily consumption the greater is the risk of vitamin deficiency resulting. Not only does the vitamin content of the diet decrease absolutely, relatively the balance of vitamin and caloric intake is also disturbed; and the progressively disordered function of the stomach, liver and other organs causes defective absorption and utilization of these essential food factors.

Trends of abnormality and instability in the personality are very apt to be aggravated by alcohol, and alcohol readily reveals the defective control which may follow head injury and accompany epilepsy, or indeed almost any kind of nervous or mental illness or defect.

The Setting and Individual Effects of Chronically Excessive Consumption of Alcohol. The incidence of alcoholism varies from country to country according to the prevailing culture, as it does amongst the individuals and groups composing each community. Lemert (1951) in his valuable review of the social aspects of alcoholism, has summarized some of the available data on the racial and geographical aspects. In the U.S.A. alcoholism, both with and without mental disorder, occurs with greater frequency among the foreign-born than among the native-born white population, the incidence being highest amongst the Irish, notably low in Jewish groups (both foreign and native born), and higher amongst negroes than whites. Urban rates for alcoholic psychoses run about three times the rural rates: and in the cities the highest concentration of alcoholics is to be found in those areas where there is high social mobility and poverty. There are also pronounced regional differences in the rates for alcoholic psychoses, which are linked with, but perhaps not wholly explained by, the incidence of industrialization and urbanization and the provision of hospital facilities.

Not only does the incidence of alcoholism vary from country to country, but so also does the sex incidence. In the U.S.A. the male/female ratio is 7:1, in Norway 23:1, in Switzerland 12:1, and in England 2:1 (Bowman and Jellinek, 1941).

Those who handle alcohol as part of their jobs (brewers, publicans, barmen) are more apt to become alcoholic than the average man. The customs of the individual's social set may also have an important influence. Week-end boozing is less damaging in the long run than steady, excessive daily drinking.

There is no doubt that persistent over-consumption of alcohol leads to serious and ultimately irreversible physical and mental damage. It is well known that persons engaged in the liquor trade have a mortality rate for alcoholism and liver disease which is far above the average. The chronic alcoholic is prone to develop cirrhosis and fatty infiltration of the liver, chronic gastritis, polyneuritis and other deficiency syndromes involving the peripheral nerves and central nervous system, and any one or more than one of the three 'alcoholic psychoses'

—delirium tremens, Korsakow's psychosis, and alcoholic dementia (see p. 357 *et seq.*). In the production of this damage the toxic effects of alcohol itself seem to be of less importance than the nutritional deficiencies, particularly of the B group vitamins, which commonly result from its consumption in excess.

Earlier this century the proportion of 'alcoholic psychoses' to total admissions to mental hospitals was placed at from 10 to 15 per cent. In the U.S.A. in 1910 alcoholic psychoses constituted 10·1 per cent. of the total admissions. By 1949 this rate had dropped to 5·2 per cent. of first admissions to State mental hospitals (rate per 100,000 population = 3·6). But in the New York State Hospitals in 1953 the rate was as high as 7·3 per 100,000 population. The French statistics for 1954 showed the highest number of deaths from acute alcoholism yet recorded.

In contrast, in England and Wales the percentage of admissions to mental hospitals on account of alcoholism has decreased from 15·99 in 1902 to 1·66 in 1956.

The discrepancies in the above figures may be because of inconsistencies in diagnosis and a too facile tendency, particularly in former years, to class as alcoholic conditions in which alcoholism was the symptom and result of pre-existing nervous or mental illness or defect. Even when clinical criteria are made stricter, the 'alcoholic psychoses' cannot be described as a sharply demarcated diagnostic group. Korsakow's psychosis may have other causes; alcoholic dementia, developing usually in the fifties and sixties, is frequently complicated by the onset of cerebral arteriosclerosis and senile changes; and it is doubtful if alcoholic hallucinosis is a clinical entity—when transient, it may be an epileptic phenomenon, and when persistent a symptom of schizophrenia. Furthermore, the rate of mental hospital admissions for 'alcoholic psychoses' does not give a complete picture of their incidence. Delirium tremens, the most characteristic alcoholic psychosis, being of brief duration, is usually treated outwith the mental hospitals.

Other Antisocial Effects of the Consumption of Alcohol. Alcohol's disinhibiting effects very frequently have seriously antisocial results, not only in those who persistently abuse alcohol. Surly and aggressive behaviour may result, or obscenity and sexual promiscuity, assaults and other crimes, dangerous driving leading to road accidents, hang-overs affecting efficiency at work.

In Britain, where beer accounts for 85 per cent. and spirits for 11 per cent. of the alcohol taken, there has been a great improvement in this situation in the past 50 years, due in part at least to improved standards of living and to restrictions in the hours of sale of alcohol and to its increased cost. In England and Wales convictions for drunkenness numbered 183,514 in 1913; 52,661 in 1938; and 62,535 in 1959. In the U.S.A. there are said to be more than four million problem drinkers, of whom more than one million are chronic alcoholics (figures from the National Institute of Mental Health, Bethesda, 1954). In 1948 the number of chronic alcoholics in England and Wales was said to be probably about 86,000 (Jellinek).

There is no doubt that alcohol's effects contribute to delinquency. In Glasgow, for example, in 1960 there were 9802 persons proceeded against for Breach of the

E

Peace (including Petty Assault), and of these 5523 were found to be under the influence of intoxicating liquor at the time of the offence. Few reliable figures are available to show how much alcohol contributes to other offences or crimes, but authorities agree that it is an important factor in the genesis particularly of sexual and aggressive crimes (including suicide and murder). Planned crimes, *e.g.* thefts and house-breaking, can be carried out usually only in the early stages of drunkenness. As intoxication increases, violent outbursts may precede the stage of 'drunk and incapable'.

An investigation of cases of attempted suicide in a Scottish city (Batchelor, 1954) showed that alcoholism, though rarely wholly or mainly the cause of a suicidal attempt, is a significant factor in about 30 per cent. of these acts, and in men about twice as often as in women. Many of the subjects had alcoholic forebears and came from homes 'broken' by parental alcoholism, and 22 per cent. gave a personal history of excessive drinking. One-fifth of the cases were under the influence of alcohol at the time of their suicidal attempts. A relatively small amount of alcohol seemed to be more potent than a large excess in releasing the abnormal behaviour; and it was unusual for there to be an amnesia for a suicidal attempt made under the influence of alcohol. This is what one would expect, since enough alcohol must have been taken to produce disinhibition but not enough to cause insensibility. Investigation of aggressive crimes directed against other persons reveals parallel findings. There is rarely a true amnesia for a crime committed when the individual is drunk.

The following general conclusions as to the influence of alcohol in the production of mental disorders seem permissible.

Alcohol is responsible for only a comparatively small proportion of psychoses. It is more commonly a symptom than a cause of mental disorder of a serious and long-standing kind; and where it is a cause of organic damage to the nervous system it acts mainly by precipitating nutritional deficiencies (particularly of B group vitamins). An inherited tendency to a certain type of mental illness is, in most cases, a more important factor than the amount of alcoholism in determining whether or not a person will become psychotic.

There are a considerable number of minor mental conditions, either of a transient or permanent nature, which do not reach mental hospitals, in the development of which alcohol is an important factor. Emotional outbursts due to alcoholic disinhibition are responsible for many homicidal and sexual crimes and for a considerable proportion of attempted suicides.

VENEREAL DISEASES

Syphilis may be congenital, or, exceptionally, be acquired at an early age, and produce subnormality (mental defect). When acquired in later life it may cause mental disease of various types.

Congenital Syphilis. A certain number of cases of subnormality or psychosis in the offspring are the result of syphilis transmitted by the parent. Those in whom the mental disease is certainly syphilitic are the uncommon cases of juvenile general paralysis (found in about 1 per cent. of cases of congenital syphilis; Stewart, 1933) and cases complicated by cerebral lesion from other gross syphilitic brain disease (gumma, meningitis, endarteritis). But there is a residuum of cases of congenital subnormality where the syphilitic origin of the defect may be in doubt.

Though congenital syphilis does not necessarily affect the nervous system and many congenitally syphilitic children grow up to be mentally normal, there is a considerable number of infected children who sustain cerebral damage with a possible outcome in subnormality. It has been stated that about one-half of syphilitic infants show a positive Wassermann reaction in the cerebrospinal fluid. Nabarro (1954) reported that of 640 congenitally syphilitic children at least one-quarter gave evidence of clinical or latent neurosyphilis. The proportion of all cases of congenital subnormality which are due to syphilis is not accurately known. Tredgold (1947) was of the opinion that the proportion of syphilitic aments is probably about 3 per cent. Reports on the proportion affected tend to vary with the age of the population studied, since with or without treatment the child's Wassermann tends to become negative as he gets older, and this reaction may be the only clue to the infection.

It is important to stress that congenitally infected subnormal children may show congenital syphilitic stigmata while the Wassermann is negative, and may not show other signs of congenital syphilis while it is positive. The subnormality may be accompanied by other signs of neurological damage (*e.g.* paralyses, blindness, deaf-mutism) and if these signs are gross the degree of subnormality is usually also severe.

Acquired Syphilis. Syphilis is the primary cause of general paralysis, which thirty years ago constituted from 5 to 15 per cent. of the total admissions to mental hospitals: with modern methods of treatment, this figure has dropped to less than 1 per cent.—the greatest triumph of our physical methods of treatment. Mental symptoms of organic type may also occur in tabes dorsalis and in meningovascular syphilis. The knowledge that syphilis has been contracted constitutes also for many sensitive individuals an intense psychological trauma, which may be overwhelming. There are few illnesses which carry a greater social stigma and are attended with more fears. In these circumstances a state of morbid depression or other form of mental breakdown may be precipitated.

Gonorrhoea. Prior to the introduction of penicillin, this form of venereal infection, which is still common, used to be responsible for a great deal of chronic ill-health, many of the major operations carried out in women's hospitals were the result of it, and its influence in producing sterility through the development of salpingitis was considerable.

Amongst those individuals who recurrently contract venereal infections the larger number are psychopathic or of dull and subnormal intelligence.

EXOGENOUS CHEMICAL POISONS

Of the chemical poisons producing mental disturbance, alcohol has already been discussed. There are many others, which will now be mentioned under the headings of metallic and gaseous poisons, and drugs. New processes in industry bring yearly new risks of poisoning, and it is a tribute to the increasing care taken of the workers that the incidence of serious illness is relatively slight. Psychosis due to a chemical poison is a rare cause of admission to a mental hospital. The mental symptoms in these cases result from direct toxic action on the nervous system.

Metallic Poisons. Lead, mercury, arsenic, silver and thallium have all produced mental disturbance, the first not uncommonly and the remainder rarely. Tanquerel recorded 72 cases of mental involvement out of a series of 1217 patients with lead poisoning.

Gaseous Poisons. The commonest is carbon monoxide, a most dangerous constituent of coal-gas and exhaust gas, and found in mines, blast furnaces, etc. Carbon monoxide poisoning, which may be accidental or suicidal, produces acute transient symptoms, and, if its action is prolonged, a chronic, irrecoverable organic disorder. The latter is rare; but it is probable that as a cause of organic dementia it is sometimes overlooked. Amongst other gaseous poisons which may affect the nervous system mention may be made of arseniuretted and sulphuretted hydrogen, methyl bromide and methyl chloride, carbon tetrachloride and carbon disulphide.

Drugs. Certain drugs are of particular psychiatric significance in their promotion of personality deterioration through addiction. The proportion of drug addicts who become sufficiently ill mentally to enter mental hospitals is, however, very small.

The following definition has been adopted by the World Health Organization (1950): 'Drug addiction is a state of periodic or chronic intoxication detrimental to the individual and to society, produced by the repeated consumption of a drug (natural or synthetic). Its characteristics include: 1. an overpowering desire or need (compulsion) to continue taking the drug and to obtain it by any means; 2. a tendency to increase the dose; 3. a psychic (psychological) and sometimes a physical dependence on the effects of the drug.'

The chief drugs which may cause addiction may be listed as follows:

1. Opium and its derivatives, including morphine, laudanum (tincture of opium, B.P.), paregoric (camphorated tincture of opium, B.P.). *Dilaudid* (dihydromorphinone hydrochloride), heroin and codeine.
2. Synthetic opiates, including pethidine hydrochloride, B.P. (meperidine hydrochloride, U.S.P.) and methadone hydrochloride, B.P. (*Physeptone, Amidone*).
3. Cocaine.
4. Marihuana.
5. Sedatives and hypnotics, including the barbiturates, bromide, paraldehyde and chloral hydrate. Alcohol also comes into this group.
6. Stimulants, including amphetamine sulphate, B.P. (*Benzedrine*), dexamphetamine sulphate, B.P. (*Dexedrine*), phenmetrazine hydrochloride (*Preludin*), and ephedrine, B.P.

One must mention also chloroform and ether which are occasionally used in this way. In the Western hemisphere opium and its derivatives and cocaine used to be the drugs most commonly abused. In more recent years synthetic opiates have also become important drugs of addiction, the barbiturates are much overused even to the extent of frank addiction, and since the Second World War marihuana, which can be grown in almost any backyard, has come into prominence in the U.S.A., particularly as a temptation to young people.

Since the addict tends to be secretive, it is difficult to get accurate figures for the extent of addiction in a community. In Britain it does not appear to be a considerable problem. According to the Report of an Interdepartmental Committee (1961), the incidence of addiction to drugs in Great Britain is still very small. The number of known addicts is 454, in a population of 52 millions. In the U.K., as in the U.S.A., the highest occupational incidence is amongst doctors and nurses, who have, of course, ready access to these drugs: of the 199 male addicts in this country in 1960, 68 were from the professions. Morphine, pethidine, diacetylmorphine and methadone were the drugs preferred by these addicts.

The drug addiction problem in the U.S.A., where control of the sources of the drugs is more difficult and less effective, appears to be both absolutely and relatively much greater. Many young people, between the ages of 14 and 25, are said to be involved in the large cities. In Canada the number of drug addicts is 3212, out of a population of about fourteen millions, but there appears to be no juvenile addiction problem in Canada.

In general, drug addiction is more commonly a symptom than a primary cause of mental illness. The addict has usually been a temperamentally unstable individual before he has become addicted; but the contributory effect of a drug habit to this constitutional instability is always great. In the later stages a physical, toxic effect on the neural elements may occur. Drug addiction does not, however, lead to outspoken mental disorder to the extent that alcohol does. The drug addict may, of course, become an alcoholic, and vice versa. He tends to undergo a moral rather than an intellectual deterioration, and may be regarded by the community more as a degenerate to be despised and perhaps punished, than as a person mentally ill and requiring treatment and protection from himself.

It is doctors who prescribe the drugs which may cause addiction, and the profession, being thus in a position of great social responsibility, must ensure that narcotics are used for the relief of pain and distress only when this is necessary, and that their use is abandoned (except of course in cases of hopeless prognosis) before addiction can be developed. Not infrequently the addiction has followed on the use of the drug for the relief of pain or sleeplessness. In this country at the present time there seems to be much laxity in the prescription of barbiturate and other drugs to those who complain of neurotic symptoms.

The manufacture, sale, possession and distribution of poisons and drugs of addiction are in Great Britain rigidly controlled by legislative enactments— notably the Dangerous Drugs Acts 1920–32, the Pharmacy and Poisons Act 1933 and the Poisons Rules 1935. The history and provisions of American legislation in the control of drugs of addiction has been summarized by Tennyson (1953).

The Phantastica. Drugs capable of producing visionary states in normal people have been called the phantastica (Lewin, 1931)—notably cocaine, cannabis, mescaline and lysergic acid diethylamide. The effects of the two latter have been frequently the subject of psychiatric research, both in healthy individuals and in the cases of those who are nervously or mentally ill. They produce similar mental symptoms: disturbances of sensory perception with illusions and hallucinations (particularly visual), synaesthesiae, distortions of time and space perception, body image disturbances, unreality feelings and affective upset (particularly anxiety). These mental symptoms are accompanied by a varying degree of clouding of consciousness (Mayer-Gross, 1951). There is considerable variation in individual sensitivity, and the personality of the subject has an influence on the symptoms elicited. The reaction-type is an organic one, due to the intoxication, and frank delirium will develop as it becomes more severe.

The giving of these drugs is one method of investigating more intensively phenomena which occur in mental illness, and a combination of pharmacological and clinical studies may be valuable. Such research should be critical and cautious, since alarming reactions may be produced: and those who talk of a 'model psychosis' should be aware that the model is of limited applicability.

ENDOGENOUS CHEMICAL POISONS

In the beginning of this century it became a fashion in general medicine to attribute to 'auto-intoxication' every disease that could not otherwise be satisfactorily accounted for: and not surprisingly practitioners of mental medicine, where the aetiology is so often obscure and where tangible physical causes have been so assiduously sought, also vigorously pursued this will-o'-the-wisp. By 'auto-intoxication' was meant poisoning by the chemical products of processes occurring within the body, usually in the alimentary canal; and it was commonly believed that the liver had failed to carry out their detoxication. Even at an early date the hypothesis had its critics, and what Taylor said in 1907 of its validity in explanation of the psychoses holds largely true to-day: 'a perusal of the literature bearing on the subject suggests that it is not the validity or natural probability of the findings that leads to the diagnosis (of auto-intoxication), but rather a conviction of the insufficiency of the previously offered hypotheses'.

Although there has been little to support the old belief that in the psychoses, breakdown products of tyrosine and tryptophane reaching the general circulation from the gut are commonly of great aetiological significance, the rôle of liver dysfunction may nevertheless be important in certain mental disorders. Recently there has been progress in the study of liver disease by physicians, and some clarification of the rôle which deranged nitrogen metabolism may play in causing abnormal mental states. Sherlock et al. (1954) reported the neurological complications found in 18 patients suffering from liver disease, and have advanced evidence that nitrogenous substances of portal venous origin, normally metabolized in the liver, may reach the systemic circulation and cause a cerebral disturbance which they have named 'portal-systemic encephalopathy'. In the production of this encephalopathy, disturbed ammonia metabolism may be particularly important. The clinical state, with its evidence of major involvement of the basal ganglia, frontal cortex and pyramidal systems, reflects a diffuse cerebral disturbance: disorders of consciousness, varying from mental clouding to coma, are in the forefront of the picture, accompanied by motor signs such as 'flapping' tremors, increased tendon reflexes in the earlier phases, muscle twitchings and disorders of speech and vision.

Similar mental symptoms (delirium and coma) may be observed in cases of uraemia and uncontrolled diabetes mellitus, and are probably also mainly due to the presence of intermediate products of metabolism.

INFECTION

General Infections. Almost any infection may produce mental disturbance. The occurrence of the latter depends not only on toxaemia, or on actual brain lesions, but on the make-up of the individual infected. Some people become mentally ill much more readily than others as the result of infection, and children and old people are more prone to react in this way than those in the middle years. The mental reactions occurring in the acute stage of infection (*e.g.* in pneumonia or typhoid fever) are most commonly of the acute type—delirium. Rarely there occur other syndromes. We have seen simply extreme talkativeness—'pressure' or 'push' of talk—in the acute stage of epidemic encephalitis. The mental after-effects of infection can be very varied. As Bonhoeffer demonstrated many years ago, there is no exact correspondence between infecting agent and type of mental illness resulting; the same specific fever may precipitate any one of the ordinary mental syndromes. The influence of the infection is in lowering the general resistance, giving mental instability or predisposition a chance to show itself, and not in any particularity in the reaction. Moreover, no novel mental disorder is produced by any specific infective agent (except, perhaps, the virus of epidemic encephalitis). Thus a depressive or manic reaction may follow an infection, or an irritable, suspicious deluded state, according to the individual's constitutional or genetic make-up. In other cases a Korsakow's syndrome may develop.

Focal Infection. Since the introduction of antibiotic remedies the aetiological importance of focal sepsis has become greatly modified. Such conditions can be successfully treated in their incipiency, but if treatment is delayed the clinical symptoms of fatigue, lack of concentration, drowsiness, apathy and headache, may be mistaken for a depressed, perplexity reaction. That is why we emphasize that physical examinations in cases of nervous and mental illness should be carried out with the same scrupulous care as in a general hospital. The offending organism may lurk in the teeth, tonsils, nasal and accessory sinuses, gastro-intestinal and genito-urinary tracts. If the clinical state should prove resistant to antibiotic remedies, then surgical measures will usually give rapid symptomatic relief.

PHYSICAL DISEASES OTHER THAN INFECTION

As with the acute infections, so with metabolic and systemic diseases; there is no specificity in the mental syndrome associated with a given physical agent. Certain systemic physical diseases play a part, not always well defined, in the production of mental symptoms. Some of them affect the circulation in, and the nutrition of, the brain, and may do so sufficiently to produce an organic type of mental disturbance, *e.g.* the delirium of heart failure. Arteriosclerosis is, however, the commonest cause of circulatory deficiency in the brain, and it can produce both the acute and chronic types of organic mental reaction.

In recent years vitamin deficiency has come to be recognized as an important and not infrequent aetiological factor in the psychiatric field. Pellagra, which is caused by a deficiency of nicotinic acid, the pellagra-preventing (P.P.) factor of vitamin B_2, is almost invariably complicated by mental symptoms which are related to tissue changes occurring in the central nervous system. It is rare in this country, but with wider knowledge of its symptomatology it has been lately more often reported. In other countries, especially Italy and the U.S.A., it is more common. Other psychiatric syndromes which may be produced by vitamin B deficiency are Wernicke's encephalopathy (mainly thiamine deficiency), and the nicotinic acid deficiency encephalopathy, characterized by delirium and stupor and first described by Sydenstricker in 1939. Vitamin B is the only one of the vitamins known to be of importance for the nervous system. Experiences in prisoner-of-war camps during the Second World War led to a considerable increase in our clinical knowledge of these deficiency states (Spillane, 1947).

Other chronic systemic diseases produce, in a more subtle, psychological way, slighter mental changes, which are partly a reaction to the victim's knowledge of the presence of the disease, and partly a result of his physical weakness and discomfort. The rôle of endocrinopathies in the aetiology of mental disorder will be discussed separately.

FATIGUE AND EXHAUSTION

The term fatigue has been applied to things as far apart as a weakness in metals induced by repeated blows, and the extra-professional duties of a soldier. As a phenomenon of human activity much about it remains vague or unknown. Little of the basic physiology even of the fatigue which follows prolonged exercise has been worked out: while in psychology it has no precise meaning and 'is applied to any of a series of states running all the way from true physiological exhaustion to psychological frustration uncomplicated by any detectable somatic disorder' (Russell Davis). Yet it is a daily experience common to us all, and probably one of the body's most important defensive regulations.

The more obvious signs and symptoms of fatigue are now well known, as the result of the work of pioneers which included Mosso, McDougall and Kraepelin, and from observations made upon factory workers by Vernon and others. Fatigue causes decreased quantity and quality of work; an increase in accidents and errors; bodily disturbances, such as eyestrain, digestive upset and muscle pains and cramps; and psychological changes both in the intellectual and affective spheres. It is most inimical to learning: memory is impaired, and powers of concentration and association are reduced. Fatigue tends also to weaken emotional control, to disinhibit, so that the tired individual is emotionally unduly labile or irritable, stubborn and less than normally self-critical. Furthermore, it may bring on feelings of depersonalization and hallucinations in the form of revived perceptual experiences (after-sensations).

Bartlett, dissatisfied with the limited results of tests involving the repetition of elementary mental operations, chose, during the Second World War, to study the fatigue following highly skilled work, and to observe not only what the fatigued man does but also how he does it. This research was carried out at Cambridge, mostly on Royal Air Force pilots, who in the laboratory (in the so-called Cambridge cockpit) were given a stringent exercise in instrument flying. Prolonged effort at this difficult task, which may also have produced some degree of mental conflict, resulted in disorganization of their skilled activities: the main factor in this disorganization was considered to be the fatiguing conditions.

Bartlett himself in his Ferrier Lecture (1943) described particularly the perceptual aspects of this disorganization, and stressed the importance of three phenomena: the raising of the threshold of range of sensitivity to stimuli calling for compensatory activity, the loss of accurate timing, and the splitting up of stimulus and response patterns. In skill-fatigue there is failure to maintain organized, co-ordinated and timed responses. As fatigue develops there is progressive inefficiency: though the skill-tired man may in fact be doing not less work but more, his performance becomes irregular and the rhythm of sequence of the activity is lost.

Russell Davis (1946) studied further the motor and emotional aspects of this disorganization of behaviour as fatigue developed in the test situation. The effects differed from one individual to another, and three-quarters of the fit men tested showed slight or no changes. But in certain individuals, two distinct responses to the test conditions could be described: an 'overactivity' reaction and a 'withdrawal' reaction. The 'overactivity' reaction was characterized by manifest emotional disturbance, the individual became dissatisfied, irritable and agitated as he made restless and inappropriate movements: he also showed bodily changes, flushing of the face, sweating and increased muscle tonus. In the 'withdrawal' reaction errors were less frequent but greater, and correction was tardy, concentration and interest failed, and there was a tendency to apathy and discouragement. Davis has claimed that the degree and type of the disorganization of behaviour he observed in the test depended on the grade and type of the neurotic predisposition of the individuals he tested: and he has suggested that the disorganization of activity shown by some individuals in the test was essentially similar to that occurring in the neurotic reactions of air-crew personnel to flying stresses; the 'overactivity' reaction, found particularly in individuals of obsessional personality, being similar to acute anxiety, and the 'withdrawal' reaction in some ways being similar to hysteria. These findings, which should be confirmed and extended, have obvious relevance to clinical problems in psychiatry:

they demonstrate the significance of fatigue as a factor in the development of nervous symptoms, and how important it is in studying behaviour to take into full account the personality of the individual.

Fatigue, of which exhaustion is the extreme case, was formerly considered to be an important cause of mental illness. 'Overwork', especially mental overwork, was thought to lead to fatigue, and fatigue in turn to mental symptoms; whereas more recently it has become customary to regard both overwork and fatigue as themselves symptoms, the outcome of mental instability or actual mental disease. There is no doubt at all that fatigue or actual exhaustion are very frequently complained of, especially by neurotic and by depressed patients. Fatigue is the classical symptom of 'neurasthenia' and it may appear as a conversion pheno-menon in hysterical reactions. The fatigue of depression is typically worst in the mornings and rest does not dispel it. Abnormal fatigability is also a com-mon complaint after head injury, and it may, of course, be a symptom of other physical diseases which give rise to differential diagnostic problems in the psy-chiatric field, for example, myasthenia gravis and vitamin deficiency. A tendency to overwork himself is characteristic of the anxious person who is not actually ill; and when his anxiety attains morbid intensity the symptom of overwork is exalted into a cause. It is a consoling thought that one's breakdown is the result of too earnest and too continuous effort.

Russell Fraser (1947) has stated that working over 75 hours of industrial duty per week is one of the circumstances associated with more than the usual inci-dence of neurosis. Such long hours of work are, of course, exceptional, and simple physical over-exertion probably rarely produces significant nervous symptoms, for the sensation of fatigue is itself a safeguard, limiting activity. It is not in uncomplicated work that sensations of this kind are frequently disregarded, but usually only in work plus emotional stress, where they are noticed either too much or too little. In peace-time, it is perhaps most often the housewife and mother of a young family who willy-nilly is chronically overworked, and amongst this group fatigue is more often a precipitant of nervous illness than has usually been suspected.

In war-time, cases of extreme fatigue are more often encountered. Sargant and Slater (1940) reported on the acute psychiatric casualties of the evacuation from Dunkirk. These men had been subjected to exceptional physical and mental stress, and exhaustion combined with loss of weight had been important factors in their breakdown. But in war-time, as in peace-time, the importance of fatigue can be exaggerated: and most psychiatrists who had experience in the recent world war would corroborate Henderson's comment made about the First World War, that he was impressed by the excellent physical condition of the majority of mental and nervous cases examined from the various seats of war, and that he had not seen a case which could be labelled 'exhaustion psychosis'. During the Second World War the label 'effort syndrome', affixed to neurotic cases with prominent fatigue and effort intolerance, gave a misleading impression that the neurotic symptoms in these cases were mainly due to activity: and Grinker and Spiegel wrote in protest, 'Operational fatigue is the euphemism by which neuroses are designated in the (U.S.) Army Air Force.'

Some individuals are undeniably more prone to fatigue than others, and we know little about the constitutional reasons for this. Sheldon considers that cerebrotonia is characterized by ready fatigability. It has also often been speculated that some endocrine anomaly might underlie a tendency to develop neurasthenic symptoms, and comparisons have been made with the fatigue which is so characteristic of Addison's disease and which may be a presenting symptom in cases of spontaneous hypoglycaemia. Probably neurotic individuals with autonomic instability are more than usually prone to hypoglycaemic symptoms, and this may in some cases be a physical basis for their complaints of tiredness.

In short, emotional conflict and perturbation lead to fatigue; while fatigue allows emotional disturbances to appear, such as anxiety symptoms, irritability and depression, especially in people of obsessional temperament.

TRAUMA

Trauma may produce mental symptoms in one of two ways. Either it causes structural injury to the brain, or it causes emotional disturbances which in one form or another are prolonged for some time. In the first instance the mental reaction is of the organic type, often with certain more subtle changes of personality; in the second the result is usually a neurosis. In the first group the injury is directly or indirectly to the head; in the second, the seat of injury may be anywhere—or nowhere. The first group are often called 'traumatic psychoses', when organic personality change or dementia has resulted from the head injury. Clinically, the difficulty arises in determining to what extent in any patient the symptoms are due to organic lesion. Wars and the increasing use of motor vehicles in this century have caused a higher incidence of these traumatic psychoses, particularly amongst younger men. Anderson (1929) found that 55 per cent. of a force of 450 motor drivers were 23 years old or younger, and that these contributed 74 per cent. of all the accidents of the force. Neuroses following trauma are much more frequent than traumatic psychoses, but they do not often enter mental hospitals. They are common in general practice and in out-patient departments of general hospitals. It seems indisputable that their incidence has increased in Britain since the introduction of the Insurance and other Compensation Acts.

MENTAL FACTORS

These may be divided into two classes, social and intrinsic. The latter are more subtle, being compounded of inner desires and the mental precipitates, as it were, of environmental influences. They will be described under 'Psychopathology'. The commonest immediate social factors are financial and business worries, domestic difficulties, dissatisfactions of all kinds, disappointments and worries in the sexual sphere and deaths of relatives. It is such situations as these that the individual, especially the susceptible individual, finds it difficult to face. He may surmount one difficulty successfully, only to go down before an accumulation of troubles. It is not the situation itself that matters, but what the subject feels about it.

SOCIAL FACTORS AND ASPECTS

There are certain social factors of a general and pervasive kind which are of particular significance in favouring mental illness, more especially of the so-called minor sort, that is to say the neurotic conditions which depend so largely on the existence of anxiety.

Insecurity, Emotional Deprivation and Unemployment. The first and possibly the most universally operative of these is emotional insecurity in early life. This can arise especially from an unsatisfactory emotional relationship between parents and child, which again is naturally influenced by unsatisfactory relationships between the parents themselves. In early life this may produce a nervous child, and the effects can persist into adult life, to produce the nervous adult prone to neurotic reactions, or, especially if there is a constitutional factor of the appropriate kind, to psychotic forms of illness. A feeling on the child's part of a lack of affection from his parents or their substitutes, and a feeling of being unwanted, can produce not only morbid anxiety, but a desire for recompense, or even for revenge, of which the result may be delinquency. Indiscriminate affection, on the other hand, induces a sheltered attitude which is apt to persist as a habit and produce a neurotic or unstable adolescence.

One of the more obvious sources of emotional insecurity of early origin is the so-called 'broken home'. This term 'broken home' is of wide reference and is often used much too vaguely and even without operative definition. It implies that the children in a home have been deprived, physically, mentally or morally, of a normal life with their parents. The deprivation may not only have many causes but may take many forms. Amongst the causes one may list illegitimacy; the temporary or permanent loss of one or other or both parents due to separation, divorce or death; alcoholism in a parent; persistent parental quarrelling; and adoption, evacuation during war-time, or rearing in a foster-home or institution. The absence of a parent, besides producing a general sense of insecurity from lack of one source of affection, means the absence of an important figure with whom a child can identify himself, as well as — what is sometimes overlooked in theoretical discussions—the absence of a source of training in sound habits. There is also the attitude and personality of the remaining parent to be considered, who may in such circumstances be unhappy or neurotic or unstable.

Bowlby in England, and Goldfarb, Spitz, Bender and others in the U.S.A., have investigated particularly the adverse effects of early maternal deprivation. The results of these researches have been brought together by Bowlby in his book *Maternal Care and Mental Health* (1951). His general thesis is that 'mother-love in infancy and childhood is as important for mental health as are vitamins and proteins for physical health', and that 'the prolonged deprivation of the young child of maternal care may have grave and far-reaching effects on his character and so on the whole of his future life'. He considers it proved that deprivation can have adverse effects on the development of children: 1. during the period of separation; 2. during the period immediately after restoration to maternal care; and 3. permanently. In particular he links early maternal depriva- tion with the later development of psychopathic states. The evidence suggests, he states, that 'three somewhat different experiences can each produce the affection- less and psychopathic character:

1. lack of any opportunity for forming an attachment to a mother-figure during the first three years;
2. deprivation for a limited period—at least three months and probably more than six—during the first three or four years;
3. changes from one mother-figure to another during the same period'.

Bowlby further states that it would appear that the more complete the depriva- tion in the early years, the more isolated and asocial the child, whereas the more that deprivation is interspersed with satisfaction, the more ambivalent and antisocial he becomes.

Bowlby's work has since 1951 been subjected to a good deal of criticism, and while not fundamentally altering his position he now (1958) states his views less categorically. He and his colleagues, amongst others, have drawn attention to the great variation in outcome which may follow a prolonged separation experience starting before the fourth birthday: some children appear to suffer great damage, others little or none. He admits that 'statements implying that children who are brought up in institutions or who suffer other forms of serious privation and deprivation in early life *commonly* develop psychopathic or affectionless char- acters are seen to be mistaken'.

Apart from predisposing to the development of psychopathic reactions, 'broken homes' may also be a factor in the genesis of many other types of nervous and mental breakdown. Madow and Hardy (1947) found that amongst soldiers suffering from war neuroses 36 per cent. came from homes which had been broken before the patients were 16 years of age: McGregor (1944), investi- gating similar case material, found 48 per cent. affected. Batchelor and Napier (1953) reported that 58 per cent. of 200 consecutive cases of attempted suicide came from broken homes: among the 42 psychopaths in the group the incidence was 74 per cent. Parental deprivation has been reported in 34–40 per cent. of cases of schizophrenia, and in 17–34 per cent. of cases of manic-depressive psychosis.

The subject is an exceedingly complicated one, requiring much detailed investi- gation and analysis. While some of the figures quoted above are clearly suggestive, they should be accepted with caution. Furthermore, their significance depends obviously on the incidence amongst controls, and the 'normal' incidence of 'broken homes' in the communities examined cannot be regarded yet as satisfac- torily established. The incidence amongst controls has been variously quoted as lying between 12 and 30 per cent. It is certain also that some deprived children make a successful adjustment and remain stable, and it would be profitable to investigate those who withstand such stresses as well as those who fail to do so. The rôle of the father, too, requires attention. In a patriarchal society the father is the figure in the home probably of chief importance for the child's super-ego development. His absence, ineffectiveness or hostility, as well as the mother's, may prejudice the child's upbringing. Andry (1957), in a controlled study of 80 male juvenile delinquents who were recidivist thieves, reported that the paternal affective relationships of the boys were less adequate than the maternal affective relationships and that the boys often felt rejected by both parents, but especially by their fathers. He concluded: 'Some form of parental rejection over a period of years rather than separation from a mother at an early age would appear to be one of the main mechanisms at work in the majority of cases in the development of delinquent behaviour.'

In summary, we may say that while childhood deprivations play an important rôle in predisposing to or causing nervous symptoms and delinquency both in the child and in the adult, it remains true that the aetiology of nervous and mental illness is usually complex, and that one cannot safely neglect or minimize either endogenous or exogenous influences. A 'broken home' in most cases can be only one adverse factor among many, and is frequently of less importance than, for example, a morbid inheritance. Looking at the figures of the incidence of broken homes in the histories of those who have become maladjusted, one may legitimately ask—were these homes not broken often because the parents were themselves temperamentally abnormal? Do these figures not demonstrate a genetic rather than an environmental effect? More research is required. We do not yet know whether an absence or distortion of parental influences (e.g. parental alcoholism) is the more important, nor at what time the greatest damage may be done to the child, nor which parent is the more essential to certain years of the child's development.

Since insecurity is a source of anxious habits of mind it might be expected that social conditions wider than the home itself would play a part, and in social conditions one has to include anything from financial insecurity to uncertainty of religious beliefs. Oddly enough, it seems that the very poorest stratum of the population is less affected in this way (Neustatter). An anxious disposition was found to be commoner among the well-to-do than among the poor, and this seemed to be reflected in nervousness among the children, which was least in the poorer classes, as if it was uncertainty rather than poverty that was important. Among the poorest children there seemed often to exist a state of mind not usually included in psychiatric literature in this connection, namely, apathy and listlessness; but bad nutrition, lack of sunshine and of the other amenities of life are as accountable for this as lack of hope of better days. Those who lose much, in social status, financially or otherwise, particularly if the blow has been sudden, are more likely to break down than those who have always been used to little.

The part played by education in the broad meaning of the word in facilitating psychological disorders in later life has received insufficient study. Education in this sense ranges all the way from upbringing in the nursery and the inculcation of sound habits to the kinds of values imparted by training at school and universities. Too often these values may instil a desire for power. The circumstances of life with power as its object may well be productive of psychological illness; in fact the Adlerian system of psychology is a study of the consequences in character and in neurotic forms of ill-health of the persistent operation of this desire. Neuroses of this sort have well been called 'cultural' neuroses, because they are the product of an essentially competitive type of civilization (Karin Horney, 1936). Such values are productive not only of despondency and depression but of chronic anxiety, fear of failure, and of inferiority feelings, which are in fact an expression of a sense of failure to achieve the desired goals, and of such characteristics as habitual criticism of others, which represents an endeavour to 'hoist oneself by one's own boot-straps'.

Apart from questions of financial security and of personal progress, mere lack of work, as well as unsuitable work, has been shown to lead to neurotic illness. There is a biological need for activity, the frustration of which alone will produce inner disturbance, certainly boredom, sometimes apathy and sometimes mental illness. In addition, work has other values by giving the worker prestige within a community, without which he becomes uneasy. Reports on the reactions of unemployed men illustrate this. It has to be remembered that unemployment, as Mannheim has pointed out, means a disintegration of the patterns of life which the individual has woven for himself. This may have a catastrophic effect on some individuals, or a more gradual undermining effect on the peace of mind of others.

Few things are more striking than the number of lonely people among the out-patients of a department of psychological medicine. Some of these are constitutionally inclined to solitariness, but others have it forced on them, with consequent limitation of interest, and dissatisfaction from frustration of natural needs. The parental deprivation which we have discussed above is one form of social isolation. Man is a social animal, and loss of contact with or rejection by the herd renders him both vulnerable and unhappy. Feelings of loneliness, the response to some loss of love or springing from feelings of being unwanted or useless, are prominent motives in many suicidal acts, at all ages. Those individuals, particularly in later life, who are not integrated in the activities of the community (for example, those who are living alone or in lodging-houses) are more prone to nervous breakdown, and particularly to depressive reactions.

Our present social organization, especially that part of it which is comprised in suburban life, does not cater adequately for these social needs. Some new housing schemes comprise community centres but many more areas of suburbia are without them; and there is a great dearth of social clubs which might offset the isolation which so many feel in our great cities.

The Epidemiological Approach. Epidemiological studies complement investigations of individual patients, and data from such mass or population surveys may throw light on the aetiology of mental diseases as well as providing the kind of social information which is necessary for the logical planning of public health services, both for preventive measures and in the provision of treatment facilities. So far epidemiological or ecological studies in psychiatry have produced few new facts of importance. The difficulties surrounding such investigations have of course been considerable: in particular, the complicated and often multiple aetiology of nervous and mental illnesses; the notorious unreliability of psychiatric diagnosis; the relative naivety of sociology as a scientific discipline; and the lack of well-trained field workers—all these factors have inhibited research. The techniques of such research and its potentialities have recently been fully discussed by Reid (1960) and by an Expert Committee on Mental Health of the World Health Organization (1960). The latter Committee considers that 'epidemiological methods can be appropriately applied to three aspects of the aetiology and pathogenesis of mental disorder: the genetic basis, the physical and psychological experiences during development which may favour the onset of clinical disease, and the social or other precipitating environmental circumstances'.

Epidemiological studies in psychiatry require the collaboration of psychiatrists and sociologists, and both must proceed with a lively sense of their limitations. From the psychiatric standpoint, where the subject of research is a biological entity, which can be both defined and readily ascertained, progress can be made, as it has been in the study of suicide. The psychoses and states of subnormality (mental defect) can be studied fairly well by epidemiological methods. It is in the field of the neuroses, character anomalies and psychopathic states that the great difficulties arise. What is socially accepted as being illness depends on the sophistication and tolerance of the society and of the various groups within each society, on the generally accepted ideas of right and wrong and of what constitutes delinquent or criminal behaviour, on how aberrant an individual's conduct can be without causing social concern or rejection, and on the readiness with which both the lay members of the society and the medical profession itself will refer problems to psychiatrists. The sociologist for his part will look at the community which it is proposed to study, to see if its social characteristics have been recently and competently defined and recorded: and if these data are not already available from census or other investigations, to see whether he has the resources in trained manpower and the access to the community's homes which will make possible a new survey of a representative sample of the population. The sociologist will also be aware that at best he will be using rather unrefined concepts and classifications in his investigations: the estimation of social class, for example, as usually recorded in this country is graded simply according to the occupation of the individual or her spouse, and satisfactory differentiation is certainly not achieved at the lower end of this, the Registrar General's, social scale of five classes.

The Prevalence of Treated Mental Illness. For several reasons, which include the lack of adequate clinical data in past years and rapidly changing facilities for diagnosis and investigation, incidence trends in the neuroses and other so-called minor psychiatric disorders cannot be computed. The psychoses which are treated in mental hospitals offer a more promising area for study. A careful and critical investigation has been made by Goldhamer and Marshall (1949) in Massachusetts, where for long mental hospital facilities and records had been at a relatively high level. These workers, using records going back as far as 1840, compared the nineteenth century and contemporary age-specific first admission rates for psychoses. Their main findings were as follows. Age-specific first admission rates for ages under 50 were revealed to be just as high during the last half of the nineteenth century as they are now. There had been, however, a very marked increase in the age-specific admission rates in the older age-groups—an increase which appeared to be due for the greater part to an increased tendency to hospitalize people suffering from the mental illnesses of the senium. In the nineteenth century there was relatively a much higher concentration of admissions in the age group 20–50; and now a relatively high concentration in ages over 50 and more particularly over 60. They concluded: 'there has been no long-term increase during the last century in the incidence of the psychoses of early life and middle life', and 'social trends probably have little influence on the incidence of psychosis'. The latter finding accords with what we know of the importance of physical factors in the aetiology of the psychoses.

Shepherd (1957) studied the admissions to an English county mental hospital during the years 1931–33 and 1945–47. He found that a large increase in the number of patients admitted took place in the latter period, but there was a quicker turnover of patients (a shorter period being spent in hospital) and there was no expansion of the hospital accommodation. The latter-day hospital population was older and included a higher proportion of female, married, voluntary and readmitted patients. The functional psychoses, particularly the affective psychoses, constituted more than one-half of all the patients admitted and were principally responsible for the changes found in the admission pattern to this hospital.

It has for long been believed that urban rates for mental illness are higher than rural rates, but this is still uncertain. Urban and rural areas differ widely in their access to treatment facilities and in their tolerance of deviant behaviour, so that comparisons are hazardous.

Influence of Neighbourhood on Mental Illness. Faris and Dunham (1939) pioneered these studies in Chicago. They plotted the residence of 20,000 patients admitted for the first time to mental hospitals and computed the rates for hospitalization in various areas or subcommunities of the city. Race differences they did not find an important factor in the incidence of breakdown, except that schizophrenia and general paralysis were reported to be commoner in whites and negroes where they were locally in a racial minority. Social conditions on the other hand were found apparently to be highly significant, mental hospital admission rates corresponding closely to the city's socio-economic structure. The highest incidence of mental illness was found in the central, densely populated slum areas: and here cases of schizophrenia (most notably), senile psychosis, alcoholism and general paralysis were concentrated. The incidence of treated mental illness in the periphery of the city was low. Cases of manic-depressive psychosis and epilepsy were randomly distributed. The central, lodging-house areas were characterized socially by high residential mobility, poverty and ethnic heterogeneity.

Other American investigators have reported similar results, and in particular the concentration of cases of schizophrenia in and around the central business districts of large cities. Two hypotheses have been advanced in explanation of these facts: the first, that the social *milieu* of these areas of social disorganization predisposes to the development of schizophrenia; and the second, the 'drift' hypothesis, that these areas are the termini for those who, due to their illnesses, have

F

deteriorated in their social adjustments. Faris and Dunham favoured the first explanation: Gerard and Houston (1953) in Massachusetts supported the second, having compared the distribution of schizophrenia in those living alone with the incidence in those living with their families, and finding that the excess of schizophrenia in the central areas 'is principally due to the fact that schizoid individuals seek to protect themselves from close personal relations by moving away from their families to the lodging-house areas, and, in addition, by frequently moving from one lodging to another'. Hare (1956) working in Bristol, England, confirmed Gerard and Houston's main findings and stated that in a quarter of his cases separation from the family appeared to have been a factor of importance in the development of schizophrenic illness.

That the social environment in which schizophrenics in cities are most typically found is more a result than a cause of their illness, is demonstrated by a more recent finding: that in England and Wales where schizophrenics preponderate among the unskilled young men of social class V, the fathers of schizophrenics are ordinarily distributed among the social classes, and that after leaving school schizophrenics seem to have been non-starters in their parental class (Morris, 1959).

Social Class and Mental Illness. The most thorough research to date on the relationship between social stratification and mental illness has been carried out by Hollingshead and Redlich (1958) in their study, in New Haven, Connecticut, of an American urban community of 240,000 people. Their investigation was concerned only with individuals under psychiatric care or treatment at the time of the investigation (1950), but they believe that they found nearly all the cases of psychosis in the community. The patient's social status was recorded in terms of Hollingshead's Index of Social Position, which, using not only the individual's occupation but also his educational record, and the ecological area of his residence, breaks the population down into five social classes not dissimilar to the Registrar General's five social classes in this country. A 5 per cent. sample census of the general population was made as a control.

Hollingshead and Redlich found, first, that the prevalence of mental illness in New Haven was related to social class. This relationship was an inverse one, the lower the social class the greater the proportion of patients in the population: and the greatest difference lay between social classes IV and V, the latter contributing many more patients than its proportion of the population.

Second, they found that the types of psychiatric disorder were related to social class: directly in the case of the neuroses, which were commonest in the higher social classes, and inversely in the case of the psychoses, which were most prevalent in the lower social classes. For the psychoses, the lower the class the higher the rate: and this inverse relationship was found in affective, schizophrenic, senile, organic and alcoholic reaction-types. Also, they found a relationship between social class and types of neurotic reaction: phobic anxiety reactions and character neuroses were most prevalent in social classes I and II, while hysteria was found predominantly in classes IV and V.

Third, these investigators reported that social class position played a part in determining the type of psychiatric treatment given, the cost of treatment, where it was given and for how long. Furthermore, social class position tended to influence the decision as to whether or not a person should be treated by a psychiatrist at all for his disturbed or delinquent behaviour: those in social classes I and II tended to be treated in such 'more gentle and insightful ways' than those at the other end of the social scale.

Similarly detailed investigations are required in this country, but it is unlikely that under the National Health Service such disparities will be found between the social classes in the availability and effectiveness of psychiatric care and treatment. The direct relationship found between class status and the rate of treated neurosis may well reflect not only the incidence of neurosis but also the greater sophistication in medical matters and the greater financial affluence of the higher social classes in Connecticut.

Hollingshead and Redlich's data on the social class distribution of schizophrenia are reported in the chapter on Schizophrenic Reaction-Types.

Suicide and Attempted Suicide. Suicidal acts are a social phenomenon of great importance and concern not only to psychiatrists but to society as a whole. Recently in Middlesex, in the economically vital group of young adults, suicide was the second most frequent cause of death—exceeding deaths due to motor vehicles. The problem can be met only by a broad programme of mental hygiene, resocialization and medical treatment, in which the psychiatric services have a key rôle since it is generally accepted that the large majority of those who attempt or commit suicide are mentally ill or suffer from serious personality disorders. Such a mental hygiene programme must be based on a clear understanding of the factors, both social and individual, which predispose to suicidal acts.

According to figures quoted by the World Health Organization in 1958, Japan has the highest suicide rate in the world—24·1 per 100,000 of the population. Amongst European countries Austria ranks first with 22·8 per 100,000 and Denmark second with 22·5 per 100,000. The suicide rate in this country is only about half as high as Denmark's (11·8 in England and Wales, 7·8 in Scotland), but the problem is still a considerable one: in 1958 there were 5237 suicides in England and Wales, 439 in Scotland.

Prior to the Second World War, apart from a period of diminished incidence associated with the First World War, the suicide rate in Britain had been rising for many years. Again the rate fell during the Second World War, but since then it has been rising, in women more quickly than in men. In an ageing population suicide is becoming increasingly a disorder of elderly people, and about 20 per cent. of suicides now occur in people over the age of 60. Men more often commit suicide than women, and more often use violent methods: but since the Second World War there has, by both sexes in this country, been an increasing use of sedative drugs or gas in suicidal acts. The suicide rates are highest in social classes I and II and professional and business men, hotelkeepers and domestic servants are amongst the occupational groups with the highest rates. Seasonal graphs for suicide show peaks of incidence in late spring and in autumn.

Undoubtedly social factors are operative in the differential incidence of suicide, and important researches have been directed towards identifying these factors. In 1897 Emile Durkheim (1951), the French sociologist, divided suicides into three aetiological types, the egoistic, the anomic and the altruistic. Durkheim claimed that there is a direct relationship between suicide and the degree of integration of social groups. Egoistic or individualistic suicides he regarded as due to a slackening of family, religious and other social ties, so that the individual was left socially isolated or unsupported. Anomic or lawless suicides occur, he believed, when the individual's needs are no longer in harmony with his means and he ceases to be regulated by the collective conscience of his society: when he is thrown on his own resources, for example, at times of economic crises, by unexpected wealth or poverty, by widowhood or divorce. Altruistic suicides, on the other hand, are due to the over-integration of the individual in his group, to his domination by what he feels the group expects of him, so that he sacrifices himself on the altar of duty.

In support of his thesis that those who are not integrated in the life of the family and the community are more likely to commit suicide, Durkheim could point to well-established facts: the higher incidence of suicide in single than in married people; the higher incidence in childless women than in those with children; the higher incidence in Protestants than in Roman Catholics (the latter seem to be more closely knit socially in their Church and less prone to religious individualism); and in time of war the fall in the suicide rate which is probably associated with the heightened sense of social purpose and the greater social integration which war brings to a threatened community. Altruistic suicide is always rare, and in our peace-time society is exemplified by the captain who refuses to leave his ship when it sinks.

Durkheim's sociological approach has been developed particularly by Halbwachs (1930) and Sainsbury (1955). The latter tested the hypothesis that differences in the suicide rates of the London boroughs would reveal their social differences. Using mainly data from the Registrar General's publications and Smith's *New Survey of London Life and Labour* (1930–35), Sainsbury correlated the suicides notified in each borough with indices of that borough's social characteristics: he also examined the case records of all suicides reported to the North London coroner during the years 1936–38. Sainsbury found that the London boroughs showed significant differences in their suicide rates, and that the suicide rates correlated with the following social characteristics; with social isolation (measured as people living alone and in boarding houses), with social mobility (expressed in the daily turnover of population and the number of immigrants), and with two indices of social disorganization, divorce and illegitimacy. Unemployment and overcrowding rates showed no correlation with suicide rates, which tended to increase in the middle class and to decrease with poverty: the unemployed, however, were found to have a significantly higher suicide rate than the corresponding employed population. 'Suicide rates were highest in the West End and North-West London where both class and spatial mobility are highest, small flat and boarding-house accommodation preponderates, shared mores are absent, and relationships impersonal. Suicide rates were low in the peripheral southern boroughs where family life and stability prevail, and in many of the working-class districts whose residents are locally born and where life is more neighbourly.'

Sainsbury concludes: 'These findings support the view that a lonely mode of life is an important adverse factor accounting for differential rates of suicide in the (London) boroughs and their subdistricts. Social isolation also provides a consistent explanation of the high incidence of suicide found in a wide variety of social groups: the aged, unemployed, divorced and among immigrants.' These important conclusions from a careful ecological study complement findings reported in cases of attempted suicide: for example, in a study of attempted suicide in old age Batchelor and Napier (1953) reported that feelings of loneliness were the commonest psychological precursors of suicidal attempts in this age group.

Attempted suicide is much commoner than suicide in Western communities: how much commoner we do not know since many cases are neither reported to the police nor even admitted to hospital. Stengel (1958) has investigated the relationship between suicide and attempted suicide and some of the social aspects of suicidal attempts. He suggests that those who attempt and those who commit suicide constitute two different populations, pointing out that the majority of those who commit suicide are males while the majority of those who attempt it are females; that the average age of those who commit suicide is higher; and that a minority of those who commit suicide have previously attempted it, while only a small proportion of those who attempt it later commit suicide. Nevertheless, the two populations overlap, and it would not accord with the facts, but lead in practice to an underestimation of the risks to life inherent in suicidal attempts, to draw any sharp distinctions between attempted suicide and suicide itself. Though perhaps less than 5 per cent. of those who have attempted suicide go on to kill themselves later, the incidence of those who do so out of this group is much higher than that in the general population. In old age those who attempt and those who commit suicide seem to come from very closely allied, if not identical, clinical groups.

In the individual case it is often difficult to be sure about the seriousness and dangerousness of a patient's suicidal intentions. No firm line can be drawn between suicidal gestures and suicidal attempts: and the circumstances of some genuine suicidal attempts indicate clearly that consciously or unconsciously there has been a wish to manipulate the environment. Stengel goes further than acknowledging this, and has drawn attention to what he believes is a marked social element in most suicidal attempts — an appeal, usually unconscious, to society for help. He calls attempted suicide Janus-faced, orientated both to self-destruction and to a revision of human relationships. Stengel believes that the majority of genuine suicidal attempts are carried out in such a way that the intervention of others is possible or even probable. This is doubtful; but Stengel's emphasis on the appeal function of suicidal attempts and on the participation of the patient's group very properly draws attention to social aspects of individual suicidal acts which must be regarded if these acts are to be prevented, and adequately treated. Suicidal talk and threats must not be minimized, since they are often both calls for help and danger-signals; and 'an understanding of the individual significance of the appeal inherent in the suicidal attempt would enable those who want to help to do so rationally and effectively and thus prevent repetition'. Hostility towards others is commonly a component in the psychopathology of suicidal acts, and this in part explains why society's response to these acts is still often itself aggressive and punitive.

RACE AND CULTURE

Our clinical psychiatry has been developed on the basis of findings made almost exclusively in Western civilization. Where the mental illness is dependent largely on organic pathology, this limitation will seldom be important. The psychoses and subnormality are probably very similar in different parts of the world; the basic symptoms at least are probably the same, though they may be variously expressed and elaborated, according to the customs and beliefs of the country. In the case of reactions more psychogenically determined we would expect the social and cultural setting to be much more important, affecting the incidence, the types of reaction favoured, tolerated or repressed, and the methods of care and treatment. The recent development of the sciences of social psychology and anthropology is enabling us to take a more balanced view of nervous and mental illness, by placing it more definitely in its social setting. Every individual is moulded by the culture in which he has been educated and by the culture in which he lives. In the culture he has a place (status) and a part to play (rôle), usually more than one, and he is subject to the stresses and conflicts peculiar to that culture. There is at least a suggestion that some of the psychological ill-health in Western communities to-day is due to the indeterminacy and rapid changing of social rôles. We know that certain types of individual are happiest if their environment is stable and their obligations defined (e.g. obsessionals), whereas others because of their temperamental instability cannot adjust themselves to any social milieu (e.g. psychopaths). The more subtle interactions of personality and culture are now a promising field of research, and important work has been done by Benedict, Mead, Linton and others.

We cannot distinguish clearly the effects of race from those of culture. We meet the old difficulty of separating effects of nature from those of nurture.

We know comparatively little about the distribution, prevalence and incidence of nervous and mental illness in Britain and in the U.S.A. We know less of conditions in most other countries, and very little indeed about any country outside Western civilization. The two main obstacles to making comparisons of mental disorder in different races are that there has been no classification of mental disorders common to different countries, and that everywhere the development of psychiatric services has lagged behind those devoted to physical disease. Our knowledge of the influence of race or nationality on nervous and mental illness is therefore very slight and insecure, and much of it has been derived from observation of foreign-born immigrants into the U.S.A. Here the situation is particularly complicated: the immigrant may not have been a stable member of the society he has left, and he has all the strains of immigration and resettlement in a foreign country to contend with. There is evidence also that migration or other rapid and extensive social changes (for example, those due to the introduction of Western civilization to a primitive society) may be associated with an increased rate of mental breakdown.

Certain reaction-types are commonly mentioned as being more or less specific to certain racial or cultural groups. For example, latah and amok have been described particularly in Malays: the former is a trance-like state with automatic obedience and coprolalia, precipitated by fright and most often found in women past their prime (Yap, 1952); the latter is an acute, clouded excitement with homicidal violence. Amongst certain North American Indians a Wihtigo psychosis has been reported, in which the individual believes that he has been possessed and transformed into a mythological beast, a Wihtigo, and may become cannibalistic (Hallowel, 1934).

The resemblances between nations and cultures as regards mental illness are, however, on the whole more impressive than their differences, which seem to be mainly of quantity and degree. Williams (1950), working in the Indian theatre of war during the Second World War, found that Indian and British soldiers broke down in rather different ways and in response to different stresses. 52 per cent. of the British psychiatric casualties developed anxiety states, but only 8 per cent. of the Indian casualties: whereas amongst the Indians hysterical reactions, often of a florid type, were much more common, comprising 31 per cent. of the breakdowns. Williams linked these variations of clinical reaction with the fact that loss of face was the basic stress factor to Indians. The maintenance of face was of paramount importance in their close-knit patriarchal society and in the maintenance of personal morale, and shame rather than guilt occurred in the event of their personal failure. Coming from martial races, they had also little guilt about killing in combat. To exhibit anxiety meant great loss of face to them, whereas hysterical symptoms such as fits were face-saving. Seligman noted among the Japanese that delusions of a religious nature with a sense of guilt were practically absent in Japan, where religion is cheerful and assumes primitive virtue rather than original sin.

In Scotland we seem to see a much larger number of cases of melancholia than is the case elsewhere, and there is some evidence that the incidence is highest in the more northern parts of the country. It is of some interest, too, to record that in cases of mental disorder occurring in the Orkney Islands transferred for observation and treatment to the Royal Edinburgh Hospital, the striking feature has been the occurrence of a peculiar dull, bewildered state: invariably these patients are more difficult to nurse and to care for than the average case in the hospital. In contrast to Scotland, Carothers has found mania in the native Africans in Kenya more common than depression. In an earlier section we have noted some racial differences in the incidence of alcoholism.

The culture is a shoe which pinches certain members of each society, and societies vary very much in the number and nature of their misfits. Malinowski, for example, believed that the neuroses are very rare among the Trobrianders in comparison with the inhabitants of neighbouring islands, on account of the sexual freedom of the former and the family organization, which is characterized by the virtual absence of anyone in the rôle of the father. On the other hand, many writers are prepared to link the prevalence of neuroses in Western civilization with the impact of the industrial revolution and the culture's encouragement of competitive, acquisitive strivings.

While the culture may elicit symptoms in certain individuals who come into conflict with it, the majority it supports. Hebb has drawn attention to this aspect, describing the culture as a protective cocoon. 'The well-adjusted adult therefore is not intrinsically less subject to emotional disturbance: he is well-adjusted, relatively unemotional, as long as he is in his cocoon.' The culture buffers the individual from emotional provocations and disturbing experiences of many kinds, tending as it does to eliminate sources of acute fear, disgust and anger, and to ensure that each member of society will not in general upset others emotionally by aberrant conduct.

The question of culture is important in assessing the import of a delusion. A delusional belief that would be ominous in a Londoner might mean little that was abnormal in a Sandwich Islander, on account of the special superstitions and folk-lore of the latter. This consideration holds, but to a lesser extent, for different cultural strata in the same population.

AGE

The part played by age in causation is in general indirect, a function of the changes in experience, in mental outlook and in the tissues which accompany the passage of the years. Of tissue changes, those affecting the endocrine glands and the brain are of greatest importance. Certain psychoses occur typically in certain age periods: hebephrenic schizophrenia between 15 and 25 years of age; chronic alcoholism, general paralysis and paranoid states in the fourth and fifth decades; melancholia in the involution; Alzheimer's and Pick's disease in the sixth decade; and, in old age, senile and arteriosclerotic dementia.

Generally speaking, the maximum incidence of mental disorder in males lies between the ages of 30 and 40, and in females between 25 and 35. After these periods there is a fall, followed by an increase at the involutional period and in the senium. The increasing age of the population has been associated with an increase in the depressive reactions and organic, degenerative mental disorders of later life. Almost 29 per cent. of the patients in the mental hospitals of England and Wales are now 65 years of age or over.

In this country suicide is becoming increasingly a disorder of elderly people, and the highest suicide rate is found in men over 65 years. Most types of crime decrease with advancing age. The age group with most offenders is 13 years, and about one-half of all crime is committed by people under 21. Nearly half of those, however, who are found guilty of indictable sexual offences are aged 30 or over.

SEX

Sex has a complicated bearing on the incidence of nervous and mental disorders, and the types of stress differ considerably in the two sexes. In the male the effects of alcoholism and syphilis are seen to a far greater extent than in women, and on them also the stress of economic competition falls more heavily. Women, on the other hand, have to face the physical and psychological stresses of pregnancy, the puerperium and the menopause. Affective psychoses and Alzheimer's and Pick's pre-senile psychoses are commoner in women. Two-thirds of the patients aged 65 or over in the mental hospitals of England and Wales are women; no doubt mainly because women live longer than men. Crime and delinquency, head injuries and most of the 'psychosomatic' disorders are commoner in men. More women than men attempt suicide, more men commit it. These sex differences in the incidence of maladjustment and disease are extremely interesting, and their full elucidation would throw much light on aetiology. Despite particular differences, however, the total incidence of mental disorder is probably about equal in the two sexes.

ENDOCRINE FACTORS

Mental diseases being as yet very imperfectly understood and their causation frequently a matter of surmise, it is not surprising that the endocrines should have been implicated in their genesis much more often than the clinical facts justified. Premature attempts to correlate endocrine and temperamental make-up, and the over-enthusiastic, though usually unavailing, therapeutic use of endocrine preparations by some clinicians have also led to rather widespread scepticism about the value of this approach to aetiology and treatment. However, the functions and dysfunctions of the endocrine system must have considerable importance in the psychiatric field. It is probable that the endocrines are among the primary factors determining personality, and that they influence considerably the individual's constitution, his physical and mental growth, and his behaviour. We know that epochs which are of particular significance in the emotional life of the individual and at which there is a tendency to mental breakdown—*e.g.* puberty, the puerperium, the climacteric, are times when profound changes are taking place in the endocrine system. We cannot yet define the mode of action of the various parts of the endocrine system in producing many of these great biological effects: but endocrinology is a young subject in which rapid advances are being made and, as techniques of investigation and assay become more accurate and subtle and as knowledge of the composition and actions of the hormones increases, we can expect more data to become available which will be relevant to the understanding of nervous and mental illness. The borderlands between endocrinology and psychiatry have been very incompletely explored.

It is important to recognize the complexity of the relationships which are involved. The endocrines are under neural control, and their hormones reciprocally affect the functions of the central nervous system. The hypothalamus acts not only as a central co-ordinating station for the endocrine system, but also as a mediator between the environment, the higher nervous centres, and that system. For convenience, we speak of the disorders of certain endocrine glands, but this is in most cases a simplification. The endocrine system functions as a whole, and is apt to be disturbed as a whole.

When one comes to link physical with mental events, the intricacy of the interactions becomes even more apparent. Endocrine disorder may be either the cause or the consequence of mental disorder, and it may be very difficult to identify the primary event, so closely do the two interact. Psychological disturbance may upset the endocrine balance: for example, when emotional shock induces amenorrhoea or precipitates Graves' disease (primary hyperthyroidism). Equally, endocrine disturbance may act as an internal stress, and precipitate mental breakdown.

With the possible exception of cretinism, there is no endocrine disease which presents an unvarying psychiatric picture: and none of the mental symptoms occurring in endocrine diseases are peculiar to them. One cannot diagnose an endocrine disorder from the mental symptoms which may be present, but must depend upon the physical symptoms and signs and the results of laboratory and other specialized investigations. Nevertheless, in certain endocrine syndromes the mental symptoms are more or less characteristic: for example, the anxiety and emotional lability of hyperthyroidism; the retardation and paranoid reactions of myxoedema; the neurasthenia of Addison's disease. Patients treated with cortisone or corticotrophin not infrequently develop hypomanic reactions. In general, and it is what we would expect, the clinical picture is conditioned both by the endocrine disturbance and by the constitutional mental make-up of the individual. Both functional and organic psychiatric syndromes may occur, the former more commonly: as examples of the latter, one may instance the delirium which may develop in severe cases of hyperthyroidism, and the confusion which may be associated with the tetany of hypoparathyroidism.

The depression of spirits which may be evident in certain cases of endocrine disease is often a very understandable reaction to the physical changes. Anyone who has seen a full-blown case of Cushing's syndrome or acromegaly or Simmonds' disease will appreciate the tremendous psychic wound which such a transformation may cause.

The endocrines influence profoundly the sexual life of the individual. Particularly is this noticeable in the case of women, who so commonly experience emotional disturbances in association with menstruation and the menopause. In the latter half of the menstrual cycle many women experience some degree of emotional irritability, a sense of physical congestion or tension, and a gain in weight: this state of pre-menstrual tension (Rees, 1953) is thought to be due largely to water retention, secondary to a disturbance of the normal oestrogen-progesterone balance. The hormonal changes of the menopause also produce both physical and emotional upset in perhaps 50 per cent. of women. It is doubtful if there is a true male climacteric: but adult castrates are known to be apt to manifest neurasthenic and anxiety symptoms, while pre-pubertal castrates are said to show schizoid trends. The endocrines may play some rôle in the genesis of certain cases of homosexuality, but the situation here is obscure: it may be said, however, that the endocrine treatment of homosexuality, as also of impotence and frigidity, usually fails. Hyperfunction of the adrenal cortices may give rise to a number of rare and dramatic syndromes of sexual abnormality— virilism, feminism, pubertas praecox, which merit fuller psychiatric investigation than has yet been made of them.

A diversity of endocrine anomalies has been reported in schizophrenics: but no endocrine anomaly occurs consistently amongst them. Kretschmer described under the heading 'dysplastic' various physical types (hypoplastic, eunuchoid, masculinism) which he found commonly amongst schizophrenics, and which he thought might be the expression of endocrine disturbances. It is a common finding that schizophrenics are abnormally insensitive to certain glandular ex-tracts, e.g. thyroid and insulin. Perhaps the most significant discovery has been Gjessing's: investigating cases of periodic catatonia, he found that in some a phasic alteration of nitrogen balance was associated with the mental symptoms, and that the mental symptoms could be relieved by the giving of thyroid [see p. 268].

There are few psychiatric syndromes which respond to endocrine treatment. Indications for prescribing endocrine preparations should be based mainly on the presence or absence of physical signs of endocrine disorder. Thus, in the management of menopausal disturbances, oestrogens may be prescribed if there are vasomotor symptoms such as hot flushes and sweats: in the absence of these physical symptoms, such treatment is likely to be ineffective. Depressions occur-ring at or after the menopause do not themselves call for endocrine treatment.

Very much more work requires to be done before any general understanding of the rôle of glandular malfunction in mental illness can be reached. In the majority of cases of endocrine disease there are no psychiatric symptoms of note, and in most cases of nervous and mental illness no clear evidence of endocrine disorder. Despite this, the study of endocrine factors should not be neglected.

PHYSIQUE

The study of the association between temperamental traits and body build goes back at least as far as the Greek physician Hippocrates. The layman too has for centuries held pragmatic opinions on this subject. When Shakespeare's Caesar exclaims, 'Yond' Cassius has a lean and hungry look; he thinks too much: such men are dangerous', he expresses not only his private apprehensions but the venerable popular belief that fat men who sleep well are more likely to be good-natured and reliable.

Ernst Kretschmer (1925) pioneered careful psychiatric studies of the problem, studying the physiques particularly of schizophrenics and manic-depressives. He isolated four main types of physique—pyknic, athletic, asthenic and dysplastic. The pyknic is the John Bull, short, thick-set with a round belly and small ex-tremities; the athletic is muscular; the asthenic is long and weedy; the dysplastic approximates to the effects of various kinds of endocrine dysfunction, for example, the near eunuchoid or infantile. Kretschmer found that pyknic physiques were more than normally common amongst manic-depressives, while asthenic, athletic and dysplastic physiques were usual amongst schizophrenics.

From the study of psychotics Kretschmer proceeded to family studies and the investigation of healthy people, and distinguished two clearly recognizable types of personality, the cycloid and schizoid. The cycloid, open, extraverted and affectionate, prone to swings of mood, is associated with the pyknic physique, and, if there is mental breakdown, tends to develop a manic-depressive psychosis. The schizoid, inhibited, introverted and cold, is associated with the asthenic type of physique and with schizophrenia. These two types were by Kretschmer vividly contrasted: 'when we come out of the psychic milieu of the schizophrene family into that of the circulars (manic-depressives), it is like stepping out of a cool shut-in vault into the open sunshine'. He emphasized rightly that cycloid and schizoid personalities 'have no foundation in disease, but indicate certain biological tendencies of which only a small proportion comes to pathological culmination'.

The finding of links between personality, physique and psychosis is in accord with genetic expectations, since they may all be expressions of the same genotype: the existence of clear-cut, discrete physical and personality types amongst the normal population is not. In nature, mixed types are far commoner than pure examples. Kretschmer's work may be criticized on the grounds that his brilliant characterizations are perhaps in their contrasts too sharply drawn, the correlations he found between physique and temperament too close, and the methods of physical measurement he used comparatively crude: but his remains a major contribution.

Sheldon (1940, 1942) has carried research on this subject further. He adopted the procedure of photographing the individual in a standardized posture from three positions, and then made detailed anthropometric measurements on the films. Examining in this way 4000 normal young men he found evidence not of discrete types, but of 'dimensions of variation' of physique. The presence of three primary components of structural variation seemed to be revealed and appeared to depend upon the relative development of tissues derived from each of the three embryonic layers. These three primary components Sheldon named endomorphy, mesomorphy and ectomorphy. Endomorphy, reflecting the predominance in development of the entoderm, is characterized by massive digestive viscera and weak development of the somatic structures; there is 'softness and sphericity'. The hallmark of mesomorphy is 'uprightness and sturdiness': somatic structures derived from the mesodermal layer—that is, bone, muscle and connective tissue, are in the ascendancy. In ectomorphy there is relatively slight development of the visceral and somatic structures, and the ectodermal predominance is expressed in 'fragility, linearity, flatness of the chest and delicacy throughout the body'.

Sheldon rates the strength of each of the primary components of physique on a 7-point scale, and his concept of the somatotype can best be illustrated by direct quotation. 'The somatotype is a series of three numerals, each expressing the approximate strength of one of the primary components in a physique. The first numeral always refers to endomorphy, the second to mesomorphy and the third to ectomorphy. Thus, when a 7-point scale is used, a 7–1–1 is the most extreme endomorph; a 1–7–1 is the most extreme mesomorph, and a 1–1–7 the most extreme ectomorph. The 4–4–4 falls at the midpoint (of the scale, not of the frequency distribution) with respect to all three components.'

Sheldon's books should be consulted for further details. He emphasizes that when the somatotype has been determined, analysis of the physique has only begun. There are many important secondary variables; for example, dysplasia, and the secondary sex characters.

In studying personality, Sheldon has used a variation of the technique of factor analysis applied to quantitative ratings on a group of traits, and claims to have standardized the description of 'sixty-traits—twenty in each of three correlated clusters—which collectively make up a scale for measuring what appear to be the three primary components of temperament'. The first component, viscerotonia, is characterized by general relaxation, sociability and love of comfort and affection. The second, somatotonia, is expressed predominantly in muscular activity and assertiveness. In the third, cerebrotonia, behaviour is dominated by shyness and inhibition. Sheldon further claims that these three components of temperament correlate closely with the three components of physique already described—viscerotonia with endomorphy, somatotonia with mesomorphy, and cerebrotonia with ectomorphy. Studying 200 young men he has reported correlations of the order of + 0·80 between the two levels of personality, the morphological and the temperamental.

This work has provided a valuable stimulus to research. Genetical factors governing bodily build are probably distributed normally in a community, and Sheldon's delineation of 'dimensions of variation' is therefore more likely to be accurate than a classification into types. It will be noted, however, that his three newly described categories of physique do bear a clear resemblance to Kretschmer's pyknic, athletic and asthenic types. Sheldon's anthropomorphic measurements improve on those employed in earlier studies. His work on temperamental traits, on the other hand, is less convincing and seems over-simplified.

Eysenck (1947) has examined neurotic soldiers, deriving an index of body build on the basis of a factorial analysis of physical anthropometric measurements. He too reports no evidence for the existence of discrete bodily and personality types. In this investigation neurotics as a whole were found to be more leptomorph (cf. Sheldon's ectomorph) than normals; and hysterics had a higher preponderance of lateral growth, as compared with dysthymics (those showing anxiety, depression, irritability), who had a higher preponderance of linear growth. The results of this carefully planned study seem considerably at variance with the reports of work already quoted, and these discrepancies point to the need for further investigation.

We are trying to correlate what we have only begun to measure scientifically, and are coming to realize more clearly the complexities of the subject. Dissatisfied with the subjective nature of Sheldon's photographic somatotyping, Parnell (1958) has developed a method which employs objective physical anthropometry in conjunction with standard photographs. Full details of his technique and results can be found in his recently published book, *Behaviour and Physique*. In his somatocharts the components are Fat, Muscularity and Linearity (in place of Sheldon's endomorph, mesomorph and ectomorph): and he describes Fat, Muscular, Linear and Central Phenotypes. Parnell has now applied his methods not only in the study of mental illness but in a wider conspectus of human matings, family relationships and education: and he reports on men, women and children. His findings in schizophrenics resemble Kretschmer's, while his results in manic-depressives seem to differ. He has obtained information about the physical constitutional influences on duration of stay in hospital and on suicide trends. Parnell has now rapidly blazed a trail, which should stimulate others to test his findings and press forward research in this promising but difficult field.

REFERENCES

Anderson, V. V. (1929) *Psychiatry in Industry*, New York.
Andry, R. G. (1957) *Brit. J. Delinqu.*, **8**, 34.
Bartlett, F. C. (1943) *Proc. roy. Soc. B*, **131**, 247.
Batchelor, I. R. C. (1954) *J. ment. Sci.*, **100**, 451.
Batchelor, I. R. C., and Napier, M. B. (1953) *Brit. med. J.*, **2**, 1186.
Batchelor, I. R. C., and Napier, M. B. (1953) *Brit. J. Delinqu.*, **4**, 99.
Bowlby, J. (1951) *Maternal Care and Mental Health*, W.H.O., Geneva.
Bowlby, J. (1958) *Brit. J. med. Psychol.*, **31**, 247.
Bowman, K. M., and Jellinek, E. M. (1941) *Quart. J. Stud. Alc.*, **2**, 312.
Davis, R. (1946) *J. Neurol. Psychiat.*, **9**, 23, 119.
Drug Addiction (1961) Report of the Interdepartmental Committee, H.M.S.O., London.
Durkheim, E. (1951) *Suicide*, Glencoe, Illinois.
Eysenck, H. J. (1947) *Dimensions of Personality*, London.
Faris, R. E. L., and Dunham, H. W. (1939) *Mental Disorders in Urban Areas*, Chicago.
Forel, A. (1900) *Amer. J. Insan.*, **57**, 297.
Fraser, R. (1947) *The Incidence of Neurosis among Factory Workers*, H.M.S.O., London.
Gerard, D. L., and Houston, L. G. (1953) *Psychiat. Quart.*, **27**, 90.
Goldhamer, H., and Marshall, A. W. (1949) *Psychosis and Civilisation*, Glencoe, Illinois.
Halbwachs, M. (1930) *Les Causes du Suicide*, Paris.
Hallowel, A. I. (1934) *J. abnorm. (soc.) Psychol.*, **29**, 1.
Hare, E. H. (1956) *J. ment. Sci.*, **102**, 349, 753.
Hollingshead, A. B., and Redlich, F. C. (1958) *Social Class and Mental Illness*, London.
Horney, K. (1936) *The Neurotic Personality of our Time*, New York.
Jellinek, E. M. (Ed.) (1942) *Alcohol Addiction and Chronic Alcoholism*, New Haven.
Kallmann, F. J. (1953) *Heredity in Health and Mental Disorder*, London.
Kretschmer, E. (1925) *Physique and Character*, London.
Lange, J. (1931) *Crime as Destiny*, London.
Lemert, E. M. (1951) *Social Pathology*, New York.
Lewin, L. (1931) *Phantastica, Narcotic and Stimulating Drugs*, London.
Madow, L., and Hardy, S. E. (1947) *Amer. J. Orthopsychiat.*, **17**, 521.
Mayer-Gross, W. (1951) *Brit. med. J.*, **2**, 317.
McGregor, H. G. (1944) *J. Neurol. Neurosurg. Psychiat.*, **7**, 21.
Morris, J. N. (1959) *Lancet*, i, 303.
Myerson, A. (1925) *The Inheritance of Mental Diseases*, Baltimore.
Nabarro, D. (1954) *Congenital Syphilis*, London.
Parnell, R. W. (1958) *Behaviour and Physique*, London.

Penrose, L. S. (1949) *The Biology of Mental Defect*, London.
Penrose, L. S. (1950) *Congrès International de Psychiatrie, Paris*, **6**, 44.
Rees, L. (1953) *J. ment. Sci.*, **99**, 62.
Reid, D. D. (1960) *W.H.O. Public Health Papers*, No. 2, Geneva.
Roberts, J. A. F. (1959) *An Introduction to Medical Genetics*, 2nd ed., London.
Sainsbury, P. (1955) *Suicide in London*, London.
Sargant, W., and Slater, E. (1940) *Lancet*, ii, 1.
Sheldon, W. H., and Stevens, S. S. (1942) *The Varieties of Temperament*, London.
Sheldon, W. H., Stevens, S. S., and Tucker, W. B. (1940) *The Varieties of Human Physique*, London.
Shepherd, M. (1957) *A Study of the Major Psychoses in an English County*, London.
Sherlock, S., Summerskill, W. H. J., White, L. P., and Phear, E. A. (1954) *Lancet*, ii, 453.
Slater, E., and Shields, J. (1953) *Spec. Rep. Ser. med. Res. Coun. Lond.*, No. 278.
Smith, H. L. (1930–35) *New Survey of London Life and Labour*, London.
Spillane, J. D. (1947) *Nutritional Disorders of the Nervous System*, Edinburgh.
Stengel, E., Cook, N. G., and Kreeger, I. S. (1958) *Attempted Suicide*, London.
Stewart, R. M. (1933) *J. ment. Sci.*, **79**, 602.
Tennyson, A. L. (1953) *Amer. J. Med.*, **14**, 578.
Thomson, G., *et al.* (1947) *The Trend of National Intelligence*, London.
Tredgold, A. F. (1947) *A Textbook of Mental Deficiency*, London.
Williams, A. H. (1950) *Brit. J. med. Psychol.*, **23**, 130.
World Health Organization (1960) Technical Report Series, No. 185, Geneva.
Yap, P. M. (1952) *J. ment. Sci.*, **98**, 515.

5

METHOD OF EXAMINATION

In the practice of psychological medicine a not infrequent obstacle enters which is not found, or very little found, in other branches of medical practice, namely a relative or total unwillingness on the part of the patient to co-operate. Co-operation may be slight or altogether lacking in many instances, for example in schizophrenia from absorption in an inner world of phantasy, in paranoid psychoses from suspicion, and in manic excitement from sheer inability to sustain attention; while in other syndromes there may be apparent willingness to co-operate, but inability to do so, for example in profound depression of spirits where thinking is so retarded that the patient may repeatedly open his mouth as if to speak and be unable to utter any more than a syllable.

It is to cases of the psychotic sort that a greater part of the following description of the manner of examination refers. It includes the method of approach to individual patients who are more or less incapable of co-operation in one or other of these ways.

But in those instances of psychological ill-health which are in the great majority, where the patient presents himself for examination and treatment, where he is morbidly anxious or excessively worried and depressed without being robbed of his volition, or still more frequently where he complains of headache, dyspepsia, palpitation or some other discomfort for which no sufficient and relevant physical cause can be found, then the procedure may be summed up as that of taking a detailed *history* along certain lines.

After obtaining a statement of the symptoms in the order in which the patient complains of them, and noting associated qualities such as time, incidence, relation to what the patient does and so on, it is necessary to trace the chronology of their development. When did the symptoms first appear, and in what circumstances? It will sometimes be found that the first statement on this point is inadvertently erroneous, and further exploration may show that in fact symptoms of a similar sort existed at some previous date. The history of the development of the symptoms is, however, of importance, principally in relation to the patient's personal history. What were his circumstances at the time the symptoms first appeared or at the time of any recurrence or exacerbation? The task, in fact, resolves itself into taking a life-history of the patient as an individual in relation to his home, the people in it, his friends, his married life, his work, his career and so forth. One looks, first of all, for evidence of external stress existing at or near the onset of symptoms, such as frank anxieties, disappointment in career, other personal frustrations, conflicts with wife or husband or work associates, jealousies and rivalries, from the nursery upwards; in fact, whatever human beings do and suffer has to be explored by the psychiatrist in relation to the occurrence of symptoms which are presumed to be signs of mental uneasiness or distress.

Where nothing of this sort appears in the history, or nothing that seems to account for the symptoms, either in the external circumstances or, what is much more difficult to ascertain, in the patient's inner attitude to his life and his fellows, then the investigation must be extended, as indeed in some degree in most cases it must be extended, for the sake of a proper understanding, into his early life, his relationship to his parents, his brothers and sisters and so forth. An attempt should also be made, primarily on the basis of the life-history, to make an estimate of the patient's temperament and character. Here the examination may follow the same lines as is discussed under 'Personality' later in this chapter.

In this way it will be possible to arrive at a provisional formulation which exhibits the symptoms as a reaction to contemporary circumstances, or shows the condition as one of much earlier origin connected with miscarriages of psychological development, starting at an early age and tending to produce feelings of insecurity and inferiority, or faulty attitudes of a more subtle kind; and on the other hand producing faults of character, such as vanity, tendencies to dodge important issues, or to bear grudges. More subtly still, emotional attitudes may be formed around certain individuals in the family and round certain episodes in the past which preclude a normal attitude to various aspects of life subsequently until these earlier attitudes have been uncovered and modified. For example, over-dependence on one or other parent may produce an apparently causeless anxiety at the prospect of marriage. More detailed exposition of topics of that kind will be found in Chapter 8.

It will be seen that what is wanted where the patient is co-operative, and especially where there is no question of mental alienation and of the existence of a radically different general attitude to the world from that of the ordinary man, is a history of the patient as a person, his character and temperament and his modes of reaction to the emotional stresses of life.

Where, however, the degree of co-operation is less than this, and where, even if co-operation is superficially good, the patient's attitude and ideas are such as to suggest that he has been developing a psychotic form of illness, then the following scheme should be closely followed, because an accurate, systematic form of examination is indispensable, and should be of material aid in the progress of psychiatry. It has seemed to us that physicians in general practice are reluctant to deal with psychological or 'mental' cases, largely because they do not know how to approach and examine them in an orderly way. No one expects a general practitioner to be fully conversant with every speciality, nor does one expect from him a detailed argument in regard to diagnosis and prognosis, but the general practitioner should be familiar with methods of examination, so as to be able to elicit the facts and present them systematically, even although he may not be able to interpret them correctly. This is fundamental. The interpretation of symptoms will only come on the basis of wide experience.

It has been unfortunate that in psychiatric case-taking there has not been a settled, uniform policy, and too often the person studying psychiatry has either had to work out methods of examination to suit himself, or has blindly followed

G

the ways of his teachers and colleagues, even although those ways were recognized to be far from satisfactory. Hence psychiatric records have often left much to be desired, and it has not been possible to correlate accurately the clinical picture with the pathological findings, nor has it been possible to compare cases occurring in one mental hospital with those in another. From this there results confusion and incongruity, where it is essential to have clearness and uniformity. One hears various excuses made for this. A common one is that the patient is so disordered mentally as to be quite unco-operative, and on that account a complete examination is impossible. How seldom is this really the case! It is true that it may not be possible to make an absolutely complete examination until after a number of attempts have been made, and certain points may not at once be elicited, but sufficient should always be obtained (whether there is complete co-operation or not) upon which to base an independent opinion. Where it is not possible to elicit all the facts, the case-record should contain an explanation of why this is so.

Although a good descriptive record of the behaviour and symptoms of the patient is of importance, it will not be of any great value unless information is collected elsewhere regarding the setting in which the symptoms have occurred, and the causes which have been instrumental in producing them. The causes are so often of a family or environmental nature that a study of the social conditions and of the family life is essential. The plan of examination, therefore, consists of two parts—the history or 'anamnesis' obtained from the relatives or friends, and the examination of the patient. The one is no less important than the other.

There are several general points which should be kept in mind in making this examination. An effort should be made to record the case in simple, non-technical language, rather than by using hackneyed terms. Further, the physician should not be satisfied with an account from any one source, but should interview several of the intimate relatives or friends of the patient.

In examining the patient a great deal depends on the method of approach. The physician should realize clearly that he is dealing with a person of disordered mentality, who cannot be treated in the same way as a patient in a general hospital, and he should therefore be more than usually tactful, very patient, understanding and sympathetic. Many medical men in examining their mental patients repeatedly fail to get hold of the essential points of the case, either because of an undue sense of delicacy, or because their manner and method do not inspire confidence in the patient. The patient should be made to feel at once that the examiner has his best interests at heart, that he is willing to do everything that he possibly can to help him, and the doctor should be quite frank in stating his position. If the patient asks who was responsible for his coming, why he was brought and so on, these questions should be answered fully at the time. The patient should be informed that all the facts will be carefully investigated. It not infrequently happens that patients are more talkative and more willing to explain their illness at the first interview than they are later on, and this time should be seized to take as complete a record as possible. Sometimes the physician feels that he may upset the patient by going thoroughly into the case at the time of admission, but this is incorrect. It is much better to make a comprehensive note at once of the patient's condition, and, at the same time, to give him any explanations which he asks for. The complete systematic examination should be conducted as early as possible. If this is not done, a change may very soon occur in the patient's attitude, and often a most valuable part of the record is lost. Until the physician has gained considerable experience in history-taking, we consider that it is advisable that the plan suggested below should be followed closely. Later, after experience has been gained, it can be changed to suit the individual case. Under these circumstances, and using this plan of examination, we believe that the different mental fields (*e.g.* behaviour, affect, intellect, personality and insight) can be examined just as thoroughly, as completely, and as systematically as any bodily organ.

The plan suggested was first formulated by Dr. Adolf Meyer when he was Director of the Psychiatric Institute, New York. In 1921 Dr. George Kirby edited for the New York State Hospital Commission a series of guides for history-taking and clinical examination, which were largely based on Meyer's original plan. We have followed these closely, but have modified them here and there, and have eliminated parts which might be considered redundant.

The form of examination which we suggest may be considered under the following headings:

1. Family history.
2. Personal history.
3. History of the present illness.
4. Examination of the patient, including the (*a*) mental and (*b*) physical condition.

FAMILY HISTORY

It is notoriously difficult to get a reliable statement of the family history. The relatives often feel sensitive about their position; they are apt to think that the patient may resent information being given, and the maternal side is apt to blame the paternal side, and vice versa. Even where evidence of definite nervous or mental disturbance is obtained, the positive statements are often glossed over, and any description of the state is usually qualified by some such phrase as 'Of course he was not insane, Doctor.'

We have already emphasized the value of the accurate study of the facts of heredity in relation to mental illness, and at this point we would merely reiterate the necessity of having as complete and as detailed information as possible, dating back for three generations. It is not always easy to get this, for various reasons, but, where the information is defective, a statement to that effect should be made in the case-record. On the other hand, where a positive history of abnormality in the forebears is obtained, then the age of onset, the duration of the illness and a description of it should be recorded. A one-word diagnosis is not satisfactory, because it is necessary to have the facts so that anyone could come to an independent opinion. This is why it is so important to avoid such vague terms as 'nervousness', 'shock', 'worry', 'melancholia' and so on. In addition to having information regarding the direct line, the collateral lines should also be closely inquired into. We not only want to have information about the occurrence of the more gross types of mental disorder, but we should also have as much information as possible in reference to subnormality in any degree, epilepsy, alcoholism, and eccentricities and peculiarities of any kind. Apart altogether from the purely nervous and mental aspects, we should attempt to obtain information about the general physique of the family, and the bodily, as well as the mental, morbidity.

PERSONAL HISTORY

This may have to be obtained from several different sources, from the brothers and sisters, or from other intimate relatives and friends. The personal history should cover the *development of the patient* from the time of conception up to the alleged onset of the illness. We want to know as much as we can about the life, habits and social circumstances of the parents at the time of conception, the condition of the mother during gestation, the character of the labour—whether it was unduly prolonged, complicated, or aided by instruments. The development and career of the individual should be followed, and such points inquired for as: whether he was strong and healthy, or sickly; the susceptibility to childish ailments; whether there were convulsions, tantrums or sleeplessness; the time of teething, of learning to walk and speak, the control of sphincters (bed-wetting) and the response to darkness, tunnels, thunder and lightning and other childish bogies.

Following this, the stage of *intellectual and social adaptation* must be inquired into, and our inquiries should concern school reports, the degree of intellectual attainment; what the patient's attitude was towards his fellows, whether he was a leader or led; how interested in, and proficient at, games; whether a spontaneous, keen, straightforward person, or cunning, a truant, untruthful. In short, we should have as much evidence as possible in regard to the individual's interests and hobbies, including such things as fondness for animals, or cruelty towards them; and interest in religion—whether it was merely formal, or had a deeper side. Special inquiry should be directed towards *sex development*, the establishment of puberty, whether much interest was taken in it, whether there was masturbation or a tendency to associate freely with the other sex; and the possibility of venereal disease. In females, one should have an accurate history of the development of menstruation, of any irregularities, of pregnancies, abortions and the response to the menopause. In this connection one should also inquire into the psychosexual interests—love attachments, perversions, and attraction or antagonism to the parents, or to various members of the family.

Inquiry must also be made regarding *general diseases or injuries*, the possibility of infection from whatever source, and the state of the endocrine and vegetative nervous system (as suggested by abnormal desire for sweets, or fats, or fluids; frequency of micturition, etc.). Addiction to alcohol and drugs and the presence of other toxic factors must be inquired for.

Previous attacks of mental disorder should be carefully investigated.

The object of the examination, therefore, is to get a description of what the individual was at his or her best, what the response was to social, business and domestic life, and what were his ambitions, dreams and hobbies. All this should be recorded in narrative form.

HISTORY OF PRESENT ILLNESS

Before attempting to take a detailed history of the symptoms, it is of even greater importance to inquire carefully about possible aetiological factors and precipitating causes. It may be that the cause is neither physical nor mental nor endocrine, but that it is a combination of all these factors, acting on a soil predisposed by hereditary and environmental influences acting over a long period of time. It is well to recognize this, because the relatives often feel that one factor is very much more important than another, whereas it is often the one which has seemed of least importance to the family that has been chiefly responsible for the break-down.

The date of the first deviation from the normal should be stated as accurately as possible, and then the development of the symptoms should be followed step by step. Such a description helps considerably in understanding whether the onset has been insidious and gradual, or sudden. It cannot be too strongly emphasized that general statements are of no value; we must get an exact description of what the patient's conduct has been, and how he has reacted to his difficulties. We must, therefore, endeavour to find what the attitude has been towards his intimate relatives and friends, whether there has been a change in mood, and whether peculiar ideas, delusions, suspicions or unusual interests have been spoken about and cultivated. It is not enough simply to have the statement, 'He is delusional', or 'hallucinated', but what is of value is to get an exact description of the delusions and hallucinations, and how the patient has reacted to them.

The memory and general intellectual faculties should also be closely inquired into. Where a variation of symptoms has occurred, it is important to give dates for the development of the various stages. In addition, one should always be quite clear whether there have been suicidal or homicidal tendencies, whether there has been an impairment of physical health, as shown by sleeplessness, disordered appetite, a loss of weight, and constipation or diarrhoea.

EXAMINATION OF THE PATIENT
(See also Chapter 6)

Personality

In 1913, Hoch and Amsden devised a guide which they recommended for a study of the personality. This guide comprised eight main groupings, as follows:
1. General intelligence, knowledge and judgement.
2. Output of energy.
3. General attitude towards environment.

4. Attitude towards self: inner mental life.
5. Attitude towards reality.
6. Mood: emotional reactions.
7. Sex instincts.
8. Feeling of inferiority.

In 1923, Amsden published a further article dealing with the 'Practical Value of the Study of the Personality in Mental Disorders', and in this he narrowed (rightly, we think) his previous conceptions under four main headings:

1. The intellectual faculties.
2. 'Somatic demands' (physical activities).
3. The individual's self-criticism and self-estimate.
4. The urgency or imperative to adaptation.

It stands to reason that such a scheme must have a definite value in helping one to come to an understanding of the individual case; for is not the colouring of the psychosis largely dependent upon the original make-up, constitution or personality of the individual? Furthermore, the prognosis of any case, no matter how serious it may seem on the surface, depends essentially on the 'stuff' of the individual, the inherent character. A person well-endowed intellectually, who has met his difficulties in his social, business and sexual relationships in a healthy, straightforward way, and who has had interests outside himself, who has been 'exteriorized' in his everyday relationships, has always much more chance of making a good readjustment than his introverted, 'shut-in' neighbour. With an exact, detailed description of the patient's likes and dislikes, hopes and fears, or of as much of them as it is possible to elicit, we are better able to guide the patient along the paths which are in harmony with his disposition, and which he can most easily accept. A study of the personality is therefore not only of importance after the development of the psychosis, but it seems to us to be particularly important in connection with prophylactic work, and in connection with the training of children. If we have clearer ideas about what the difficulties of make-up are likely to lead to, then we may be able to prevent the development of serious break-downs. The scheme which Amsden formulated is difficult to improve upon, and we would summarize it as follows:

1. In a description of *intellectual activity*, the points which we specially desire information about are: (*a*) the readiness with which knowledge is acquired; (*b*) the power of retention; (*c*) the ability to be guided by past experience. These points can be elicited by having a detailed account not only of the patient's schooldays, but also of his business and family life. We want to determine whether the well-endowed type is able to co-ordinate his activity in a healthy-minded, constructive way, whether he is in touch with things as they are, or whether he is apt to be diffuse, absent-minded, lacking in purpose and easily side-tracked. The questions to elicit these various points must be left to the individual examiner.

2. The *somatic demands* concern themselves especially with motor activities and the demands of sex. Motor, or, better, psychomotor, activity involves the questions whether the patient was lively or sluggish, *i.e.* whether there was push

and energy as evidenced by talkativeness and enthusiasm, or whether he was inert and lacked initiative; whether there has been much interest in sports, games, hobbies, or whether there has been idleness and lassitude. Regarding sex, it is important to know how much the topic has interested the patient, whether the reactions to it have been hygienic or unhygienic, whether there have been unhealthy habits, actual and mental masturbation, prudishness or its opposite. Some importance has been attached to vaguer matters, such as nail-biting, and response to mucous-membrane stimulation—eating, drinking, smoking.

3. *Self-estimate and self-criticism* depend largely on comparing ourselves with others. Such comparison may bring with it a feeling of satisfaction, or a feeling of failure, according to whether the comparison is favourable or unfavourable. If the comparison is favourable, the reactions are likely to be capable and adequate, but if unfavourable, a variety of responses may be elicited. Either the individual may realize his deficiencies, and attempt to correct his shortcomings in a healthy way, or else the individual may shrink, become sensitive, self-effacing and dependent. Again, evasions and compensations may be called into being. A sidelight on these various aspects may be obtained by the knowledge of whether the person is greatly influenced by the opinion of others, whether he is proud, fussy and makes much of discomforts. Other important sidelights are the individual's ability to make friends, the degree of easiness or uneasiness in the presence of strangers and the tendency to jealousy. The questions of over-conscientiousness, and the ability to take advice, also come in.

4. *The urgency or imperative to adaptation* centres round the question why we need to adapt ourselves at all. This, as Amsden says, is the crux of the whole study, because it is just these tendencies which favour or impede adaptation which are so important. A constructive assertion of it is seen in ambition, courageousness and vigorousness generally. Where we find a diminution of such tendencies we must attempt to get some explanation for it.

Mental Examination

We will attempt in the chapter on 'Symptomatology' to describe the great variety of mental symptoms which commonly occur, so that the plan of examination as here laid down will be put as briefly as possible. It will concern itself mainly with the order to be followed, and the method of eliciting the required information. Where a technical term appears of which the meaning is not evident from the context, an explanation of it will be found in the chapter on 'Symptomatology'.

General Behaviour

The general behaviour of the patient is usually the first indication to the relatives that all is not well. The facial expression, the dress, the attitude, often tell at a glance the underlying state of the patient, and we note at once whether there is depression, or elation and talkativeness, apathy and listlessness, co-operation or resistance, stupor or undue suggestibility. We must note whether the activity is free or constrained, changeable or stereotyped, whether there is anxiety and agitation, with scratching and picking at the skin, and whether there is any reaction to imaginary sense-perceptions. A good deal can be learned from the way the patient adapts to a new environment, as, *e.g.*, on admission to hospital, and it is always wise to get a description from the nurse of how the patient accepted the formalities of admission, *e.g.* having clothes taken and marked, the bath, and the association with other patients. The description should be made as vivid and telling as possible, but it should be couched as far as possible in non-technical language, and it is perhaps best written at the end rather than at the beginning of the examination, because facts will be observed during the examination which were not at first apparent.

The Stream of Mental Activity

This is easily and quickly determined by a number of simple questions, *e.g.* 'What is your name in full?' 'Are you married or single?' 'How old are you?' 'What is your occupation?' 'What do you complain of?' 'Do you know why you are here?' The response to such questions will demonstrate at once whether there is any formal disorder—that is to say, whether there is over-talkativeness or mutism, whether questions have to be repeated, whether the answers tend to go into too much detail, with flight of ideas and distractibility, whether there is a considerable pause before a reply is given (retardation), or whether there is an element of suspicion, *e.g.* 'Why do you ask me such questions?' Again, questions may be answered promptly and to the point, or there may be irrelevance with incoherence, verbigeration, perseveration, echolalia, neologisms, stereotypies. On the other hand, the response to questions may indicate a total lack of understanding, and point towards some organic change. It is a most excellent plan to take, if possible, a verbatim report of the patient's spontaneous talk.

Emotional Reaction (Affect)

The superficial manifestation of the patient's affect (facial expression, etc.) will have been noted already under general behaviour, but we want to analyse more deeply not only the affect, but also the situation producing it, whether it is dependent on domestic, social or business difficulties. We have to depend a great deal upon what the patient himself tells us regarding his feelings. We note at once what his general attitude is, and we point our more specific questions in accordance therewith. It is a false move, and a great insult, to ask a patient obviously depressed whether he is happy; in consequence, it is always best to ask some such general question as 'How do you feel?' and then, according to the reply, this can be followed up with such questions as, 'Are you happy?' and then, 'Why?'; or, 'Are you sad or melancholy, or out of sorts, or worried?' and, again, 'Why?' Where possible, the mood should be described in the patient's own words. After these more or less formal questions, the patient should be asked to tell his story from the beginning, and should be kept to the topic with a minimum of questioning, until the condition has been thoroughly detailed. If the patient is allowed to tell his story in this way, it usually means that a satisfactory basis of co-operation is established, which permits of not only completing the examination expeditiously, but also gives a foundation for future work. Furthermore, the patient at once recognizes that a real effort is being made to understand him. This produces gratitude, and establishes confidence. Our questions must largely be dictated by our common sense, and must simply suffice to keep the patient to the topic in hand, without unduly suggesting things. The points which have particularly to be kept in mind are the intensity of the affect, whether it varies, the response to reassurance, and the question whether it is in harmony with the ideas expressed. The affective state can be approximately gauged even when the patient is unresponsive and mute, by noting such things as pallor, flushing, perspiration, the respiration rate and the pulse.

Mental Trend: Content of Thought

It often happens that when a patient is describing his 'feelings' he will express ideas pointing to a disordered content of thought, and at this point he should be encouraged to detail the development of his ideas. This may be done quite spontaneously, and without much urging, but, on the other hand, there may be evasion and hedging, and more direct questions may have to be asked. The narrative, however, does not read so tellingly when questions are interposed, and it is usually best to omit them, and to continue the story as it is given. In case of necessity, however, we must ask such questions as, 'Do you believe that you have been watched, laughed at, or spoken about?' 'Have people been behaving strangely towards you?' 'Do they seem to take undue notice of you?' 'Have attempts actually been made to persecute and injure you?', and 'With what motive?' 'Does it seem as if your mind or your body is being influenced by electricity, wireless, drugs?' 'Do your thoughts seem to be read?' 'Have you been influenced by hypnotism?' 'Do you feel as if you had a mission?' It must be determined whether the patient is convinced that all this is being done for some special purpose, and whether these ideas occur in a setting of complete intellectual clearness. When it is evident that hallucinations play a prominent part, one should not hesitate to put direct questions, as 'Will you describe your imaginations to me?' 'Do you hear voices or noises?' 'Are they imaginary?' 'Do they occur in one ear or in both?' 'Do you see things?' 'Have you ever had visions?' 'Is this condition worse at night-time?' 'Have you noticed whether your sense of taste or smell is affected?' One should determine whether these experiences appear real (lack of insight), or whether they are regarded as being something strange and peculiar, and the result of imagination. When a positive history either of illusions or hallucinations is elicited, a detailed account should be obtained of how, why and when such disturbances appear. With regard to the condition described as 'compulsive' thought or action, or obsession, inquiry should be made whether thoughts come with insistent force into the patient's mind, and dominate completely. Have actions to be repeated? Is there 'a ritual' in regard to any of the daily tasks?

Orientation

This can be determined by the following simple questions: 'What day is it?'

'What time of day is it?' 'What month is it? 'What year is it?' 'Do you know the date?' 'What place is this?' 'What kind of place?' 'Who am I?' 'What is my occupation?'

Memory

The most convenient way to test the memory for remote events is to ask the patient to give a chronological account of his life from the date of birth. The patient should be asked for the date and place of birth, the age on going to and leaving school and what standard was reached. After leaving school what was the further development in occupation or training, the first place of employment and the subsequent career? If the patient is married, one should ask when the marriage took place; and the names and ages of the children. Where is the patient presently employed; what has been the longest time in one job; was he ever previously ill? It is wise to get as exact dates as possible of the various important events of the patient's life, in order to determine whether or not they are properly correlated.

The memory for recent events can be tested by such questions as 'When did you come here?' 'Where from?' 'What were you doing yesterday?' 'Who came with you?' 'How many meals have you had since you were admitted?'

Retention (Immediate Memory)

In order to test the power of retention, the patient is given verbally and asked to remember a street address, a person's name, a colour and some object such as a cabbage, a table, a house, and then, after a period of one to five minutes, or an hour, or several days, is requested to repeat what he was asked to remember. More specialized tests can be given, such as the memory for digits or letters or words. Franz, in his book on Examination Methods, gives these various tests in detail. We would particularly mention the test by word-pairs. The patient is asked to repeat five or ten word-pairs, and after this has been done, the stimulus word is given again, and the patient has to supply the second word, *e.g.*:

Head	—	hair	Window	—	door
Room	—	hall	Book	—	pencil
Chair	—	table	Lake	—	river
Grass	—	tree	Apple	—	pear
White	—	red	Pipe	—	tobacco

Recent attempts to give more precision in tests for failure of memory and of intellectual capacity in general are described on pages 418–19.

Apperception (ability to assimilate and comprehend impressions)

Franz's second useful test is to give the patient a short story or paragraph to read, and then ask him to give the gist of what he has read. The cowboy story is a good test for this purpose:

A cowboy from Arizona went to San Francisco with his dog, which he left at a friend's while he purchased a new suit of clothes. Dressed finely, he went back to the dog, whistled to him, called him by name and patted him. But the dog would have nothing to do with him in his new hat and coat, but gave a mournful howl. Coaxing was of no effect, so the cowboy went away and donned his old garments, whereon the dog immediately showed his wild joy on seeing his master as he thought he ought to be.'

The following two stories are taken from Bleuler's *Textbook of Psychiatry*:

THE DONKEY LOADED WITH SALT

'A donkey, loaded with salt, had to wade a stream. He fell down, and for a few minutes lay comfortably in the cool water. When he got up he felt relieved of a great part of his burden, because the salt had melted in the water. Longears noted this advantage, and at once applied it the following day, when, loaded with sponges, he again went through the same stream.

'This time he fell purposely, but was grossly deceived. The sponges had soaked up the water, and were considerably heavier than before. The burden was so great that he succumbed.

'The same remedy does not apply to all cases.'

NEPTUNE AND THE LABOURER

'A day labourer worked along a stream. By accident his axe fell in, and as the stream was so deep that he could not get it out, he sat on the bank and bemoaned his fate to the river god.

'Neptune took pity on the man's poverty, dived down and brought up a golden axe. "Is this yours?" he asked the labourer. The latter honestly answered "No". Suddenly Neptune dived down again and appeared before the woodcutter with a silver axe. To this one, too, the labourer made no claim. For the third time the god dived and brought up the right iron axe with the wooden handle. "Yes, that is it. That is the right one. That is the one I lost", the labourer exclaimed joyfully. "I only wanted to test you", replied Neptune; "I am glad that you are as honest as you are poor. There, take all three axes; I present them to you."

'The honest man told this story to several acquaintances. One of these wanted to misuse Neptune's goodness, and for this reason he purposely threw his axe into the stream. Hardly had he begun to bemoan his fate to the river god when the latter appeared with a golden axe. He asked, "Is this the one that fell into the stream?" He quickly exclaimed, "Yes, that is it", and grabbed for it. But Neptune denounced him as a shameless liar because he wanted to deceive even a god, and turned his back on him. With him disappeared the golden axe, and the labourer had to go home without even his own axe.

'Honesty is the best policy.'

The *thinking capacity and the power of attention* are important topics. In order to test these a series of digits or letters are read aloud to the patient, who is required to tap each time a certain digit or letter recurs. Or the lists may be given to the patient with the instruction to cross out the designated digits or letters.

Other tests to illuminate the same topics are the Heilbronner test, where familiar objects are drawn with varying degrees of completeness and the patient asked to indicate their defects; and the Ebbinghaus test, which tests the patient's ability to fill in blanks in a short story:

'Once upon a time —— heard a —— chirruping in the ——. "Ah," he said to himself, "if I could —— like that, how —— I should be." So he bowed low to the ——, and said, "Kind friend, what —— do you eat to make your —— so sweet?" "I drink the evening dew", replied the ——. The foolish —— tried to live on the same ——, and died of ——.'

School and General Knowledge

It is necessary in testing school and other knowledge to keep in mind the nationality, the educational level and the general experiences of the individual. School and general knowledge can be tested by giving simple questions in arithmetic, in history and geography, as follows:

     7 times 9?   3 times 17?   63 divided by 7?

     Subtract 7 from 100 consecutively and aloud (*i.e.* 93, 86, 79, etc.).

If the patient is able to accomplish these satisfactorily, then such questions as the interest on £200 at 4 per cent. for a year and a half can be asked, or such simple problems as—If 6 times X equals 18, how much is X?

In regard to history, one can ask questions in reference to the two World Wars. Who fought at Waterloo? Who was Napoleon? Wellington? Caesar? Name the oceans. Where are Brussels, Rome, Vienna, Berlin, Melbourne? What is the capital of France? of U.S.A.? Name the chief rivers in England. What is the highest mountain in the world? the largest lake?

Approximately correct replies to such questions in some instances would of course stand, and a number of failures must be allowed for.

General Intelligence

This can be gauged by the general character of the responses, or in special cases by tests for intelligence described on pages 460–1.

Sometimes it may be useful to ask more abstract questions, or to read a fable to the patient, and ask what is implied by it. One can put such questions, for instance, as the difference between a lie and a mistake, idleness and laziness, character and reputation.

Insight and Judgement

The questions here relate to the amount of realization the patient has of his own condition; does he realize that he is ill, that he is mentally ill, that he is in need of treatment in a mental hospital? Does he acknowledge that his ideas have been due to his disordered imagination? Does he show poor judgement regarding the question of discharge, plans for the future, family responsibilities, and ethical standards?

The foregoing outline applies more particularly to patients suffering from a psychosis. For modifications in cases of subnormality, and of neuroses, see the corresponding chapters, as well as the first part of this chapter.

Physical Examination

A thorough physical examination is absolutely essential in every mental case. This follows the ordinary lines.

REFERENCES

Amsden, G. S. (1923) *Amer. J. Psychiat.*, **11**, 501.
Hoch, A., and Amsden, G. S. (1913) *Rev. Neurol. Psychiat.*, **11**, 577.

6

SYMPTOMATOLOGY

An attempt will be made to define the terms used in clinical psychiatry, and this in the order in which they occur in the scheme of mental examination. Their discussion in the categories of the usual type of normal psychology, which has not proved fruitful in psychopathological practice, is thus avoided. Although the observation of individual symptoms is very important, it is only in connection with the whole life-history and the general clinical setting that they have their full meaning.

In the great majority of psychological illnesses there is little or no outward change; but in others there are alterations in demeanour, especially in the psychotic reactions, where the changes in social attitude and behaviour are sometimes both conspicuous and persistent. In most instances, however, we meet mainly or entirely subjective discomforts which may, however, be as great a handicap as the disability of physical disease, which indeed they often resemble, in the form of pains, 'indigestion', palpitation, headache and the like, without discoverable physical basis. The commonest type of subjective complaint is fear of something, whether it be of crowds, of open places, of being alone, of anything resembling dirt, of certain thoughts or of disease.

BEHAVIOUR

Behaviour will be used here in the general sense of the conduct and deportment of the patient as seen by the physician, and as related to him by the patient's friends. A change in behaviour can be one of the earliest and most striking indications of mental disorder. A man of hitherto ordinary normal habits becomes different from what he was previously. The change may be evidenced predominantly either in his emotional (affective) manifestations, in his activity, or in his intellectual performance. If previously cheerful and capable, he may become dull, morose and lacking in initiative; or, on the other hand, he may become unduly optimistic and enterprising, undertaking much more than he is fit to do. Another type of individual, with different characteristics, becomes an idler, unable to concentrate, dreamy and sensitive. Often with these changes goes lack of care of the person—slovenliness in dress and in habits of personal cleanliness. A good indication of the general condition is obtained from the facial expression and the general bodily posture, both of which may help to portray the prevailing affective state.

Intellectual disorder, e.g. of memory, may profoundly influence conduct by the resulting failure to carry out the ordinary everyday tasks, and, further, by the depression, restlessness or irritability which may result from the patient's realization of his inefficiency.

A definite delusional or hallucinatory condition is apt to reveal itself in a bizarre type of conduct, entirely out of keeping with the person's known habits.

The degree of *co-operation* which the patient displays towards those who wish to help him is of considerable importance. An attitude of suspicion, or even actual antagonism, will show itself either in speech or in gesture.

In general, these are indications of the kind of information that can be obtained from observation at first meeting the patient. Disorders of behaviour will be considered in greater detail in the general and special sections.

Motor behaviour comprises: 1. bodily movement; and 2. stream of talk.

1. Bodily movement may be abnormal either in degree or quality. *General over-activity* may consist in a rapid succession of purposive acts, with few of them carried to a conclusion, and not directed to a continued objective ('psychomotor excitement', 'push' and 'pressure' of activity). The over-activity is said to be playful when accompanied by a tendency to mischievousness, the whole having an 'infectious' character. On the other hand, over-activity may consist of a repetition of movements, with little or no diversity, *e.g.* wringing of hands, pacing up and down. Such an oft-repeated movement is known as a *stereotypy*.

Stereotypy shows in several types of motor behaviour. It includes stereotypy of attitude, of movement and of speech. An action, or group of actions, or words monotonously repeated, or a posture maintained long after fatigue would ordinarily have caused relaxation, is a stereotypy. Such monotonous activity may begin as an expression of emotional perturbation, or may have at first a special complex-determined significance; but in either case it gradually becomes a habit, from which meaning has partly or wholly departed.

Perseveration, or the repetition of a recent movement in spite of the patient's effort to produce a new movement, is to be distinguished from stereotypy. It is in its particular instances transient, requires a stimulus and is associated particularly with cases showing changes in the brain substance.

Stereotypy of attitude is excellently exemplified in the 'Egyptian mummy' position maintained sometimes for years—the patient sitting with head bowed, palms downwards on the thighs. Stereotypy of speech consists in such phrases as these, which were questions asked by a patient day after day for years: 'Is the door open yet?' 'Is the conveyance at the door?'

A *mannerism* differs from a stereotypy in that it is not so monotonously repeated, and is more in keeping with the personality.

Partial over-activity may take the form of isolated movements such as the tics or habit spasms, which are to be differentiated by the relatively simple nature of the movements involved, by the general setting in which they occur and by the fact that the subject is acutely aware of them, and complains of them.

General reduction in activity shows all gradations up to complete immobility. It may be associated with diminution in initiative, or with actual resistance to movement (negativism, *vide infra*). Slowness of initiative and slowness of execution ('psychomotor retardation', initial and executive) usually accompany each other, but may be found apart.

Negativism, like stereotypy, shows itself in various spheres of activity. In general, it consists in responses exactly opposite to those normally elicited by a given stimulus. In the muscular field, it may show itself either as an actively opposite performance to that asked for—*e.g.* shutting the mouth when told to open it—and as a resistance to passive movement. In speech it forms a variety of mutism. Negativism is seen also in the retention of saliva, urine and faeces, and in lack of general co-operation.

Contrasting with negativism is the so-called *automatic obedience*, showing itself in echopraxia (repetition of actions seen), echolalia (repetition of words heard), and flexibilitas cerea (the maintenance of imposed postures).

Automatic movements or automatisms occur in a pathological sense, without the subject's being aware of their meaning, and even without his being aware of their happening at all. They have not the full co-operation of the personality; they may, in fact, when generalized, occur in the complete abeyance of the normal personality. Automatism may be local, *e.g.* automatic writing, or general, as in the fugues and somnambulisms. Stengel restricts the term fugue to describe a state of alteration of consciousness combined with an impulse to wander. He has drawn attention to the relationship between vagrancy in childhood and episodic wandering in adult life, the common factor being a broken or disturbed home life. Very frequently a fugue occurs in a state of depression, and indeed the going away or wandering is often symbolic of suicide. An epileptic disposition is also often associated.

The significance of *impulses* varies with the clinical setting in which they occur. The term impulse has usually been applied to sudden outbursts of activity which are supposed to occur with little or no deliberation. Formerly 'impulsive insanity' was spoken of as an entity (*cf.* Clouston's 'Remarkable Case of Impulsive Insanity'), whereas it is at most only a symptom. Our experience is that the great majority of impulses, although apparently sudden, are the outcome of a long preceding period of mental unrest. Hence it is impossible to make clear differentiation between impulses and compulsions. The latter have been supposed to arise against the subject's wishes, and to make him uneasy until they are carried into effect. The term compulsive is also used in a similar sense which will be dealt with under obsessional neurosis.

Posture may be defined as static motor activity. It is often a telling expression of the general condition, physical and mental, and especially of the emotional (herein called 'affective') state. The bent head, furrowed brow and drooping shoulders of sadness are well known. The over-erect attitude of the vain and proud man is sometimes seen in an exaggerated form in mental disorders, associated with phantasies of self-importance. Strained and unnatural positions may be maintained ('fixed positions') over long periods of time. These may be produced by the observer by virtue of the 'flexibilitas cerea' already mentioned. The absence of apparent fatigue in such cases is remarkable. 'Catalepsy' is a term sometimes used for any form of sustained immobility.

2. In the stream of talk a distinction has to be made between content and form—the content meaning what the patient says, and the form, how he says it. Form only will be discussed here. Content is more appropriately dealt with under

'thinking'. Talk may be more copious than normal ('pressure' or 'push' of talk), but still perfectly coherent and logical. This is mere *volubility*, and is spontaneous, irrespective of the asking of questions. In *circumstantiality* there is much unnecessary detail and great spontaneity, but the object in view at the beginning is ultimately reached. Mrs. Nickleby is the classical example. In *flight of ideas* the stream is continuous but fragmentary, the connections being determined by chance associations between the fragments. The connections can be followed—there is a certain coherence—but the direction is frequently changed, often by chance stimuli from the environment (*distractibility*), and the original objective is quickly lost sight of. *Punning* and *rhyming* (sound or 'clang' associations) are not infrequent in a flight of ideas.

Slowing of the stream of talk shows itself, like slowing of activity, in initial and executive retardation. In certain states of emotional exaltation the utterances may be slow and stately; but this is a deliberate slowing—an affectation. There may be no utterance at all, even in response to repeated questioning—*mutism*. This may be associated with one of several conditions—as an accompaniment of extreme depression, an expression of complete indifference to the environment, a form of negativism, the result of a hallucinatory command, of a complex-determined belief, or of an extreme degree of difficulty in thinking. When mutism is an expression of negativism, it may be only partial, occurring in response to questions, while spontaneous utterance takes place.

Blocking is a sudden stoppage of the stream of talk, occurring apart from any environmental influences, and without the patient's being able to account for the stoppage.

Deprivation of thought is an extreme degree of blocking, when the stream is arrested for a time, and there is no longer any apparent content whatsoever.

Relevance of the patient's answers is an important point. In the types of disorder of the stream of talk so far mentioned, the answers, when given, are relevant; but there are many other types where the disorder of thought shows itself by an answer not in harmony with the question, or even conveying no meaning at all. This irrelevant type of answer is closely related to *disconnection*.

Disconnection may be of all degrees up to complete *incoherence*. The minor degrees of incoherence are known as 'scattering' and 'dilapidation'. The most complete disconnection has been called verbigeration—simply a flow of unconnected words, some of them often repeated. A 'word-salad' is a string of substantives poured out in a similar manner.

To be contrasted with these disorders of the stream of talk which result from disorders of thought are the paraphasic disorders depending on a focal organic lesion. These, too, consist of a jargon, and on this basis Stransky applied the term 'intrapsychic ataxia' to the incoherent types of talk found in certain purely psychogenic disorders. *Perseveration* is often associated with a true paraphasic disorder, and consists of the persistent repetition of one word or group of words, in spite of the patient's attempt to change the topic, and the observer's attempt to introduce other stimuli (in contrast with stereotypy).

Neologisms are words of the patient's own making, often portmanteau condensations of several other words, and having originally had a special meaning for the patient.

EMOTIONAL REACTION

'Affect' and 'mood' are both used to denote the emotional condition. 'Affect' is the term of preference, for it has none of the popular connotations of 'mood'. Affect is difficult to define. The language of emotion is in any case very inadequate. Affect can, perhaps, be called the subject's inner feeling at a given moment, but this is not a definition. The automatic (*i.e.* self-regulating) nature of affect is well known. The commoner normal affects are those of sadness, elation, fear and their variants—joy, happiness, gladness, sorrow, anxiety, etc. Pathological states show exaggeration or mixtures of normal moods, or apparent complete absence of affect (apathy). The chief criteria of abnormality are depth, duration and setting—*i.e.* how great the affect is, and under what psychological and material conditions it occurs. *Incongruity or disharmony* of affect—inappropriateness of affect to thought-content—is very important, and should always be looked for and noted.

Elation is a joyful affect, and is used for sheer happiness. It is pathological when out of accord with the patient's actual circumstances. *Exaltation* means something in addition to elation—an element of grandeur and pomposity is usually implied. In pure elation and in exaltation, everything that could not harmonize with the general emotional condition is shut out. Pure elation is generally 'infectious', the observer having a sympathetic sense of the patient's happiness. *Ecstasy* is a less robust happiness, usually with a mystical colouring. *Euphoria* is a generalized feeling of well-being, not amounting to a definite affect of gladness.

Affective depression or sadness is pathological when not warranted by the patient's condition or surroundings. The patient may say that he feels 'downhearted' or 'sad'; but often no statement of affect can be elicited, and a conclusion has to be reached from posture, facies and other sources.

Anxiety as a technical term is a fear of danger usually from within, *e.g.* impending physical illness. It may occur either as a continued state of fear, or (more commonly) in episodic attacks. The episodes have the well-marked physical manifestations usually associated with fear. It is said that a typical anxiety attack has nothing but somatic symptoms: there is usually, however, a conscious fear, generally of illness, sometimes undefined.

Apprehension is usefully confined to the fear of external danger.

Apathy is an absence of affect, and can only be inferred from the patient's statement, or, failing that, from his failure to respond to stimuli which would otherwise call forth an affect of some kind. It carries no subjective sensation with it, and should thus be differentiated from sadness. Apathy may exist in a setting of depression—the patient complains that he cannot respond with any feeling to incidents which should arouse emotion of some kind. 'Indifference' and 'dullness' are used almost synonymously, and are descriptive of the lack of objective response, while apathy refers specifically to a lack of feeling.

H

Irritability, as a description of affect, is used in the ordinary sense of response elicited with undue readiness. It is usually associated with some other prevalent affect, and is a symptom of lack of harmony of the subject with his environment, and especially with a feeling of 'subjective insufficiency'—*i.e.* inability to perform ordinary tasks with the usual facility.

Morbid anger is an unprovoked angry outburst. It occurs in children, and in states of subnormality, and is then designated as 'tantrums'. The striking features are the lack of provocation, the violence, and the transient nature of the outburst.

It is disputed whether *suspicion* is an affect. Bleuler considered it more an intellectual than an affective condition. It is best included among the affects for practical purposes.

Emotional instability or *lability* is characterized by fluctuations in the affective condition without external cause. It occurs especially in gross organic lesions.

Emotional deterioration is a progressive failure to show the normal emotional responses, and is usually characterized by a childish, easily suggestible (facile) state.

THINKING

The general characteristics of thinking are altered in mental disorders. Phantasy assumes large proportions—*i.e.* there is less correction by reality than in the normal; and thinking passes but little into action. These are the two chief characteristics of 'autistic' thinking (Bleuler, 1950).

It follows that the content and course of thought are much more at the mercy of the affects and wishes of the mentally ill than in the case of healthy persons. Disorders of thought have to be inferred from the patient's utterance, including his own statements about his thinking, and from his conduct. Disorders of the form of thought have, for the most part, been discussed in disorders of the stream of talk. In certain conditions the patient makes complaint of *difficulty in thinking*. This may be due either to difficulty in concentration on one topic from preoccupation with another, or to actual slowing of the thought processes.

In *preoccupation*, the patient continually reflects on one topic or group of topics, to the exclusion of environmental interests, and to the detriment of useful activity.

Obsessive thoughts (or obsessions) persist with full realization on the part of the subject that they are abnormal, and in spite of his endeavours to rid himself of them. In these two respects they differ from simple preoccupation.

Autochthonous ideas are 'thoughts coming to the patient in some unaccountable way, strange but not dependent on hallucination' (Meyer). In other cases the patient believes that someone reads his thoughts. This condition is an example of 'passivity' (*v. infra*).

The *idea of reference* consists in the subject's being acutely aware that something in the environment is intended to have a meaning for him, when, as a matter of fact, no such personal reference is intended. The idea of reference is thus partly based on some external circumstance, and is open to argument, whereas a fully developed delusion more often arises with apparent spontaneity. Moreover, the idea of reference is usually transitory, and is an example of a general tendency. It is based on personal sensitiveness, and is easily understood as an exaggeration of the normal; the abnormality lies rather in the source and acuteness of the sensitiveness—the source being affective in origin, and depending, for example, on feelings of exaltation or of guilt.

Ambivalence is a term coined by Bleuler to denote the co-existence of two contradictory ideas or feelings in consciousness, both of which cannot be true, but which are allowed to co-exist without rejection by the patient of either one. *Double orientation* is a case in point—the patient, for example, stating almost in the same breath that he is in Glasgow and in London. But ambivalence is also used by the Freudian school in a somewhat different sense to denote the entertaining of two opposite feelings towards the same person, *e.g.* both love and hate of a parent by the child.

The term *katathymic* has been used to characterize thinking along the lines determined by some complex.

DISORDERS OF THE CONTENT OF THOUGHT

A *delusion* is a belief which: 1. is not true to fact; 2. cannot be corrected by an appeal to the reason of the person entertaining it; and 3. is out of harmony with the individual's education and surroundings. As Mercier pointed out: 'The delusion is not an isolated disorder. . . . It is merely the superficial indication of a deep-seated and widespread disorder. . . . As a small island is but the summit of an immense mountain rising from the floor of the sea, so a delusion is merely the component part of a mental disease, extending, it may be, to the very foundations of the mind.'

The type of individual most likely to have delusions is one who normally shows a suspicious, argumentative attitude.

The nature of the delusion is important—to what extent it displays judgement or lack of it. There are degrees of reasonableness even in delusional beliefs, and their unreasonableness varies directly as the degree of impairment of judgement and as the depth of the affect which supports them.

Insight in the form of the patient's own criticism of the fact of his holding delusional beliefs is a related problem of even more significance. A person who entertains a false belief, but at the same time admits that it may be unjustified, and who may spontaneously talk of it as a delusion, is, as a rule, more amenable to treatment than one whose beliefs admit of no criticism.

Systematization denotes that the delusions are well knit, and that they form a fairly coherent system, logical within itself, if the premises once be granted. In other instances, the delusions are not correlated with each other; they are more or less isolated, and little or no attempt is made at logical correction.

Delusions have frequently been classified, but this is a matter of convenience only. A delusion has its full meaning only in the setting of the whole mental state of the individual possessing it. There are, however, certain uniformities which enable us to mention certain general types.

Delusions of grandeur and *delusions of persecution* are very common varieties, which are frequently found together. They result from the projection of instinctual trends. They are sometimes obviously compensatory for failure in some direction. For example, a girl deformed from poliomyelitis believed that she was descended from Royalty, was married and had a family. In other instances their foundations are not so clear, and for the persecutory type psychoanalysts have postulated a repressed homosexuality.

Another general type is formed by delusions of *sin*, delusions of *poverty* and *nihilistic* delusions. In the nihilistic variety, the patient declares that he does not exist, that there is no world, etc.

Hypochondria consists in a settled conviction of physical disease in the absence of any evidence thereof. As a symptom it occurs in many forms of mental illness. It is most common in depressions, especially in the depressions of the involutional period. It also occurs as part of a schizophrenic syndrome, when the hypochondriacal ideas are of the most grotesque kind. Sometimes hypochondria is hysterical in origin, and not infrequently what appears on superficial examination to be hypochondriasis is actually a chronic anxiety state. But a hypochondriacal conviction and preoccupation is sometimes found in which it is impossible to demonstrate that it is part of one of the larger syndromes. This occurs sometimes, for example, in elderly men, whose whole life centres round their supposed ailments—a withdrawal of interest, perhaps never strong, having occurred from the outer world, with a corresponding intense concentration on their bodily functions. Hypochondriacal delusions are closely connected with disordered bodily feelings. For example, delusions that the bowels are obstructed, and the stomach cancerous, are associated with dyspepsia and constipation.

Ideas of unreality are probably sometimes psychologically related to nihilistic delusions, but they are not usually delusional, the patient recognizing their abnormality, and complaining of the distress which they occasion. Everything is expressed as seeming different—the streets and houses look unusual, the patient wonders whether his friends are the same people as they were, or whether indeed they exist at all ('derealization'); he feels differently in himself, and may wonder whether he himself exists ('depersonalization'). Such ideas, and the feeling associated with them, are not at all uncommon in older children, especially the more intelligent, and as neurotic or depressive symptoms in adults. But even strong, healthy, normal people may experience such disturbing sensations. Sir Walter Scott in his *Journal* under date 17th February 1828 at Abbotsford writes as follows: 'Yesterday at dinner time I was strangely haunted by what I would call the sense of pre-existence—videlicet, a confused idea that nothing that passed was said for the first time, that the same topics had been discussed, and the same persons had stated the same opinions on the same subjects. It is true there might have been some ground for recollections, considering that three at least of the company were old friends, and kept much company together; that is Justice-Clerk (The Right Hon. David Boyle), (Lord) Abercromby, and I. But the sensation was so strong as to resemble what is called a *mirage* in the desert or a calenture on board ship, when lakes are seen in the desert, and silvan landscapes in the sea. It was very distressing yesterday, and brought to my mind the fancies of Bishop Berkeley about an ideal world. There was a vile sense of want of reality in all I did and said. It made me gloomy and out of spirits, though I flatter myself it was not observed. The bodily feeling which most resembles this un-pleasing hallucination is the giddy state which follows profuse bleeding when one feels as if walking on feather-beds and could not find a secure footing. I think the stomach has something to do with it. I drank several glasses of wine but these only augmented the disorder. I did not find the *in vino veritas* of the philosophers. Something of this insane feeling remains to-day, but a trifle only.'

Hallucinations are mental impressions of sensory vividness occurring without external stimulus. They are distinguished from *illusions*, which are similar im-pressions, depending, however, on a misinterpretation of an external stimulus.

The psychopathological basis of hallucinations is usually stated as follows: a wish is disowned by the ego and is repressed and so becomes unconscious, when it assumes independent activity, and forces its way back into the consciousness by the only method permitted to it—in disguise. The disowning by the ego makes it necessary that the disguised wish should appear to come from outside; it is accordingly projected, assuming an external sensory appearance when presented to consciousness.

Hallucinations may of course be physiogenic and not psychogenic in origin. Hallucinations occur in toxic states as the result of physiological disturbances, and brain lesions are responsible for hallucinations of a special type. Mechanical irritation of the uncus may cause hallucinations of taste and smell; and the same cause in the occipital lobe may produce flashes of light apparently before the eyes. The content of the hallucination is to some extent determined by individual psychological experience. In the case of at least one toxic substance, however, namely mescaline, the hallucinatory content is often entirely novel, and may even, in an apparently normal person, have characteristics that belong to schizo-phrenic experience.

Hallucinations occur even in normal people on rare occasions. William James gave several interesting instances in his *Principles of Psychology*.

The evidence for the presence of hallucinations is various—the patient may state frankly that he hears voices, but he more usually does so only after some time and trouble have been spent in obtaining his confidence. He may be seen in a listening attitude, or he may talk aloud as if answering someone, or his lips may be seen to move. The subject's response to hallucinations may be that of a passive listener, or he may reply to them. More active responses may be made to hallucinatory commands, which are often obeyed. Hallucinatory insults may lead to attacks on bystanders. In any case, hallucinations entail a certain amount of preoccupation.

The general setting in which hallucinations occur is of great significance, espe-cially in relation to the question whether the setting is one of mental clearness, or of disorientation (*v. infra*).

Hallucinations may occur in any of the sensory fields. Auditory hallucinations are the most common. The simplest form is 'buzzing' or ringing in the ears.

More usually hallucinations are of the nature of voices, the spoken words being distinguished as a rule. They may occur in one or both ears, and sometimes appear, like hallucinations in general, to be determined in their incidence by local disease or irritation (*e.g.* chronic otitis media). It is their *content* that is of special interest—and it has to be remembered that their content is just as much a part of the patient's mental life as his ordinary thought, however foreign in origin they appear to be. Illustrating their affective basis and their dependence on factors similar to those producing delusions is their similar colouring—grandiose, persecutory or accusatory as the case may be. Thus the voices may be those of exalted personages, conversing with the patient, who derives therefrom much satisfaction; or they may call him unpleasant names, or accuse him of vile practices. Occasionally the voices seem to the patient to come from inside his body.

Visual hallucinations occur in their simplest form as flashes of light and colour. More complex visual hallucinations commonly occur in a setting of general disorientation, but they also appear in states of ecstasy. Organic disease of the optic connections in the central nervous system is a cause of hallucinations either of the simple or of the complex type.

Toxic factors such as alcohol and morphine produce complex hallucinations often of a terrifying kind, more commonly associated with withdrawal of the drug; and they may or may not be accompanied by disorientation. When of purely psychological origin, the hallucinations are usually in accord with the prevailing affective tendencies, *e.g.* the religious ecstatic sees angels in his visions.

Hallucinations of smell may (rarely) be the result of irritation of the uncus from organic disease. When they occur in a psychosis, they are usually unpleasant odours, *e.g.* a patient stated that there was a skunk in bed with him. Odours may be interpreted by the patient as gas being pumped into the room to annoy him. There is evidently a frequent relation between hallucinations of unpleasant odours and a sense of guilt with reference especially to masturbation.

Hallucinations of taste are often associated with those of smell, and, like them, may rarely be the result of organic disease. They occur infrequently in psychoses. Illusions of taste are more common, and are related to affective conditions (usually suspicion)—the food tastes queerly, and is inferred to be poisoned.

Hallucinations of touch (haptic hallucinations) and other skin sensations are common—for example, in the form of creeping sensations under the skin (*formication*—the 'cocaine bug'). Sensations 'like electricity' are related to sex-feelings, unrecognized as such by the patient. All kinds of paraesthesia—numbness, tingling, pains, etc.—occur, and are sometimes used as part of a delusional scheme, the persecuted patient inferring that some injury to him is being attempted. Sensations in the genital or anal regions help to substantiate delusions of assault.

In *pseudo-hallucinations* the patient has the vivid sensory experience, but realizes that it has no external foundation.

Reflex hallucinations occur in one sensory sphere as the result of irritation in another. An auditory sensation may in this way arise from irritation in the region of the inferior alveolar nerve (carious tooth).

In *Lilliputian* or *microptic hallucinations*, the objects seen appear much reduced in scale. They are usually of very pleasant content and bright in colour. The patient is amused at seeing diminutive women and children in bright clothing. They have been observed in cases of scarlet fever (Hall, 1922), in typhoid and in intoxications by alcohol, chloroform and ether (Leroy and de Fursac, 1920).

Hypnagogic hallucinations occur in the state between sleeping and waking. They can be recognized from the conditions under which they occur, including the accompanying sensation of drowsiness, and from their dream-like nature, as well as from the fact that the subject who experiences them usually realizes their hallucinatory nature.

Impressions that part of one's body is being moved are sometimes described as *psychomotor hallucinations*. These are better understood under ideas of passivity.

Ideas and feelings of passivity or influence include such diverse ideas of the patient as that his thoughts are being read, his limbs moved without his control or consent and without visible agency, or even that he is entirely under the control of someone in the environment. Such ideas, or less well-defined feelings, may be associated with motor phenomena—flexibilitas cerea, and the main-tenance of fixed attitudes. They are then expressions of a general attitude of passivity, and are sometimes the reflection of a wish, not consciously formulated, to be under another's control. From the psychoanalytic point of view, such ideas and signs have been interpreted in certain conditions as part of the attitude of the passive homosexual. In some conditions, especially where the phenomena are less generalized, the ideas of influence are more probably the interpretation of certain automatic motor acts—automatic because occurring without the co-operation of the personality, and dependent, it is supposed, on the activity of certain dissociated tendencies. The idea that one's thoughts are being read may in some instances rest on an affective basis of guilt.

ORIENTATION

Orientation is the appreciation of one's temporal, spatial and personal relations at the present moment. It may be deranged on either a psychogenic or a physio-genic basis. It is important to know whether the disorientation is complete or partial. Simple inattention, from distractibility or from general lack of interest, may cause partial disorientation. Strong affects may also do so, causing a patient to give for the actual date an erroneous one in which he is particularly interested. The answer in these cases must be judged from the general setting of memory, orientation in other respects and general clearness. Inattention and lack of interest may also cause random answers to be given, when closer questioning may elicit the correct information.

It is in organic conditions (toxins, arteriosclerosis) that orientation is most frequently lost, wholly or partially. In cases of this kind, a false orientation is often given, and this statement of orientation itself changes rapidly.

MEMORY

Disorders of memory are commonly divided into *amnesias, paramnesias* and *hypermnesias.*

Amnesia, or absence of memory, may be complete or partial, continuous, periodic or circumscribed. Complete amnesia, *i.e.* for the entire previous existence, is rare. Amnesia, confined to recent events and progressive (*anterograde*), is characteristic of senile cerebral degeneration. In the gradually extending amnesia of advancing degeneration, rote memory tends to be retained better than other kinds. *Retrograde amnesia* involves only past events, and is not progressive.

Circumscribed amnesia involves some isolated event, or group of events, which usually have had a strong affective meaning; but in many cases of brain trauma there is a localized amnesia which persists for events immediately before and immediately after the accident.

Paramnesia denotes false recollection—the patient relates with conviction and circumstantiality events which never took place, or gives a false colouring to those that did happen. *Confabulation* is the term applied to the fabrication of memories in this way, and *retrospective falsification* to the adding of false details and meanings to a true memory. *Pseudo-reminiscence* covers both these meanings. An outstanding example of fabrication of memory occurs in *pseudologia phantastica* (*pathological lying*).

Hypermnesia or excessive retention of memories, especially of detail, is found in certain prodigies, and in certain mental disorders, especially paranoid psychoses and hypomania. In the former of these two conditions it is related to the general affective tendencies, and any detail is remembered which might possibly have a bearing on the delusional topics.

A variety of paramnesia, known as the *déjà vu* phenomenon, refers to the not uncommon experience of seeing something (or hearing it) with the feeling that one has seen it before, but does not know when or where. Such an experience occurs sometimes in epilepsy, as well as in normal persons. The basis may lie in some real experience, which has been forgotten; something which one has read and does not clearly recollect; or in some previous phantasy, conscious or unconscious, of waking- or dream-life. Where the feeling of *déjà vu* is continuous, as in an epileptic recorded by Kinnier Wilson, the term 'reduplicative paramnesia' has been applied. Zangwill (1941) has made a careful study of a case of paramnesia from a volume of English memoirs entitled *Our Old Home*, by Nathaniel Hawthorne. Zangwill points out that theories regarding *déjà vu* fall into two broad groups. On the one hand the phenomenon is explained in terms of transient inability to distinguish old from new and past from present. This difference is not considered to be dependent on the external setting, the condition being regarded as endogenous and due to a momentary disorder of mental synthesis. It has been thought that there may be an associated organic predisposing condition, such as fatigue or constitutional inadequacy. On the other hand, the phenomenon is regarded as reactive or determined by some specific peculiarity of the setting or environment in which it occurs. This theory suggests the possibility of a psychological linkage between the constitution in *déjà vu* and some previous experience or disposition in the history of the individual. The matter is one which may be determined by unconscious trends and, in consequence, this theory stresses the psychogenic factors. On the basis of the study of the particular case of Hawthorne, Zangwill concluded that Hawthorne's experience of *déjà vu* was a reactive state co-determined by an early (and probably unconscious) phantasy and an accident of circumstance.

ATTENTION

This is sometimes loosely called 'mental tension', or regarded as a manifestation of that ill-defined entity; it may be increased or diminished. Decreased attention to the environment may be the outcome of lack of interest, or of a more deliberate shutting-out (in its extreme form a manifestation of negativism). A patient's attention varies inversely with his preoccupation with his own problems. Hence any affective disturbance may cause a diminution in useful attention.

Inability to attend, in spite of the wish to do so, is seen in organic diseases (toxins and in structural cerebral lesions). 'Fluctuation of attention', in which the attention varies to a much greater extent than in the normal, is a fairly characteristic disorder in these conditions, in which also perseveration of previous impressions is sometimes an interfering factor in attention, new impressions being hindered by the persistence of old ones. It has been pointed out by Bleuler that active attention is often good in organic cases, while passive attention is poor; and that in 'functional' disorders (*e.g.* schizophrenia) the reverse is true. *Blunting of attention* is an extreme form of inattention, and occurs in stuporous states, when even nocuous stimuli, *e.g.* pin-pricks, fail to elicit a response.

Increase of attention (*hyperprosexia*) is less common, and is sometimes associated with a sensory hyperaesthesia, *e.g.* auditory hyperaesthesia, and with certain excitements (hypomania). But increased attention is usually affectively and selectively determined. *Distractibility* is a disorder of the attention in which the patient gives attention to every passing stimulus; consequently his attention passes very rapidly from one object to another.

Comprehension (or *apperception*) is impaired by organic (cerebral) disorder, whether from toxins or from grosser lesions. Comprehension may be modified in certain directions by affects—misunderstandings occur in line with them, or comprehension may suffer from the inattention that comes from apathy.

JUDGEMENT

Judgement depends on the ability to bring together two contrasting propositions, and to discriminate that one which is in closer accord with the general body of the subject's knowledge. Anything which interferes with associative processes will therefore impair judgement; hence toxins, organic lesions and congenitally defective cerebral organization lead to defective judgement. But it is now also generally admitted that judgement is much more dependent on affect than was formerly believed. A delusion is the result of a judgement in which affect has had excessive weight. It is not, however, difficult as a rule to distinguish the affectively perverted judgement from a judgement defective from the other causes mentioned; the latter will be displayed in a wide variety of general topics of indifferent interest.

SUGGESTIBILITY

This becomes abnormal when the patient habitually conforms with unusual readiness to suggestions made to him. It is common in neurotics, and Babinski attempted to make suggestibility the fundamental factor in hysteria, on which all the wide variety of symptoms depends. Suggestibility is very much influenced by the relation of the patient to the person making the suggestion. A suggestion is much more likely to be effective if coming from someone whom the patient likes and trusts. Crude examples of suggestibility, not seen in neurotics, are the forms of automatic obedience—echopraxia, echolalia and flexibilitas cerea, already described.

Negative suggestibility, in which the subject habitually does the opposite to what is suggested to him, is seen in spoiled children, even in early infancy—the infant refusing the bottle offered by the over-solicitous mother, but taking food readily if the mother's fussiness is corrected. It is seen in more obvious and more direct form in certain mental disorders as the so-called negativism, already described.

Suggestibility plays a part, among other factors, in the genesis of *folie à deux* or 'communicated insanity', which is the term applied when two persons closely associated with one another suffer a psychosis simultaneously, and when one member of the pair appears to have influenced the other. The condition is not of course necessarily confined to two persons, and may involve three or even more (*folie à trois*, etc.). It is commonest in persons living secluded lives. Husband and wife, brother and sister, or parent and child, or friends of the same sex living closely together are the usual subjects of the condition. It is usually either a paranoid or manic-depressive state. Craike and Slater (1945) have drawn attention to a case of *folie à deux* in uniovular twins reared apart. The twins were separated at nine months, were brought up in different families in different parts of the country, met for the first time at the age of 24, never lived together or had any close contact with one another, but each in due course developed a paranoid psychosis, each involving the other in her own system of delusional ideas.

CONSCIOUSNESS

Under disturbances of consciousness are usually included sleep, various psychogenic disturbances (*i.e.* produced and removable by psychic means, and occurring without demonstrable physical basis), such as the multiple personalities, transformations and depersonalizations, somnambulisms, twilight states, trances, hysterical deliria and stupor; and the physically determined disorders such as deliria, stupor and coma.

SLEEP

All kinds of disturbances are possible. Sleep may be diminished, abolished or increased in quantity (hyposomnia, insomnia and hypersomnia), or the sleep rhythm may be inverted, so that the patient sleeps by day and is awake by night. Diminution in sleep may be due to delay in falling asleep (from preoccupation, anxiety, habit or physical disease), to early waking (from depression), or from interruption, *e.g.* by terrifying dreams.

The most nearly complete deprivation of sleep occurs in certain psychotic patients (manic-depressives). Experimental deprivation of sleep in man for three days has failed to show any change in metabolism of any kind. The subjective symptoms produced by artificial insomnia are quickly abolished by permitting sleep. Many normal people, including intellectuals, require comparatively little sleep. William Hunter habitually slept only four hours per night.

Apart from mental disorder arising from demonstrable physical disease, of the brain or of the body generally, there are few mental disorders accompanied by increase in the amount of sleep. Of physical disorders, increased intracranial pressure from whatever cause, tumours and inflammatory disease of the base of the brain, and general toxaemia are the commonest causes of increase in the amount of sleep. The drowsiness that appeared in some cases was the reason for the term 'lethargic' applied to what is now known as epidemic encephalitis. In epidemic encephalitis inversion of the sleep rhythm is not infrequent.

A *somnambulism* is a general automatism occurring in the course of, and interrupting, normal sleep. In this condition the patient rises from sleep, disregards the ordinary significance of his environment and those in it, and behaves as if he were living in an environment conjured up by himself. If spoken to, not brusquely, he may reply in terms of the phantasy which he is enacting. If roughly stimulated, he may regain full consciousness, or pass into a trance state of immobility, muscular flaccidity and total lack of response of any kind. Patients in somnambulic states have sometimes met with unfortunate accidents, *e.g.* scalding, or even death from drowning.

STUPOR

In stupor the subject's activity is reduced to a minimum. There is no response to any stimulus, external or internal. In the deepest variety, not only is there no muscular activity even with regard to nutrition and evacuation, except (in some cases) that involved in the maintenance of posture, but there is no response to external stimuli, whether these be supplied by questions or actual pain. Stupor may be either of psychogenic or organic origin, or both. The maintenance of postures with resistiveness occurs more characteristically in cases of psychogenic origin, but it may occur, *e.g.*, in uraemic stupor.

In the lesser degrees of stupor, the patient may sometimes be partially roused for a moment or two to pay some attention to, or even to answer, simple questions. A very striking feature of the stupor (so-called 'lethargy') of epidemic encephalitis is the ability of the patient to answer questions to the point when roused for a time. In psychogenic stupor, the suddenness with which the patient may pass from stupor to considerable activity is in contrast with the gradual recovery from the stupor of physical disease.

Coma is but the profoundest degree of stupor; all consciousness is lost; there is no voluntary activity of any kind.

DELIRIUM

Delirium is a symptom-complex consisting essentially in disorientation and hallucination, and very commonly having an accompanying affective disturbance, especially of fear. It is in its typical form the result of a toxic process, but psychogenic deliria are not unknown. These are apt to be characterized by a certain grotesqueness, or by the appearance of a certain preponderant affect (other than fear) running through them.

TYPE OF PERSONALITY IN PSYCHOSES

Personality, as used in clinical psychiatry, is the integrated activity of all the reaction-tendencies of the daily life of the individual. It is, in other words, the person as he is known to his friends. This is the simple clinical connotation of the word. It has lately been the custom to use the term also in a much wider sense, regarding personality as the total integrated expression of the various 'levels' of which the individual is constructed—the lowest, or vegetative level (endocrine-autonomic), the sensorimotor level (central nervous system) and the psychic level.

Certain personalities in this sense are less adapted to meet environmental influences adequately than others. This may be the result of inherited handicap or of faulty training and habit. The result is a malintegration, in the sense of biological inefficiency. It has been found that personalities of this kind are specially prone to develop mental illness (which is, by our definition, a phenomenon of maladaptation). Thus a 'psychopathic personality' is recognized in individuals who habitually display excess or defect of emotional reactions, together with impaired judgement and inadequate or anti-social behaviour, and in whom there commonly occur transient or permanent mental disturbances, which are merely exaggerations of their normal condition. In other instances mental illness appears to be not simply an exaggerated development of the personality, but implies also a qualitative change in it. In schizophrenia it is found that in a strikingly large percentage (51 to 60 per cent.—Hoch) the personality that existed before the disease occurred or was recognized was of the so-called 'shut-in' type (see Chapter 11, 'Schizophrenic Reaction-Types', p. 259). This is similar to an extreme degree of introversion (Jung) and to the 'schizoid' personality types of Kretschmer. The type of personality that is prone to manic-depressive illness is the so-called syntonic (Bleuler) or cycloid (Kretschmer) or cyclothymic personality. This type represents an extreme degree of extroversion, and is characterized by its affective lability and responsiveness. It has been found that anxious, gloomy people are prone to develop depressions of the manic-depressive variety (Hoch, MacCurdy). In epileptics, long before convulsions develop, it is sometimes possible to observe an overwhelming egoism, with moodiness, irritability, and sometimes a shallow hypocritical religiosity (Pierce Clark). Preceding the onset of paranoid psychoses, there is often a long-standing history of sensitiveness, tendency to suspicion, and inability to take criticism. These are the principal types of personality related to the development of mental illness which have so far been recognized. The importance of further work in this direction is obvious, not only from the point of view of prevention, but also for the prognosis of mental disorder—it is probable that the outlook in many psychoses depends as much (or more) on the type of pre-existing personality as on the type of psychosis.

MULTIPLE PERSONALITY

'Double' and 'multiple' personality are the terms applied when the same individual at different times appears to be in possession of entirely different mental content, disposition and character, and when one of the different phases shows complete ignorance of the other, an ignorance which may be reciprocal. Each 'sub-personality' (for the personality in these conditions at least is compounded of a series of sub- or partial personalities or 'monads', as McDougall called them) is said to be 'dissociated' from the total personality, and from the other sub-personalities, on each occasion when its activities are fully conscious and control the motor apparatus of the individual. (See further under 'Hysteria', p. 152.)

PERSONALITY IN MENTAL SYNDROMES

The phrase 'preservation of the personality' is used in clinical work to denote that, in spite of some disease process, the previous traits of personality are clearly recognizable, and especially in a narrower sense when the patient preserves his ordinary social decorum and keeps his clothes, etc., neat and tidy. Thus, general paralysis, which is a sweeping disorder, and involves complete and rapid disintegration of the personality, contrasts with arteriosclerotic brain disease, where in the early stages at least the patient has complete insight for his illness, feels it keenly and endeavours to preserve his previous social appearance.

Depersonalization

Depersonalization or a feeling of unreality is a subjective state which may occur in any morbid psychological reaction, but it is especially common in depressive states either in young people or in those at the involutional period of life. For convenience, this state of depersonalization can be described as occurring in the allo-, somato- and auto-psychic fields, e.g. the flowers do not look real; my legs are not legs at all; I am not I, I cannot die. Mapother suggested that in those cases in which the environment is implicated the term derealization is preferable to depersonalization; the two conditions, however, frequently occur together. For instance, a young lady talked as follows: 'Life is so funny, I look at things and I cannot realize them; I am not real, I am nothing, nothing at all, I go about in a dream, I feel I do not know who my husband is or who my baby is; I feel that I am not a person at all; the wool I knit with seems strange, and as for reading I don't know that I can read.' A somewhat similar case has been quoted by H. K. Johnson: 'I have not a moment of comfort and no human sensations, surrounded by all that can render life happy and agreeable, still to me the faculty of enjoyment and of feeling is wanting—both have become physical impossibilities. In everything, even in the most tender caresses of my children, I find only bitterness. I cover them with kisses, but there is something between their life and mine, and this horrid something is between me and all the enjoyment of life.'

It should be emphasized that such cases often show a marked fluctuation in mood. Even when describing the most extraordinary sensations and feelings they may themselves be amused by their own descriptions and may talk with considerable animation and vehemence. It is this paradoxical situation, this apparent incongruity between mood and thought which has led some observers to relate such states to a schizophrenic process. That, however, is more apparent than real, because in Shorvon's (1946) review of a group of 66 cases he remarked on the frequency of an acute onset, and the close relationship to migraine and obsessional states. Irrespective of the time factor, the course of the disorder is towards spontaneous recovery.

Transformation of the Personality

This is a phrase sometimes used to designate the not uncommon condition when the patient has a delusional belief that he is some other person, and to some extent acts upon that belief—for example, an epileptic patient periodically believed himself to be Christ, allowed his beard to grow and wrote letters to the newspapers protesting against his detention, and signing himself 'Yours truly, Jesus Christ'. Another type of periodic personality transformation, but not of this bizarre type, is that furnished by the multiple personalities already referred to. More lasting and more bizarre transformations are seen in the schizophrenics, who believe themselves to be Napoleon, or a king or some similar dignitary. In schizophrenics these transformations are often fairly sudden, and the rôle is very poorly sustained—a 'princess of the blood royal' will scrub the floor without protest. A gradual transformation of the personality, where the behaviour shows more consonance with the delusional beliefs, is characteristic of paranoid psychosis.

A certain vagueness and diffuseness of the concept and feeling of personality is common in schizophrenia. There is a 'suspension of the clear distinction between the ego and the environment, in which, for the ego, the clear presence of the external world vanishes' (Jaspers). In this way a schizophrenic woman came to say, 'Sometimes I cannot tell myself from other people' (Storch). There results an identification of the self at different times with different people. Another of Storch's patients felt himself to be eight separate persons at once.

The most extensive, and at the same time most profound, of all personality changes is the 'splitting of the personality' that occurs in advanced schizophrenia. This consists not simply in a disintegration of the personality, so that the latest acquired reactions crumble away and leave only the primitive functions, but there is rather a fragmentation or splitting-up of the entire personality, with apparent independent activity of the individual split-off functions, with the result that all kinds of incongruities of thought and action are possible. Hence the schizophrenic's conduct lacks coherence and purpose, and often appears utterly bizarre, and he may appear happy when his thought content is tragic, or apathetic when he believes himself the recipient of untold wealth. He may perform actions which he does not want to perform, or feel that his thoughts belong to someone else. Some of the split-off reactions are projected and appear as hallucinations, or as delusions.

REFERENCES

Bleuler, E. (1950) *Dementia Praecox*, New York.
Craike, W. H., and Slater, E. (1945) *Brain*, **68**, 213.
Hall, J. C. (1922) *Brit. med. J.*, **2**, 1146.
Leroy and Rouges de Fursac (1920) *Encéphale*, i, 189.
Shorvon, H. J. (1946) *Proc. roy. Soc. Med.*, **39**, 779.
Zangwill, O. L. (1941) *Character and Pers.*, **13**, 246.

7

GENERAL PSYCHOPATHOLOGY

Mental development occurs in response to the needs of adaptation. The mind grows in complexity as the necessary adaptations multiply. The adult mind is far more complex than that of the child; the European's more complex than that of the native of Borneo. Adaptation implies originally conflict, the conflict in human beings between certain forces inborn in them and the environmental circumstances. It will be convenient, therefore, to consider mental development under three heads: 1. the nature and working of the inborn forces; 2. the nature of the environmental influences; and 3. the methods and means of mental adjustments between them. The discussion of the genesis of symptoms (maladjustments) will then be possible.

INSTINCTUAL DEVELOPMENT

The inborn forces are commonly called *instincts*. They are primary data, being given in the innate equipment of the organism. A common confusion occurs in failing to distinguish between instincts in this sense, and the innate paths or patterns which they utilize for their expression, and which are probably fewer in man than in any other animal. The prevailing instinctive forces, however, are the same in man and animals. There are probably only two, *self-preservation* and *sex*. Some add a third—the so-called *herd* instinct. At birth in man the instincts have but few patterns of expression, but these multiply (under environmental influences) as the age of the individual increases, so that there are two varieties of pattern of instinctive expression—inherited and acquired. It is in the number and complexity of his acquired patterns that man surpasses the lower animals. Some of the patterns which are actually inherited do not mature till after birth— the myelinization of the brain is not complete. The patterns of expression of the self-preservative instinct are adequate from an early age (although they continually multiply), while those for sex are much less developed, and do not begin to approach completion till puberty is reached. The process of unhindered satisfaction of an instinct—*i.e.* where the reaction-patterns are in full play—is accompanied by a conscious feeling of pleasure, and frustration of the process by unpleasure—a kind of pain. In early life all the activities of the organism are concerned with the immediate increase of pleasurable, and the reduction of painful, stimuli (the so-called *pleasure-principle*). Later, the increasing demands of reality make necessary a postponement of pleasurable attainment until certain mediate conditions have been fulfilled—this has been described as obedience to the *reality-principle*. Instincts are in themselves not conscious, but the feelings that accompany their processes of satisfaction or frustration are conscious. The self-preservative instinct attains satisfaction fairly readily from birth onwards, although not without repeated and increasing effort on the part of the organism. The sexual instinct is much more persistently frustrated. The conscious expression of an instinct seeking satisfaction is a *wish* or desire. This wish or desire by virtue of the representative-imaginative function of consciousness can have a definite conscious *object*, through which the general *aim* of the instinct can be fulfilled. The sexual instinct has a development peculiarly its own, in that its object normally changes at various stages of life although its general aim remains the same (Freud). First of all it attains satisfaction in the body of the individual himself—the *auto-erotic* stage. In this auto-erotic stage, satisfaction giving a pleasurable feeling akin to sexual pleasure is attainable by stimulation of almost any part of the body surface, but especially of certain *erotogenic* zones (mouth, anus, etc.). Thus, for example, stimulation of the mouth area is associated with pleasurable sensuous feeling—an association which persists in adult life. Similarly stimulation of the zone of the anus is, at least in some individuals, associated with pleasurable feeling, and this persists in adult life in a few of them as 'anal erotism'. In the later stages of development of the sexual instinct, these regions usually lose most or all of their pleasure-giving possibilities, which are now largely confined to the zone of the genitals. In the second or *homosexual* stage, the object of the sexual instinct becomes another individual, but of the same sex, and in the third or *heterosexual* stage, of the opposite sex. This is probably the normal development in which the stages overlap. But it may be arrested ('fixated' is the technical term) at any stage—one of the erotogenic zones may continue to afford sensual pleasure to as great an extent, or greater, than the genital zone; or the development with reference to the object may not go beyond the auto-erotic or homosexual stage. Further, 'bi-sexuality' has to be taken into account. The individual's sexual instinct is capable of expression and satisfaction in two opposite ways—with the individual as active or the individual as passive. In either case the process of satisfaction gives pleasure, but in the passive rôle the general feeling-tone involves a certain amount of pain; while in the active rôle evidently a certain amount of the pleasurable feeling may be derived from the inflicting of pain on the sexual object. These are called respectively the 'sadistic' or active and 'masochistic' or passive part-expressions of the sexual instinct.

A later psychoanalytic theory came to regard these tendencies as expressions not of the sexual instinct but of an aggressive or destructive instinct. According to this view there are two broad groups of instincts; the life instincts or 'eros', using a collective term, and the death instincts. Most instinctive manifestations are held to be the results of the fusion of these two broad groups. Hence the appearance of sadistic and masochistic elements in sexual relationships. This distinction cuts across the distinction formerly made between self-preservative and sexual instincts. Instead we have a life instinct which directs itself either to the aims and objects of self or those of sex, and on the other hand an aggressive instinct or group of instincts which find their object more usually in the external world but sometimes turn back from that on to the ego itself, producing, according to Freud, such phenomena as automatic

I

self punishment, *e.g.* in patients with whom everything seems to go wrong all their lives.

Affect

'Affect' or emotion arises in consciousness when an instinct is prevented from attaining easy complete satisfaction. Emotion and feeling-tone (pleasure and unpleasure) are not the same. Pleasure occurs during the process of satisfying an instinct; emotion probably only if there is some obstruction to the process of satisfaction. All emotions can be divided into two classes—those with a pleasant and those with an unpleasant, feeling-tone, the latter occurring when obstruction is for the moment complete.

Consciousness

Consciousness (sensations, feelings, emotions, wishes or desires and ideas) arises when instincts, themselves unconscious, are in action, requiring certain complicated adaptations to the environment for the satisfaction of the instinct. Consciousness is not an otiose creation. It has a function, the representative-imaginative function, especially when satisfaction has to be delayed in accordance with the so-called 'reality principle', in facilitating the satisfaction of instinctive needs. The instinct is represented in consciousness by a wish, and its object by an image. The wish and the image are in some way associated by a tension furnished by the instinct, and this tension brings about the motor adjustment necessary for the fulfilment of the wish (satisfaction of the instinct).

In the course of the individual's experience, certain mental events have a peculiar intimacy; such events become welded together to form the ego or self. Another group of mental events is attributed to the environment—'projection' is the attributing of subjective impressions to external causes. But their conscious representations form part of the experience of the self. Mental events are retained (memory), but do not persist in consciousness unless they continue to minister to an immediate need. They are said to become *unconscious*. Thus one's knowledge of French, say, remains unconscious while one is talking English. Although the content of consciousness is small at any moment of time, previous conscious events, being retained (memory), can be revived (recollection or recall). Many of these revivable unconscious events have had the peculiar intimacy mentioned and have been incorporated in the ego; hence the ego or self is composed of certain conscious facts of the moment together with a great many revivable mental events. The latter are, at any moment of time, for the most part unconscious, *i.e.* not conscious. 'Preconscious' is the term often used for this easily accessible type of unconscious fact.

But there is another type of unconscious fact—one which has proved distasteful to the ego and has been disowned by it. The forgetting of such facts occurs in an automatic way, and this process is known as repression. The percipient ego may or may not be aware of the occurrence, the repression itself being done largely by a part of the ego which is jointly the product of the ego's conception of the environmental demands and, on the other hand, of the instinctive urges. The joint product is the super-ego which Freud believed to be composed fundamentally of the introjected images of persons, especially the parents and those on whose conduct the child has modelled himself.

The super-ego is therefore the result of a process of identification with the parents and of wanting to be like them. The nature of the super-ego, it should be noted, is held to be coloured very much by the component it contains from the aggressive instinct. The aggressive component is derived in this way: the child projects his own aggression on to one or other of the parents, picturing the rival parent as having the same aggressive impulses as himself. Therefore when the parental image is introjected the aggressive aspect is introjected along with it. Thus the super-ego is felt to be severe as well as kind. This aspect of severity is supposed to be responsible for the feeling of guilt so commonly encountered. It is recognized that the super-ego is to a large extent an unconscious formation and consequently the repression carried out by it occurs unconsciously and therefore automatically.

Yet another type of unconscious content has never reached consciousness. Such are many feelings and tendencies closely connected with the instincts. This unconscious reservoir of instincts and feelings and attitudes connected with them has been subsumed by Freud under the term 'Id'. Many of the items of the conscious content, and of the repressed unconscious content, were by Freud regarded as originally derivatives of this primal reservoir.

Strictly speaking, 'unconscious' feelings, emotions, wishes and ideas are a contradiction in terms. But particular aspects of the instincts of which feelings, etc., are the conscious representations can persist in an 'unconscious' form. The term 'unconscious' is itself a bad one, since it defines something in terms of what it is not.

That part of the individual's unconscious which is inherited, including the 'instinctive' part, has been called the racial unconscious (Jung).

The inherited and the acquired possibilities of reaction—the instinctive re-action-patterns—have something associated with them (something designated above, instinctive forces), which converts them from mere possibilities of reaction to actual functioning elements, and the reactions they subserve must occur if life is to be sustained at all. The something which forces these patterns into action it is usual to regard as analogous to the 'energy' of physics. This psychical 'energy', if we may call it so for brevity, is commonly labelled 'libido'. The libido is regarded as being at the disposal of any reaction which subserves an instinct. In Jung's original sense of the term, the energy designated 'libido' was of a general kind, and applied to any instinctive force; but in Freud's usage libido was always associated with the sexual instinct. It is to a certain extent transferable from one reaction to another. When it is transferred from the service of a reaction which fulfils the ordinary instinctive aim more or less closely to one which fulfils that aim in a less direct way, the libido is said to take part in a reaction of 'sublimation' of the instinct. Freud had a special theory of the libido, of which the barest outline follows. In early life, as we have seen, instinctive satisfaction is largely obtained from the individual's own body. The libido at the service of the instincts is then pictured as directed inwards—the auto-erotic direction of the libido. As development proceeds, instinctive satisfaction is obtained increasingly from without; and the libido is directed to external objects. The libido is then said to expend itself partly in keeping the mental representation of these objects in consciousness: it is 'attached' to these mental representations and is spoken of as 'object-libido'. By this time self is not only a succession of experiences with a common feeling of intimacy: it is a developed concept. Sometimes it happens that very little of the total libido is attached to object-representations, and most to the concept of the self. That part of the libido which is attached to the concept of the self is called 'narcissistic libido'. 'Regression' is the return to an earlier stage of development of the individual personality, and, in the language of the libido-theory, consists in a withdrawal of libido from its present object to objects characteristic of an earlier stage of psychosexual development.

A distinction is made in Freudian theory between the *aim* and the *object* of the libido, the aim being the mode of satisfaction and the object the person with whom satisfaction is desired. The aim may change with reference to the same object according to the developmental stage.

The aim is believed to be concerned first with the satisfaction of oral cravings and then with anal. Each of these stages is divided into two; satisfaction is obtained first by sucking and later by biting in the oral stage; and in the anal stage of libidinal organization first by expelling or annihilating and then by retaining, possessing or holding fast. These aims are sought with reference to an object in the environment, usually one of the parents or a parent substitute. It will be seen that in the second and third phases the aggressive aspect predominates and this aspect is directed towards an object otherwise loved, *i.e.* an example of ambivalence. In this way the foundations of guilt feelings are supposed to be laid in the pre-genital stages of libidinal organization. In the next stage, the so-called phallic stage, satisfaction is concerned with the genital zone, still with incomplete investment of the object with libido. The final stage is said to occur when the female genitals receive for the first time the recognition that the male genitals have previously obtained, and complete object-love is now said to be possible.

Phantasy

We have seen that an important mental function is the conscious representation of an object or end with which a desire is associated. The occurrence of this conscious representation creates a state of tension (furnished by the instincts whose end is the conscious representation) which issues in bodily activities adequate to attain the desired end. Sometimes, however, these activities are not permitted to take place, and satisfaction of the instinct does not then occur. But in such an event the representation sometimes continues to be held in consciousness, and even to be elaborated, the energy which should have actuated the necessary bodily movements dissipating itself instead in the elaborative process. This is the development of phantasy and the achievement of phantastic wish-fulfilment at the expense of application of energy and activity to reality—at the cost, in other words, of adaptation to reality. The state of conscious pre-occupation with phantasy is called *introversion*, to distinguish it from the normal adaptation, which is the direction of the energy or libido outwards to reality (*extroversion*).

Phantasy is an important part of normal mental life, and it can serve a useful purpose if kept in sufficiently close conformity with reality to form the basis of a scheme of future action. Ambition, for example, is a phantasy, and is patho-logical only if real striving is abandoned for indulgence in the phantasy alone. The child's formulations of reality are phantastic in nature. His father is a great man, his mother the personification of goodness. He may identify himself very closely with these *imagines* (embellished concepts not in strict conformity with reality), and when these illusions which lapse more or less into unconsciousness are encroached upon in later life by contact with reality, he will feel the encroach-ment keenly, although unconscious of the source of this feeling, since the source has lapsed long ago into the unconscious. The resulting emotional perturbation leads to much thinking—an obsessive preoccupation, which is really an attempt to reconcile the real with the unconscious ideal. Since the motivation of this continued thinking is unconscious, the thinking appears in consciousness as a 'symptom' and forms one type of the obsessional neuroses (see Chapter 8).

ENVIRONMENTAL INFLUENCES

In early infantile life the child remains in the closest association with the mother. The child being still in a primary undifferentiated phase of conscious-ness, the associations of the earliest days are entirely subjective, *i.e.* there is at this stage no objectivation, no differentiation of the mother from himself; and his interest follows the direction of his mother's interest—namely, his own body. At this stage and later, his slightest gestures are followed by satis-faction of his instinctive nutritional needs—the stage of omnipotence (of 'magic' gesture and 'magic' words—Ferenczi). Soon, however, this primary subjective phase begins to pass, reality makes increasing demands on his con-sideration and he has to conform increasingly to it if he would compass the satisfaction of his instincts. His consciousness increases in extent, and a distinc-tion arises mentally between self and objective reality—his conscious experience is divided into self-consciousness and object consciousness. Both are experiences of the self, but the source of the second is projected. Object consciousness is at first a vague affair, the details of which are poorly differentiated among them-selves. For example, objects are assumed to have a kind of organic connection with the persons to whom they belong—a connection which in later life is recognized not to exist. This stage of object-consciousness corresponds to one which primitive man never completely passes—the stage of sympathetic magic or participation. The most prominent objective facts for the child at this early stage are his parents, and so they become the objects towards which his interest is chiefly directed. But here a complication occurs, in that one parent becomes more important for the child than the other. Furthermore, each parent has a place in the interests of the other, as well as having a place for the child; and so the latter meets what is probably his first great environmental obstacle of a personal kind—his first rival—and the germs of hate may grow in association and contact with the group of emotions and feelings comprising the conscious expression designated love. Thus love and hate are said to begin that association which persists throughout life. Prohibitions and punishments also can produce a feeling of antagonism and play a part in the genesis of hateful emotion. The attachment of the child to his parent of the opposite sex is conventionally called the Oedipus situation or complex. The early identification with the parents has a formulation partly conscious, partly unconscious, in the creation of an ideal to be like the parents. The ideal is the *imago* already mentioned. The parents thus serve as an example to the child, and so unknowingly train him in the formation of habits. Deliberate training begins with example and later proceeds with pre-cept, in earlier days from the parents, and later from school influences and the influence of companions. Morbid reactions, as well as healthy ones, may be impressed in this way, and not only specific reactions but general attitudes with emotional components—*e.g.* morbid gloom or anxiety. Training also makes use not only of rewards but of punishment and threats of punishment. Punishment implies either the frustration of some conscious wish and the production of unpleasant emotion, or the infliction of actual pain of physical origin. There is no doubt that the inflicting of pain in one of the erotogenic zones may be accom-panied by a certain amount of pleasurable feeling, and frequent arousal of pleasure in this way may cause a desire for it to become fixed. This desire may appear as a sexual perversion in later life, just as any other premature fixation of the sexual libido may appear as a perversion. When the primary parental stage of the environment begins to be less important, and the child's mental environ-ment widens and his contacts with it increase in number and complexity, a group of tendencies come into play which have been included under the term 'herd instinct'. The use of this term connotes that certain reactions necessary for adaptation to society in general are inborn. It seems doubtful whether it is necessary to make this hypothesis, rather than to attribute the more primitive less differentiated reactions to the social *milieu* as reactions derived from personal contact with it. In any case, it is in connection with adaptation to the require-ments of the herd that the ego-ideal is further built up, and that the most powerful repression is exercised.

THE MENTAL RELATIONS OF INSTINCTIVE MANIFESTATIONS AND ENVIRONMENTAL INFLUENCES

The infant, receiving its first sensory impressions, treats them in the beginning as part of itself—'introjects' them—they have a purely subjective reference. But from his motor activity and the different quality of sensations arising in his own body from those not so arising, he learns to differentiate those of the external world and to attribute them to influences external to himself and less within his control—*i.e.* to 'project' them. Not only does he do this with his sensations, but he projects also his emotions. The emotions he experiences in certain situations, *e.g.* in beholding anything large and new to him, he attributes to the thing itself, so that what fills him with awe has an awesome quality attributed to itself. Furthermore, all his projections are of the personal type; he endows external objects with all his own conscious properties. This is comparable to the stage of animism in primitive man.

Imitation

Imitation of example, especially of parental example, is a training method which is used early. It is one of the modes by which suggestion operates. *Suggestion* seems to depend on a particular relation of operator (suggestor) and subject, analogous to but not identical with the active-passive relation in the play of the sexual instinct. Suggestion operates only in an affective relationship.

Intelligence

Intelligence is phylogenetically the last-developed of all the adaptive functions. It appears in rudimentary form in the highest apes, at least. Intelligence is said to grow in the individual till the age of sixteen. After that its apparent growth is mostly a matter of experience and consequently improved judgement. In the growth of intellectual processes which deal eventually with the adaptation of means to ends, not merely the end is consciously represented, but the means to it, and so *symbolization* plays an important part.

Symbolization

This consists in the conscious representation of experiences derived from the environment by something mental which *stands for* that experience. Language is made possible by symbolization. For example, a certain sensory experience of roundness and depth and colour and consistency becomes represented by the vocalization 'ball'. The word 'symbolization' has unfortunately attained many meanings. In ordinary life it has come to be specially used where some simple object has become endowed with great affective meaning, *e.g.* a country's flag as a symbol for patriotic feeling. A very similar use is now made of the term in psychopathology; but the object acting as a symbol is invested with a very strong personal affective meaning instead of a general one, as in the case of the flag. Symptoms are often symbolizations in this sense when the meaning is unconscious (repressed).

The association of one idea with another, or of an emotion or feeling with an idea, is an important adaptive function subserving both practical (real) and phantastic thinking. It works in a way analogous to the conditioning of reflexes in physiology, in that once a certain feeling has become associated with a certain idea the revival of the idea (or, unlike the conditioned reflex, of some similar idea) may revive the feeling. For example, if an article of food has accidentally been associated with a feeling of nausea, the same or a similar article may on a later occasion revive nausea simply by virtue of the previous accidental association.

Adaptation

Adaptation is not at all a matter of pure reason. It is eventually and at all times a matter of modifications of instinctive trends, which have a very much closer association with emotional than with intellectual processes. But wherever an adaptation is consciously made or results in conscious experience of some kind, an intellectual formation tends to occur, which by virtue of its conscious nature, contrasting with that of the instinctive reaction which is wholly unconscious or only indirectly conscious, is apt to masquerade as the reason for the particular adaptation. This substitution of an intellectual conscious 'reason' for the actual instinct-derived (unconscious) basis of a reaction, is known as *rationalization*. It is usually a formulation more closely in accord with herd or ego-ideal requirements than was the primary instinctive trend.

The gradual building-up of an ego or self has been stated to arise from a continuous synthesis of certain experiences having a peculiar intimacy, while at the same time a 'not-self' or external world has been mentally constructed (represented). There is here a contrast, which results, among other things, in the formation within the experiences of the ego of an idealized representation of the self, or ideal ego, of which the unconscious part is called by Freud the super-ego (*v. supra*). It is a very gradual growth, and consequently not at all fully conscious at any time. It gives rise to an important subservient reaction, in that where the attributes of the self are conceived as lacking in some of the qualities of the ideal self, the self makes an attempt to *compensate* in one direction what is lacking in another. These deficiencies which it is attempted to compensate may be of either physical or intellectual attributes.

The more intimate part of the environment constituted by the body has important relations to the mind. In the first place, the mental representations of bodily activities are regarded as part of the self. Secondly, mental events (ideas) are followed by bodily (physical) events in so regular and invariable a way that a relationship of cause and effect is universally assumed to exist, and the relationship is called a process of 'will'. Thirdly, mental events which have an emotional accompaniment have a bodily reverberation also, not in the form of directly adaptive movement as in the case of 'willed' sequences, but in the form of disturbances of function of a special kind, especially visceral disturbances, but involving also movement of the limbs of an apparently useless sort, *e.g.* tremors. Fourthly, most visceral functions go on without any conscious accompaniment, and the intervention of conscious accompaniment usually betokens malfunction. Conversely, in the absence of spontaneous malfunction, conscious attention to the working of the viscera tends to derange the latter. Attention alone would not do so, but such attention is usually accompanied by emotion (usually anxiety), which has visceral reverberations. Attention of this sort arises only when the normal direction of interest towards the environment is frustrated and turns towards the self. Frustration of any instinct causes emotion of some kind, emotion produces palpitation, etc.; palpitation draws the attention, already failing to find an environmental object, and a vicious circle is set up, since attention makes the palpitation, etc., loom larger, and so the emotion increases.

For the individual the combined result of the innate endowment, of the environmental impressions, and of the reactive-tendencies arising out of the conflict between them, is what is customarily called the *personality*. This is a more or less completely synthesized group of reactive tendencies, including not only all those that the ego acknowledges as its own, but some of which it is unaware, *i.e.* unconscious but not repressed tendencies. Certain mannerisms are a simple example of this latter class of components of the personality. No two individuals ever have exactly the same history, from the zygote stage onwards, and so no two personalities are exactly alike. But there are certain general types, representing different types of adaptation. Some of these are more successful than others, reality being more adequately dealt with. Those personalities that are less successful are *ipso facto* apt to develop substitutive reactions (Meyer) for healthy ones, *i.e.* to have symptoms of mental illness.

THE PRODUCTION OF SYMPTOMS

The very important part played by unconscious factors in normal conscious mental life has already been emphasized. Normally the unconscious factors co-operate harmoniously in facilitating conscious reactions. But in some cases the unconscious factors break through indirectly (symbolically in the second sense given above) into consciousness in a manner out of harmony with the conscious mental life of the individual; in other cases, the unconscious factors usurp the whole realm of consciousness (dreams and dual personalities, for example). In either instance, symptoms of mental disorder become apparent. It is obvious that to do this the unconscious factors must have an activity that is independent of consciousness; they are said to be *dissociated* from the rest of the mental content, and the field of consciousness to be 'restricted' with regard to them. This lack of connection between conscious and unconscious may result either from a simple failure on the part of the conscious ego to recognize a connection, or it may be due to a refusal of the ego to do so ('repression').

The first case (of simple failure of recognition) is not at all uncommon. A patient may have a great deal of emotional perturbation which is associated with visceral disturbance. The latter attracts his attention, and as its subjective accompaniments (symptoms) are the same as those of some organic disease, and as he fails to recognize their connection with emotion, he concludes that he has that disease. Then because affects are easily displaceable from one idea to another the emotional perturbation which originally arose from other factors becomes attached to the idea of disease—and in this way an anxiety state is set up.

In the second instance, where the dissociation depends on repression (the result of conflict of the repressed material with the ego ideal), the dissociated material has had originally a strong affective accompaniment. The formation of a symptom denotes a partial or complete failure of the ego to repress the affectively accompanied material ('complex'), the degree of failure being proportional to the directness of expression of the latter. The symptom may take a bodily (physical) form: in the motor field, a muscular movement (tremor, tic) or a paralysis; in the sensory field, an anaesthesia or amblyopia, or some other sensory disturbance. The particular form is a matter of minor determinants. In other instances the symptom may have a psychic form—a fear or an idea, either being apparently meaningless for consciousness. The commonest conscious emotional symptom is 'fear' in the special form of distressful expectation usually designated 'anxiety'. Conflict of any kind, whether self-preservative or sexual, may lead to anxiety. The anxiety tends to attach itself to an idea, since affects can hardly remain unrelated in consciousness. This idea to which the anxiety attaches is apt to be one consciously very far removed from ideas associated with originally repressed material—this is the so-called 'displacement of affect'. Whatever the idea to which the affect (of anxiety) attaches, an attempt may be made to ward off the anxiety in a way reminiscent of the magic acts of infancy. Thus a school-boy had to touch everything twice in case he should not pass a forthcoming examination. This is the genesis of some compulsive acts—a wish, a fear and a magic act to overcome the fear. A similar mechanism accounts for certain obsessive ideas (magic words).

Another fashion in which the ego may deal with an imperfectly repressed complex (of idea plus emotion) is by *projection*. The complex material is permitted to appear in consciousness but projected as external reality, so forming a delusion (*e.g.* a belief that other people are watching the patient wherever he goes), or as a hallucination (*e.g.* a voice accusing him of vile practices). The method of projection is more seriously pathological than the preceding modes, since it involves a distortion of reality.

The projected complexes are often considerably elaborated, being originally the phantasy-formations already mentioned. Phantasies may, however, appear directly as part of the conscious ego, instead of being projected, in one of two ways: 1. either the phantasy is not one involving the emotions of guilt or other emotions such as would cause the ego to disown it; for example, a delusion of grandeur may involve simply a turning to phantasy from disappointment with reality, as in an individual with inflated self-regard; or 2. the ego-ideal is so disintegrated that repression is not exercised at all, and any complex which involves material, no matter how distasteful originally to the ego, is admitted into consciousness. This occurs only in the most serious forms of illness, *e.g.* in schizophrenia.

Frank conscious indulgence in wish-fulfilling phantasies when disintegration of the ego is not too profound, is accompanied by the appropriate affect, viz. elation. In many patients in whom elation occurs there is, however, little conscious evidence of a wish-fulfilment; and it appears that elation may also colour the consciousness while the wish-fulfilment associated with it remains unconscious but active (dissociated).

The emotional state which we are accustomed to consider as the psychological contrast to elation, namely depression, reaches pathological intensity in several ways. When a wish is not fulfilled—when frustration occurs—depression results. Depression is more likely to occur when the aim of the frustrated tendency is abandoned: anxiety when there is frustration with continued striving. This is a normal occurrence, but the depression attains pathological significance, magnitude and duration when the frustration occurs in relation to some conscious but very much overvalued end, the depth of depression being proportional to the degree of overvaluation. Overvaluation of the end is common in 'neurotics', especially as this overvaluation is derived from an exaggerated ego-ideal. Hence the continual striving of neurotics (Adler's 'masculine protest'). Depression is also pathological when the frustration is in relation to some unconscious object. In the latter instance the depression appears pathological, because there is nothing in consciousness to account for it. Depression may also be the conscious accompaniment of a feeling of guilt or remorse, which itself may be derived from an unconscious trend imperfectly repressed. A conscious rationalization of the feeling of guilt may be produced in the form of self-accusatory ideas, which may reach delusional intensity. Guilt is particularly apt to be felt in connection with sexual trends, on account of social prohibitions.

The methods of symptom-formation which have just been described are used in response to contemporary environmental influences, and may or may not imply any developmental defect hindering adaptation. In some individuals the development of the libido's object-direction may be arrested at an intermediate stage (*e.g.* the auto-erotic or the homosexual). This hinders adaptation to adult reality, which is heterosexual in organization, and brings the individual into contact with social prohibitions, *e.g.* in fixation at the homosexual stage. If he accepts his homosexuality in a matter-of-fact way, no mental disorder results, but if he represses his tendencies from consciousness because of the socially induced feeling of guilt, and if the repression fails, depression or anxiety or projected wish-fulfilment occurs as a symptom.

Failure of adaptation at any level of development implies dissatisfaction. The individual may revert in phantasy to a previous level of development, *e.g.* the infantile stage of helplessness, and obtain a phantastic satisfaction which may be dramatized, *i.e.* the patient lies helplessly in bed, uttering baby talk, and having to be fed. 'Regression' is not an unimpeachable description of this state, since there is no recapitulation, and the reinstatement of the previous terms of existence is never an identical one.

All these reactions can be described as substitutions for healthy adaptations. Their general tendency is to lead the patient away from reality. Some are more pernicious in this respect than others; the further away from reality, the more symptomatically pronounced the mental disorder, and (on the whole) the worse the prognosis for recovery.

DREAMS

Dreams are the representations, in the disturbed state of consciousness called sleep, of unconscious mental states, based on experience of both the lapsed and repressed kinds. It is customary to call the dream-content as remembered by the dreamer the 'manifest' content, and the unconscious processes which give rise to the latter the 'latent' content. This distinction is of considerable importance when applied to psychopathology, for it is held in Freudian theory that the manifest content is produced from the latent content in the same way that symptoms ('manifest') are produced from unconscious ('latent') factors. The latter are said, on the basis of the theory of repression, to be made palatable to the ego by various methods of transformation by which the manifest content is finally manufactured. It would perhaps be more generally correct to say that in a state of lowered consciousness such as occurs in sleep, more primitive mental processes occupy the field. Visual imagery, for example, which was shown by Galton to be much more used by children and the uneducated than by educated adults, plays a large part in dreams. Nevertheless, it also can subserve repressive ends, on account of the distortion involved in clothing everything in visual images.

The methods of transformation which unconscious material undergoes before constituting the 'manifest content' are chiefly condensation, displacement, secondary elaboration and symbolization. By condensation is meant that the manifest dream is a kind of abridged edition of the latent content, this result being obtained especially by the blending into one whole of several latent elements with some characteristic in common, *e.g.* one person in a dream may represent several people actually known to the dreamer. *Displacement* consists in the transfer of the emotional setting of one idea to some other apparently insignificant idea, as has already been explained for symptoms. *Secondary elaboration* consists in welding the dream-content transformed in the other ways described into something like a coherent whole. By *symbolization* is meant that certain objects which occur often in the manifest content of dreams have a fairly constant symbolic value—they stand regularly for the same unconscious content or latent dream thought. In Freudian theory the standard symbols have usually a sexual significance. Symbolizations of a more general type occur, *e.g.* a man recovering from a neurotic illness, anxious to get well and finding the way hard, dreamt that he was crossing a bridge, that it progressively narrowed, so that he had to clamber along the parapet, but that finally it widened and he could proceed safely and easily.

Dreams in general, like the one just related, are considered to be fulfilments of wishes, conscious or unconscious, and often of the repressed type.

Jung emphasized a purposive aspect in dreaming and also in the neuroses—an attempt to solve an immediate problem.

REFERENCES

See section on 'Neuroses and Psychopathology' in the Bibliography (p. 564).

8

NEUROTIC REACTION-TYPES

Neurotic forms of reaction are the commonest kinds of manifestation of psycho-logical ill-health. The specialist in psychological medicine encounters conditions of this kind much more often in that part of his work which lies outside mental hospitals, while for the general practitioner they constitute no small proportion of his practice.

Meaning of the Term 'Neurosis'

The term neurosis has, from the standpoint of classification, two connotations. In the first and historical connotation its meaning is purely *descriptive*. It is a term referring to conditions characterized by certain mental and physical symp-toms and signs, occurring in various combinations. The most usual of these combinations or syndromes have been distinguished as sub-types of neurosis called respectively anxiety neurosis, hysteria and obsessional neurosis. None of these is dependent on the existence of any discoverable physical disease. They are not mutually exclusive categories so far as individual symptoms are concerned, but they signify certain recurrent patterns of symptoms commonly occurring together.

'Neurosis' has, however, another connotation, more fundamental, since it is an aetiological one. This is to the effect that the existence of a neurotic reaction is an indication of mental conflict. Neurotic reactions are the commonest modes of faulty response to the stresses of life, and especially to those inner tensions that come about from confused and unsatisfactory relationships with other people, whether they are a legacy from the past or from early childhood onwards, which remain to hinder future adaptations; or arise in the present in relation to hopes, ambitions, jealousies and so forth. The constitutional factor, where it does operate, seems to facilitate the development of inner tensions, but this factor is less conspicuous than it is in the psychotic forms of illness, such as manic-depressive and schizophrenic conditions. The pathology of neurotic reactions, in other words, is essentially a pathology of interpersonal relationships.

On this view the existence of mental conflict is the commonest reason for the existence of neurotic symptoms, but because the individual is unconscious either of the conflict within him, or at least of its connection with his symptoms, the neurotic symptoms appear in the ordinary sense to be irrational. Although they may consist for the most part of ideas, no rational explanation exists for them in terms of the rest of the patient's thoughts so far as he is able to give an account of them; or if the mental conflict expresses itself as physical disturbances, such as blindness or paralysis or tremor, no physical disease can be found that can be regarded as causal. A neurotic patient may be disconcerted by a morbid fear of travelling in a train or a bus, or he may be unable to go more than a few yards from his own door, but he does not have the faintest notion why; yet this fear may be so impelling that the attempt to walk a few yards in the open may prove utterly beyond him.

The irrationality is confined, however, to the account that he is able to give of his symptoms. If enough of his thoughts and feelings are known, what has seemed mysterious becomes logical and coherent with the rest of the contents of his mind. It has been demonstrated many times that there are undercurrents of feeling and thought, and connections between thoughts and feeling, of which the individual himself may be quite unaware until the connection is exhibited to him·

A complication must be considered here, in that neurotic reactions resulting from mental disturbances in earlier life may be perpetuated as habits of behaviour and attitude and so become part of the personality. Even simple stresses, such as fatigue, may allow these characteristics to appear in such exaggerated form as to constitute an inadequacy of adaptation in the symptomatic form of a neurosis.

Disturbances of constitutional origin, especially depression, may have a similar effect, and this probably accounts for some of the instances where symptoms of neurotic form cover an underlying depression.

Incidence

It has been reported that about one-sixth of the ordinary run of hospital out-patients in the departments of general medicine, about a third of those receiving benefit under the National Health Insurance Act for a month or more, and a similar proportion of patients in general practice, are not suffering from physical disease, but have some psychogenic disorder, usually of the neurotic type. Watts and Watts (1952) stated that in their general practice there was an average of 12 per cent. of people who were functionally ill, and a further 10 per cent. who were suffering from a psychosomatic illness. Labels like 'insomnia', 'gastritis', 'anaemia', 'rheumatism' and so forth commonly attached to minor complaints which are nevertheless often responsible for absences from work for weeks, rather than days, at a time, usually cover neurotic reactions.

Precise figures of morbidity are difficult to obtain because diagnosis is often not precise in this field: neurotic reactions border on the one hand states of tension and unhappiness which can be considered to be within the range of the normal, and on the other hand 'psychosomatic' syndromes of still uncertain aetiology. There is no doubt also that many illnesses are diagnosed as neurotic by general practitioners which are in fact affective psychoses. In England and Wales a joint survey by the General Register Office and the College of General Practitioners (1958), based on the returns of 171 general practitioners, reported the patient-consulting rate (the number of patients suffering from an illness, regardless of the number of consultations) for various illnesses in general practice. Whereas the number of patients consulting for malignant disease was found to be 5·2 per thousand, the patient-consulting rate for neurotic and allied disorders was 45·7 per thousand: that is, about one in twenty of the population apparently came under the care of their doctors in one year for minor psychiatric disorders.

It is uncertain whether there has been a real or only an apparent increase in these neurotic forms of illness in recent years. They are certainly now much more widely recognized, whereas they passed formerly for other things. Mythical diseases, such as 'mucous colitis', 'dropped kidney' or 'spinal neurasthenia' have been debunked: they were the labels formerly attached to the patients' complaints, *faute de mieux*, by doctors of generations who had not been taught that physical disease is often simulated by mental disturbance. The public themselves are now also much more knowledgeable about nervous and mental illness, and of the out-patient and other facilities available for early treatment.

That there has been a real increase has been difficult to prove, but figures obtained by Halliday (1948) from statistics of the Department of Health for Scotland have tended to show that an increase had in fact occurred between the world wars. If this is so, then the increase has probably been related to one or more of the general factors favouring neurotic forms of illness, namely insecurity in one of its many forms, whether due to social isolation, changing social mores, financial stress or an absence of mental values of the sort that transcend purely material issues.

General Clinical Features and Groupings

Clinically, a neurosis implies either a bodily disturbance without structural lesion and dependent in a way unknown to the patient on mental causes; or a mental disturbance, not the result of bodily disease, in the form of morbid fears of many different kinds, or episodic disturbed mental states such as losses of memory and trances, or persistent troublesome thoughts, or acts which the patient feels compelled to do—all of which the patient realizes to be abnormal but the meaning of which he is at a loss to understand. The bodily disturbances may be sensory and subjective, or motor and therefore directly observable, or visceral. The sensory disturbances may occur in any of the physiological systems of the body; disturbances which are emphatically real, not 'imaginary'. A hysterical pain is a real pain, and causes genuine distress. The motor and visceral symptoms are also multiform.

Whytt of Edinburgh, as far back as 1765, distinguished three types of neurotic reaction—neurasthenia, hysteria and hypochondria. About 1880 Charcot's use of hypnotism focussed attention on the symptoms of hysteria, in particular on those cases where the patient's neurotic reaction was expressed in physical disabilities of a rather bizarre kind. About the same time Beard popularized the diagnosis of neurasthenia, drawing attention to a syndrome of which the nucleus was complaints of mental and physical fatigue. Janet recognized two groups, hysteria and psychasthenia; in the latter group placing obsessions and compulsions, fears of all kinds and feelings of fatigue. Later Freud divided states of morbid anxiety into two varieties, anxiety neurosis and anxiety hysteria. In anxiety neurosis there was supposed to be a primary physical disturbance expressed in the form, for example, of tremor or palpitations, with a mental content of discomfort or vague fear. In anxiety hysteria there was a fear of some definite external object or disease, and the physical disturbance was said to be less important. This differentiation proved to be unhelpful: the first variety did not appear to exist in a pure form, while the second, which was common, seemed to have been given a designation which was both confusing and incorrect: these patients showed usually no evidence of hysteria clinically, and psychodynamically no unusual 'capacity for conversion of psychic excitation into bodily innervation'.

The most acceptable clinical grouping of neurotic reactions now seems to us the simple one of describing them under the heads of anxiety neurosis, hysteria and obsessional neurosis. The criteria for the diagnosis of hysteria are given on p. 144: the term should not be used just in the sense that the patient is over-emotional or acting-out his or her emotions. When there is much mental perturbation in the form of fear, and when any bodily symptoms seem to be the outcome of this, the best term probably is anxiety neurosis (anxiety state). The term obsessional neurosis includes obsessive-ruminative and obsessive-compulsive states, and the central feature here is a feeling of subjective compulsion, so that the patient has fears or preoccupations or carries out motor acts of an apparently trifling or meaningless kind, against his better judgement. We will give our reasons later for doubting whether there is now any point in considering neurasthenia a clinical entity, among the neurotic reactions.

We make no distinction between the terms psychoneurosis and neurosis: they reflect psychodynamic theories which have been abandoned, and the shorter term seems preferable.

Differentiation from Psychosis

There are few clearly defined boundaries in nature, and there is many a case of mental illness which it is difficult to assign definitely to the neurotic or psychotic group. But between a well-developed psychosis on the one hand and a full-fledged neurosis on the other there is a world of difference, from the descriptive as well as from the therapeutic aspect. Transitions also occur; so that a patient who reacts neurotically at one time may react psychotically at another. We have, for example, seen a patient who began with neurotic anxiety symptoms subsequently develop obsessive compulsive ones and finally enter a paranoid psychosis, as if these were successive stages of mental disintegration. But such transitions are the exception and not the rule. The neurotic who has among his other topics of anxiety the fear of insanity can usually be reassured with statistical certainty that he will not 'go out of his mind'.

The distinctions between neuroses and psychoses are symptomatic, psychopathological and therapeutic. The symptoms of the neuroses will be enumerated later, when the divergences from the clinical pictures presented by the psychoses will be evident. Considered biologically, that is, regarded as types of reaction to environment, the neuroses are distinctive in several ways. A psychosis involves a change in the whole personality of the subject in whom it appears, while in the neuroses it is only a part of the personality that is affected. With the development of a neurosis there is often no outward change of personality of any kind. As

Meyer put it, a neurosis is a part-reaction, while a psychosis is a total one. Furthermore, in a psychosis reality is changed qualitatively and comes to be regarded in a way very different from the normal, and the patient behaves accordingly; in a neurosis reality remains unchanged qualitatively, although its value may be quantitatively altered. But the neurotic acts always as if reality had the same kind of meaning for him as for the rest of the community. Psychopathologically the psychotic change in reality-values is partly expressed as projection, which consists in attributing an experience in origin entirely subjective to some external personal agency, *e.g.* an externally unfounded belief that one is being continually watched often depends on a sense of guilt, subjective but unconscious. Projection of this sort does not occur in the neuroses.

Language is the symbolizing function and the latest developed function for social adaptation. In the neuroses, language as such is never disturbed, whereas in the psychoses it often undergoes distortion. From the psychoanalytic viewpoint, the unconscious comes to direct verbal expression in the psychoses; whereas in the neuroses it never attains more than symbolic expression in some physical or localized mental disturbance. The reactions in the psychoses are of a much more primitive type on the whole than in the neuroses: there is often a regression to an infantile level of activity in the psychotic. For example, wetting and soiling without shame are not found in neurotics in the presence of clear consciousness.

AETIOLOGY—GENERAL ASPECTS

We have stated already that neurotic reactions develop most commonly as faulty responses to the personal problems of everyday life. Stressful situations of a great many different kinds, instead of eliciting an out-going and constructive response, may precipitate a state of continuing anxiety and mental conflict, with the development of neurotic symptoms. There are two variables: the stress, and the strength of the human material tested. The stresses which precipitate breakdown vary greatly from case to case in their nature, quality, intensity and duration: they may be either psychological or physical (or both combined), but the former are usually of first importance and predominate. Physical illness or injury or fatigue may reduce an individual's resistance to psychological stress. If the environmental stress is severe enough almost anyone may break down with anxious or depressive symptoms, as has been demonstrated repeatedly in war-time; in the sequelae, for example, of long-continued trench warfare or combat flying. The stresses of civil life which are most commonly important arise from personal relationships and social and sexual difficulties. These stresses are as various as the personalities which encounter them: if they elicit emotions of fear, guilt and hate which have to be repressed, they are particularly likely to produce mental conflict and neurotic responses. For facing these stresses the individual may be weakened or wholly disabled by his inherited constitution and the incidents of his personal biography: the personality traits which he has developed out of the interaction of his inherited constitution and early environment may, in other

K

words, have predisposed him to neurotic breakdown. Hence the aetiology of neurosis is a multiple aetiology, of great individual variety and complexity. We are still far from understanding it fully.

During the Second World War it became particularly important to select for specially arduous combat duties men who would not be likely to suffer neurotic breakdown under very severe stress. Attempts were made therefore to identify at examination and to eliminate those liable to breakdown. Four groups of characteristics were found (Gillespie, 1944) to indicate neurotic predisposition and to correlate with neurotic breakdown: 1. pronounced morbid fears; 2. traits pointing to timidity and lack of aggressiveness; 3. 'nervousness'; and 4. 'physiological instability'. 'Nervousness' was defined to include proneness to instability of mood, obsessional characteristics, inferiority feelings and solitary habits. 'Physiological instability' was thought to be shown by habitual restless sleep and sleepwalking, stammering, nail biting, bedwetting, and fainting at the sight of blood. A concentration of five or more 'neurotic' traits in one individual was considered to be significant of predisposition. Selection along these lines proved effective: those thought to be resistant to stress proved to be so—for example, less than 5 per cent. of bomber aircrew in the Royal Air Force became neurotic casualties, though the casualty rate for killed and missing rose to 48 per cent.

As we shall see later when discussing the different neurotic reaction-types in more detail, psychodynamic formulations deriving from Freud have proved of much value in understanding how a great variety of mental and physical symptoms may arise from the anxiety and tension which are fundamental in neurotic illness. There is also another kind of aetiological explanation which has few points of contact with psychoanalytic hypotheses, and is based on Pavlov's concepts of the conditioned reflex. An emotional reaction first aroused by a certain mental event tends afterwards to be aroused by any other mental event which has become associated with the first one. This secondary mental event may be without emotional significance in itself, but by virtue of its association it becomes capable of arousing the emotional reaction without the presence of the primary event in consciousness, or (perhaps and more often) in the absence of any conscious connection between the primary and secondary events, which may both nevertheless be fully conscious. The signs of emotional disturbance, physical or mental, aroused in this way, without adequate conscious reason, are reflected upon by the subject and mistaken for signs of disease. Thus the necessary conditions for the formation of neurotic symptoms are reproduced—the presence of localized bodily or mental disturbances without adequate conscious explanation of their occurrence. A simple example of this type of conditioned response was that of soldiers returned from battle areas who jumped at the slightest sound—not because the sound brought back memories of warfare into full consciousness, but simply because sudden sounds had become associated with reactions of fear.

Pavlov's work has been the starting-point for the contemporary development of 'learning theory', of which Eysenck (1960) has become the leading protagonist in the psychiatric field. Eysenck considers all neurotic symptoms to be either surplus or deficient conditioned reactions.

Constitutional Factors

Brown (1942), from a study of the relatives of neurotic patients, produced evidence that neurotic syndromes of the anxiety, hysterical and obsessional types have in some instances at least a constitutional basis, that the inherited constitution may be specific in each group, but that there is also some common factor which shows itself in an anxious personality.

Brown found that 21·4 per cent. of the parents of patients with anxiety states had a similar disorder, while 17·5 per cent. had either an anxious, depressive or obsessional personality. The anxious personality was described as timid, apprehensive, given to excessive worry or to mild phobias. Five per cent. of the parents of patients with anxiety neuroses had had depressions. In a control group the proportions of relatives affected were significantly less. It appears likely therefore that there are inherited constitutional factors in anxiety neuroses, and that these factors may in some instances be related to the depressive constitution.

In this sample also 19 per cent. of the parents of hysterical patients had themselves had hysterical reactions, while 14 per cent. of them exhibited an anxious personality. 7·5 per cent. of the parents of obsessional patients had suffered from obsessional syndromes, and the same percentage had had depressions: 19·6 per cent. of the parents had anxious personalities.

The same tendencies were confirmed by a study of the sibs and first and second degree relatives of patients with neuroses, the differences from controls being in all groups significant.

Slater (1943) investigating the relationships between personality traits and subsequent neuroses, found significant correlations between pre-existing traits and types of neuroses developed: the neurotic symptoms appeared as exaggerations of the personality traits. In the obsessional group in particular the correlation was high. A positive correlation was also found between hysterical traits of personality and hysterical symptoms; between anxious characteristics and subsequent symptoms of anxiety; and between depressive traits, such as mood swings, and subsequent depressive illness—in that diminishing order of relationship. If one assumes that these personality traits are inherited rather than acquired, this is additional evidence of a constitutional predisposition to neurotic types of reaction. The correlations were not high enough to indicate that constitutional predisposition is an essential factor in all cases. Slater (1944) proceeded to develop 'a heuristic theory of neurosis': that the neurotically predisposed individual represents one of the extremes of normal human variation, having more than average susceptibility to environmental stresses, and that this constitution is preponderantly determined by a very large number of genes of small effect. 'The effects of these genes, at least in so far as they are qualitatively similar, may be additive; and they become manifest by producing a reduced resistance to some form of environmental stress, and so facilitate the appearance of a neurosis. In so far as the effects of the genes are qualitatively dissimilar, the type of stress effective in producing breakdown, and the neurotic symptoms produced, will tend to differ.'

What is further required is a collaboration between the psychopathologist, the student of personality traits and the statistician in an attempt to establish what the fundamental and presumably inherited characteristics may be, and how they may produce in the course of psychological development in secondary fashion the traits which we recognize as predisposing to the development of certain types of symptom. In the obsessional type of character, for example, does the inherited factor essentially consist in an excessive degree of aggressiveness, which by happy accident and happy upbringing may result in a dominant and forceful personality in the one case; or which, on the other hand, as a result of a miscarriage of psychological development, may produce reaction formations, such as extreme scrupulousness devised to keep the aggressiveness in constant check, leading in the long run to the development of inner tension and ultimately of symptoms; or does the obsessional possibly inherit a nervous system which is distinctively organized? How far is the habit of anxiety, which appears to favour the development of anxiety symptoms, based on inherited emotionality; how far a mere infection, as it were, from an anxious parent; and how far an inner conflict, never properly resolved? Some of these are questions to which there can be no general answer. Studies of inheritance and constitution must be blended with studies of the life history of the individual and if possible with that of his parents. Probably only in this way can a true understanding be obtained, and at the same time scientific methods of prevention and treatment be gradually devised.

In the meantime it can be said that the individual constitution alone may be enough in some instances to determine the onset of an obsessive-compulsive state; while in the case of the hysterical, anxious and depressive syndromes much more depends upon accidents of experience and upbringing. It appears, in effect, that if an experience is severe enough these latter forms of reaction may appear in anyone, whereas it would be difficult to develop obsessional symptoms without a relevant constitutional predisposition.

Intelligence plays a part in determining the occurrence of neurotic reactions as a whole, which are relatively commoner among people of superior, than among those of inferior, intelligence. Intelligence also has an effect in determining the form of reaction, hysterical symptoms being commoner amongst dull individuals.

Environmental Factors

The environmental situations which may elicit neurotic reactions are multiform and may occur at any time throughout the individual's life. Each person has his own peculiar vicissitudes as he develops and ages: and at certain periods, in infancy, at puberty and in adolescence, in middle and old age, he is subject to stresses which he shares with all his coevals.

The earliest adverse environmental situation is a disturbed relationship with, or separation from, the mother. The infant's mind is dominated by the need to retain the mother, the primary source of love and food and protection, and in a state of nature vital of course to the offspring's survival. At the age of 83 Thomas

Carlyle wrote, 'It was the earliest terror of my childhood that I might lose my mother and it has gone with me all my days.' Later the infant develops emotional bonds with his father and siblings, and, as he grows, with people outside the family circle, so that he becomes dependent on others not only for his material existence but for love and satisfaction in its many forms. The seeds of neurosis are sown often in these early relationships, when they are disturbed or distorted. How this may occur is described in Chapter 19, where problems arising from the child's emotional development are considered in greater detail.

Some of the social factors which may influence the incidence of neurosis, and the relationships between neurosis and social class, have already been discussed in Chapter 4, in the section on 'Social Factors and Aspects'. Here we wish in addition to draw attention to aspects of the life of the suburban areas of our large cities, which may be inimical to mental health and productive of neurosis.

Taylor (1938) described 'the suburban neurosis' of young women with anxiety states. He thought that these neurotic reactions developed because the environment had failed to interest, sustain or inspire these young married women, and they seemed to have little to live for. He thought the immediate causes were: 1. boredom occasioned by lack of friends, not enough to do and not enough to think about; 2. anxiety about money, the house and having another baby; and 3. a false set of values, due to the decline of religious faith and its replacement by the values of the advertisers and fetish-worship of the home. This paper of Taylor's was impressionistic. Martin and his colleagues (1957) have studied the incidence of neurosis in a new housing estate in Hertfordshire and found a relatively high incidence of psychological disorder: their findings in fact suggested that the prevalence of neuroses in this environment might be as high as 77 per cent. in excess of the national rate. Tentatively they suggested that two adverse social factors might be operating: the effects of rehousing in producing family and social dislocation, and the loneliness of life on the estate, where each family tended to 'keep itself to itself'. Further information about these situations is obviously required, since it appears that here we may have a public health problem of some magnitude and one which may offer opportunities for preventive medicine.

Finally, we must take note that few persons are more suggestible than those who are anxious from any cause. Physical illness in other members of a family, or in near relatives may suggest symptoms to neurotic patients and focus their fears. Their suggestibility also makes the handling of neurotic patients or those potentially neurotic a delicate matter. We doctors, by mistakes in diagnosis and the injudicious handling of neurotic complaints, ourselves foster and fix neurotic reactions. Over the years there have been very many iatrogenic disorders, whose prevention has been wholly in our hands.

THE CLINICAL SYNDROMES

The main neurotic reaction-types have no hard and fast boundaries, and the classification we employ here—anxiety neuroses, hysteria and obsessional neuroses—is essentially a clinical one. Certain symptoms are held in common by each group—anxiety, for example. A given case may sometimes change so much that now it falls within one group, now in another: and cases showing admixtures of neurotic symptoms are commoner than those which exhibit the classical features of only one of the sub-types. Phobias can be classified either with the anxiety neuroses or with the obsessions: we have described them with the latter. There is also a considerable number of cases which may be difficult to classify definitively either as neuroses or affective psychoses: these are the so-called 'neurotic depressions', in which reactive emotional features are prominent and the symptoms are often clearly the response of an unstable personality to a situational problem. Some of these reactions are hysterical—it has indeed been suggested that this is the most typical contemporary form of hysteria: others, the majority we believe, are to be considered as belonging to the manic-depressive psychoses, the distinction between reactive and endogenous depressions being an arbitrary one.

Neurotic reactions may occur at any age, but are commonest in adolescence and in early adult life: women are more prone to them than men.

ANXIETY NEUROSES

These are the commonest of the neuroses, and fortunately the most responsive to treatment. Anxiety may occur as a symptom in almost any psychiatric syndrome: here it is the leading and predominant feature. It goes beyond any normal reaction of fear and worry: it is more intense, more persistent and more disabling. It is, however, always precipitated by some environmental situation or problem. A very similar syndrome may appear with no discoverable psychological cause, and subside spontaneously: in these cases anxiety has probably masked an underlying depression.

Clinical Features

Symptoms of morbid anxiety commonly develop in people of *anxious personality*—tense, timid, self-doubting, worrying people, who tend to expect the worst to happen and 'to cross their bridges before they come to them'. They often set high standards, there is a gap between their expectations for themselves and what they can in fact achieve, and this leads to feelings of insecurity and inferiority.

The symptoms of an anxiety neurosis are both mental and physical.

The mental symptoms take the form usually of a state of persistent anxiety, tension, apprehension and worry. The patient describes himself or herself as 'strung up', 'on edge', constantly expecting trouble or calamity: there is restlessness, impaired concentration, 'absentmindedness' and forgetfulness in day-to-day affairs, jumpiness, irritability and intermittently depression of spirits. The patient's tension makes him feel fatigued and he has difficulty in falling off to sleep at nights because worries and forebodings crowd his mind. His sleep may be broken by unpleasant dreams or nightmares, of pursuit perhaps or attack or falling or failure.

The patient's anxiety may be unfocussed, 'free-floating' it has been called, a nameless dread, or attaching itself to obvious trifles: or it may become specific, channelled into fears of many kinds, especially of insanity and cancer and other bodily illness. The locus of fears of bodily illness is often suggested by the bodily symptoms of the neurosis itself: palpitations and praecordial pains will be interpreted as evidence of heart disease, for example (a situation often given the unnecessary label of 'cardiac neurosis').

In some cases the apprehension recurrently rises quickly to a crisis in the form of acute attacks of anxiety or panic, which may last for a few minutes to half an hour or longer. The patient may describe these panics in physical terms, calling them feelings of dizziness or faintness; or may even not mention them, out of a fear of mental illness or of being thought a weakling. The attacks begin often with unpleasant sensations in the epigastrium, feelings of unease or tension or nausea which may resemble the aura of an epileptic fit. Then the symptoms mount towards the throat and head. The patient may feel his chest so constricted that he cannot get a full breath, and he pants for air. Palpitations, choking sensations, sweating, tingling of the limbs, feelings of lightheadedness, are accompanied by a fear of collapsing, fainting or dying: a terror, often, quite plainly of impending death. Then gradually the fear recedes, leaving the patient shaken and limp and afraid of being left alone. These panic attacks may occur both during the day and at night, in bed, and the patient may understandably feel afraid to leave his house because of them. The German poet Rilke, in his autobiographical *Notebooks of Malte Laurids Brigge*, described his own attacks: 'Why should I pretend that these nights had never been, when in fear of death I sat up, clinging to the fact that the mere act of sitting was at any rate a part of life: that the dead did not sit. . . . One wakes up panting. . . . Higher it mounts, here it passes out over you, rising higher than your breath, to which you flee as to your last stand. . . . Your heart drives you out of yourself, your heart pursues you, and you are almost frantic. . . . Your slight surface hardness and adaptability go for nothing.' And Rilke, a grown man, would call for his mother, remembering how she had come to him as a child when he had had a night terror, saying 'It is I, do not be afraid'—and his fear had gone.

The somatic symptoms of an anxiety state may involve any one or all of the bodily systems: most cases complain of a number of physical symptoms with the emphasis usually on one or other bodily system. Rapid heart beats, breathlessness, lack of appetite, a lump in the throat, flatulence, fullness in the stomach, water-brash, constipation, diarrhoea, frequency of micturition, twitching of muscles, weakness of limbs, tremors, pains and other paraesthesiae, blurring of vision, tinnitus, general fatigability—all these are common symptoms. There is evidence both of sympathetic and parasympathetic over-action: the former displayed, for example, in dilated pupils and rapid pulse, the latter in diarrhoea and frequency of micturition. Pains derived from muscle tension are very common and are often miscalled rheumatism: they may occur anywhere in the patient's back or at the back of his neck (so that he 'can't get his neck comfortable'), in his scalp muscles, his face and jaws, the left side of his chest and his limbs.

Praecordial jabbing pains, due to spasm of intercostal muscles, draw the patient's attention to the state of his heart.

The patient suffering from an anxiety neurosis may exhibit no abnormality on physical examination; or he or she may show some of the somatic signs of anxiety, as described above—dilated pupils, tremors, cold and clammy hands, a raised systolic blood pressure, and very brisk tendon reflexes. There may be some loss of weight.

Aetiology and Psychopathology

In the genesis of an anxiety neurosis there are to be found some or all of the following factors. There is commonly an inherited predisposition. Frequently also, there is what in its effects may be mistaken for heredity, namely, a morbid family environment such as may be produced by maternal anxiety or much parental quarrelling or some other form of 'broken home' situation. These are the predisposing factors. The immediate factors include any source of dissatisfaction, whether in personal relationships, domestic, sexual or social, or in connection with employment or financial stress, or elsewhere. Exposure to some overwhelming, and usually sudden, external stress, for example a terrifying experience involving threat to life, can produce an anxiety syndrome in the absence of mental conflict, especially in people of timid temperament.

Anxiety neuroses may originate from any type of collision between individual needs and reality. These needs may be sexual, but are not necessarily so: and childhood conflicts which had been incompletely resolved (for example, an Oedipus complex) may or may not be reactivated, so that consciousness is threatened with the return of repressed material. Freud maintained that excessive anxiety, even when attributed to obviously reasonable objects of concern such as business difficulties, would not arise in the absence of faulty organization of the libido; and that in these cases the libido had remained partially attached to an infantile and incestuous object-choice. The result was that in face of a situation producing conflict, libidinal regression would occur in an infantile and still forbidden direction, with the production of anxiety. This hypothesis, that the basis of an anxiety neurosis is always in the sexual life, while valid for some cases is too narrow to be generally applicable, even if 'sexual' is interpreted in a very wide sense. One encounters sometimes a more straightforward connection between the sexual life and morbid anxiety, in the cases of women whose failure to obtain satisfaction in sexual intercourse (as a result, for example, of coitus interruptus) is expressed directly in heightened physical and emotional tension, in vague aches and pains and ill-defined fears.

When anxiety arises from any situation which arouses intense feelings either of fear or hate or guilt and which is not squarely faced, it diffuses itself generally throughout the mind, and in the course of its diffusion tends to become concentrated again (in a manner determined by the individual mental history) around some special topic in itself apparently of more indifferent emotional value. Fears, vague or 'free-floating' at first, may thus become attached to some particular idea or situation, remote from the original source of the anxiety: that is, displacement of affect occurs. This displacement has the result of enabling the patient to escape from the painful contemplation of a personal difficulty. It should be noted that displacement of affect does not necessarily involve repression into the unconscious: the original difficulties may remain in consciousness, on the fringe as it were, while preoccupation is focussed elsewhere. The individual usually rationalizes this preoccupation, thus making the displacement of affect more effective. Displacement and rationalization are the two main mental mechanisms employed.

The symptomatic form of an anxiety neurosis, in its somatic aspects, is determined by the influence of emotional perturbation on the functioning of various bodily organs. Emotional disturbance produces bodily symptoms: these bodily symptoms may then attract the affect displaced from other problems, and become the patient's chief complaints and apparent source of worry. Alternatively, displacement of the anxiety may take place in the mental sphere without bodily reference.

That general problems—for example, of business or other material circumstances—may be an adequate cause of an anxiety neurosis by displacement or diffusion of affect is well shown by the following case histories.

CASE NO. 1
A commercial traveller who had suffered some deafness from middle-ear disease since childhood did not seek advice till he was aged 41, when he complained of tinnitus and inquired anxiously what was wrong. It transpired that his business had recently failed, that his partner had been committed to prison for fraud, that his new employers were expecting him to produce more than twice the financial result he could hope to obtain and that he had a wife and family to support. Reassurance about his tinnitus, and discussion and advice on his difficulties, gained the patient's confidence and he thereafter confined his anxiety to his business and to ordinary dimensions.

CASE NO. 2
A married man of 47, who complained especially of attacks of diarrhoea in trains, of sweating of feet and hands, of dizziness, tremblings, irritability, insomnia and poor memory. He was a conscientious, hard-working man of artisan stock who had worked his way up to a position of responsibility in a large business. Most of his symptoms had begun three months before, when he was transferred by his employers from an indoor to an outdoor job, another employee being discharged to make room for him. The latter had been in the business for thirty years, and the patient felt very 'heavy and miserable' at usurping this man's position. The new post involved much travelling by train, and the patient began to suffer from diarrhoea from the very start of his train-journeying. He became so weak that after ten days he had to stay at home, where he remained till he entered hospital, after 'convalescence' at the seaside had failed.

Investigations showed that some of the symptoms—insomnia and irritability—had existed for some time before the diarrhoea began, that he had attributed them to overwork and had actually resigned from his previous (indoor) post. His resignation had not been accepted, but he was hurt nevertheless at the small amount of attention that was paid to him. Further, he divulged that he had been afraid of supersession by his employer's son, who was coming to years of discretion. His fear was to some extent justified, for his removal to an outdoor traveller's position, although ostensibly for his health, was carried out to allow of his former post being taken by his young rival. He was a quiet, unaggressive man, who disliked a traveller's work intensely and embarked on it with great reluctance. It seemed likely that much of his regret for the dismissal of the other employee was a reflection of his feeling about his own supersession. The connection between his mental perturbation and his symptoms was pointed out. He accepted the explanation willingly and his symptoms ceased with dramatic rapidity, and did not recur. He said that he now felt confident, and that he never had understood his symptoms previously, having thought he had some physical disease.

The foregoing patient illustrates several points. The diffusion of affect from his own plight to that of his fellow-employee, showing itself as an unusual degree of regret, is an example of 'displacement'. The bodily symptoms were all those that are associated with fear; and he had a fear of his new job, plus a reluctance to leave his old one. He was also jealous—although he would not permit himself to feel it—of his employer's son, and he had a grievance towards his employers for their apparent lack of commiseration. His symptoms could be viewed as: 1. the result of his fear; 2. a protest against leaving his former post; and 3. retaliation against his employers, since he, as a matter of fact, proved their most efficient traveller, in spite of his handicaps, and his incapacity through illness penalized them financially. This threefold origin is a good example of 'overdetermination' as Freud has called it. The kind of process seen in this patient is one that is not uncommon in everyday life, perhaps especially in children and young persons. There is a grievance: the child is sorry for himself, he finds an ache or a pain easily enough, and he complains about it, either for sympathy or as an excuse from duty or for both. The process is not far removed from full consciousness. In the above case it was so near full consciousness that the patient quickly saw the explanations that were put to him, and laughingly, but a little shamefacedly, admitted their truth.

Differential Diagnosis

An anxiety neurosis must be differentiated from other abnormal mental reactions, and from physical disease. The commonest mistake is to call an agitated depression an anxiety neurosis. It is a serious mistake since the former is accompanied by a suicidal risk which may thus be ignored and the proper treatment of the two conditions is very different. A man or woman who develops symptoms of morbid anxiety for the first time in middle or later life should be suspected of suffering from a depression rather than a neurosis. The depressive symptoms associated with an anxiety neurosis are not so persistent, nor does the neurotic patient complain of early morning wakening nor of being at his worst in the first half of the day. One's clinical sensitivity is called fully into play in deciding whether the patient is more anxious than depressed, and how deep may be his depression: and the differential diagnosis may be really difficult, since particularly in the involutional melancholia type of depressive reaction anxiety is often in the forefront of the clinical picture and there is no retardation. Before the diagnosis of neurosis can be established, one must be able to demonstrate an adequate cause of the neurotic reaction. But psychoses may be reactive too, and it is all too easy to find a spurious psychogenesis.

Discrimination between the symptoms and signs of anxiety, and physical disease, also calls for good clinical judgement. The autonomic upsets of anxiety may suggest disease in any of the bodily systems, and the neurotic patient is often referred initially to the medical departments of a hospital, suspected of suffering from heart disease or peptic ulcer, rheumatism or endocrinopathy; or to the ophthalmologist to have his eyes examined or to the orthopaedic surgeon for relief of the pains in his back. Perhaps the most difficult differential diagnosis on the physical side lies sometimes between an anxiety neurosis and primary hyperthyroidism. The anxious neurotic patient may have a rapid (waking) pulse, a raised systolic blood pressure, slightly enlarged thyroid gland and some upper-lid lag. Radio-iodine estimations may be necessary to establish the correct diagnosis in these borderline cases.

HYSTERIA

Hysteria has been known since antiquity. In Hippocratic times it was supposed to occur only in women and to result from 'wandering of the womb' into another part of the body. Later, the more dramatic aspects of hysteria—the convulsions, for example, were for a long time attributed to demoniacal possession. Many of the dramatic cures by exorcism and other preternatural methods recorded in popular and religious history occurred in hysterical patients. The study of neurotic symptoms was on the whole haphazard until Charcot, who was primarily a neurologist, began a systematic study of them, confining himself to the hysterical type of manifestation. Applying the methods of clinical observation which he had used for organic nervous diseases, he succeeded in formulating a group of clinical pictures, of paralyses, contractures and convulsions which constituted a graded series of increasing complexity, and all of which together he called 'hysteria'. The one causative factor which he found uniformly in his patients was a morbid inheritance, and he considered hysteria a malady of degeneration. A relatively minor observation of Charcot's had far-reaching effects in the hands of certain of his pupils. He reproduced paralysis in his patients by means of hypnotism, proving that hysterical paralysis could be the result of specific ideas existing in the patient's mind. But Charcot believed that such paralyses could be hypnotically reproduced only in hysterics and in *grande hystérie* at that. It remained for his successors to develop and modify his views. These modifications were on very divergent lines, and the principal varieties of theory and practice were associated with the names of Bernheim, Dubois, Dejerine, Janet and Freud.

Bernheim gradually came to the opinion that all the phenomena which Charcot had described as hysterical were capable of being produced by suggestion. He declared that not merely hysterical patients were hypnotizable, but that practically everyone could be hypnotized. 'Suggestion', said Bernheim, 'consists of the influence exercised by an idea that has been suggested, and has been accepted by the brain.' Hysterical symptoms were therefore in Bernheim's opinion the result of suggestion. Babinski went further and stated that nothing is hysterical which cannot be produced by suggestion and removed by persuasion. The views of Dejerine, Janet and Freud will be discussed later, when we deal more fully with the psychopathological aspects.

Not only have there been many changes in the theories elaborated to explain hysteria, the clinical features also of the reaction have changed over the years. Patients displaying the features of Charcot's *grande hystérie*, women resting on their shoulders with their bodies and legs in the air, or in opisthotonos, are no longer seen. Cases of multiple personality have become very rare since Morton Prince was interested in them. Gross physical symptoms, in the nature of paralyses or bizarre gaits, have also become very uncommon in civilian practice. Perhaps the most frequent hysterical complaints are now 'blackouts' and bodily pains of one sort or another, which present more subtle problems in differential diagnosis. Both the public and their doctors have become more sophisticated.

Definition of the Reaction-type

Hysteria is more than a symptom or collection of symptoms: it is a special type of reaction to difficulties displayed in a number of syndromes which are distinctive both clinically and psychopathologically. It has a relationship with anxiety states in that an anxiety state may in certain circumstances replace hysteria in a given patient, and a case may begin as an anxiety neurosis and end as a hysteria. But these are not usual transitions. On the whole, in any one patient the type of reaction tends to remain fairly pure. It is important to distinguish between anxiety in the sense of mental conflict and its accompanying distress, which is a normal reaction, and an anxiety neurosis which is a clinical syndrome, is abnormal and has already been defined. In the former sense hysteria always begins with anxiety.

If the symptom or sign produced in hysteria is a physical manifestation such as a paralysis or anaesthesia the result is called *conversion hysteria*, the psychic energy derived from the repressed drives, emotions and ideas being said to be 'converted' into a physical symptom or sign.

Clinical Features

Commonly, though by no means invariably, the previous personality is an unusual one. An aggregation of traits is found which comprises what has been called the '*hysterical or histrionic personality*'. Such people tend to be highly egocentric and immature, both in talk and appearance, and to be conspicuous for the demands they make on people around them. There is a lifelong theatricality of behaviour and a desire to impress and gain sympathy, a contrast between actual shallowness of the feelings and the intensity of the expression of them and between external shyness and intense erotic interest, a lack of persistence of emotion and of effort, and much compensatory day-dreaming. Most often they are women, though adult still to a great extent dependent on one or other parent, sexually frigid, prone to react with sudden spites and piques and to try to dominate others with their tempers, whims or suicidal threats. They seem to have carried with them into adult life the infantile need for exclusive love and attention. There is an excellent description of such a personality in Lord David Cecil's biography *The Young Melbourne*, where the author reconstructs the character of Lady Caroline Lamb.

All neurotics are suggestible, and it has for long been held that hysterics are the most suggestible of all and show in fact an exaggerated suggestibility. Eysenck (1947) formulated the view that there are different types of suggestibility and distinguished a primary suggestibility of an ideomotor kind. 'The main feature of the tests which go to define this trait is the execution of a motor movement by the subject consequent upon the repeated suggestion by the experimenter that such a movement will take place, without conscious participation in the movement on the subject's part.' The test most commonly used to demonstrate this primary suggestibility is Hull's Body-Sway Test, in which the subject stands still and relaxed, with eyes closed, while the experimenter suggests to him that he is falling forward: the amount of sway is measured and a suggestibility score can be constructed. Using this and a number of other tests Eysenck found that primary suggestibility is closely related to hypnosis; that suggestibility is strongly correlated with neuroticism—'both when comparing neurotics with normals and when comparing the more seriously ill with the less seriously ill it was found that degree of neuroticism was reflected in the suggestibility test scores'; and that hysterics are not more suggestible than other types of neurotics.

According to Rivers and MacCurdy environmental factors in the way of training and education are of importance in determining the hysterical form of a neurosis. A training in implicit obedience, such as occurs in soldiers, is said to heighten suggestibility to an extent that makes hysterical symptoms more easily produced; while lack of education makes possible gross signs, such as a paraplegia, the arbitrary appearance of which an educated mind would not tolerate.

Hysterical symptoms may be found as secondary features in both 'functional' and organic psychoses. One may, for example, find stuttering or an hysterical weakness of the legs in a psychotic depression, or aphonia in the course of a schizophrenic illness. A brain tumour or other organic nervous system disease may release hysterical symptoms.

Symptoms and Signs

Both mental and physical symptoms are developed, but usually one or other type of symptom predominates in the individual case. These symptoms may mimic closely those of other diseases and the greater the patient's medical knowledge the closer will be the resemblance: it is advisable therefore always to ask the patient what he thinks or fears his illness is. The particular symptom chosen depends on a number of factors which vary from case to case: it may clearly have symbolic meaning (hysterical vomiting, for example, may symbolize rejection of an unwanted pregnancy); or it may be based on the residuals of some earlier injury or disease; or it may be suggested to the patient by previous medical examinations or the recent illness of a friend or relative.

Hysterical signs and symptoms have certain general characteristics. Taking those with a physical reference first, it may be said almost universally that there are no physical signs or symptoms in hysteria that could not be produced in the beginning either by volition or by emotion, although they could be so sustained only for a short time. Long-standing contractures, for example, which may persist during sleep and anaesthesia, require some additional explanation to account for their continuance. It can also be said that the physical aspects of hysteria correspond strikingly with the usual concepts of disease entertained by the lay mind. Thus a paralysis is always of an entire limb or of a movement, and never of an individual muscle; a tic is always a co-ordinated movement of synergic muscles, never a chaotic movement of muscles not functionally associated; and an anaesthesia does not follow a segmental or peripheral nerve-distribution, but is of the 'glove' or 'stocking' variety. Hysterical symptoms in general are readily produced and removed by suggestion in the waking state or in hypnosis.

Hurst showed that if a group of normal medical students in the pre-clinical years were asked to suppose that they had suffered from some bodily injury, the signs and symptoms they developed upon suggestive questioning had the characteristics of hysterical symptoms above described.

Physical Symptoms. These may be conveniently considered as motor, sensory, visceral and trophic.

The *motor symptoms* which are in the nature of some incapacity, partial or complete, involving the voluntary musculature, include pareses with or without contracture, mutism, aphonia, tremors and tics. The incapacity is often sudden in onset, variable, and only superficially like that of neurological disease. If paresis exists, it may affect the proximal muscles of a limb more than the distal ones, which is the reverse of what commonly happens in organic paralysis; and the muscles may be used in some movements and not in others. When asked to make the movement that is paralysed, the patient only succeeds in producing a spasm of the antagonistic muscles. Thus an artisan of 63 when asked to walk faster (his right leg had a hysterical paresis) threw his body into such strenuous jerkings that he was very breathless in two minutes and perspired freely. There is no reaction of degeneration in hysterically paralysed muscles. The reflexes are not grossly disturbed; but they may be much increased in amplitude. Not infrequently one notices a certain amount of what seems like voluntary exaggeration —the patient either jerks his limb before it is struck, or he jerks it again immediately after the true tendon-jerk has occurred. In hysterical flaccid paralysis the tendon reflexes may be very much diminished, but they are not lost. The plantar reflex is always flexor. If atrophy occurs, it is usually secondary to long disuse. Hysterical hemiplegia may involve the face on the same side, and may involve speech as well, even when left-sided.

Mutism and *aphonia* are distinguished from similar conditions resulting from organic disease: 1. by their completeness—every phonated word and sound is lost; 2. the absence of any intellectual disorder; 3. the preservation of the ability to communicate by writing or by signs; 4. the absence of paralysis of the lips and tongue; and 5. the vocal cords can be seen to be fully adducted in inspiration. The mute individual may be able to cough normally. These features are not always all present.

Hysterical *tremor* is usually coarse and often involves the whole limb. It may occur at rest, but commonly only when attention is drawn to it, or when the patient makes a voluntary movement.

Motor *tics* involve a co-ordinated group of muscles. They range from an occasional jerking of a limb to choreiform movements. Hysterical movements are apt to be more co-ordinated than those of true chorea and to be less varied, involving the repetition of a comparatively few movements. Rapid jerking movements of the head occur, and may be indistinguishable from spasmodic torticollis: the latter, however, is probably in the majority of cases due to organic disease of the extrapyramidal nervous system. A respiratory tic, for example, hiccough, may be hysterical; but it has frequently been difficult to distinguish the respiratory disorders of epidemic encephalitis from those of hysteria. The encephalitic or post-encephalitic tics have often had some of the marks of an hysterical disorder. For example, post-encephalitic tics may be influenced by emotional factors and may come on at precisely the same hour each night. But it does not of course follow that hysterical and encephalitic tics are identical.

A good example of the production of a rhythmical hysterical rotary movement of the head on the neck of rapid phase occurred in:

CASE No. 3
A youth of 20 had recently left home after a quarrel with his father. He intensely regretted doing so, and slept badly, but was too proud to communicate with his home. One evening at 9 o'clock while returning from his work to his lodgings, his head suddenly began to jerk violently. It continued to do so, interfering still further with his sleep for three days, during which time he was sent by his employers to consult one of us. At an interview he related his troubles and said hopefully that he thought his employers would get into touch with his father. They did so, and he recovered on the evening of the day in which he received the news that his father knew of his condition. The recovery took place at exactly the same hour as his symptoms had begun, ninety-six hours previously.

Curious gaits of all kinds may occur. The patient may attribute them to pains in the back or to loss of power in the lower limbs.

It is understandable that in pilots and other members of aircrews manifestations of hysteria should affect the eyes rather than the limbs, for what his legs are to an infantryman, his eyes are to a pilot (Ironside and Batchelor, 1945). Many hysterical signs were reported—coarse tremor of the eyelids, blepharospasm, nystagmoid jerkings, all degrees of heterophoria, convergence weakness and dissociation between convergence of the visual axis and contraction of the pupils. Variable convergence spasm and spasm of accommodation were also recorded.

Sensory Symptoms. Anaesthesias, paraesthesias and hyperaesthesias are common. It has been said that they are produced by suggestion from the physician, but this is certainly not true of all. They are commonly distinguished by their distribution, which is not that of an organic disturbance; by their variability at successive examinations; and by their susceptibility to suggestion. In the case of anaesthesias also, the lack of sensation is much more sweeping than in organic lesions, all kinds of sensation being abolished in a given area; it is also deeper, pain not being felt at all; and its margin is much more sharply defined—there is no gradual transition to a normal area as in neurological lesions.

The susceptibility to suggestion can be shown very easily in certain patients with a hemianaesthesia. This can be transferred to the other side of the body by suggestion in the waking state. In a chronic hysterical patient in whom this was done, the anaesthesia could be very readily transferred from the left to the right side of the body, so that she would tolerate the passing of safety-pins through her skin; but it had invariably returned to the left side the following morning.

Hyperaesthesias most commonly are localized in the head or the abdomen, and may be described as pains of any type or in bizarre terms, as constant (even during sleep) and as unassuageable.

The special senses can be affected also. A concentric diminution of the visual field is not uncommon. If the perimetric examination is continued through 360 degrees a spiral field may be obtained. Amaurosis and amblyopia also occur. There may be a bizarre contradiction in the symptoms—the patient may be able to read a paper and yet may be unable to see to get about. Hysterical blindness is often sudden. The bilaterally blind hysteric commonly avoids obstacles placed in his path. Hysterical unilateral blindness can be detected in various ways. For example, pressure on one eye may produce double vision. Specially coloured spectacles to read correspondingly coloured types can also be used for its detection, the patient reading type of a colour which can only be seen by the 'blind' eye. Subjective disturbances of vision are usually associated with intact pupillary reflexes and intact extra-ocular movements, but the light reflex may actually be lost, to return when the blindness is cured.

Visceral Symptoms. Anorexia, bulimia (excessive appetite), vomiting, air-swallowing, hiccough, fullness or pain in the abdomen, flatulence and regurgitation may occur as hysterical symptoms. Since gastric functions are so readily affected by emotions, it is easy to see why they should so often be disorganized in hysteria and why they should so readily have a symbolic significance: vomiting, for example, may signify a repressed disgust. Hysterical vomiting is rapid and easy, often occurring just after a meal and usually without nausea.

Anorexia nervosa, an uncommon, interesting and puzzling condition, is commonly classified with the hysterical reactions but it is not certain that it is correct so to describe it; it is a syndrome which is not fully understood, either from the psychological or the physical aspects, and whose boundaries have not yet been clearly delimited. Valuable studies have been made by Nemiah (1950) and Kay (1953), amongst others.

Anorexia nervosa occurs typically in girls in their teens and in young unmarried women: it is doubtful if the same syndrome is found in men. The typical triad of symptoms is anorexia, amenorrhoea and loss of weight. The illness has an emotional basis and begins often with a voluntary restriction of the diet. One young woman said afterwards, 'It was a silly idea to get into my head' (to starve herself), 'but I thought I was too fat, and then I couldn't get rid of the idea. I just wouldn't eat.' The girl may have been teased by her friends about putting on weight or have become unduly sensitive about the development of her breasts. Appetite is gradually lost and is replaced by a repugnance for food. Amenorrhoea may precede, be contemporaneous with or follow the anorexia. The patient becomes markedly constipated and as a result of not eating loses weight; the resulting emaciation may prove fatal. A remarkable feature that these patients sometimes display is tireless activity in spite of their emaciation. The B.M.R. is low and the patient may show a fine downy hair (lanugo) on her back.

It is usually the mother who brings the patient to the doctor. The patient herself may declare that she is perfectly all right and that she does not know why people are fussy and worrying over her. In this she may exhibit the *belle indifférence* of the hysteric, but this is by no means always the mental state. Depression of spirits may be prominent, with feelings of guilt and isolation and suicidal thoughts. Nor is the previous personality by any means always hysterical, though it is usually immature, with evidence of neurotic predisposition. Several other personality types are encountered, the obsessional, the anxious, the hypochondriacal—and of these the obsessional is probably the commonest. There may be a history of previous food fads and alimentary preoccupations. Insight is minimal and co-operation in treatment often poor, the patient covertly disposing in various ways of the food given her.

The psychogenesis of these cases is complex. There may be a severely disturbed mother-daughter relationship, the patient at one and the same time being unduly dependent and rebelling against maternal domination: or a preoccupation with phantasies of pregnancy and birth. From some of these immature girls one elicits fears of oral impregnation, and they appear to have identified growing fat with being pregnant.

Some of these patients recover mentally, marry and have children: many do badly. Kay (1953), who doubted whether anorexia nervosa is a specific clinical entity, has pointed out the difficulties of treatment and reported a follow-up study of 37 patients. He came to the following conclusions: 1. these patients tend to have a poor prognosis; 2. when clear-cut psychotic features are not present from the outset, there is little tendency to develop a psychosis; 3. only 10–20 per cent. recover to the stage of good adjustment, the majority continuing to show neurotic symptoms. Many patients still show weight fluctuations, and menstrual disturbances, even after five years or more. About 15 per cent. die.

Trophic Symptoms. The *vasomotor* disturbances of hysterically paralysed limbs are well known. The limb is often blue and cold. This is partly the result of disuse and of posture (the dependent position of a paralysed arm, for example), but there is possibly another element, since the vasomotor changes may be rapid and considerable.

The spontaneous appearance of *skin lesions*, blisters, erythemas, etc., has usually been considered an artifact (dermatitis artifacta): but it has been known for more than 50 years that skin blisters, localized urticaria and oedema could be produced hypnotically at specified points on the body surface. Moody (1946) reported a striking case of bodily changes during the abreaction in a somnambulist of an incident when many years previously his hands had been tied behind his back during sleep to restrain him from violence. During abreaction this man developed on both forearms deeply indented weals like rope marks. However,

L

many such lesions are undoubtedly more properly regarded as simulation than as hysterical. Some cases respond fairly readily to suggestion:

CASE NO. 4

A single woman of 25, subnormal (mental age 8 years), was referred from the skin department where she had been treated for three months with little result. She had an erythema with much desquamation of the entire extensor surface of the left hand and left forearm. She was submitted to light hypnosis in which suggestions were made that the skin would become intact. Improvement set in at once and continued until the erythema and desquamation had gone (in about six weeks), but in the meantime she developed brownish discoloured patches on the right leg and arm. Further hypnotic suggestion that all her skin would be free from lesions was rapidly successful in removing them.

In other cases of dermatitis artefacta we have seen there has been a depressive, masochistic, exhibitionistic or erotomanic basis.

CASE NO. 5

For example, one young woman when she admitted that she had inflicted the lesion upon herself, exhibited great anxiety and related how she had had to nurse an invalid mother and sacrifice her career for her, how she had come to hate the mother and to desire to injure her and had at last felt she could only avoid this by turning the injury against herself. Discussion of this situation was followed by a cure.

Mental Symptoms. The symptoms of hysteria which are obviously from the first of a mental kind are chiefly amnesias, somnambulisms, fugues, trances, hallucinations, dreamlike states and fits. They are all of dissociative type; that is, they are all to be regarded as the result of detachment and independent functioning of a part of the mental content. *La belle indifférence*, the typical mental attitude, is by no means always found. It tends to be a late feature, developing when disabling symptoms have become established. The lack of insight may then be striking. The patient denies any worries and insists that his symptoms are purely physical.

Amnesia is commonly of a circumscribed series of events in the patient's memory. It is as if a part of his life had dropped out, although the hysteric may not be aware of the gap in his recollection till it is pointed out to him. This amnesia usually hides some incident about which the patient has felt guilty, and he has forgotten what it would be painful for him to remember. Henderson recorded that amnesia sometimes served as a defence for desertion in war-time.

In some cases the amnesia is for the entire life up to a certain recent point. The patient may forget his own identity, the names and faces of his friends, even his wife and children. The amnesia is always for something with which a strong emotion has become associated. For example:

CASE NO. 6

A young flying officer who complained of insomnia and a terrifying dream of an aeroplane crash, with which he always awoke, could remember nothing of the events of a period of three days which began while he was at his flying depot, but ended with his finding himself in a hotel in London in mufti. In response to persuasive insistence, he reconstructed the period little by little. Asked to begin with the events preceding the first day of the amnesia, he gradually gave a consecutive account, although with many pauses and transient inability to recall, which were overcome by encouragement. It appeared that he had been for some time under stress, as he disliked and feared flying, and was at the same time engaged to be married. If he stopped flying, it meant breaking the engagement, for financial reasons. Finally his fear became so intense that he deserted. The amnesia was for the episodes connected with his desertion, including the exchange of some letters with his fiancée, announcing the step he had taken. The recovery of the lost memory was followed by disappearance of the insomnia and anxious dreams.

Fugues and Somnambulisms. In a hysterical fugue the patient suddenly leaves his previous activity and goes on a journey which has no apparent relation to what he has just been doing, and for which he has more or less complete amnesia afterwards. The lost memories may be recalled under hypnosis.

CASE NO. 7

A boy of 17, attending a military academy in the Southern States of America, repeatedly was found miles from his school (where he boarded) clad sometimes only in his pyjamas. On one occasion he was found at a place sixty miles from school, in a 'dissociated state', *i.e.* he was walking, avoiding obstacles, but with his eyes half closed, and unable to say where he had come from, or where he was going, or to give anything but his name.

He was in a condition identical with that occurring in somnambulism. Under observation he continued to have similar attacks, which occurred suddenly by day or night, the condition sometimes beginning with his falling on the floor (although he had been a few minutes before in ordinary health) in a state of complete flaccidity.

In a few minutes he would get up in the condition described above, and endeavour to leave the hospital. He did not reply to questions, but given a pencil and paper he wrote with his eyes closed a remarkable statement. This was to the effect that he had been hypnotized by a travelling showman many months before, who told him while he was in the hypnotic state that if he returned six months later to the place at which he had been hypnotized he would be released from his (the showman's) power. Otherwise, he said, the boy would remain under his influence. Later, while in the 'trance' state (flaccid paralysis with apparent oblivion to his surroundings), the patient related verbally the same story as he had written ('automatic writing') with a few more details, and still later he repeated it under hypnosis (he was easily hypnotized). The memories (which may well have been phantasies) revealed in hypnosis were brought into consciousness, but he continued to have attacks.

Somnambulisms are dissociated states identical with the above except that they begin during sleep. They are common in childhood, when their motivation often appears on the surface. For example, a boy much attached to his mother and antagonistic to his father, who treated him badly, in his somnambulisms would make for his parents' bedroom and endeavour to get in at the side of the bed on which his mother slept. Janet described 'monoideic' and 'polyideic' somnambulisms according to the poverty or wealth of mental content of the dissociated state. He pointed to the regularity of the development of each attack, the same features repeating themselves each time or (more rarely) each attack beginning as far as mental content is concerned where the other left off. Janet distinguished fugues from somnambulisms chiefly on the ground that the former last longer, and consequently require for their continuance more rapport with the surroundings. During the somnambulism the patient commonly lives through a vivid experience, little or not at all related to his surroundings, and therefore hallucinatory in character. By talking to him, not insistently, but in a persuasive attempt to enter into his experience, the patient may be got to describe the nature of the experience while he is still in the somnambulistic state. Although such patients appear to be 'walking in their sleep', they are not really asleep. Their perceptions are often acute. The Virginian schoolboy above described had his eyes apparently closed, but when one door was shut he turned away without hesitation and chose another which allowed him to pass from the hospital ward into a corridor.

Fugues occur in conditions other than hysteria: in epilepsy, for example, as post-ictal automatisms or as ictal phenomena in psychomotor seizures; and in depressions, when they may be suicidal equivalents.

Stengel (1941, 1943) has made interesting contributions to the understanding of fugues. Of the 25 cases reported in his earlier paper 10 were related in some way to epilepsy, 1 was a schizophrenic and the remainder were typical manic-depressives, hysterics and psychopaths. There appear to be, Stengel stated, 'three essential conditions without which fugue states do not develop: the tendency to indulge in periodic changes of mood, a disturbance of home conditions in child-hood, and a tendency towards the production of twilight states, the last factor being most prominent in epileptics'. He drew attention to the similarity between fugues and wandering states in children with disturbed home circumstances. Stengel's second paper reported 11 further cases in detail. In all these a tendency to depressive reactions of the constitutional type was noted, and in a number the transformation of a suicidal impulse into the impulse to wander was demonstrated.

Berrington and his colleagues (1956) reported findings in 37 cases. The following were the diagnostic categories: psychopathic states 24, hysteria 6, reactive depression 4, involutional depression 2, schizophrenia 1. They stressed the common factor of a depressive mood, and the rôle of head injury: severe head injury was found in 16 cases and doubtful head injury in 3 cases, as against 3 in controls. Ten of the patients were also alcoholic. Hysterical mechanisms were found to be fairly common and compulsive features rare. With regard to the rôle of head injury these authors concluded: 'We are not of the opinion that the organic trauma produced the fugue directly, but rather that it produced impairment which facilitated the occurrence of a psychogenic fugue, or that the concussion and subsequent amnesia formed the basis for the suggestion of a psychogenic amnesia at a later date. We incline to the latter viewpoint.'

A fugue should therefore not too hastily be diagnosed as hysterical. Detailed psychiatric and neurological assessment is required.

In *double or multiple personalities* there is a further elaboration of the process occurring in fugues and somnambulisms. The groups of dissociated functions are now so extensive that any of the dissociated groups is capable, when fully conscious and in charge of the motor functions, of appearing superficially as a complete personality. Stevenson's *Dr. Jekyll and Mr. Hyde* is a fictitious instance of this kind. William James recorded a case which has become famous:

CASE No. 8

A clergyman, the Rev. Ansell Bourne, disappeared from a town in Rhode Island. Eight weeks later a man calling himself A. J. Brown, who had rented a small shop six weeks previously in a town in Pennsylvania and had stocked it with confectionery, etc., woke up in a fright and asked who he was. He said he was a clergyman, that his name was Bourne, and that he knew nothing of the shop or of Brown. He was subsequently identified as the Rev. Ansell Bourne by his relatives, and remained terrified by the incident and unable to explain it.

In Morton Prince's patient, Sally Beauchamp, there were not two but several distinct personalities, which alternately occupied the field of consciousness.

Hysterical Fits. Hysterical fits can usually be distinguished from epileptic seizures, although there is an intermediary group very hard to assign definitely to one or other class. A true epileptic seizure can be provoked by emotional factors; and an epileptic may have hysterical fits.

The typical hysterical fit usually occurs only in the presence of others, and in the daytime, does not involve any but very minor injuries, is often provoked by an emotional situation, has a very variable duration and does not show the tonic-clonic succession, but consists of irregular movements, which have been supposed to have sometimes a symbolic significance, representing some emotional episode which the patient is re-living. Attempts to restrain the patient usually result in increased struggling. Tongue biting, incontinence and reflex changes do not occur: nor is the hysterical seizure followed by confusion, headache or nausea.

There are numerous anomalies in hysterical fits. Thus an elderly woman bent her head on her chest, screwed up her eyes (especially on an attempt to examine her pupils, which reacted normally during the fit), extended her right arm and rotated her forearm to and fro. She resisted both passive flexion and extension of the arm. The 'aura' was of a peculiar, visual hallucinatory kind in which she saw her mother's grave.

Hysterical *trances* and *stupors*, '*twilight states*' of altered consciousness, states of ecstasy, and hallucinations, are rarely encountered; and these types of reaction are much more often psychotic than hysterical. Much more common are dramatic scenes, in which the patient becomes acutely excited (usually following some frustration), 'acts out' and may threaten or attempt suicide.

Hysterical Pseudo-dementia. In situations in which a lack of mental responsibility, if recognized by the authorities, would bring some advantage, gross hysterical mental symptoms of a clearly purposeful nature may be developed. In prisoners awaiting trial, for example, and in persons still at large who have committed some illegal act, a state *non compos mentis* may excuse, or be conceived to excuse, the misdoer from the immediate legal consequences of his acts.

The patient may be unable to answer very simple questions: for example, he cannot tell the date. He cannot give a coherent account of himself and behaves in a simple, childish way. As Bleuler pointed out: 'What is characteristic is the disappearance of the memory for elementary knowledge and experience, which remains intact in the organic disturbances.'

The *Ganser syndrome*, or 'syndrome of approximate answers', was described first in prisoners. The patient gives bizarre replies to questions; for example, asked how many tails a sheep has, he will reply 'two', or if asked how many legs a horse has, he may say 'five'. Similarly asked to multiply 5 by 6, he will say (perhaps) 32. If requested to perform some simple action, the patient goes about it clumsily. Thus given a key and asked to lock a door, he will fumble and use the wrong end of the key. Dates will be given only approximately. We have seen the Ganser condition also in an acute hallucinatory paranoid state in one patient, and among the residuals of such a condition (probably alcoholic in origin) in another.

In some instances a much more elaborate attempt is made at dramatization, and in these the voluntary (simulated) element is much more clear.

Case No. 9

A banker from one of the Southern American States furnished a good example of an elaborate reaction which was very probably simulated. His bank had failed at a time when he had utilized, for investments in companies in which he was interested, money from the funds of the bank in excess of the 10 per cent. permitted by the laws of the State. When admitted to hospital he was mute, shook his head in answer to questions and refused food. An hour later he took supper, and answered some questions relevantly and coherently. Then he became mute again, and the same evening he got out of bed, lay on his back on the floor and propelled himself towards the wall with his feet. He next proceeded to make a show of 'climbing the walls'. He mildly but firmly resented being put to bed, smiled, showed his teeth and moved his lower jaw rapidly up and down. When being carried to another ward he held himself rigidly, so that he could almost have been supported horizontally by his head and heels. For the following two weeks he alternately was mute and talkative. When he did talk it was in a disconnected fashion with sometimes a peculiar verbigeration, as 'Mother—Mary—Mary—Mother —All Marys—All Mothers'. After two weeks he recovered suddenly. He denied that any legal trouble was pursuing him, but some weeks after he left hospital, completely well, a telegram was received from his lawyers asking for a certificate that he had been in a mental hospital, as the patient had been arrested for irregular dealing with the moneys of his bank.

There is a *hysterical puerilism* which is related to this 'pseudo-dementia'. In this there is a return to the behaviour of early childhood. McDougall (1926) cited a good instance, which he regarded as an example of regression to an ontogenetically earlier mode of behaviour.

Case No. 10

An Australian private, aged 22, after a series of experiences, including a bombardment and an air raid, 'reverted to the mode of life, bodily and mentally, which is normal to a child of some months of age'. With certain exceptions he showed no trace of comprehension of spoken or written language, and had little or no apparent understanding of the use of ordinary objects or utensils. He walked jerkily with feet wide apart, and, when allowed to do so, crawled on his buttocks. He had to be spoon-fed, and would take only milk and slops; if he took anything else, he complained of belly-ache and curled up in bed. A doll was his chief toy. Fears of animals, sudden noises, etc., were prominent. However, there were some aspects of his behaviour which were of a more adult kind—he smoked a cigarette when offered it, showed some knowledge of finger speech and swam well. From time to time he showed progress in learning, especially in handwork, and the use of gesture-language, but he repeatedly relapsed after small frights. Once he wrote his own nickname spontaneously, and he sometimes tried to kiss his nurse. He recovered gradually 'to an approximately normal condition'.

Hysteria and Simulation. The differentiation of these uncommon pseudo-dementias from simulated mental disorders is often difficult. To distinguish sharply between hysteria and simulation is in fact arbitrary. Simulation is the voluntary production of symptoms by an individual who has full knowledge of their voluntary origin. In hysteria there is typically no such knowledge, and the production of symptoms is the result of processes that are not fully conscious. Kretschmer rightly pointed out, however, that the criteria 'conscious or unconscious?' will not serve to distinguish simulation from hysteria, for not all the motives of a healthy mind are conscious, and not all hysterical ones are unconscious. There are all graduations between hysteria and simulation.

We would emphasize the importance of contradictions in the patient's story, discrepancies between his subjective account (of pain, for example) and his behaviour (whether he knows himself to be observed at the time or not), the presence of marked hysteriform symptoms with great profession of concern about them and clumsy unwillingness to be cured, *e.g.* complete forgetfulness for what has been told him at previous interviews. All these strongly suggest simulation.

Estimation of the aim of the illness, and of discrepancies between the loss occasioned by it and the apparent gain, is often not easy. The patient conceals the gain—if he is a hysteric, he conceals it from himself as well as from others—and there may be objects other than avoiding justice or gaining pecuniary advantages from disability, of which the value for the patient is difficult to assess.

Aetiology and Psychopathology

Despite intensive research over the past century by psychiatrists, neurologists and psychologists of great ability, hysteria remains in many of its aspects mysterious. Neither its aetiology nor its psychopathology has yet been fully worked out. The relationships between suggestibility, hypnosis and hysterical symptoms are complex. Hypnosis is a state of heightened suggestibility. Hypnosis can remove hysterical symptoms and induce phenomena akin to hysterical symptoms: but the hypnotic state, which can be induced in many normal individuals, is not an illness.

According to Dejerine (1911), hysteria resulted from emotional disturbance, but only in subjects with a peculiar emotional constitution. The emotional constitution of the hysteric was, he believed, shown in his or her tendency to react much more intensely than the normal to an emotional stimulus, and to react in a specific region, that is, in a particular organ or group of organs: the psychic representation of the function had a distinctive tendency to become dissociated from the seat of consciousness, and there was a peculiar passivity in the patient's attitude to the dissociated function. Dejerine performed a considerable service in stressing the part played by emotions and preoccupation with their bodily results, but his explanations of hysterical reactions lacked the precision and detail which were to be supplied by Freud.

'Hysteria', said Janet (1911), 'is a malady of the synthesis of the personality.' It is a form of mental depression characterized by restriction of the field of personal consciousness and a tendency to dissociation (that is, independent functioning) and emancipation of the systems of ideas and functions that constitute personality. There are two kinds of psychological functions, according to Janet—easy ones, requiring the co-operation of only a few elements; and difficult operations, which require the systematization of an infinite number of elements, involving a very new and intricate synthesis in each operation. When the 'nervous tension' or 'psychological force' is lowered by puberty, disease, fatigue or emotion (the last named involving great expenditure of nervous strength and therefore approaching fatigue) there is a general lowering of the level of psychological performance. Hence only the simple acts can be performed. In hysteria the lowering of psychological tension is localized in one particular function, which disappears in consequence from consciousness; it is 'dissociated' from the rest of the conscious personality. This dissociation is mainly of a function which has been weak or disturbed, especially if the function has been in activity at the moment of a great emotion. The function that disappears is commonly one that is very complicated and difficult for the subject: in this way, for example, professional and social paralyses are developed.

The objection to Janet's views is that they are a matter not so much of explanation as of description in terms of doubtful physical analogies. Except that the hysterical dissociation is said to occur at moments of great emotion, his hypotheses offer no explanation of what brings about the dissociation.

Freud, also a pupil of Charcot, began where the latter left off. Following up a discovery made by his colleague Breuer, that a hysterical patient became apparently well after a forgotten event of a personal and emotional nature was recalled under hypnosis, and after establishing further in some cases that the forgotten event had been of a sexual kind, Freud formulated the generalization that hysterical symptoms are memory-traces of sexual traumata—'the hysteric suffers from reminiscences'. Soon he modified this view to include among memories of aetiological importance not only those of actual traumata, but those of sexual experiences which had existed only in the patient's childish phantasies. He developed the concept that this sexual trauma (real or imagined) was the Oedipus complex, that it was repressed in early childhood, that this repression failed in later life only if some contemporary event reactivated by association the early repressed memories, and that a repressed Oedipus complex was in fact the necessary condition for the development of hysteria in later life. Sexual frustration in adult life led to an infantile type of (forbidden) love-object being again sought out. The hysterical symptoms are the result of a conflict between the super-ego and wishes not palatable to the super-ego which seek expression. Repression is only partially successful: the forbidden wishes succeed in gaining a disguised expression by 'conversion' into the symptom, which is therefore in a sense a symbol. The localization of the physical sign or symptom is determined by various factors—especially the appropriateness of the particular sign or symptom to symbolize the repressed wish, but also by accidental factors such as a previous physical disability.

The Freudian explanation can hardly be accepted as having universal validity; it is probably true only for a proportion of hysterics. It is impossible, for example, to see anything sexual in the aetiology of hysteria occurring in the soldier on the field of battle, or in peace-time as the result of injury involving questions of compensation. The purposive aspect of hysterical dissociations is particularly evident in the hysterias of war-time, the hysterical disability making further service in the danger zone impossible. The reaction is to observers obviously purposive and self-protective, but the hysterical individual is not himself consciously aware of his evasion. Therefore he is not malingering.

A case history will serve to bring out the more frequent complexity of the situations in which hysterical symptoms are developed, the emotions involved, the influence of both heredity and environment, the part played by patterns of reaction acquired in childhood, the unconscious determination of the locus of the symptoms, the purpose of the individual symptoms and the aim of the illness, and its unsatisfactory nature as a solution of the problem.

CASE No. 11

The patient, a married man of 40, complained of exhaustion, tremor of right side of body, giddiness, pain in right side, photophobia (right eye) and jerking of body and limbs.

A maternal uncle had had a brief episode of elation followed by depression. A maternal aunt died in a mental hospital of 'religious mania' at 45 years. The maternal grandfather died from jumping out of a window. The patient had no children, his wife being 'delicate'.

Personal History—He was always 'very nervous' of his father, who was very severe in his punishments. In his boyhood the patient was thrashed every day for a week, put on dry bread and water and deprived of his clothes. While at school (from 5 to 15 years) the father made his son work in the garden before school hours from 4.30 a.m. The father was a very large man physically, and the patient was terrorized. His ambition was to be an engineer, but his father frustrated him, and he took up clerical work. He remained at this and has been fairly successful.

After the war he returned to his previous business, not from a strong desire to do so, but ostensibly from a sense of obligation because his employers had treated him very well during his absence.

He was a very ambitious man, fond of decorations and of social distinction, and was somewhat ashamed of the fact that he did not occupy an executive position in the office. His general attitude was one of some superiority, but this was not marked, and tinged with a good deal of uncertainty about himself and his position. His financial position was an unusually good one, largely from his own efforts.

Present Illness—In October the patient was transferred to work of a type which displeased him in several ways. He was told that excess of work had been deliberately added to his predecessor, 'in order to make or break him'. His predecessor had succeeded in doing it, although he had had a 'nervous breakdown' previously. Further, the work was much less congenial than the patient's previous work, and involved much more writing. It also savoured of degradation in rank. His immediate superior was domineering, and the patient disliked him, and, on account of his position, feared him. The superior had the reputation of being unable to keep assistants. The patient decided to make the best of it and to give the new work a three months' trial. Soon he found the work very difficult to overtake, and on most days he was exhausted even in the mornings. He began to sleep badly and obtained sick leave in the following May. In the previous November his father had had a stroke, and the patient for three months thereafter made a special journey every day to shave him. He 'couldn't stand being at work all day and then doing this'. While on leave he received a letter asking him to resign. This 'hurt' him very much, and he 'got such terrific pains', especially on his right side, that tears ran out of his eyes. He felt he was very badly treated. The pains in his right side were so bad that he could not lie on it for a time. Right-sided tremor began also at this time. His doctor reproved his superior for sending such a letter, and the patient returned to work. Four days before his return, however, his right hand swelled, with shooting pains in it. He thought, 'Am I getting some creeping paralysis?' He subsequently remembered that many years previously at business he had noticed his hand numb after much writing, and still earlier after writing impositions at school. His hand had been swollen for some time in France (frost-bite?). This painful swelling of the hand incapacitated him for anything except the type of work he had done before his transfer in October. On his return to work he was in consequence placed on an easy but menial task, which hurt his dignity still more. His condition did not in any way improve, and when his chief ultimately told him he was slacking, he felt this was the last straw, and practically did not sleep at all afterwards till he finally abandoned work two weeks later.

He was slightly depressed, and displayed considerable subdued resentment towards his business superiors, mingled with a fear of them and of their opinion, although he had no reason to fear the financial consequences of losing his job. He recovered rapidly with psychotherapy.

One of the most striking aspects of this patient's make-up was his ambition for the outward signs of success. Another was his timid, schoolboyish attitude to his superiors. Both these characteristics were marks of an underlying feeling of inferiority; and the manifestations of both of them entered largely into the foundations of his illness. His ambitious vanity produced an intense emotional revulsion from the new conditions of his work (which was a preponderating interest despite his financial independence), while his juvenile attitude helped to prevent his taking any action. Even verbal expression of his resentment he found difficult. If it is attempted to trace the origin of his feeling of inferiority with its special manifestation of timidity towards his superiors, it is difficult not to suppose that his remarkable early experiences at the hands of his father were responsible for it. Furthermore, his father's denial of an education to him while it was given to his younger brother added to his inferiority in another direction.

This patient exemplifies also the transition from a condition of conflict with anxiety into hysteria with 'conversion' symptoms (paralysis of arm, pains, right-sided tremor). The hysterical solution, however, was an unusually poor and incomplete one. The patient remained uncomfortable in mind for the greater part of the time. He was much too ambitious to be pleased with such an unsatisfactory compromise. The unsympathetic attitude of his immediate superior, while it helped to produce the illness, also seemed to shorten it, since the symptoms were not permitted to achieve their object—resignation was suggested and not reinstatement. The case is interesting also in that it shows with unusual directness the symbolic nature of certain bodily pains—the receipt of a letter whose contents were painful to his self-respect was followed at once by 'great pain' in his right side. The relation of the paresis of his right arm to his reluctance to do his new work has to be inferred, but with considerable certainty, from the connections of the facts recorded.

Hysteria seems to occur chiefly or entirely in persons particularly predisposed, either by inheritance or the effects of their early environment, to mental dissociation. The actual occurrence of this dissociation depends on the problems which the individual encounters on his or her way through life. The symptom developed is symbolic in the sense that it has a meaning for the patient. This meaning is eventually purposive, the symptom being a solution, however unsatisfactory, of some problem of everyday adaptation. The patient is unaware of the real meaning. If he thinks about it at all, he believes the symptoms mean simply an illness in the ordinary sense. From these two facts—that the symptom is a solution of a problem, and that it is misinterpreted by the patient's consciousness—arises the patient's *belle indifférence*. The onset of the symptom may not always involve repression, but only a mental conflict without repression. The conflict leads to emotion and its physical manifestations. These are misinterpreted as the outcome of physical disease, and physical disease suggests disability of the part affected. Suggestion operates powerfully where there is mental conflict, and as the suggestion of disease is in harmony with one side of the conflict—the desire to escape— the suggestion is accepted and the symptom results. There is a gain of mental composure, since the conflict is solved, but at the expense of part of the personality, since suggestion operates primarily at the mental level, and can isolate a function only at that level. The actual problem may remain in the patient's mind; but it is no longer acute, since the symptom has provided a solution of an indirect kind. But the connection between the problem and the symptom is not seen by the patient. The connection cannot so much be said to be repressed as to be neglected. Only in some such way as this can it be explained that in many a psychological analysis of hysteria nothing that was not conscious before— although it may not have been clearly defined, or alluded to—may be brought out, and yet the symptoms disappear as their causations and connections are exhibited.

Where repression does occur, the same processes will serve to explain the occurrence of symptoms. For the production of symptoms at all means a partial failure of repression: if repression has partly failed, conflict conscious or unconscious exists, and conflict is the condition that led to the formation of symptoms in the way already set forth. These theories hold for the physical symptoms of hysteria.

With the mental symptoms of hysteria a similar process occurs. In hysterical amnesia, for example, there has been a period of conflict; then emotional preoccupation prevents the subject's noticing events in the ordinary way, consequently the memory of them, when the conflict has died down (they are registered marginally), is vague; vagueness of memory suggests complete failure of it, the patient does not wish to remember in any case—again the emotional symptom coincides with the wish—we accept what we wish to believe, and so does the hysterical patient—and an amnesia results.

An exactly similar process will account for fugues—the patient starts out on his fugue simply with a consciousness whose clearness is disturbed by emotional conflict, and ends with an amnesia. In a fugue there need not be repression at the beginning—the amnesia is an end-product. Where a fugue-habit has once been established, however, dissociation appears to occur at the beginning of each fugue.

Differential Diagnosis

In every case a careful physical examination is essential either to exclude physical disease or injury, or to define it if it is also present. There may of course be no physical disease and this is the usual situation: but on the other hand there may be hysterical aggravation of an existing injury (for example, a hysterical paralysis of an arm with a flesh wound), or organic nervous system disease may have released hysterical symptoms. Hysteria is often mistaken for physical disease, and physical disease is often called hysteria. Central nervous system disease is not infrequently miscalled hysteria in its earlier stages: cases of brain tumour, encephalitis and disseminated sclerosis may be thus misdiagnosed. Myasthenia gravis may be thought to be hysterical weakness. It is helpful to remember that the hysteric does not usually look physically ill (anorexia nervosa is, of course, an exception), and that hysterical symptoms in young people are often of dramatically sudden onset—which is unlike physical disease at that age. Hysterical-seeming symptoms occurring for the first time in middle age or later should always be suspected of being organically determined.

Hysterical fits may be difficult to distinguish from epileptic fits. A careful description of the attacks is essential. A full examination will include electro-encephalography.

To establish the diagnosis of a neurotic reaction, it is essential not only to exclude physical disease but to demonstrate that the illness is psychogenic. There must be positive as well as negative grounds for diagnosing hysteria. One must be able to link the hysterical symptoms understandably with a life-situation which has presented difficulties to the patient. His or her previous personality must, of course, be taken closely into account in assessing these environmental factors.

If the reaction is clearly neurotic, then the doctor must assess the importance of the hysterical features and determine whether they are primary or secondary. Hysterical symptoms may, for example, be developed by a patient with an anxiety neurosis, or anxiety appear in a reaction which is predominantly hysterical. Too much should not be made of these distinctions, but they may have some bearing on treatment.

Hysterical reactions rarely appear like psychoses. Fugues and stupors here present the chief problems in differential diagnosis. The personality of the individual, and the development and whole setting of the symptoms, must be taken into account. A stupor in a young person is more often schizophrenic than hysterical.

OBSESSIONAL NEUROSIS

Definition of the Reaction-type

In common usage the terms obsession, obsessed and obsessional signify that an individual is in some way preoccupied or harassed or haunted. In delimiting an obsessional neurosis the term obsession must be used with more precise meaning. Schneider proposed the following definition of obsessions—'contents of consciousness, which, when they occur, are accompanied by the experience of subjective compulsion, and which cannot be got rid of, though on quiet reflection they are recognized as senseless'. This was later modified by Aubrey Lewis, to give a definition which is now widely accepted—'Whenever a patient complains of some mental experience which is accompanied by a feeling of subjective compulsion, so that he does not willingly entertain it, but, on the contrary, does his utmost to get rid of it, that is an obsession.' The three essential elements are the feeling of subjective compulsion, the resistance to it and the retention of insight.

Obsessional symptoms may occur in many different kinds of nervous and mental illness, neurotic and psychotic, 'functional' and organic. In an obsessional neurosis they form the kernel of the illness and its presenting and predominant symptoms. The patient's peace of mind is seriously disturbed by these symptoms and his daily life is to a lesser or greater extent hindered and disrupted by them.

The term obsessional neurosis includes both obsessive-ruminative and obsessive-compulsive states.

Clinical Features

Obsessional neuroses are the most constitutionally determined and the least common of the neurotic reaction-types, comprising less than 5 per cent. of the total of cases.

The majority of those who develop an obsessional neurosis have shown previously personality traits which are conventionally described as constituting the *obsessional personality*. These traits are an unusual conscientiousness and adherence to method, order and cleanliness. Their possessors are described as fastidious, meticulous, fussy and tidy, punctual, persistent, painstaking and hardworking, prone to recheck rigorously what they do, liking to have everything 'just so' and 'cut and dried', rigid and often pedantic. Samuel Pepys said of himself—'My delight is in the neatness of everything, and so cannot be pleased with anything unless it be very neat, which is a strange folly.' Though these characteristics are commonly called obsessional, it is obvious that very many normal people who never become nervously ill exhibit these traits. Also, if the possessor of these traits is subjected to stress and breaks down, he is more liable to develop a depression or a 'psychosomatic' syndrome than an obsessional neurosis. Furthermore, some of those who develop an obsessional neurosis have not had obsessional personality traits: Pollitt (1960) in a review of 115 cases found that 34 per cent. had had no obsessional traits before breakdown. It may be said therefore that the grouping of these particular traits together and the giving to them of the title 'obsessional' does not have a faultless theoretical basis.

Lewis (1935) described, in the nuclear group of chronic severe obsessionals, two types of previous personality—'the one obstinate, morose, irritable, the other vacillating, uncertain of himself, submissive'.

Psychoanalysts, notably Freud, Abraham and Ernest Jones, have called these obsessional traits 'anal' or 'anal-erotic' (constituting the *anal-erotic character*'), believing that these traits preponderate in persons whose instinctual life has been anally orientated, and that these traits are partly reaction-formations against anal-erotic activities and partly sublimations of them. The main anal-erotic traits are held by psychoanalysts to be orderliness, frugality and obstinacy. Frugality is considered to be a continuation of the anal habit of retention, orderliness an elaboration of obedience to the environment's requirements about excretion, and obstinacy a continuing rebellion against these same requirements. The instinctual conflicts are commonly fought out around problems of money and time—'no compulsion neurotic can handle time and money rationally'—he is stingy or prodigal or both alternately. Psychoanalytic explorations of these anal-erotic traits have been carried out in fascinating detail and many acute observations have been made (they are summarized by Fenichel, 1946). Attention has been drawn to the irritability and frequent bad temper of the obsessional, the evidence of aggression and sadism he often reveals and his reaction-formations against these trends. Ernest Jones (1948), in a classic exposition of anal-erotic character traits, demonstrated the complexity of the interrelations of the different anal-erotic components with one another and with other constituents of the whole character.

Like the other neurotic reactions, obsessional neuroses develop usually in early adult life. In Pollitt's (1960) series of cases the mean age of onset of the main illness was 28 years, but about half the patients had previously suffered from obsessional symptoms, either very transiently or in attacks which had cleared up after some months: many had had their first obsessional symptoms between the ages of 11 and 15 years. An obsessional neurosis may be a single illness, lasting only months, or it may take a phasic or cyclic course; but there is a marked tendency for it to become insidiously established and to develop in severity over a period of many years.

Symptoms and Signs

Obsessional symptoms may take several forms—phobias; intrusive ideas or images or rumination; impulses and compulsive acts.

A *phobia* is a recurrent intense, unreasonable fear associated with some situation or object or idea. The external focus of the fear varies according to the individual sufferer's history. The patient realizes that his fear is irrational, but he is dominated by it. If he enters the fear-producing situation, anxiety, acute tension or panic assail him. Previously various Greek and Latin names were assigned to these phobias—agoraphobia—fear of open spaces, claustrophobia—fear of closed spaces and so on. The phobia may be a fear of a recurrence of an attack of anxiety with pronounced somatic symptoms which has once previously occurred, for example, in a crowd (agoraphobia) or in a railway compartment or in Church (claustrophobia). Or the phobia may be of dirt, or disease, or animals, or sharp instruments—or many other things. The relationship with anxiety states is close, but the fear has the typical obsessional quality.

CASE NO. 12

A man of 39 complained that he had fear of open spaces, of large rooms and of meeting people. The reason he gave was that such situations produced 'panics' in which he felt giddy, trembled, had curious sensations in his legs and saw everything as if through a mist. The panics lasted sometimes for many minutes, and in the intervals he was more or less always apprehensive of them. He had been subject to occasional panics in open spaces or large buildings since later childhood, but this had not interfered with his work until four months before he came for advice. They had increased in frequency until he was entirely disabled. The first panic of any kind had occurred in a schoolroom when he was 11 years of age, when there was an epidemic of mumps in the school and the patient feared he might be infected. Suddenly he felt a lump in his throat, and wondered if it meant mumps. A schoolmate said, 'You look pale—are you ill?' and the patient promptly became very much afraid and had a panic similar in all respects to those from which he suffered in later life. The patient was a married man, with one child. For some years he had suffered from premature ejaculations and his wife in the last eighteen months had seemed very cold towards him. He had a feeling of guilt with regard to her, because he had flirted a good deal about a year ago. He had a recurring dream of missing a train, sometimes accompanied by an emission. In addition to this, he gave in response to inquiry the information that he was in business or partnership with his father-in-law. Business had not been going well for two years past. He was in some awe of his father-in-law, feeling that he was inferior to him, and was afraid to discuss business with him. Another relative was in the same business and the patient did not get on well with her. His financial affairs were in a serious muddle. Speaking of his family and financial affairs, and not the specifically sexual ones, he said—'I never talked to anyone like this before. . . . They were subconscious. . . . I had always shelved these things.' He gradually lost all his fears, except that of open spaces; dissolved partnership; went to work elsewhere; was divorced, and married again.

Obsessional ideas and images are disturbing and often very distressing: they may be frightening, blasphemous, disgusting or obscene. Their intrusive nature is characteristic. One patient described it as—'it is like being chained, my mind is gripped by the thought, it is torture to me': another said, 'If I try to divert my attention from the thoughts, the more I seem to get back to them. If I keep trying to tell my mind to forget about them, I seem to remember them all the more.'

A few examples may be given. A man aged 39 complained that his mind seemed to follow the same pattern all the time, certain words ('vivid thoughts') went persistently through his mind—'cancer, heart attack, mouth'. Sometimes these words were grouped into a phrase, 'I won't have a heart attack worrying about cancer in the mouth.' Then he had the thought that if he worried about this, he 'wouldn't go wrong in the mind'. Another young man had recurrent frightening thoughts about violence, about how he would react in an emergency if he were attacked, thoughts of fighting and being killed, of being buried alive or drawn into machinery. A single woman aged 38 was tortured by blasphemous thoughts: 'God is ——', the thought would come into her mind, some obscene epithet being used. Then she tried to fight this thought by doing or saying something before the obscene thought was complete: she would repeat to herself, 'Nobody's a ——', or in order to prove that she did not mean it she would perform certain movements, lifting her arm sideways or forwards.

The characteristic feature of *obsessional rumination* is the continuous pre-occupation with some topic or group of topics, to the exclusion of most other interests and to the distress of the patient. The relationship of some obsessive-ruminative conditions to anxiety states is close. Nevertheless there is a clear clinical difference between an anxious preoccupation and a true obsessive one: in the former it is the anxiety that is objected to by the patient, in the latter the thought-content itself is seen by the patient to be morbid. The topic of the rumination is commonly religious, philosophical or metaphysical, something that permits interminable, inconclusive thought, the origin of the universe or the destiny of man. The subject of one young man's rumination was—'we are all like that, the animals of the forest are like that, creedless and without thought and we were like that once'. Dan Leno proposed an ideal subject: 'Ah, what is man? Wherefore does he why? Whence did he whence? Whither is he withering?' It may take the form of an internal debate or catechizing, the pros and cons stated again and again and argued without cease, or be like, as one patient described it, a trial in a Court of Law. 'I must analyse my thoughts and must repeat them but I'm always aware they are my own thoughts. Its like a prosecuting counsel. He gets up to say something and the defence counsel makes an objection. It may be shouted down but he has planted a thought in the jury's mind. The prosecuting counsel makes the suggestion to me and I'm the jury.'

On the borderland of obsessional rumination are those states of obsessive thinking where the ideas themselves are not meaningless nor of indifferent interest or irrelevant—they are on the contrary legitimate subjects for reflection: but 1. their persistent obtrusiveness is inexplicable; and 2. the patient does not regard them as pathological intruders. In such cases the subject with which the individual is preoccupied has a clear relation to the rest of the content of consciousness and an obvious affective relationship. The following case was an example of this type:

CASE NO. 13

A tall, very thin young man of 20, who had recently been unable to follow his occupation because his mind was totally occupied by speculations about religion. To his friends he had seemed to think and talk of nothing else. He explained that for two years he had been very much troubled by the divisions he saw existing in the Church, and said, 'I can't get them out of my mind. I can't assimilate the attitude of religious meetings.' At one of these where a woman evangelist had spoken, the patient was 'very much upset'. 'She laid down the law. It made me feel very uncomfortable. There always seems to be some sort of mystery about the Church. . . . What is Christianity?—that is the point. Why are some people so religious?—There is something funny about their appearance. . . . The different religions—that's what bothers me.' Hymns in church disturbed him: 'They seem so ruthless, sweeping everyone aside.' He spoke of the awed feeling with which he looked on a king as similar to his feeling towards religion generally. He had also a feeling of 'suspicion' regarding his choice of profession, as he felt he had been pushed into it. But it was significant that he designated his attitude to the world generally as 'suspicious'. It transpired that his feeling of being upset at a religious meeting was closely paralleled by an emotional experience which he had when 12 years of age, when he had listened to a difference of opinion between his parents and had sided with his father. The patient came to define his attitude to religious matters and to the world as one of fear, which made him physically sick and his mind a blank. This attitude was closely similar to the attitude he had held towards older boys when he first went to school. 'It goes very far back—those young boys at school.' In other words, it appeared that in facing the problems connected with emancipation from home he was reproducing in part and more intensely the affective attitudes belonging to an earlier age, and further that the obsessive preoccupation with religious matters depended on a discrepancy between religion as he found it in the world and his preoccupations regarding it. The discrepancy reanimated the fearful type of affect which had characterized his childish attitudes, and the fear supplied the motive power for the obsessive thinking.

In the case of this young man there was an obvious conflict between his childish concepts and reality, and an inability to modify the former in the light of real experience: the rôle of the unconscious concepts was not realized by the patient. He ceased to be preoccupied after three months' psychotherapy.

Another form of obsessional thinking is *persistent doubting—'folie du doute'*: the individual is never sure that he has completed a certain action, and may have to go back repeatedly to assure himself that he has done so. He may have to look several times to see if he has turned off the gas downstairs, or check repeatedly his addition of sums or measurement of lengths of material, or he may feel unsure whether or not he has behaved wrongly. A woman, who had impulses to strike children in prams, would when a pram had passed her wonder if she had in fact hit or killed the child. She would then become intensely and painfully preoccupied with trying to reconstruct in her mind exactly what had happened, becoming in the process more and more certain that she had killed the child, requiring repeated reassurance that she had not, but never quite reaching certainty either way, always doubting. The obsessional may be continually vacillating, like Mr. T. S. Eliot's J. Alfred Prufrock, who found that 'In a minute there is time for decisions and revisions which a minute will reverse.'

Some obsessional patients become preoccupied with numbers and have, for example, to count letters in words or do or avoid doing certain things a certain number of times. A patient under our care recently was obsessed with the number two. He delayed his admission to hospital because he had noticed that it had been arranged for the second day of the second week of the fourth month. He refused his night sedative because it consisted of two capsules, and would not make a rug in the occupational therapy department because he was given two colours and a pattern which he saw in multiples of two. He carried this avoidance of the number two into every sphere of his life, even in tying his shoelaces.

Obsessional Impulses and Compulsive Acts. The impulses of the obsessional are often aggressive—to attack, injure or kill. They may be directed against other people, for example, a puerperal woman may have impulses to strike or kill her baby; or the patient may have a recurrent and strong urge to kill himself, by throwing himself from a height, it may be, or under a moving vehicle. A young unmarried woman, to give another example, had recurrent impulses to kick, beat or otherwise interfere with children and other defenceless people: this caused her to keep her hands in her pockets when she was outside or to carry a shopping bag to keep her hands engaged. An impulse to injure is commonly associated with a phobia of weapons or potential weapons, razors, knives, scissors, etc. The impulse can be on the other hand to commit some social aggression—to laugh or swear aloud in church, for instance. The obsessional aggressive impulse nearly always remains an impulse; it is not carried out. The exception to this generalization is that the individual with obsessional impulses

M

to self-injury may, if he or she becomes depressed, commit suicide. The obsessional's illness does not drive him to crime.

Compulsive acts are stereotyped, usually innocuous behaviour, which the patient feels compelled to carry out. The urge to carry out these acts is pressing, even imperative, and if the patient resists this urge he becomes tense and anxious. Many of these compulsive acts resemble the superstitious observances of everyday life, but the latter are much more easily resisted; they can often be understood as prohibitions or penances. One of the classic examples is compulsive handwashing, which is accompanied often by a phobia of dirt or contamination, and which may readily be interpreted as a symbolic cleansing of impulses and memories of which the patient feels guilty. Lady Macbeth is an examplar.

A few further examples may be given. A man aged 41 had had for eleven years a compulsion, when he passed any scrap of paper in the street, to return and pick it up: he felt that if he did not do this, his parents would die. This caused him to be seen in many ridiculous situations as well as to be constantly late for work, appointments and his meals. Another man, 31 years of age, always an extremely neat and tidy person, could not bear to see things unfinished or in disorder, and had to straighten out creases and wrinkles wherever he observed them. He had also the compulsion to touch things with his right thumb. He would pass a telegraph pole and try to avoid touching it, and then have to turn back to touch it ('*folie du toucher*'), feeling that if he did not touch it something would befall himself or the people he loved. He also felt compelled to cross the road at a certain point so that he could step over a manhole, and he was often unable to resist the urge to stand for a certain period of time on the manhole cover. A man in his twenties developed a phobia of infection and connected this with a cousin whom he resented. He felt compelled to wash money because this had been in contact with his clothes which in turn may have been in contact with a door handle via his hands or with furniture in his mother's house, and this furniture had been touched by his cousin or his cousin's father. This chain reaction became almost unending, so that there was scarcely a thing in his house or on his person that he could not have reason for washing and which he had not in fact at some time washed.

In all his symptoms the obsessional shows a great tendency to perseveration and repetition, to rituals and protective devices, to self-doubt and self-torment: and he is prone to become more and more involved in a tangle of fears, impulses and compulsive acts. He cannot argue himself out of his preoccupations, nor banish his phobias by trying to drive himself through the situations in which they occur. He is usually tense and anxious, and very often becomes intermittently depressed in spirits. His insight is maintained, except at times of crisis when it may temporarily be swamped in his emotional upset. Usually he manages, though with great difficulty sometimes, to carry on with his daily job: rarely does he become quite disabled or even immobilized by phobias and rituals.

Aetiology and Psychopathology

The main aetiological factor in obsessional neurosis appears to be heredity.

Obsessional traits and obsessional illness are found in significant concentration in the families of obsessionals—in about one-third of the parents and one-fifth of the sibs. Lewis (1935), in a review of 50 cases of obsessional neurosis, found that 37 of the parents showed pronounced obsessional traits, and in a number of instances both parents were obsessional: 43 of 206 siblings showed mild or severe obsessional traits.

Perhaps one should say, at a time when our knowledge is still very incomplete, that the main causal factor appears to be the individual's constitution, since the effects of heredity and early environment are so difficult to separate and we do not have findings from any large group of twins to guide us. The obsessional child or adult may either have inherited these trends from an obsessional parent or parents, or been drilled into obsessional modes of behaviour by them. Certainly one frequently obtains the history of an unusually strict or puritanical upbringing, with much insistence on rectitude and cleanliness.

The obsessional personality may shade into the illness, by the insidious aggravation of the pre-existing trends. In many cases, but not in all, some emotional stress, some situation producing major worries or conflict, may be seen to have precipitated the illness.

Physical factors may also be of aetiological importance. An obsessional neurosis may be precipitated by physical illness or prolonged fatigue. Encephalitis lethargica may produce obsessional symptoms, with or without forced movements, in an individual who has not been obsessional before.

The mental mechanisms most prominent in the development of obsessional symptoms are repression, displacement and substitution. Repressed earlier drives and memories gain symbolic representation in the symptoms. The writings of Freud and his school should be consulted for a full exposition of the complicated psychoanalytic theories of the illness's genesis. If one may paraphrase very briefly and superficially the analytic viewpoint, it can be stated somewhat as follows. There is in the obsessional neuroses regression to the anal-sadistic stage of libido development, at which there has been a developmental fixation. Memories of early traumata and difficulties at that stage, either spontaneously or because they are revived associatively by some contemporary experience, tend to return to consciousness. The ideas and emotions, often aggressive, are of a kind intolerable to the patient's super-ego and in relation to this the affect is usually one of reproach. The ego has to defend itself and tries to keep the intolerable ideas out of consciousness by substituting other ideas, indifferent in themselves. In the compulsive variety of the illness, not ideas but acts are substituted. What maintains the substituted ideas or acts in consciousness is the affect of reproach, which the patient does not succeed in getting rid of when he treats the intolerable ideas in this way: the reproach attaches itself to the substituted ideas or acts.

In the case of phobias there is a displacement of the fear from its real source to some associated object. For example, a girl had such a persistent phobia of bichloride of mercury tablets that she remained confined to her room for two years. Such tablets were associated in her mind with an illicit pregnancy, which had been both desired and feared. Aggressive impulses may be displaced into a phobia of knives, forbidden sexual drives into a venerophobia. The phobia serves as a defence against realization of the real problem.

A simple type of obsessive thinking is initiated by a desire to keep some unpleasant thought out of one's mind by thinking continually of something else. The obsessive idea continues as long as the necessity for repression of the unpleasant thought lasts, and sometimes to all appearances longer, as a habit. Freud recounts the case of a woman who was continuously brooding over such questions as, 'Why must I breathe?' She had been afraid of becoming insane, and to reassure herself she had begun to catechize herself on serious problems. This quieted her at first, but soon her fear was completely replaced by the habit of speculation, which lasted for years.

A very frequent basis of an obsessive rumination is an opposition between a desire and a fear. There is a desire, more or less unconscious, for something which the ego itself cannot permit, and a conscious dread as a reaction to the desire. This conflict may be fairly simply expressed. Greenacre quoted the case of a clergyman, who had distressing impulses to sing 'Dim-dam-dimmity, dammity' to the tune of some hymn. Even here, however, the matter was not simple, for there was a certain amount of symbolization. The obsession to use profane language symbolized his desire to be rid of the burdensome restrictions of his calling. An extension of this principle of the basis of obsessive preoccupation in the conflict between a wish and a fear enables us to understand the following case, in which there was an obvious wish followed by fears of homicide.

CASE No. 14

A Russian Jewish tailor, aged 35, married, and with three children. He complained that for six months he had been obsessed, to his immense distress, by a desire to kill his wife and children and to commit suicide. If he saw a river he wanted to jump in; a window would tempt him to jump out. He had had to leave work, and suffered from insomnia, his obsessive thoughts being worst during the night. It transpired that six months before the development of obsessive symptoms business had become very bad, and he was worried and mildly depressed. One evening he read in the newspaper that the Home Secretary advocated the deportation of aliens. This angered him and he 'wished he were the Lord that he might dismiss the Home Secretary'. Then it occurred to him that such thoughts portended madness. At this he felt 'hot all over', left his room and went out of doors, where he felt he wanted to assault a bystander, just as he would have liked to assault the Home Secretary. This alarmed him still more, and he became afraid that he would assault his wife and children in the same way.

The transition from an obsessive-ruminative condition to an obsessive-compulsive state is easily understood. The compulsion is a method of mastering the fear. The act chosen as a defence against the desire is usually mentally connected with the latter in some way—as a simple association, or as a symbol. The origin of certain compulsive acts is well seen in children, where they are motivated by a fear of some impending disaster. This is exemplified in the next case, where the fear was that of scholastic failure.

CASE No. 15

A boy of 13 was brought by his mother because he 'had to touch everything twice'. He would often go back to a door which he knew to be closed, reopen it and close it again.

He frequently was seen to smell his cap. All these symptoms had existed for six months. He had had a scholastic examination three months after the symptoms began, which, however, he had successfully passed. With considerable reluctance and some tears, the boy, who was a fresh-complexioned well-built youngster, related how he had been dreading the examination, that he wanted very much to pass, but was afraid he would not do so, and that he had begun to touch articles twice and go through the other ceremonials mentioned because he feared he might be 'unlucky' if he omitted them. The compulsive acts had persisted as habits after the occasion for them had passed, and his fear of bad luck became generalized. With this confession, which he had refused to his mother, and some simple reassurances, he quickly improved.

In the obsessive-compulsive states of adult life the mechanisms may be similar, but they are not usually so superficially clear as in the case just quoted.

Differential Diagnosis

We have already pointed out that many normal people show obsessional traits in their personalities, and under the influence of fatigue or physical ill-health these traits may become more prominent: the individual may indulge temporarily, for example, in an unusual amount of obsessional re-checking (going back to see if the light has been switched off, the back door shut and so on). But these minor things do not amount to a neurosis.

Many children, too, have ritualistic activities, and apparent obsessive-compulsive traits, but these are not usually to be taken very seriously unless they are unduly marked or persistent: some of these repetitive activities the child obviously enjoys, which is quite unlike obsessional neurosis. It is recorded of the poet W. B. Yeats that when he was a boy, before he had any knowledge of Latin, he loved to repeat the phrase 'Magna est veritas et praevalebit', and that he went about for days repeating a phrase which he had heard from a village boy, 'I saw thee and the little brothers and the maids at church.'

Occasionally the severe obsessional's rituals seem so bizarre and his trains of thought so far-fetched, that he is diagnosed to be schizophrenic. Much more often, the differential diagnosis lies between an obsessional neurosis and a depressive psychosis with secondary obsessional symptoms (a common conjunction of symptoms). The differentiation may be very difficult. Some obsessional neuroses, in their lack of external precipitants, in their recurrent attacks or cyclic course, closely resemble manic-depressive depressions, and some of these apparently obsessional illnesses may in fact be masked depressions. But not all these cases, where the illness is of more acute onset and the course limited, are depressed. It is only by close scrutiny of the history and of the patient's whole behaviour and symptomatology that one can determine whether the illness is fundamentally affective or obsessional.

Transitions to Psychosis. Rarely an obsessional neurosis passes into a psychosis.

CASE NO. 16
A man, aged 50, complained at first that he could not stop worrying about such apparently senseless topics as where he had thrown a match, and could not sleep for wondering whether the house door was closed. He was also much preoccupied with his anal zone. He remembered that he had had much itching there, and that he had scratched himself

to the effusion of blood. Although no interpretations were given him of any kind he contemplated with horror the possibility that he might have scratched himself for pleasure. Soon also the fear occurred to him that he was thinking of his anus and his masseur in conjunction. These fears and homosexual thoughts took the place of his earlier obsessive preoccupation with indifferent topics, and drove him to avoid completely the company of men. He used such phrases as 'It's *not* a wish; it's a fear that the dread will turn into a wish.' Then he began to believe that he had been homosexually assaulted. There had been a gradual clearly evident transition from obsessive preoccupation with indifferent topics to obsessive sexual ideas, and finally to delusions of assault, with the development of a paranoid psychosis.

Gordon (1926) described 6 cases in which an obsessive-compulsive state had been followed by a psychosis: in 4 of the 6 patients the development was to a paranoid psychosis. It may be noted that both obsessional and paranoid states show a marked tendency to systematization and chronicity, and that the previous personality is characteristically rigid. Stengel (1945) found no report in the literature where the psychotic reaction occurring in an obsessional neurotic was of the hebephrenic or catatonic variety, and commented that schizophrenic reactions occurring in obsessionals show a tendency to remission and that if deterioration does set in it develops slowly over many years. Stengel's paper, in which 14 cases are presented, gives a comprehensive review of the relationships between obsessional neuroses and psychotic reactions. He draws attention to the prevalence of aggressive-destructive obsessional ideas and compulsions during depressive states occurring in obsessional patients, and to the suicidal risk in this type of case: and expresses the opinion that the obsessional personality structure, by exercising a strong integrating influence, is capable of subduing and aborting schizophrenic reactions.

OTHER NEUROTIC AND ALLIED REACTIONS

Neuroses following Trauma

The terms 'traumatic neurosis' and 'traumatic psychoneurosis' should be abandoned. The neuroses which follow trauma differ in no essential way from the neuroses which have other precipitants.

The trauma may be psychological or physical: and when it has been of primary importance in the aetiology, it has usually been sudden and intense. In the cases where physical trauma has occurred, the effects of physical injury may complicate the emotional reaction, and after head injury in particular it may be difficult to separate physical from emotional sequelae. Post-concussional syndromes are discussed on p. 414. In all these cases questions of compensation may arise.

A psychologically traumatic, terrifying experience may produce an immediate response of extreme anxiety or wild panic: or there may be apparent calm with development of symptoms after a latent period. The symptoms that follow the fright are usually insomnia with terrifying dreams from which the patient wakes time and again—these dreams representing the accident in more or less distorted form. Anxiety symptoms occur during the day, especially lack of concentration and uneasiness of mind, and the bodily discomforts of anxiety, such as tremor or palpitation. Such symptoms may appear even in the most stable individual if the experience is severe enough; but they usually diminish and ultimately disappear, although it seems likely that they are readily revived by subsequent analogous experience.

The following is an example of a neurosis consisting in acute anxiety at the time, subsequent anxiety symptoms and prolonged associative or conditioned revival of the symptoms amounting to panic when the situation encountered reproduced, after nearly twenty years, more closely than ever before, the circumstances of the original experience.

CASE No. 17

An air gunner, aged 33, who had previously flown without symptoms, occupying the rear turret of a bomber for the first time was seized with acute panic on a practice flight. When he was released from the turret his breathing was observed to be deep and noisy. It was remarked by his medical officer that on the ground he had shown no symptoms at all. His history revealed that at the age of 14 he had a particularly disturbing experience when he found himself one Saturday afternoon shut in the vaults of the office in which he worked; moreover, soon after he found the exit closed against him, the lights went out and the watchman went off for the week-end. He became increasingly uneasy, and the intensity of his anxiety can be gauged from the fact that it was only after many hours that he noticed in the darkness a little red bulb which had the word 'Pull' printed on it. This set off the burglar alarm throughout the building, which after nearly 24 hours' incarceration brought people to his rescue. The air had become increasingly hot and dry, or so it seemed to him, and his prevailing fear during his imprisonment was that of being suffocated. The door was opened and he ran out in a state of extreme tension. He was off work and in bed for the two days following. For nearly two years afterwards he had nightmares in which usually he was in a tunnel which caved in on him. He remarked, apropos of the episode in the rear turret, that his breathing when he left the turret was very much the same as he recollected it when he got out of the vault. His pilot remarked that he 'sounded like a steam engine'. He was a man of stable character and temperament, and in the intervening years he was apparently well; but closer investigation showed that he had had mild claustrophobic symptoms all the time since the original trauma. When he drove a car it was always with the windows open, and he chose to drive a tourer rather than a saloon. On the first occasion in which he travelled in a tube train he had the thought that it was a risky business, but he was reassured by the lights and the open platform. For some time after his original experience he refused to take the elevator to his place of work, which was on the fourth floor—he walked up the stairs. This phobia he ultimately surmounted.

The period which normally elapses between an acute emotional trauma and the onset of neurotic symptoms is of considerable interest, both from the point of view of differential diagnosis from organic conditions as well as psychologically. Evidently the latent period is filled with ruminations, but the memory of these is usually difficult to recover—they were probably ill-defined in the first instance and underwent repression with the development of the symptoms.

It is reported that after a Vesuvian eruption all the survivors were at first emotionally upset; after three months only a few—and those obviously predisposed—showed neuroses; and after six months no one showed any ill-effects. There was no question of compensation in this instance, and the short duration of the neurotic phenomena, even in those predisposed, is an interesting contrast to what very frequently occurs in cases where monetary compensation is concerned—in workmen after accidents in their work, in railway passengers after a rail smash, and the like, when the symptoms tend to remain till compensation is settled. In some cases following trauma a sense of grievance, and even a desire for revenge, help to sustain the symptoms until compensation or some other satisfaction is obtained. This will obviously be more common where an employee is dissatisfied with the general conditions of his employment, or where the employer does not make satisfactory arrangements for rehabilitation. It is claimed that in large organizations where the disabled workman is given some kind of job as soon as he is fit to do any at all, and is gradually restored to as near his previous status as possible, compensation neuroses virtually do not exist. Sometimes an accident impinges upon an individual who is in the throes of a mental conflict on some personal issue and the symptoms may then be exploited unconsciously as an escape, however temporary, from an apparently insoluble problem.

Neurasthenia

This syndrome classically comprised the following symptoms—complaints of mental and physical fatigue, associated with sensations of pressure in the head, poor memory, inability to concentrate, irritability of temper, poor sleep and various aches and pains. It was first described by Beard in 1880 and quickly became so popular a diagnosis that by 1894 Muller was able to furnish a bibliography of fourteen pages. Now it is rarely recorded by clinicians, though the individual symptoms of the syndrome are of course still commonly complained of by both neurotic and psychotic patients. Being suggestible, neurotic patients mirror medical preoccupations. Neurasthenic symptoms were common while physicians were interested in fatigue syndromes, expected them frequently and sought them diligently: and they became much less common when medical interest in them waned.

Overwork being obviously related to fatigue, it was assumed by many that neurasthenic symptoms were identical with fatigue and must have an identical cause. On this assumption was based Weir Mitchell's treatment by absolute rest, in which the patients were not allowed even to feed themselves, lest they incurred unnecessary expenditure of energy. Overwork is an aetiological theory sometimes offered by neurotic patients because overwork is a creditable thing, but a closer investigation of the history does not often reveal that the hours worked have been excessive. It is emotional disturbances which produce fatigue, much more often than physical fatigue initiates illness.

Fatigue and allied complaints may, in our experience, be the expression of one of several types of emotional perturbation. They may be the simple result of conscious mental conflicts. If the conflicts persist, the symptoms also persist, and the latter may come to be autonomous, the patient observing them and dwelling upon them and shifting this preoccupation from the original problem to his physical health. Or fatigue may be the expression of some less conscious difficulties: it is then often a conversion phenomenon and really a hysterical symptom. Again, affective depression is commonly accompanied by fatigue; not uncommonly it is the fatigue rather than the depression of which the patient complains; or fatigue may wholly replace depression and is then a symptomatic equivalent of the latter. Finally, fatigue symptoms may arise in the course of any psychosis, 'functional' or organic.

Unreality States

Feelings of unreality may take two forms—the patient himself feels unreal (depersonalization) or the world around him seems unreal (derealization). The affected individual may complain of both types of change, but derealization is very uncommon without depersonalization.

Reactions in which unreality is a leading symptom do not comprise a distinct clinical entity. Mild feelings of unreality may be experienced by the normal individual in the setting of unusual fatigue. Feelings of unreality may also be symptoms of almost any neurotic or psychotic illness, occurring in anxiety and obsessional neuroses more often than in hysteria, in depressive psychoses and in schizophrenia, in cases of temporal lobe epilepsy (in close association with *déjà vu* phenomena) and in other organic reaction-types. The abnormal feelings may be very transient, or recurrent, or persist for months or years.

As presenting symptoms feelings of unreality are commonest in young adults of anxious or obsessional temperament: but many patients with unreality do not complain of it spontaneously, either because they find it hard to put their experience into words, or are not sufficiently introspective, or are afraid of being thought insane. The abnormal feelings are unpleasant and distressing.

The onset is often sudden, with sensations of faintness or dizziness, followed by a fear of impending collapse or insanity—the latter often persists. The patient complains of feeling unreal, emotionally dull or flat, mechanical and like an automaton; his voice or his face in the mirror may seem strange to him, and his experience of time may be altered, so that for example the recent past seems remote. If he experiences derealization too the outer world may seem far away, indistinct, misty, drained of colour. Sometimes the patient says that it is as if a shutter or glass screen had come down between him and the outer world, from which he has become shut off in some subtle but frightening way. The patient retains his insight, realizing that he is nervously unwell; he has no delusions that he or the world has altered fundamentally, it is 'as if' there had been a great change. Neither the psychological nor the possible physiological basis of these feelings is fully understood.

Shorvon (1946) gave a comprehensive and valuable review of 66 patients with depersonalization (46 females, 20 males), and suggested that these cases could be considered to form a distinct clinical entity, the depersonalization syndrome. He drew attention to a 'constellation of constitutional deviations', which included obsessional personality, migraine and mild non-specific cerebral dysrhythmia; and to the tendency of the syndrome to occur in more than averagely intelligent but emotionally immature individuals, with a history of unsatisfactory parent-child relationships. Thirty-eight per cent. of his cases suffered from migraine, and in 21 per cent. there was a family history of migraine: many ceased to have migraine attacks with the onset of depersonalization. Shorvon also noted that the onset is often related to relaxation following intense or prolonged stimulation or stress, and that a few cases are helped by stimulation by ether abreaction. This study increased our knowledge of depersonalization symptoms, but Shorvon did not make out a convincing case for accepting depersonalization as a separate syndrome: his patient material was selected, being drawn from out-patients and those seen at a neuropsychiatric unit, and excluded obviously psychotic patients.

Ackner (1954) reviewed the literature, and concluded that depersonalization should be used as a generic term for a number of different syndromes, often related only by a loose similarity of complaint.

TREATMENT OF THE NEUROSES

Psychotherapy is the main form of treatment of neurotic reactions. It developed out of the 'moral treatment' of the nineteenth century, and there are now numerous methods of psychotherapy, superficial and deep, eclectic and special-ized by the various schools (Freudian, Jungian, Adlerian and others). It may take the form of counselling, support, abreaction, analysis, conditioning, sugges-tion or hypnosis, or be a mixture of these techniques. It may be conducted individually, that is with a single patient, or in groups large or small.

The neurotic patient should usually have psychotherapy as an out-patient, individual treatment sessions lasting up to one hour and being spaced (daily, weekly and so on) according to the individual patient's needs. These needs range from good advice at one end of the scale to prolonged and detailed analysis of a complex illness at the other. Successful treatment takes usually a matter of months: it may be quicker, and if it is taking longer than six months or so the situation should be very carefully reviewed. The initial diagnosis and approach may have been mistaken, or the patient be so limited constitutionally that psycho-therapy could be interminable and still unavailing.

The general practitioner should be competent himself to carry out the simpler forms of psychotherapy, and is best placed to treat neurotic symptoms quickly, before faulty habits of reaction have become entrenched. If his psychotherapy is not successful within a few months, he should refer the patient to a psychiatrist for more detailed assessment and investigation. It is better to refer to a specialist too soon than too late.

Much depends in psychotherapy on the quality of the attention which the doctor gives to these unhappy and bewildered people, and therefore on his own personality, insight and wisdom. He must be interested, sympathetic, patient and above all a good listener. If he is critical or censorious, these timid people will shy away from him: and unfortunately many doctors, despite the improvements which have taken place in both professional and lay education in the field of mental health, still feel irritation at the sight of personal failure and still too often tell the patient to 'pull himself together'. On the other hand, if the doctor is over-sympathetic and paternal, he may foster a dependence which will be as unhealthy for the patient as it is likely to be inconvenient and embarrassing to himself. It is probably true that the outcome of psychotherapy depends more on the personality of the therapist than on the particular technique employed. Furthermore, the successful therapist is usually modest enough to allow that much depends on time and changing circumstances, and on the patient's native powers of readjustment and recovery. One's attitude should be melioristic rather than too ambitious, aiming at an improvement in happiness and efficiency rather than at dramatic cures.

Two preliminaries are essential to psychotherapy—the taking of a detailed chronological history and a careful physical examination.

It is advisable, before proceeding with any explanation or reassurance (and these are frequently asked for by the patient even before the end of the initial interview), to find out what the patient himself thinks is wrong with him. Usually he has his own views and theories about his symptoms defined to some extent, and the longer he has been ill the better defined and elaborated they will be. It is also useful to know what he has been taught by other doctors, so that one may not be unsuspectingly led into the position of contradicting another man's opinion. The other physician may be, at least in the patient's eyes, a greater authority than you are: in which case, unless you are forearmed, your dicta may not avail much if they should chance to be in opposition to his. Views that the patient has already formed of his illness are commonly of a physical aetiology, and acceptable to his ego-ideal. If these views are discovered by the doctor beforehand, they can be dealt with much more effectively.

The doctor, whether he be general practitioner or psychiatrist, should carry out the physical examination of the patient himself. It is nonsense to say, as some psychoanalysts have claimed, that to do this is to prejudice one's psychotherapeutic relationship with the patient. The opposite is true: not to carry out a full and painstaking physical examination is both bad medical practice and poor psychotherapeutic strategy. If physical disease is found, this should be fully investigated and dealt with at the outset: it may of course have played some part in causing the neurotic breakdown.

The next step is to inform the patient that his symptoms are not due to any physical disease. The doctor must be able to reassure his patient on this point, with confidence; any hedging or hesitation may be fatal to one's ability to help the patient. Occasionally this reassurance is curative: the anxious patient with fears of heart disease, loses them, or the patient of low intelligence with hysterical symptoms recovers when following an impressive physical examination he is informed authoritatively that recovery is imminent. In the vast majority reassurance is not enough. The disclosure to the patient that he is not, as he had thought or feared, physically ill, must be done very tactfully: it is a critical moment in handling the patient's problems. The patient is liable to react acutely, with the feeling 'He thinks there's nothing wrong with me, that I am imagining it all or putting it on.' The doctor must therefore go on immediately to say that the absence of physical disease is a matter for congratulation, and that it does not mean that the patient's symptoms are imaginary. He should say that he realizes that the patient's symptoms are real and distressing, and that all doctors recognize that the symptoms caused by nervous and emotional upset are as unpleasant and as painful and disabling often as those caused by physical disease. He must then explain how anxiety, worry, depression or other emotional upset can produce both nervous and physical symptoms: how anxieties tend to be repressed into a subconscious part of the mind, with the production of inner tension, and how this inner tension gains expression in symptoms. He may tell the patient how, for example, emotional tension is accompanied by muscle tension, and how tense muscles become painful and fatigued; how excitement makes the heart race and may cause frequency of micturition or looseness of the bowels; and how anxiety may be expressed alternatively in panic attacks or phobias or obsessions. In this way the patient is brought to an understanding that there have been good reasons for his symptoms, but reasons probably of a kind quite different from what he had believed.

The general nature of psychotherapy and its objects must now be explained to the patient: and here we must add that the patient's relatives should not be left out of the treatment situation—normally the nearest relative should be interviewed, not only for the purpose of obtaining a full history of the patient's illness, but also to be told in general terms what is wrong with the patient and by what method of treatment it is hoped to help him. The patient himself is told that, with the doctor's help, the influence of various events on his mind and feelings will be explored, that there may have been important events and connections which he has forgotten or of which he has not been fully aware, and that it will be an essential part of the treatment that he talks freely of his memories, feelings, motives, attitudes and so on. If the doctor fails to give this explanation of the treatment, the patient is liable soon to conclude that he is getting no treatment, that there is just talk; and he may well cease to attend for something so esoterically different from the kind of medicine he had expected. The patient may ask how long the treatment will take. The doctor should on no account commit himself in reply, but say only that they will both have to see how quickly progress can be made. The patient may be reassured, if he asks, that this kind of treatment is likely to be helpful, but he should not be promised a cure. It is very important from the beginning to make it clear that the treatment will be a co-operative effort, and that success will not depend on the doctor alone.

At this stage one goes back usually to the patient's history. A detailed account must be obtained, not only of the illness but of the patient's life generally: and usually a number of exploratory interviews are given over to this. It is a good rule to accept almost nothing that seems at once important in the history, at its face value. Reports of previous physical illnesses, especially if they have borne such equivocal labels as influenza, anaemia, rheumatism or debility, must be investigated closely. It is desirable to survey the patient as widely as possible, and to regard the symptoms as arising not usually as an isolated response to one factor but as part of a wide problem of adaptation. Any mental unrest forms a fertile soil for the development of neurotic reactions. There is often fairly easily traceable an immediate cause which has precipitated the symptoms: but behind this there is usually a predisposition, the nature and determinants of which are much less easily ascertained.

It is now the task of the physician in collaboration with his patient to collate the chronological development of the patient's symptoms with the events of his life, or more strictly with the mental events which have accompanied them, so that the reasons for his present behaviour and symptoms can be found. It is best to take the most prominent symptoms first, and to take the patient back over his mental history to their onset. Then he is asked to recall as far as possible all that happened at that time, and what his thoughts were about the events and about himself. If he cannot reconstruct sufficiently what was going on in response to ordinary questions, or preferably as a narrative in response to a vague general question, the method of free association may be tried: but this latter is a method that works well only with a minority of patients.

By this time the chronological relation of most of the symptoms, and the relation of their first onset and their recurrences to events in the patient's life and to his phantasies (ambitions, reflections upon events), will be fairly clear to the physician. They will also have begun to be clear to the patient. Often at first he will deny that anything occurred at the time of onset of a given symptom. He will assure his doctor that nothing whatever took place at that time. But often a little later he will remember and will communicate what he has recollected— fragmentarily at first, more fully later. This may occur without pressure, the original question having set a train of thoughts going. For example, a woman of 35 complained that she had suffered from abdominal symptoms (nausea and discomfort) since she was 19. She at first denied altogether that anything had happened at that time. Two days later, without further reference to the subject in the meantime, she volunteered that she had been disgusted at that age by an assault from a very ugly man. Another patient who had recurrent attacks of trembling (at first associated with being called up for military service) had an attack in November 1923, which had lasted till he came under observation, and had disabled him from work. He at first denied that anything whatever had occurred in November 1923; but finally, in response to a general question, and after much reflection, saying he knew of nothing important at that time, he said— 'Why, I got married then!' He saw the point, and laughed. His tremors disappeared, and he returned to work.

This, the development of insight, is one of the most important elements in successful psychotherapy. The more the patient can be allowed gradually to see things for himself, and the less direct explanation given to him in consequence, the better and the quicker in the long run. The more the patient contributes to his own recovery, the more permanent that recovery is likely to be. There is a considerable difference between the demonstration by the doctor of a cause and the patient's acceptance of a causal explanation. There is often some reluctance ('resistance') on the patient's part to accepting it, which is not surprising since a neurosis is an intensely personal affair and is usually in some degree a defence against unpleasant truth.

During the exploration of the patient's mental history, the objective is to bring back into full consciousness, against more or less 'resistance' on the patient's part, the mental events and conflicts which have been associated with the development of symptoms. The recall of these events and the uncovering of forgotten memories may be emotionally very disturbing to the patient, especially if these events have been associated with strong and painful feelings (of guilt, for example). The patient should, however, be helped always to recover both the memories and the feelings associated with them, and to experience these feelings again intensely. The release of pent-up, repressed emotions is often a vital part of the therapeutic process: it is known as abreaction or catharsis. It may be necessary to take the patient back again and again to the memories of a period of great unhappiness: and to give barbiturate drugs, by mouth or intravenously (so-called 'narco-analysis'), to disinhibit the patient and make recall and emotional expression easier.

It must always be kept in mind that the exploration and revival of past mental events is designed to be part of a process of re-education. The repressed material which is recovered must be used constructively, to increase the patient's self-awareness and to help him to deal more adequately with his life's problems. Like surgery, psychotherapy must have a plan of action, and sewing up must follow opening up. Neither the patient nor his therapist should lose touch with the realities of the patient's everyday life. Successful psychotherapy should strengthen the patient's ego, as well as relieving his symptoms: it should make him by re-learning a more self-reliant human being.

When the symptoms are not found to be accounted for satisfactorily in terms of external situations, and when consequently they appear to be mainly constitutionally determined, the investigation has to be carried further back into the early formative influences of the patient's personality—his relation to parents, brothers and sisters and companions, his reactions to dangers real or imaginary, and to sexual experiences, his ideals, aims, religious attitudes and the like. Something of this kind is desirable in practically every case. How far to go in this deeper exploration depends upon the requirements of the particular patient. One aims to help the patient to unravel the tangle of childhood memories, phantasies and feelings, and at the same time to realize more comprehensively his personal assets and liabilities, to bring the former into use and to mitigate the latter by understanding how they have arisen and how they may be compensated for.

There are patients whose resistance to becoming well is considerable, who leave all effort to the physician and believe stultifyingly in his miracle-working powers; and it is necessary to discover why the patient wishes to be so dependent and to lead him to independence away from his or her childlike or actually erotic attitude to the physician. Other patients who are among the most difficult to make well are those with a general attitude of superiority. Their symptoms are even more with them than with others an emblem of their attempts to preserve their self-respect. To teach them a new attitude to life is the task of the physician. This new attitude may not be necessary for the disappearance of the symptoms: these patients may rush off to some spa or special nursing home where they are treated with ultra-violet rays, or radiant heat, or colonic lavage or what not, and these treatments, implying as they do a physical and therefore objective or even heroic aetiology of their trouble, may bring about symptomatic relief. But the illness is not cured in these physical ways, and the patient's liability to breakdown is as great as, perhaps greater than, before.

The deeper exploration of a patient's personality concerns itself much with unconscious factors, and is the province of the specialist. Special techniques are used, the discovery of which we owe almost entirely to Freud and to his development of psychoanalysis. The main psychoanalytic techniques, which will only be outlined here, have been free association, dream interpretation and analysis of the transference. They are now used to a greater or lesser extent, with numerous modifications, by most psychotherapists and not only by those who have been trained by other analysts.

The technique of 'free association' consists in asking the patient to relate without reserve whatever comes into his mind, no matter how irrelevant it may seem or how personally objectionable it may be. The doctor may intervene seldom, except to urge the patient when the flow of his talk becomes temporarily arrested. Where an arrest of this kind occurs, it is said to be due to 'resistance', which may be either a more or less conscious desire to withhold some unpalatable piece of information or may be due to influences that are wholly unconscious— those of the super-ego. At suitable junctures interpretations of the material offered by the patient are given by the therapist, who bases these interpretations on the general theory of psychoanalysis and makes use of such concepts as repression, displacement, sublimation, rationalization and other 'defence mechanisms'.

Similarly, to obtain an account of the patient's dreams is often useful, both for suggesting topics for investigation and especially for throwing light on unconscious factors: but interpretations have to be very carefully based upon the patient's associations and not the physician's, and the time for unveiling them has to be carefully chosen.

Between a doctor and his patient there is normally rapport, and a feeling on the patient's side of trust and confidence. This rapport becomes heightened during any prolonged psychotherapy, and the feeling which then springs up in a patient towards the doctor with whom he or she is closeted for so long a time has been called the 'transference'. It is usually a mixture of affection and dislike. There are two aspects of transference. In the first place, it is held that the psychotherapist is made to occupy in the patient's mind various rôles formerly played by the patient's parents, brothers, sisters and others, in early life. Secondly, in accordance with this, the patient feels with regard to the analyst the emotions of love, hate, fear and so forth, which he once experienced towards those other people in his infancy and childhood, some of which he sooner or later repressed. Undoubtedly something of this kind happens, particularly when psychotherapy is lengthy or pushed deeply: and the therapist must be sensitive to the complexity of the emotional situation. Later psychoanalytic theory and practice has gone further, and by many analysts the analysis and interpretation of the transference is now considered the essential therapeutic process. The task of the analyst is said to be to employ this transference of emotion to overcome the patient's 'resistances', and to take advantage of the revival of the old situations to have them dissected consciously, and the reason for their repression clearly exhibited. This process also gives the patient an opportunity to abreact the original feelings connected with these early situations.

Psychoanalysis as a Therapeutic Measure

Any well-founded psychotherapy will employ some at least of the principles so fruitfully emphasized, if not always first propounded, in psychoanalytic theory. As a theory, or congeries of theories, there is no doubt of the epoch-making importance of psychoanalysis not merely in the field of mental disorders but in normal psychology. It was of course founded by Freud on his observations of neurotics. But when it comes to assessing the value of classical psychoanalysis as a method of treatment of neurotics we are on much more uncertain ground. There can be no doubt that wrongly used psychoanalysis can be dangerous, and at best it is a therapeutic method of limited applicability.

'Psychoanalytic therapy was created through and for the treatment of patients permanently unfitted for life.' Freud himself mainly restricted his treatment to chronic neurotics, and we are of the opinion that this restriction is a very proper one. He considered that the conditions peculiarly favourable for psychoanalysis are hysteria and obsessional neuroses. But probably most analysts would now agree that whatever may be the theoretical justifications for treating obsessive-compulsive states analytically, they are peculiarly resistant to psychotherapy.

Freud also laid it down that the patient must be intelligent, and that he must have a certain amount of education, and a certain degree of 'ethical development —deep-rooted malformation of character, traits of a degenerative condition . . . can scarcely be overcome'. Further, the patient must not be too old: if his age is 'near or above the fifties . . . the mass of psychical material can no longer be thoroughly inspected, the time required for recovery is too long and the ability to undo psychic processes begins to grow weaker'. The patient must also be co-operative and desire help in this way. Finally, as far as the patient is concerned, he must have considerable resources of time and (usually) money, since psychoanalysis is long, arduous and expensive. The patient may have to devote an hour five days a week to the treatment, over a period of two or three or more years. The expense of the treatment is usually considered to furnish a valuable motive to benefit from it. It should be added that neuroses complicated by compensation issues are not suitable for psychoanalysis.

The limitations of psychoanalytic therapy appear, therefore, on Freud's own showing to be considerable and to narrow the field so as to exclude the great majority of those who attend our psychiatric clinics. We consider that there are further limitations which may arise in individual cases. It seems necessary to estimate beforehand the possible effects of submitting to a prolonged analysis even a patient who conforms to all the above requirements; whether, for example, persons of a sensitive, idealistic type who have met their difficulties by interest in social, philanthropic and religious works should be submitted to the profoundly disturbing influence of psychoanalysis rather than be treated by the simpler methods described earlier in this chapter. The physician must also have a clear view of the circumstances surrounding the onset of a neurosis: where immediate material circumstances, for example disappointment in a career, financial difficulties and the like, play a large part, it is superfluous and often harmful to enter upon a course of psychoanalysis.

For details of psychoanalytic treatment the reader is referred to the volumes of Freud's complete psychological works. He was a most lucid expositor of his own methods.

Jung was the most important analyst to diverge from Freud's theories and methods. Laying less emphasis on the sexual interpretation of symptoms, he regarded each neurotic illness as an attempt at solution of the general problems of the patient's life. Symptoms and symbols generally he interpreted in a more abstract way than Freud did, in terms of an unconscious which is not only individual but collective (an inheritance of the experience of earlier generations), and of archetypes, which are mythical ideas and images of particular importance and at the same time of esoteric significance. Jung found his technique of analytical psychology of most value with older patients.

Group Psychotherapy

In group psychotherapy the individual patient is the subject of treatment and the group itself is the main therapeutic agency. Psychotherapeutic groups consist usually of less than a dozen individuals, with a therapist who acts the rôle of 'participant observer'. Free, uninhibited discussion is encouraged amongst the group, and interpretations are offered by the therapist, usually along psychoanalytic lines with elucidation of interpersonal relationships and dynamics: but methods vary as much as do those of individual psychotherapy. In the group the patient shares a social experience with a substitute family. His social isolation may be overcome and his social readjustment effected. Group psychotherapy can certainly be justified on economic grounds, since psychotherapists are few and patients many: and it is claimed that it has beneficial effects of its own which cannot be obtained from individual psychotherapy. Foulkes and Anthony (1957) have given a comprehensive account of it.

Conditioning Therapy

Wholly distinct from analytic psychotherapy are the methods of treatment derived from Pavlov and learning theory, and advocated recently by Eysenck (1960) and others. Unconscious conflicts are disregarded and treatment is symptomatic, a conditioning therapy employing methods which are described as reciprocal inhibition, positive conditioning, and aversion therapy *inter alia*. Success has for some time been claimed for the aversion therapy (by emetine or apomorphine) of alcoholism, and the positive conditioning (by electrical pad and

N

buzzer) of nocturnal enuretics. This type of treatment is still, however, largely experimental, tentative and unproven.

Physical Methods of Treatment

The neurotic patient's general health must be cared for, and if there has been a considerable loss of weight, admission to hospital for a short period and the giving of modified insulin treatment to bring about a gain in weight, may be very helpful.

Drugs should be used very sparingly in the treatment of neurotics: and it is better, if possible, to do without them. The neurotic patient easily becomes dependent on tension-easing drugs, and addicted to them. It is also bad therapeutic tactics to make the patient too comfortable, since the discomfort of his symptoms acts as a spur to drive him through their psychological treatment. If the patient's tension is relieved by drugs, all too often he feels that this is sufficient; and he goes on taking the drugs because when he ceases to do so his symptoms return in full force. He is like the patient in cardiac failure who manages fairly well while he is digitalized: but compensation is never properly achieved and the neurotic usually needs his drugs in increasing doses.

The drug most effective for the relief of neurotic tension is amylobarbitone sodium, in 1 to 2 gr. doses given twice or thrice a day. It is particularly effective in the relief of anticipatory tension and in the treatment of acute anxiety attacks. Other barbiturates may be prescribed instead, and it is often advisable to ring the changes on them, if sedation is necessary for a prolonged period. Three of the most useful, quickly acting sedatives for those who cannot get to sleep at nights because of their anxiety, are pentobarbitone sodium, $1\frac{1}{2}$ to 3 gr., quinalbarbitone sodium in the same dosage, and cyclobarbitone, 3 to 6 gr.

The newer tranquillizing drugs have not been of much assistance in the treatment of neurotics. Euphoriant drugs should be avoided, again because of the risk of addiction: so should alcohol.

Environmental Adjustments

Where adjustments can be made in the domestic circumstances, or in the conditions of work, and where such adjustments are justifiable, the circumstances and conditions being positively morbid or disadvantageous, the physician derives much indirect therapeutic aid from whatever changes in this direction he is able to effect. The services of a psychiatric social worker are often of great value in this respect. In the case of hysterical patients in particular, to take the patient out of the stressful environment—whether this be a school where he is unhappy, or a job which is disliked, or a situation of war-time danger—may be sufficient for complete relief of the symptoms. But this is the easy way out, and it must be kept in mind that to follow such a course of action may be demoralizing. The neurotic patient commonly himself or herself suggests changing the environment, often in a dramatic way—a different spouse is wanted, or a new house, or a move to a new country, and the physician has in most cases to say that this will not do, that difficulties must be faced and overcome, not burked.

Cases following trauma when a legal action for damages is pending, or compensation is involved in some form or another, are very refractory to treatment. Such cases should be assessed by a consultant. A lump sum settlement of compensation claims has been shown to be a very unsatisfactory method of dealing with these situations. Dr. Carl Norcross, examining 321 cases three years after their settlement for a lump sum averaging 3000 dollars, found that 67 of his 321 cases had some form of neurosis, and that of the 67 only one case had made a complete recovery, the remaining 66 being divided into three equal groups: the first 22 had returned to work, but their average weekly earnings were down by over 40 per cent.; the second 22 had not improved but were back at work, with their average weekly earnings down by over 60 per cent.; while the last 22 were none of them at work, 2 being dead and 17 on the rates. Several of the original 321 had developed neuroses since the settlement of their claims. Too much is hoped often from the settlement of claims: it seldom results in a rapid cure. There are some cases in which the persistence of symptoms depends on a dread of return to the particular class of work at which the accident occurred, and in these the remedy of transfer to other work is obvious.

Treatment of Hysterical Symptoms

Suggestion plays some part probably in all psychotherapy: it may have to be used deliberately in the treatment of hysteria. Like other neurotic patients hysterics are suggestible, and their symptoms will often be influenced by therapeutic suggestions: but one of the dangers of treatment by suggestion alone, is that the disappearance of one hysterical symptom is apt to be followed by the appearance of others. Treatment should therefore not be confined to suggestion and to a superficial, symptomatic level, but should include exploration and explanation along the lines already described in the general discussion of psychotherapeutic procedures. The cause of the symptoms must be found and dealt with. The peculiarly disabling nature of certain hysterical symptoms may however mean that they have to be treated before a deeper psychotherapy is possible: deafness, mutism and amnesia are obvious examples of this.

In the great majority of cases it is possible, by gaining the patient's confidence and by the exercise of firmness as well as tact, to persuade him that the lost function is recoverable, that he can move his hitherto rigid arm, or walk upon his seemingly powerless legs. For this kind of treatment, immediate complete success is necessary and the doctor must believe it can be achieved. Piecemeal improvement is tedious and often temporary. The doctor should choose a day when he can devote, if necessary, an hour or more to the patient. The patient must be informed that the doctor does not intend to leave him until the limb is moved. The doctor then shows (often against actual physical resistance) that the movements can be done passively, and this being done he orders the patient to walk or to use the arm as the case may be. In walking, support is given at first, but the patient is told that if he tends to fall the support will be insufficient. Complete function must be restored at one sitting by this method. Incomplete restoration means the perpetuation of an incomplete function for weeks or months. In a proportion of cases the symptom is a hysterical habit which has outlived its usefulness, and which the patient would gladly be rid of, if he knew how. Such patients are easily amenable to treatment. The difference between 'trying' to move a limb—which involves a fear or a belief that it will not—and belief that it will move must be explained to the patient. Baudouin put it crudely but cleverly when he said that for the removal of symptoms the power of the imagination is inversely as the square of the will.

Mutism can be dealt with at a sitting by a determined attempt at persuasion and re-education. The patient is told to place his mouth and lips in certain positions. He readily does so. He is then shown that by placing them in certain positions and making sudden movements of them he can whisper consonants. Soon he can whisper sentences. It should then be pointed out that he thought he could not whisper, whereas it is proved that he can. He has then to be told with assurance that he can put his voice into it. He usually responds by doing so. Aphonia is usually a more difficult symptom to treat, partly because it causes less inconvenience than mutism.

If simple persuasion and suggestion fail, recourse can be had to intravenous barbiturates (amylobarbitone sodium or thiopentone) or hypnosis. In patients who have already shown a decided tendency to dissociations (in amnesias, trance-states, fugues, etc.), hypnosis is usually easy and may be the simplest method of recovering the content of episodes for which there is amnesia. Barbiturate narcosis is perhaps to be preferred, since hypnosis tends to make the patient unduly dependent on the therapist. By neither method are memories likely to be recalled unless the patient is willing that they should be. Amnesias which involve the whole of the individual's past life, with loss of identity, clear up spontaneously.

Cases of anorexia nervosa should be admitted to the psychiatric unit of a general hospital. Special feeding and close nursing supervision should begin at once. Meals, light and nutritious, should be supervised until everything is being eaten, and the patient must be given no opportunity to conceal food instead of consuming it or to vomit immediately after meals. Chlorpromazine in large doses, soluble insulin in small appetizer doses and testosterone to aid nitrogen retention, may all be helpful, and some cases are helped by E.C.T. When the patient's physical state no longer causes anxiety, psychotherapy should commence. Even superficial exploration may reveal some of the originating ideas—they may be fully conscious, and such an approach will also serve to show the patient that at last there is some understanding, and so gain her confidence. Where the basis is a fear of fatness the patient should have it pointed out to her that she will not be expected to eat so as to become too fat, and that, since she has been able to make herself so thin this time, there is no fear of adiposity. Whether a deeper exploration of the psychodynamics of the illness is possible and advisable, depends on the features of the individual case.

Other gross hysterical symptoms, such as blindness or fugues, or the poor general physical health of the patient, may make admission to hospital necessary; but it should be avoided if possible. Hospital tends to become a refuge which the patient may be very reluctant to leave. Admission to hospital should be a part therefore of a constructive plan of treatment. Otherwise it is apt to lead to therapeutic stalemate and when the doctor in frustration decides to discharge the patient still not symptom-free, there may be emotional outbursts, recriminations and suicidal threats.

It is essential in all these cases that the patient's relatives should clearly understand the therapeutic situation. If they do not, the patient may manipulate it so that the relatives come to blame the doctor for any lack of progress. The relatives must be taught also how at home to handle the patient's problems so as to give him understanding and encouragement but not too much solicitude.

Treatment of Obsessional Symptoms

Many phobias respond reasonably well to psychotherapy. While an understanding is being obtained of the determinants of the phobia, the patient should be advised to avoid phobia-eliciting situations. A vicious circle development is thus broken. When the patient has lost some of his apprehension and gained some confidence and understanding of his symptoms, he may be advised to re-enter the situations which had previously caused him distress, fortified by a sedative such as amylobarbitone sodium. He should be told he can leave again as soon as he feels uncomfortable, and that he is not being weak in doing so. Gradually he is likely to find that he can tolerate the difficult situations for longer, the sedative becomes a standby which he carries with him, and then if all goes well he can dispense with it altogether.

Where obsessive rumination depends on an inability to reconcile objective facts with desires, or facts with childish preconceptions, discussion and modification of the desires helps to bring relief. Also, where the motive power of the obsessional preoccupation is remorse—and much of the malignancy of obsessional states may depend on their basis in feelings of guilt and remorse—discussion of the foundations of the remorse, when they are discoverable, and readjustment of the mental attitudes to them, may be of considerable assistance: but this deeper exploration has to be carried out with great care, and too much analytic probing may precipitate greater distress and a depression of spirits with a suicidal risk.

One cannot hope to rid the obsessional of his obsessional personality, but he can be taught how best to live with it by understanding both its strengths and its disadvantages. Obsessionals drive themselves very hard, and they may have to be guided about taking adequate rest and holidays, and advised against overloading themselves with duties and too many responsibilities. Promotion is sometimes better avoided by the obsessional. He is more than normally sensitive to major changes in his way of life and upset by them. Many obsessional patients are helped very much by the opportunity now and again of a talk with their doctor, when they can ventilate their problems and get his reactions and encouragement.

Environmental readjustments may be all that is required in the case of the child who has developed obsessional symptoms under stress at school, for example, or is being brought up too strictly at home.

The patient with obsessional impulses will want to know whether or not he should give in to them. Usually he is forced to do, because not to give in to them creates intolerable tension: the doctor therefore in his reply should accept the *fait accompli*. But he cannot advise the patient not to withstand his impulses, if these are to antisocial actions or so frequent that he cannot get on with the business of life.

Treatment of the classical obsessive-compulsive type of case is a matter often of great difficulty. In those cases which are particularly resistant to any form of psychotherapeutic treatment and where the person's life and conduct is entirely dominated by obsessive symptoms, the operation of leucotomy should be seriously considered—particularly if the illness has been for some years disabling. In our experience leucotomy has proved very effective in certain malignant cases, and has made life much more bearable.

PROGNOSIS

There are great individual variations in the outcome of these illnesses, which is easily understandable since the reactions themselves range from transient responses to stress to states of chronic invalidism. In general, the prognosis depends not so much on the specific symptoms developed, as on the adequacy of the personality for the demands made on it by the circumstances of daily life. The prognosis may therefore be seen to depend on at least four factors:

1. The type and duration of the neurotic reaction.
2. The previous personality of the patient.
3. The circumstances of his life.
4. The treatment given.

Usually, the shorter the duration of the illness the better the outlook, since some neurotic reactions have a tendency to become habitual and the longer they persist the more likely is it that the development of hysterical symptoms may complicate the issue. Anxiety states usually clear up satisfactorily over a period of months; hysterical reactions may be very superficial and short-lived, or longer lasting, and in a few cases become so ingrained that they may be said to be malignant; while obsessional neuroses (which are more endogenously determined than other neurotic reactions), except for those which run a cyclic course or present as phobic states, tend to be persistent. We must stress the individual variations, and how unwise it is to generalize dogmatically. Anorexia nervosa, for example, is a serious condition, often intractable, sometimes fatal: but a considerable number of cases respond well to treatment, menstruation becomes re-established, and they remain well. Again, while obsessionals have in general the poorest prognosis, the outlook here is also very variable and usually not unsatisfactory. Lewis (1935) reported that in an unselected sample of obsessional patients roughly one-half may be expected to do well. He followed up 50 cases ('a good sample of the obsessionals of London'), five years or more after they had been treated at The Maudsley Hospital. Sixteen were then quite well (free of symptoms), 7 were much improved, 5 had been well but had relapsed, 5 were a little improved and 17 were no better or worse. Lewis noted that many obsessionals show a late improvement, after years of illness. Pollitt (1960), reviewing the published reports of follow-up studies, found that 43 per cent. of obsessional patients have a good prognosis.

The more stable and mature the previous personality, the better the outlook; except for those cases where the obsessional personality shades over into the obsessional illness. The neuroses are illnesses of young adult life, and there appears to be a general tendency for people to grow out of them. The immature, hysterical personality, after many alarms and excursions, may mature late and become much better adjusted. On the other hand, if neurotic symptoms are essentially an expression of the persistent maladjustment of an inadequate psychopathic personality, the outlook is far poorer.

Obviously the circumstances of the patient's life play an important part in determining the prognosis. These illnesses are responses to environmental stresses, as well as to inner conflicts. If these external stresses are relieved, either spontaneously or by deliberate manipulation of the environment, psychological healing can take place and the patient tends naturally to recover. On the other hand, circumstances which have been the main cause of the illness, may be irremediable; for example, a woman unhappily married to a drunken husband may on account of her children be unable or unwilling to leave him: in such a case the neurotic reaction will tend to chronicity, and it can be seen often to be to some extent self-protective and adaptive, a way of diverting and dulling the distress of the domestic predicament.

So individual are these reactions and so various, with in many cases a spontaneous tendency to readjustment, that the effects of psychotherapy and other methods of treatment are difficult to gauge. There is a good deal of evidence that, whatever the form of treatment employed, about 70 per cent. of neurotic patients may be expected to recover or become much better within a year or two. Ross (1936) in a follow-up study of 1186 cases treated at the Cassel Hospital, found a year after discharge that 40 per cent. were well and 25 per cent. improved. The more or less corresponding and contemporary figures from the Berlin Psychoanalytic Institute were 40 and 18 per cent. The Berlin cases were treated by psychoanalysis in its strictest sense, for an average of 17 months: the Cassel Hospital cases were treated by hypnosis, explanation, persuasion and sometimes by a modified form of analysis, for an average of 4·1 months. The results of treatment in these two groups were remarkably alike, in spite of considerable differences in methods and duration of treatment. Similar results have been reported by other workers since then. Denker (1946), investigating 500 cases of neurosis treated by general practitioners with superficial psychotherapy, found that 72 per cent. had recovered in 2 years.

This suggests that there are biological factors present in neurotic illnesses which promote improvement, independently of therapeutic efforts. On the other hand, the experience of individual cases and of watching the relation of their progress to the steps in treatment carry to the clinician conviction of the efficacy of psychotherapeutic methods. Statistical surveys of the results of treatment in large groups involve the lumping together of individual differences where the differences themselves may be of great importance, and the very varying standards by which improvement is measured make comparisons of dubious worth.

Eysenck (1960) has reviewed the most recent literature on the effects of psychotherapy and comes to challenging conclusions. He states that 'when untreated neurotic controls are compared with experimental groups of patients treated by means of psychotherapy, both groups recover to approximately the same extent'; and he goes on to say, 'We have found that neurotic disorders tend to be self-limiting, that psychoanalysis is no more successful than any other method, and that in fact all methods of psychotherapy fail to improve on the recovery rate obtained through ordinary life experiences and non-specific treatment'. These conclusions should not be considered as final, but they point very clearly to the need for more research, and research carried out with control groups (however difficult this may be).

The quality of the recovery which the patient makes can only be fully gauged by his ability to withstand the strains of life over the subsequent years.

PSYCHOSOMATIC DISORDERS

The word psychosomatic has been used with two main meanings: first, to describe a method of clinical approach to all patients; and second, to delineate a group of physical diseases or syndromes.

In its first sense, the term has much the same connotation as Adolf Meyer's psychobiological. It expresses a holistic approach to clinical problems, an interest in the vicissitudes of the whole organism rather than in the activity of single organs, a belief that psychic and somatic are two complementary and equally necessary angles of observation, understanding and management. So far as it assists to promote such an approach, the term is unexceptionable. It calls attention to the close relationship of mind and body, and especially it impresses upon doctors in general that many of the symptoms that they have been accustomed to treat along physical lines are really of psychological origin. Psychogenic, especially neurotic, conditions as a whole present themselves more frequently in a somatic guise than a mental one. Patients come more often with a complaint of palpitation or headache than with irrational fear of crossing the road. But in the past it has commonly happened that symptoms referred to by the patient as indigestion were accepted as such by the doctor and labelled 'dyspepsia', which was then treated as a disease *sui generis*, although no physical lesion had been demonstrated. Similarly, vague pains were labelled 'rheumatism'; complaints of fatigue were attributed to a 'weak heart' or 'anaemia'; breathlessness was called 'asthma'; localized pain was often disposed of as 'neuralgia' or 'neuritis'; and complaints both general and vague without discoverable physical causes were labelled 'debility'. The attachment of the diagnostic label gave form and substance to the syndrome in the patient's mind, and in this way neurotic invalids who were always complaining, improving a little and relapsing, were created in considerable numbers. Such chronic conditions might well be called iatrogenic, fostered, if not produced, by the doctor's failure, arising from shortcomings in his medical education, to recognize or even to look for the emotional factors that were upsetting digestion or causing pains or fatigue or what not.

It seems to take a war to bring home these principles in a comprehensive way, since war produces fear or anxiety in most people at some time or another, and it is emotions such as these that are among the commonest causes of the physical discomforts for which medical advice is sought.

The term psychosomatic has also been used with a much more limited reference to describe a certain group of diseases or syndromes. These are physical illnesses, in which one physiological system is predominantly affected, autonomic disturbance is usually apparent, and emotional factors are believed to be of decisive importance. The following list includes many, though by no means all, of the syndromes commonly described under this heading: vasomotor rhinitis, asthma, essential hypertension, coronary thrombosis, duodenal ulcer, ulcerative colitis, primary dysmenorrhoea, persistent enuresis, primary hyperthyroidism, diabetes mellitus, rheumatoid arthritis, migraine, and various forms of urticaria, pruritus and neuro-dermatitis. It will be readily appreciated that this list comprises many syndromes with no obvious similarities, but there are certain facts which suggest that its heterogeneity may be more apparent than real and that there is some justification for a tentative grouping of this kind.

Halliday (1948) has pointed out that a striking feature of the public health of this country in the present century has been a rising incidence of these psychosomatic affections. He links this rising incidence with socio-environmental changes which he believes have led to an increasing proportion of the population developing physiological dysfunctions and obsessional modes of behaviour. These affections appear to be commoner in urban than in rural areas, and in certain social classes and occupational groups: for example, doctors seem to have a lamentable tendency to coronary thrombosis. With regard to the sex incidence, most of these disorders are commoner in men and the rate of rise in incidence appears generally to be greater in men. Ehrström (1951), investigating Eskimos in Greenland, has reported such illnesses as being five times as common amongst those acquiring the mode and thought of Western civilization. All this demonstrates the need for further epidemiological studies: though the evidence available hardly justifies the conclusion of those who believe that these affections can now be labelled the diseases of civilization.

Most of the earlier psychiatric investigations in this field took the form of enumerations of the traits of character and temperament, or delineations of the personality profiles, associated with the various physical syndromes. There was a notable uniformity in the findings reported. In different affections the same type of personality seemed to occur with great frequency—described as typically anxious, over-conscientious and covertly aggressive, it was often loosely called 'obsessional'. These were superficial observations, and the suggestion that a specific predisposing personality had been demonstrated was open to many objections. The traits reported, easily recognized and perhaps also rather readily extracted from the patients' accounts of themselves, were not shown to have any inevitable connection with the physical symptoms. Those of apparently similar personality may develop quite different somatic lesions or, even more significantly, remain physically fit. A complementary study is certainly required of different groups of people arranged according to temperament and of the physical disorder to which they are prone. Later studies have been less superficial in their psychopathological approach, but theory has still tended to outrun established fact.

Various explanations have been advanced as to why one system of the body should be involved rather than another, if emotional trauma or continued emotional tension can in fact facilitate the appearance of certain organic diseases. It is very possible that an already existing organic defect, due to previous injury, can determine the locus of symptoms: for example, the sufferer from dysentery may be left with bowels more sensitive to emotional stimuli. It may also be readily supposed that an individual can have a specific, systemic weakness or locus of lower constitutional resistance. Most of the psychosomatic disorders appear to show a familial incidence, and the study of possible genetic factors should have attention. The sufferers from psychosomatic affections may inherit abnormally labile autonomic nervous systems, and their temperamental traits may also have an inherited foundation.

There have been many explanations in terms of psychopathology. Some workers have sought symbolic meaning in the symptoms and others have delineated emotional constellations or conflicts which seem to have pathological results. The Chicago group of workers headed by Franz Alexander (1952) have suggested that certain unconscious emotional conflicts tend to affect the functions of certain internal organs, producing specific vegetative responses, and that such chronic functional disturbances ('organ neuroses') may lead to irreversible organic disease. This theory has been elaborated somewhat as follows: if competitive, aggressive, hostile attitudes are blocked, the sympathetic nervous system may be thrown into sustained excitation and hypertension, for example, or hyperthyroidism or migraine may result: whereas if gratification of help-seeking, regressive tendencies is denied, parasympathetic over-activity may lead to peptic ulcer, colitis or asthma. According to these workers, psychosomatic disorders which develop under parasympathetic preponderance show a more complete withdrawal from the solution of external problems. In contrast, Grace (1951) believed that he could in several of these affections identify a particular, often conscious and clearly expressed, attitude towards certain situations precipitating the symptoms. Such theories, in the present state of our knowledge, are clearly very provisional.

Studying these disorders in a wider biological context, Harold Wolff (1953) considered them as purposive, though inappropriate, protective responses to stress, *i.e.* to problems and challenges in day-to-day life; and he emphasized that biological protective devices, elicited by danger or threats of danger, are for short-term use, and that bodily disorder or disease may arise if the threatened individual sustains such patterns of response unduly long or as a way of life. This is a stimulating formulation and it may be brought into relation with the work of Selye who, studying particularly the complex interplay of nervous and hormonal mechanisms in the individual's adaptation to stress, has also proposed the concept that when normal adaptation breaks down certain physical disorders ('diseases of adaptation') may result. Other American research workers (Massermann, Gantt, Anderson and Parmenter) have produced evidence which suggests that dogs, cats and sheep may under stress develop disorders of behaviour, with emotional and physiological accompaniments, which bear some resemblance to the psychosomatic disorders found in man.

This delineation of a limited group of 'psychosomatic' physical affections implies that bodily lesions may be psychogenic in origin. How direct and explicit is the evidence for this? The skin was one of the first organs to get detailed attention, and over the past 50 years many investigators have claimed that skin blisters, localized oedema and petechial haemorrhages can be produced at particular points of the body surface by hypnotic suggestion or during abreaction. In 1943 Wolf and Wolff, examining an apparently otherwise normal man who had a gastric fistula, were able to observe a sequence of events beginning with emotional upset (*e.g.* resentment), accompanied by prolonged hyperaemia of the gastric mucous membrane, increased acid secretion and increased motility of the stomach, leading to haemorrhages and erosion of the gastric mucosa, and culminating (in the absence of protecting mucus) in the development of gastric ulceration. This group of workers at the New York Hospital have more recently made similar detailed investigations of the nose and of the colon. Though the mechanism of these events is still obscure, a great many other findings have been reported which lend more or less plausibility to the concept of psychogenic lesions. This extensive literature has been summarized by Flanders Dunbar (1954).

Research has taken four main directions:

1. The study of cases where the symptoms referred by the patient to one or other of his physical systems are purely the result of emotional disturbance—as in neurotic reactions; *e.g.* muscle tension pains ('fibrositis'), headache.

2. The determination of the frequency of incidence of emotional events (emotional precipitants), or the occurrence of emotional tension at, or just before, the onset of a physical ailment—in cases of, *e.g.* peptic ulcer, primary hyperthyroidism, asthma.

3. The study of the patient's emotional attitudes to illness, injury or mutilation, which may influence the course of the physical illness and determine the degree of disablement. Studies of this kind have been made, *e.g.* in cases of blindness, pulmonary tuberculosis, amputation.

4. The analysis of personality types or emotional constellations which are

associated with or seem to predispose to certain types of physical illness. Most of the psychosomatic affections have been frequently investigated from this angle.

Further research is required, particularly into the constitutional factors which may be hereditarily determined (twin studies would be applicable here), and into the detailed physiology of the emotions involved (along the lines developed by Wolff and his colleagues).

The psychosomatic concept in therapeutics implies that each patient must be treated with many-sided understanding, both as an individual and as a member of a community, in all the aspects of his sickness, suffering or maladjustment. Attention to these principles will ensure a broader, more humanitarian and effective handling of all medical problems, and will avoid the reproach voiced by the philosopher Amiel in his Journal (Aug. 22, 1873):

'Why do doctors so often make mistakes? Because they are not sufficiently individual in their diagnoses or their treatment. They class a sick man under some given department of their nosology, whereas every invalid is really a special case, a unique example. How is it possible that so coarse a method of sifting should produce judicious therapeutics? Every illness is a factor simple or complex which is multiplied by a second factor, invariably complex—the individual, that is to say, who is suffering from it, so that the result is a special problem, demanding a special solution. . . . The principal grievance which I have against the doctors is that they neglect the real problem, which is to seize the unity of the individual who claims their care.'

These therapeutic principles apply also of course to the limited group of so-called 'psychosomatic' disorders; but it is proper to add that at present the psychiatrist has a modest rôle to play in their management. Many of these conditions are associated with prolonged emotional tension, and tend to run a chronic and relapsing course. The psychiatrist who claims too much in this field does his speciality no service. A fuller knowledge of aetiology is essential if we are to make progress.

REFERENCES

Ackner, B. (1954) *J. ment. Sci.*, **100**, 838.
Alexander, F. (1952) *Psychosomatic Medicine*, London.
Berrington, W. P., Liddell, D. W., and Foulds, G. A. (1956) *J. ment. Sci.*, **102**, 280.
Brown, F. W. (1942) *Proc. roy. Soc. Med.*, **35**, 785.
Dejerine, J., and Gauckler, E. (1911) *Les Manifestations functionnelles des psychonévroses*, Paris.
Denker, P. G. (1946) *N.Y. St. J. Med.*, **46**, 2164.
Dunbar, F. (1954) *Emotions and Bodily Changes*, New York.
Ehrström, M. C. (1950) *Finska LäkSällsk. Handl.*, **93**, 3.
Eysenck, H. J. (1947) *Dimensions of Personality*, London.
Eysenck, H. J., ed. (1960) *Behaviour Therapy and the Neuroses*, London.
Eysenck, H. J., ed. (1960) *Handbook of Abnormal Psychology*, Chapter 18, London.
Fenichel, O. (1946) *The Psychoanalytic Theory of Neurosis*, London.
Foulkes, S. H., and Anthony, E. J. (1957) *Group Psychotherapy*, London.
Freud, S. (1955) The Complete Psychological Works of, London.

Gillespie, R. D. (1944) *Psychological Effects of War on Citizen and Soldier*, London.

Gordon, A. (1926) *Amer. J. Psychiat.*, **5**, 647.

Grace, W. J., Wolf, S., and Wolff, H. G. (1951) *The Human Colon*, New York.

Halliday, J. L. (1948) *Psychosocial Medicine*, London.

Holmes, T. H., Goodell, H., Wolf, S., and Wolff, H. G. (1950) *The Nose*, Springfield, Ill,

Ironside, R. N., and Batchelor, I. R. C. (1945) *Brit. J. Ophthal.*, **29**, 88.

Janet, P. (1911) *The Mental State of Hystericals*, London.

Jones, E. (1948) *Papers on Psycho-analysis*, 5th ed., London.

Kay, D. W. K. (1953) *Proc. roy. Soc. Med.*, **46**, 669.

Lewis, A. (1935) *Proc. roy. Soc. Med.*, **29**, 325.

McDougall, W. (1926) *Outline of Abnormal Psychology*, New York.

Martin, F. M., Brotherston, J. H. F. and Chave, S. P. W. (1957) *Brit. J. prev. soc. Med.*, **11**, 196.

Moody, R. L. (1946) *Lancet*, ii, 934.

Nemiah, J. C. (1950) *Medicine (Baltimore)*, **29**, 225.

Pollitt, J. D. (1960) *J. ment. Sci.*, **106**, 93.

Ross, T. A. (1936) *An Enquiry into Prognosis in the Neuroses*, London.

Shorvon, H. J. (1946) *Proc. roy. Soc. Med.*, **39**, 779.

Slater, E. (1943) *J. Neurol. Psychiat.*, **6**, 1.

Slater, E., and Slater, P. (1944) *J. Neurol. Neurosurg. Psychiat.*, **7**, 49.

Stengel, E. (1941) *J. ment. Sci.*, **87**, 572.

Stengel, E. (1943) *J. ment. Sci.*, **89**, 224.

Stengel, E. (1945) *J. ment. Sci.*, **91**, 166.

Taylor, S. (1938) *Lancet*, i. 759.

Watts, C. A. H., and Watts, B. M. (1952) *Psychiatry in General Practice*, London.

Wolf, S., and Wolff, H. G. (1943) *Human Gastric Function*, New York.

Wolff, H. G. (1953) *Stress and Disease*, Illinois.

9

SEXUAL ANOMALIES

The social and medico-legal problems which arise in cases of sexual anomaly present many perplexities of an intricate nature involving both aetiology and treatment. But it is usually only after the social, ethical and legal codes have been transgressed that the advice of the physician or psychiatrist is sought. Otherwise the sexual deviate remains secretive, either because he does not wish to change his nature in the belief that it gives him a certain superiority over his fellow-men or, on the contrary, if guilt feelings predominate, he lives in the vain hope that some time or other he may reach an adequate solution for himself. A psychiatric opinion may only be requested when he has fallen foul of the law and been arrested for lewd and libidinous behaviour. Then it becomes essential to reach a decision as to whether the offence was committed during the course of some form of mental or nervous disorder, or whether it arose *sui generis*. In the former instance the sexual anomaly is regarded as one of the symptoms of an otherwise disordered mind which requires the care and treatment a hospital provides; in other cases of a neurotic nature with obsessive-compulsive symptoms the Court may sanction probation with the proviso that the individual co-operates in medical supervision and treatment.

In the absence of nervous or mental illness the position is more complex; if the psychiatrist can, with justice, emphasize any mitigating factors, which may have influenced the conduct of the individual, he should not hesitate to do so, but he must be most scrupulous in his ascertainment of all the relevant facts so that the Court may be given every assistance to come to a fair decision. The cordial relations which now exist between the medical and legal professions has led to a greater emphasis on treatment and rehabilitation rather than on an arbitrary prison sentence. The better understanding of the man himself is aimed at rather than the quality of his act. But even if the sexual offender is sentenced to a term of imprisonment, specialized medical facilities for treatment are now available.

Anomalies of sex conduct affect all ranks of society and all age groups. Our case records show that we have been consulted in relation to members of the aristocracy, lawyers, doctors, professors, clergymen, scoutmasters, business executives, and manual workers; the young, middle-aged, and elderly have all been implicated. Alcohol has been one of the most outstanding precipitating agents. Even a small amount, given the particular circumstances and opportunity, may be sufficient to trigger off impulsive and instinctive conduct which otherwise would have been controlled. That of course is by no means invariably so for there are many sex deviates who are total abstainers. The fact that the person may be deeply under the influence of alcohol at the time of the offence does not, necessarily, excuse his conduct.

In the great majority of cases which have been referred to us the accused has been found to be of sound mind and fit to plead to the charge against him; in a considerable number there were extenuating circumstances which the Court took into consideration in assessing punishment or treatment. Our examinations showed that the offence was rarely an isolated one, it had been repeated on many occasions, but surprisingly enough it had not interfered with the person's ability to pursue his duties, or to lead a happy life at home; his employer, and his wife and family, often, had no knowledge of his incongruous conduct. For the accused, arrest and court appearance came, sometimes, as a blessed relief. There was no need for further duplicity, an opportunity had been provided whereby the secret life which had dominated his conduct and his conscience could now be fully disclosed, and a restart made to reach a higher and more mature level. The younger the person the greater the chance of readjustment. The older group, many of them married men with families, presented tragic situations jeopardizing their careers and their homes. Their history often showed that they had been hard-working capable persons occupying positions of responsibility, happy in their homes, kind to their children, but who for one reason or another, *e.g.* predisposition, drink, sexual deprivation, impotence, sought relief from their inner tensions by lewd conduct, irrespective of the inherent risks. Many admitted their guilt, expressed remorse, and did not know why they should have behaved in such a way, but others took refuge in specious excuses or pled amnesia.

In this sophisticated age when the sexes mix with so much freedom it is surprising that so many remain profoundly ignorant of the facts of life. Inborn constitutional factors influencing or retarding normal sexual development may be one element, but parental over-solicitude, prohibition, threats of punishment, *e.g.* castration, are even more likely to inhibit the onset of the natural instinctive biological urge. Sex becomes taboo, a sense of shame and guilt is generated, and a mature heterosexual level may never be reached. We meet such situations in civil cases, as apart from criminal, where non-consummation of marriage due to impotence, of a physical or psychogenic nature, may lead to nullity proceedings. E. B. Strauss (1950) in his impressive and detailed account of this topic writes as follows: 'No medical practitioner can afford to be ignorant of the aetiology and nature of this sexual disability, and should always be prepared to give a sympathetic hearing, and informal advice to his unfortunate patients'. We concur entirely with that point of view for its full acceptance might be the means of preventing many disastrous marriages. For instance, a general practitioner had advised a sensitive, prudish, middle-aged schoolmaster to marry in the hope that his impotence and sense of inferiority would thus be cured. The result was disastrous. Investigation showed that a strong Oedipus situation existed, and even despite all the willing help his wife gave him he was unable to consummate the marriage. In contrast the powerful sexual reactions he experienced when he gave a boy a thrashing caused him the most intense alarm. The deep-seated nature of the psychogenic factors, and his age precluded the possibility of successful psychotherapeutic treatment and led to nullity proceedings.

(For a detailed, factual study of sexual behaviour as it affects male and female we refer readers to the authoritative investigations of Dr. Alfred C. Kinsey.)

Masturbation

This is the most frequent sexual habit which the family doctor and psychiatrist may be consulted about. In infancy and early childhood it is more correctly regarded as an instinctive search for a pleasurable sensation rather than as an overt form of sexuality. Even the normal warmth and security of the mother, sucking, rhythmic movements, cuddling and accidental stimulation of the sexual zone, during bathing and cleansing, may produce it. It is only when puberty or adolescence is reached that the child becomes conscious of sexual feelings as such, and may experience alarm, horror, shame and fear. The investigations of Havelock Ellis, Kinsey and many others have shown that practically all persons of both sexes have practised masturbation during some period of their lives, and it can therefore be regarded as a normal stage in one's sexual development. It is something to be lived through, and to be replaced at a later stage by heterosexual interests. This, however, may not always occur. There are some unfortunate people who remain stuck at the narcissistic level, and who learn to accentuate their erotic feelings by phantasy thinking (psychic masturbation). Sooner or later anxiety, shame, guilt, rear their ugly heads, and the victim may believe that he has done himself irreparable harm, committed the unpardonable sin, and deserves to be punished. An attempt at self-mutilation may seem to be the answer to his problems. Such persons are of a shy, sensitive, introspective make-up, they shun company, are sure that people can tell by looking at them that they are guilty of sinful conduct, and believe that bodily, mentally and spiritually they are doomed to failure and defeat. Some attempt to sublimate their problems by burning the midnight oil, by having recourse to philosophy and religion, and it is only when they are near breaking point that they seek advice and assistance. Others of stronger fibre—and they are the majority—pass through this ordeal of development unscathed.

The habit may be continued into adult life but gradually becomes less insistent, and does not, necessarily, interfere with the prospect of marriage, or ability to carry out one's marital duties. It does not lead to insanity or moral deterioration, as was at one time supposed, but if it has been practised excessively (several times a day) over a period of years it may produce a state of lessened potency. It is, therefore, of importance in relation to one's biological development to put away childish ways and habits at as early a date as possible—and strive for more healthy and mature outlets.

Scoptophilia and Exhibitionism

Scoptophilia and exhibitionism have been described by Clifford Allen as the counterparts of one another. Scoptophilia is the state of sexual excitement and pleasure derived from viewing sexual scenes, or the genitalia of a member of the opposite sex. Exhibitionism or 'indecent exposure' is the habit of displaying the sexual organs to persons of the opposite sex; it is probably the most common of all sex offences.

The above tendencies or anomalies are part of the play-life of the normal child. Most of us have indulged in them in one way or another, and have gained physical and moral satisfaction by comparing ourselves with others; even in later life our sexual gratification and curiosity may be satisfied by pornographic literature, drawings and pictures of an erotic nature, tailor's 'dummies', statues, e.g. Pygmalionism, rock 'n roll dances, strip-tease acts, glamorous young women in theatre or on television. It has been interesting to note, when 'star' prisoners are allowed to decorate their cells, the prominence given to the 'pin-up' girl. All such actions are harmless enough, but when they become of such a compelling nature as to inhibit or prevent further biological development they can produce dangerous situations.

The so-called *voyeurs* or 'peeping Toms' are usually emotionally immature persons who, in their search for satisfaction, travel alone (sometimes in disguise), and constantly court recognition and disaster, by repeating their offence time and again. The risks they run are amazing because during the day as well as at night they are driven into behaviour which, in their inmost being, they may despise. It is in complete contrast to the mask of respectability they present to the public.

They frequent public parks, playgrounds, or other places where they are likely to observe loving couples; even seeing them walk hand in hand, or kissing may be sufficient to stir their erotic fancies by identifying them with the participant. They go on holidays by themselves, seek secluded spots where there may be better opportunities to observe. We have known some who have made a habit of lurking in hotel corridors, of listening at bedroom doors, of peeping through the key-hole; others emulate the exploits of the cat-burglar by climbing up to windows in the hope of seeing people undressing, in the nude, or indulging in sexual intercourse.

Such persons do not lead dissociated lives, there is no absolute split in their personality, they are fully conscious of their actions, and know they are unbecoming to their pride and prestige. The conflict of forces between their conduct on the one hand, and their inability to control their perverted desires on the other gives rise to intense psychosomatic symptoms which not infrequently show themselves as nausea, abdominal discomfort and vomiting, symbols of overwhelming disgust. When such is the case, and when it becomes accentuated by phantasy thinking, then business efficiency and power of concentration may be seriously interfered with; appropriate treatment, however, can solve many such problems.

Exhibitionists also demonstrate the frailty and ambivalence of human nature. They, too, prefer the by-ways, the secluded places, the dimly lit streets where they may display themselves, with less chance of detection, to women and children. The light, however, on occasions, does not daunt them. For instance, a man who had been brought up by an over-solicitous, possessive mother obtained his revenge and a false sense of freedom by exhibiting himself from a window

O

in his mother's house to a group of girls who were employed in a factory opposite. The Court accepted the suggestion that he should be placed on probation in the hope that he would benefit from psychotherapeutic treatment. Even a happy marriage may prove no barrier to such conduct as was exemplified by the case of a man, 50 years old, the father of several children, who, during several years, had been in the habit of, repeatedly, behaving in this indecent manner. He acknowledged his guilt, was co-operative in treatment, and received the whole-hearted support of his wife and employer in effecting a readjustment.

Another man who had taken a prominent place in public affairs and been interested in charitable schemes was not so fortunate. He was found guilty of many acts of gross indecency with children and sentenced to two years' imprisonment. The prosecuting counsel, in his plea for sentence, remarked that the main consideration in such a case was not what would benefit the accused but what punishment he deserved, and how the community could be protected. Such cases occurring in the middle-aged and the more elderly illustrate a compensatory phenomenon whereby their exhibitionistic endeavours become indicative of their dwindling potency; the regression to a more primitive instinctive level is not so strange as it might appear. In certain cases it may be an indication or symptom of a beginning organic deterioration of the central nervous system. As a case in point and as an unusual outcome of psychosurgery a man, 47 years old, who never previously had committed sexual offences was charged with exhibiting himself, and interfering with a child aged 5 years. He had undergone a leucotomy operation ten years previously on account of paranoid symptoms. He was the type of person who required to be under constant medical supervision.

It is far from easy to understand the mental mechanisms which can influence and dominate people so dangerously. The ordinary standards of social conduct are thrown aside, ugly facets of the personality seem to take on individual activity and precipitate situations which can be alarming and tragic. The psychoanalytic school postulates the view that all such conduct is determined at an unconscious level, and that its root is embedded in castration fears (the denial of castration). No doubt there is much truth in that opinion but there is no specificity about it as in matters so complicated we can never think in terms of one underlying mental mechanism; there are always extraneous, accidental, unpredictable factors which also play a part. It is our opinion that many emotionally distorted, biologically inferior persons continually strive for dominance and power by the use of over-compensatory mechanisms.

Transvestism

The wearing of clothes of the other sex for sexual gratification.

This condition like so many other sex anomalies may start naturally and innocently as a state of make-believe, of play acting, of a 'lark' which has no apparent or obvious relationship to sexuality at all. The roots must be deep in our unconscious. Most of us have had fun in dressing-up, in pretending that we are different from what we really are, and of reverting to an earlier period of our development. Flag days for charity conducted by students provide many examples. It is only when the practice is continued into manhood and womanhood and becomes established as a mode of life to produce sexual gratification that a dangerous state of abnormality is reached. It can, however, have its romantic aspects as well: James Barry (James Miranda Steurt Barry) was a little woman, barely five feet high, who assumed male clothing and was successful, in 1812, in becoming a doctor of medicine of Edinburgh University. In 1813 she joined the Army Medical Service, and after 46 years achieved the rank of Inspector-General of Army Hospitals. Only at her death in 1865 was the secret of her sex revealed. She seems to have carried out her duties admirably and was such an accomplished surgeon that in 1815 when stationed at the Cape of Good Hope she performed a Caesarean section on a Mrs. Munnik and delivered her of a son who, appropriately enough, was christened James Barry Munnik. A daughter of James Barry Munnik married a Hertzog, and their son became the Prime Minister of South Africa—James Barry Munnik Hertzog.

Miss Russell (1943), to whom we are indebted for the story of James Barry, also records that in 1904 an article written by G. E. Marvel and published in the *Cape Times* throws some light on the unconscious motivation which may have determined James Barry's remarkable sex impersonation.

She is supposed to have been an illegitimate daughter of the Prince Regent, and her real name was Joan Augusta Fitzroy. After learning the story of her birth and bringing up, and of her mother's seduction she rejected the name of Joan Fitzroy, and became James Barry—a dominating aggressive personality who was a law to herself, and in her mental attributes over-compensated for her small stature and physique.

The story of another lady who was well known to us has certain points in common. Before she was born her mother had anxiously anticipated the birth of a boy. In consequence she was brought up as a boy, became interested in boyish sports and games and despised her femininity. When 5 years old she was sexually assaulted by a man in the family's employment. Later in life, during her adolescent period, she identified herself closely with soldiers who were being trained for service overseas. When she read of the casualties the regiment had sustained she passed into a delirium during which she identified herself with them and believed that she also was serving in the trenches. When she resumed her ordinary life she became conscious that other women seemed to be attracted to her, wrote her passionate letters, expressed undying affection, and said they did not know how they could live without her. She was so pestered by these attentions that she contracted a marriage in the hope that she might escape from the fatal attraction which she appeared to exercise. If she had fully realized what marriage meant, she said, she would never have undertaken it.

In *The Diary of a Country Parson*, Parson Woodforde tells how on May 21, 1778, he walked up to the White Hart with Mr. Lewis and Bill to see 'a famous Woman in Men's Cloathes, by name Hannah Snell, who was 21 years as a common soldier in the Army, and not discovered by any one as a woman. Cousin Lewis has mounted guard with her abroad. She went in the Army by the name of John Gray. She has a pension from the Crown now of £18 : 5 : 0 per annum and the liberty of wearing Men's cloathes and also a cockade in her hat which she still wears. She has laid in a room with 70 soldiers, and not discovered by any of them. The forefinger of her right hand was cut by a sword at the taking of Pondicherry. She is now about 60 years of age and talks very sensible and well, and travels the country with a basket at her back, selling buttons, garters, laces &c. I took 4 pr. of 4d buttons and gave her 0 : 2 : 6.'

The reverse situation, whereby men may desire to reject their sex and become registered as women, is more common but by no means frequent. Such states may involve fathers of families who throw up successful careers, and commence a new life; their wives may never discover the motive of their actions. After finding a new home such persons dress as women, wear extravagant jewellery, and occupy themselves with feminine pursuits, e.g. knitting, embroidery and cooking. Often they may wish to adopt a woman's name, to undergo a surgical operation, if permitted, so as to transform their sex organs, and to become registered officially as women. After attaining even a part of their purpose it is astonishing how their states of restless tension are replaced by contentment.

There are, of course, many much less clearly defined cases of men who from an early age have identified themselves with girls rather than with persons of their own sex. Usually they are of sensitive, artistic, aesthetic dispositions, refrain from team games of a robust nature, and derive their main pleasure by employing themselves in tasks of an essentially feminine nature. They love to dress themselves in women's clothing, bedeck themselves with jewellery, use lip-stick, scent and powder, and try to imitate the graces of beautiful women. If they do form friendships with other men they prefer those with a similar effeminate nature to their own. Some have expressed a desire to become pregnant so that they might undergo the experience of giving birth to a baby. Usually, however, they are inclined to shun physical contact, and sexual gratification may only be obtained in their phantasy and dream life. There are many who realise that they are living dangerously, that they may involve themselves in unsavoury episodes and be arrested by the police. We have known others, however, who have been able to learn to conduct their lives at a more mature and responsible level.

Fetishism

In all such cases the normal sexual act may not reach attainment in the absence of some accustomed stimulus. A particular scent, hair, fur, silk underwear, slippers, high-heeled shoes, garters, handkerchiefs, may all be necessary accompaniments. It is only when the particular fetish becomes completely detached from the person, and is itself utilized as the sexual object that we regard the condition as pathological. A youth described his irresistible desire to purchase women's shoes or slippers (he had accumulated a considerable quantity) which he had to fondle and kiss before he attained complete sexual satisfaction. A man, 42 years old, described how when he was 4 years old he used to obtain pleasurable excitement from swinging on his mother's foot. In later life he had a compelling desire to touch the feet of women with whom he might be associated, *e.g.* the chambermaid in an hotel. Sexual satisfaction was only attained when a foot was visualized.

The possible psychopathology underlying such conditions will be discussed at a later point.

Bestiality

This unnatural sexual offence is usually perpetrated by farm workers of low intelligence, by psychopathic personalities, or those who are of unsound mind. It may be associated with aggressive sadistic tendencies. Fortunately it is not common. A man 25 years old of average intelligence, who had never been able to adjust to a normal social life, was accused of homosexual offences. His history showed that he had a hypersexual nature so that he indulged indiscriminately either with men, women, or animals.

Homosexuality

The growing public concern in relation to the prevalence of homosexuality and the commitment of homosexual offences was expressed in 1954 by the appointment of a Departmental Committee under the chairmanship of Sir John Wolfenden to inquire into Homosexual Offences and Prostitution; it is only the former aspect which concerns us here. The remit to the Committee was to consider: the law and practice relating to homosexual offences and the treatment of persons convicted of such offences by the Courts. In 1957, after an exhaustive analysis of the many issues involved, the Committee published its report and recommendations. It is a most important and valuable document which serves the purpose of informing the public regarding a medical and social problem of outstanding national significance. While we endorse the careful manner in which the Report has been prepared, yet we are doubtful whether the specific recommendation (one member dissenting) that 'homosexual behaviour in private between consenting adults, 21 years or over, should no longer be a criminal offence', can be supported. It is not the law's business, the Report argues, 'to settle questions of morality, to interfere with the private lives of the citizens; it is only when public decency is offended that the law is entitled to step in and institute criminal proceedings. The need to do so is especially necessary in those cases in which children have been victimized.' While the law is not concerned with morality in a narrow sense, yet it is deeply implicated in the dispensation of social justice and human rehabilitation. Such aims are the duty of any properly constituted authority whether vested in the law, medicine, the Church or public opinion. The Committee's viewpoint, however, is evasive and leaves the impression that anyone can behave as he likes so long as nobody knows about it. Instead of arguing in favour of a dubious proposition we believe that a more constructive approach would have been for the Committee to state that the prevention of homosexuality, a condition which serves no biological purpose, was a matter in which all social scientists might unite their resources for the public weal. Homosexual tendencies develop during childhood, they may be susceptible of cure if children are trained in more hygienic habits, and if parents and educators are familiar with the dangers associated with unhealthy relationships. It appears to us that the recommendation made by the Committee may lead to the growth of homosexuality and homosexual offences rather than to their decrease. It fails to take into account the underlying emotional or affective factors which underlie homosexuality, its inherent immaturity whether due to genetic or environmental anomalies. There are many men and women of 21 years and over who have never reached emotional maturity even although intellectually they may surpass their neighbours. It is, therefore, in our opinion, a grave mistake to fix an arbitrary age level in an emotionally or instinctually developed state such as homosexuality. A selfish individualism is approved rather than the wider aspect of the duty of the individual to society.

We have considered it essential to make these critical comments before proceeding to the more detailed discussion of the subject, as the matter is one of great social importance which demands the most careful scrutiny.

Homosexuality is a sexual propensity or attraction between members of the same sex, and does not necessarily lead to overt sexual conduct which is offensive to public decency. We all know 'the man's man' type, the person who is happier and more at ease with other male companions than in female company. Where the relationship is maintained on a purely platonic basis we should not read more into it than is warranted. All of us probably have a latent homosexual component in our make-up. We may, in our youth, have passed through a homosexual phase so that we must be discreet and sensible in our outlook, and not read meanings into friendships between members of the same sex unless we have substantial proof that the relationship is a prejudicial and injurious one. Those men and women who do not marry until late in life may have many reasons of a personal, family or economic nature which prevent them from doing so, but the factors may be more complex, and may be concerned with unresolved doubts in relation to potency, latent homosexuality and so on which make them play safe in a companionate marriage than in one involving heterosexual intercourse. The same mechanisms may determine the marriage of partners where the age difference is quite remarkable. These matters were clarified by Freud (1910); he explained how the narcissistic, auto-erotic phase of development is replaced by a homosexual one which in turn is supplanted by a heterosexual one. Some persons are unfortunate enough to remain fixed at an immature level, and may never develop any heterosexual instincts at all; indeed a person of the opposite sex may be viewed with such repugnance that no possibility exists of normal sexual relationship. On the other hand there are persons of a bisexual nature who are indiscriminate in their choice of a partner whether man or woman.

Kallmann (1953) affirms, as a result of his investigation of 95 predominantly or exclusively homosexual twin index cases of the male sex, that homosexuality may be dependent on a genetically oriented 'imbalance' between male and female maturation (hormonal) tendencies, but that more evidence is required fully to support that view. He found that nearly 60 per cent. of dissimilar co-twins of homosexual subjects showed no evidence of homosexual behaviour, but in a series of 44 one-egg pairs there was concordance of homosexual conduct.

Homosexuality is no respecter of persons; it involves all manner of men and women drawn from all ranks of society. For the most part they are sensitive, artistic, aesthetic types who seek an outlet in poetry, music, the theatre, dress designing, interior decorating, etc., but doctors, lawyers, professors, clergymen, youth leaders, business executives and manual workers are by no means exempt. The majority are capable efficient persons who in every other respect lead their lives at a responsible and highly successful level. That may be the reason why in certain countries such as Belgium, France, Denmark, Sweden, Netherlands, Norway, Italy, homosexual conduct is no longer regarded as punishable unless it offends against public decency. In Great Britain we have no accurate statistics regarding the prevalence of homosexuality—no detailed investigation has ever been carried out—but we may be able to draw deductions from the investigations of Dr. Kinsey which were conducted in the United States. He concluded that 4 per cent. of adult white males are exclusively homosexual throughout their lives after the onset of adolescence. He suggested that 10 per cent. of the white male population are more or less exclusively homosexual for at least three years between the ages of 16 and 65, and that 37 per cent. of the total male population have at least some overt homosexual experience to the point of orgasm between adolescence and old age. The above statistics are difficult to accept, they appear to be on the high side, but they give more than an indication of the prevalence of sexual anomaly and experience.

Sweden's statistics are more modest. In that country it was found that 1 per cent. of all men were exclusively homosexual, and 4 per cent. were bisexual.

Many of the cases we have examined have been proud of their homosexuality; it has given them a sense of superiority so that they have rejected, with scorn, the suggestion that medical treatment might be made available. Some prefer a prison sentence for a defined period rather than the indeterminateness of psycho-therapeutic treatment. That holds true even in cases of gross indecency involving sodomy with boys or adults and accompanied by sado-masochistic components:
1. A professional man said that he did not wish to change his mode of life;
2. A man, 68 years old, who had held a distinguished position but had developed the unfortunate and dangerous habit of inviting boys to his own house, ex-claimed: 'This is what you get for being kind to boys.'

In some cases the legal viewpoint has seemed unnecessarily harsh and incon-sistent, *e.g.* a judge said he was not going to pay attention to the medical report, that it was his duty to administer the law, and that the sentence would be eighteen months' imprisonment; but on the whole any medical evidence submitted meets with consideration and respect. This was demonstrated in the case of a school-master who, on account of homosexual offences with boys, had already had prolonged psychotherapeutic treatment. On being re-convicted for another series of similar offences the Court referred him for a psychiatric examination 'so as to determine whether any mental imbalance existed which could be susceptible of treatment in terms of Section 3 of the Criminal Justice (Scotland) Act, 1949, and also as to whether residence for observation was necessary in order to decide whether treatment was possible or desirable'.

In contrast to those who refuse medical help we have met others who seek, urgently, for all the assistance they can get. The poignant distress contained in the following letter requires no emphasis: 'Once upon a time I had a will to fight, there were times when I felt that religion, art, literature, music were all that mattered to me, that no other things, particularly wrong things, had any hold over me. Now I have no such moments, my whole life is becoming one horrible obsession. . . . I have no longer any will-power with which to fight; no diversions, no refuge in the arts . . . they are being killed by this one disease. . . . Do try to help me, please. . . . If it be true that with God all things are possible, then it is also true that men may rise over stepping-stones of their own dead selves to better things.'

Another became alarmed at the great change which seemed to be occurring in his disposition. The homosexual tendencies which had existed since he was 8 years old became, while he was in the Services, acutely intensified. He had proved to be a most capable officer, reached a position of responsibility, but was insecure in his personal relationships with his subordinates; he recognized that his tyrannical, impatient and inconsiderate behaviour was closely related to his underlying homosexual tendencies.

The above brief extracts illustrate the various reactions to which homosexual persons are prone, and demonstrate the conflicting, ambivalent feelings and compensatory mechanisms which influence the conduct of many men.

PSYCHOPATHOLOGY

To give adequate help to the patients who consult us, and to aid the Court in dealing fairly with the sexual offender, we must have a far greater understanding of the forces at work, instinctive or conditioned, which produce the disturbing, dangerous and sometimes tragic states which we have described. Only rarely can we be content to accept such matters at their face value, to differentiate black from white is not enough; there are always ever-changing shades and hues which must be inquired into; by doing so we may find the key to an enigmatic situation. Freud taught us how to carry out such investigations. His imaginative concepts, developed through the technique of free association and dream analysis, enabled us to get behind the scenes, to penetrate into the depths of the unconscious and to relate our findings to the actual situation. We learned that behaviour patterns did not form in a haphazard manner but that they were centred round our loves and hates, our fears and guilt feelings which are the ultimate expression of the fundamental needs and reactions of our personalities. Most people, from infancy onwards, pass through their psychosexual development without too much trauma, but others fall by the wayside, sometimes never to rise again; even if they do they may continue to be dominated by malignant traits which exercise a stranglehold on further emotional development. It may be an Oedipus complex, castration fears, anal or oral tendencies which are the unconscious motivating forces. One or all of such trends may be present in any particular case. They can be uncovered without too much difficulty but their treatment may require the special skill of the well-trained psychotherapist to disentangle them, and render them more innocuous. Facile symbolic interpretations should be avoided at all costs; they merely complicate the picture and lead to an assumption of knowledge which is unwarranted.

It is when the patient tries to break through his own bonds, to emancipate himself, that the compensatory phenomena such as a striving for power and dominance, or the acting out of deep-set emotional crises (katathymic crisis), become prominent.

TREATMENT

The sexual anomalies we have described have usually developed insidiously and innocently during childhood and if not overcome may persist as fixed habits which exercise a profound influence over the psychosexual life. The essence of successful treatment is to prevent or anticipate their occurrence, and to deal with them in their incipiency. This may not be a matter for the doctor only; it may require the co-operation of parents, social workers and schoolmasters, all of whom must be able to produce in the child a sense of security. Love, kindness, understanding, plenty of sleep, good nutrition and a training in hygienic habits of a bodily and psychological nature are essential. Such qualities and habits may not be easy to attain because of the interrelationship with domestic and economic problems, unemployment, crowded living conditions, poverty, alcoholism and other social evils. Contrariwise wealth and luxury and sheltered conditions may not provide the bed of roses they are supposed to do, because too great wealth, over-indulgence, non-understanding and over-solicitous parents can be as great a menace as those who are negligent. They produce selfish, self-willed, individualistic children who indulge in tantrums, flout authority and seek new pleasures and sensations—often of a sexual nature—out of a feeling of ennui. There may be no objective reason to explain such deviations from accepted social conduct— the other children in the same family group may be healthy and normal—so that in addition to possible conditioning factors we require to think of bio-genetic influences resulting in 'throw-backs' so constitutionally ingrained as to be almost impossible to modify. We cannot afford, however, to be too pessimistic and must utilize all the medical, social and educational advantages available to off-set, at least to a certain extent, what has been bred in the bone. There is much that can be done. A complete physical and mental examination should be made, and while doing so the opportunity should be taken to inquire into the sexual life as naturally as one asks about other bodily functions. It can be done in a delicate and sensitive manner. To avoid it merely surrounds the topic with greater mystery and secretiveness and adds to the perpetuation of sexual habits which are better avoided. The explanation that the sexual function constitutes a fundamental biological need, that it is not wicked, obscene, taboo, brings comfort, trust, confidence and co-operation. It is tact and understanding which help to obtain satisfactory results; arbitrary prohibition, blows and threats lead to resentment, and a feeling of not being understood. An attempt should always be made to sublimate unhealthy sexual activities and interests by directing them into more constructive channels, and by avoiding those things which may, inadvertently, lead to greater sexual stimulation. For instance, over-solicitous mothers who constantly cuddle their children, allow them to sleep in their beds even when they are past puberty, are too possessive, disapprove of their children's friends, and Olympian fathers who create terror rather than friendship, can be advised to alter their ways because of the danger of provoking attitudes and fixations which can be devastating. It is the fretful, sensitive, rejected children, the artistic, aesthetic ones who indulge in phantasy thinking of a sexual nature and who require all the help we can give them. Emancipation, however, is a slow process, it should be allowed to develop gradually otherwise emotional crises may be precipitated which are better avoided. It is a matter of timing, of choosing the appropriate psychological moment rather than trying to force a person into a situation before he is fit to cope with it. At a later stage of development explanatory psycho-therapeutic interviews are indispensable. Forebodings and fears can be dispelled, reasons and arguments can be advanced to show that sexual anomalies are not unique experiences but are common to all mankind, and need not be regarded too moralistically. The assurance that they do not lead to insanity, that they can be cured—especially when the person is anxious to be cured—that they are the aftermath of childish habits, and that they need not interfere with a normal married life, constitutes a great comfort, and lessens the tension and fear which have been prominent.

When public offences have been committed and Court proceedings have been instituted we must appreciate that, medically, we have a duty to protect society as well as to do the best we can for the offender. Sometimes it may be the offender's first appearance in court, the first time he has been found out, but investigation almost invariably shows that the sexual offences which are charged against him have been committed over a period of months or years; his whole personality has to be inquired into before we can present a fair, unbiased report to the Court as to whether or not he is likely to benefit from medical treatment. We must try to ascertain all the facts on the basis of such questions as: Is this man willing to co-operate in treatment in the hope of being made better? or does he merely wish to escape a prison sentence? Has he sufficient intelligence to understand what psychotherapeutic investigation attempts to do? Is he of an age (under 40 years) when treatment is likely to prove successful?

We must always be careful not to promise more than is likely to be accomplished. If, however, we can answer the above questions affirmatively then we are justified in asking the Court to consider the advisability of probation on the understanding that medical supervision and treatment would be instituted. The crowded conditions which prevail in most prisons militate against successful therapy there, but prison doctors with psychological insight can accomplish a great deal.

In certain cases we have advised psychoanalytic treatment, but after explaining the time it may take and the uncertainty of the final result, the Court usually takes the view that a prison sentence should be served in the first place, and that afterwards any treatment may be undertaken that is considered advisable.

Apart from psychoanalytic treatment we suggest that much can be accomplished by suggestion, education, persuasion, injunction and encouragement so as to aspire to a greater sense of personal pride and prestige. The mere fact that someone is anxious to help is a tremendous relief from the secret, losing personal conflict which has been waged for so long.

While we have stressed the psychogenic aspects of sexual anomalies yet the possibility of physical impediments to normal sexual intercourse should always be investigated, and if endocrine deficiency or abnormality is present it should be treated with the appropriate hormone.

The understanding and treatment of sexual anomalies is a most complex matter, medicine and law should co-ordinate their approach, but that will never be accomplished so long as angry judges thunder moralistic platitudes from the Bench, and indiscreet psychiatrists indulge in optimistic theorizing; there is much common ground between such extremes.

REFERENCES

Allen, Clifford (1949) *The Sexual Perversions and Abnormalities*, 2nd ed., London.
Ellis, Havelock (1933) *Psychology of Sex*, London.
Freud, Sigmund (1910) *Three Contributions to the Sexual Theory*, New York.
Kallmann, F. J. (1953) *Heredity in Health and Mental Disorder*, London.
Kinsey, A. C., Pomeroy, W. B., and Martin, C. E. (1948) *Sexual Behavior in the Human Male*, Philadelphia.
Kinsey, A. C., Pomeroy, W. B., Martin, C. E., and Gebhard, P. H. (1953) *Sexual Behavior in the Human Female*, Philadelphia.
Russell, M. P. (1943) *Edinb. med. J.*, **50**, 558.
Strauss, E. B. (1950) *Brit. med. J.*, **1**, 697.
Wolfenden, Sir John (1957) Report on Homosexual Offences and Prostitution, London, H.M.S.O.

10

AFFECTIVE REACTION-TYPES

MANIC-DEPRESSIVE PSYCHOSIS

The term manic-depressive psychosis was introduced by Kraepelin to characterize disorders of affect consisting either of elation or depression—disorders which had previously been termed mania and melancholia in the belief that they were quite separate diseases.

The first attempt to formulate a clearer conception was made in 1854 by Falret senior and Baillarger, who independently described recurring attacks of mania and melancholia in the same patient. This was followed in 1879 by certain observations by Falret junior, who published a paper on what he termed *folie circulaire*. This he described as 'a hereditary affection generally found in a similar form both in ascendants and descendants'. His paper contains a detailed description of the typical alternation of mood from periods of excitement to periods of depression. In addition, he specifically mentioned the existence of 'mixed states', which he considered were transitory stages between attacks of mania and depression. In 1882, Kahlbaum spoke definitely of the phases mania and melancholia not as two separate types of mental disorder, but as two stages occurring in the same disease. He used the term cyclothymia to designate the milder, recoverable types, while the more grave, lasting types he called 'vesania typica circularis'. Hecker likewise used the term cyclothymia, and drew attention particularly to the non-dementing features. These observations preceded the observations of Kraepelin, who made a further advance when, in 1896, he formulated his conception of the manic-depressive psychosis. In this group he included the whole domain of periodic and circular insanity, simple mania, the greater part of the morbid states termed melancholia and also a considerable number of cases of confusion or delirium. He considered that all these conditions were representations of a single morbid process, and he showed that the different phases might succeed and replace one another in the same case—mania might lead to melancholia, with transition stages. His contribution was a stimulating and important one, because it not only conduced to a more careful analysis of symptoms in the individual case, but was of even greater importance from the point of view of prognosis; for Kraepelin declared that such attacks might occur throughout the life of the individual, and would never lead to profound dementia. He stated: 'Usually all morbid manifestations completely disappear, but where that is not the case, only a rather slight, peculiar psychic weakness develops, which is just as common to the types here taken together as it is different from dementias in diseases of other kinds.' The deterioration is characterized chiefly by a shallowness of mood, an acceptance of the situation and a readiness to be guided—it is more a state of invalidism, which the patients themselves appreciate, than a true deterioration.

AETIOLOGY

Hereditary predisposition is the most important predisposing aetiological factor. Kraepelin and numerous others have stated that 60 to 80 per cent. are hereditarily predisposed. When this type of disorder exists in the parents, the same type is likely to show itself directly among the descendants, but other types of mental disorder may also occur, *e.g.* schizophrenia. It is probable that manic-depressive psychosis is due to a single dominant gene, transmitted by an affected parent to one-half of the offspring, but with incomplete penetrance so that many who possess the gene do not develop the illness. Rosanoff, Handy and Plesset (1935) reported that of monozygotic twins both were affected in 69·6 per cent., and of dizygotic twins both were affected in 16·4 per cent.: a finding which clearly confirmed the importance of the hereditary factor. Kallmann (1953) confirmed these findings in a study of 27 monozygotic and 58 dizygotic twin pairs. In this series he found that the expectancy of manic-depressive psychosis varied from 16·7 per cent. for the half-sibs to 22·7 and 25·5 per cent. for the sibs and dizygotic co-twins, respectively, and to 100 per cent. for the monozygotic twin partners. The corresponding rate for the parents of index cases was 23·4 per cent. The perfect concordance in the one-egg twin pairs is explained by Kallmann as probably due to the fact that only hospitalized manic-depressive patients were chosen as index cases. There is certainly no evidence that the usual degree of expressivity of the genotype is 100 per cent., or any figure near to that. In Kallmann's sample there was no twin pair with a schizophrenic psychosis in one partner and a manic-depressive psychosis in the other.

Kallmann states that amongst Western peoples the average general frequency of manic-depressive psychosis does not exceed 0·4 per cent. in the population: if involutional cases are included the risk rises to about 1 per cent. Women are more liable to the disease than men; it is estimated that 70 per cent. of the patients are women.

Kretschmer has attempted to differentiate mankind on the basis of their physical state. He has termed the short, stocky people with thick necks his 'pyknic' type, in contrast with the thin, visceroptotic 'asthenic' or leptosomatic type, and the long-limbed, muscular 'athletic' type. The former group-type is usually associated with people showing a manic-depressive psychosis, while the latter types are more frequently seen in cases of schizophrenia.

From the purely mental side, Meyer, Hoch, Kirby and Bleuler have pointed out that the mental make-up which frequently characterizes the individual in whom a manic-depressive psychosis occurs deserves close study. The manic-depressive disposition is one in which the affect swings from states of elation to states of depression in people who are generally recognized to have frank, open personalities. They are either bright, talkative, optimistic, aggressive people, who make light of the ordinary affairs of life, or else they take a gloomy outlook, bewail the past, make mountains out of mole-hills; or there is a combination of the above moods, rendering the person emotionally unstable and variable. Reiss gives his cases in percentages:

Type of pre-psychotic temperament	Psychoses		
	Depressive	Manic	Combined forms
Depressive temperament	64·2	8·3	27·5
Manic temperament	35·6	23·3	41·1
Irritable temperament	45·5	24·4	30·1
Cyclothymic temperament	35·3	11·7	53·0

Quoted from Kraepelin.

The variability of affect may never go beyond normal limits. The mood of most people does swing to a certain event, but such changes are transitory, and interfere little with daily activities. Some 'gastropaths', some sexual 'neurasthenics', and many who suffer from obsessions, are probably closely related to the manic-depressive groups.

When manic-depressive disorders arise from a clear sky, without any definite precipitating factor, they are termed constitutional or endogenous. There are cases styled *reactive depressions* (and there are also, but more rarely, reactive excitements) because the condition follows upon some obvious exciting cause. These are often illnesses of the classical manic-depressive variety, in which the precipitating factors are unusually clear (the 'psychically produced melancholia' of Lange). Others with similarly obvious precipitants show an ability to react to intercurrent stimuli (such as the doctor's visits), combined sometimes with attacks of weeping, or of anxiety, various hysterical symptoms, and a tendency to blame others rather than themselves—or if they are self-accusatory, it is in a tentative manner, seeking reassurance for their blamelessness. These are the so-called 'psychogenic depressions' of Kraepelin, and they are more properly classed with the neuroses.

PSYCHOPATHOLOGY

A number of suggestive indications of the psychopathology of these conditions will be derived from a study of the case-histories to be given below. The following general account is largely derived from MacCurdy (1925).

Manic States

The elation that is so prominent a symptom of manic states is to be regarded as the mood appropriate to the fulfilment of a wish; its pathological intensity is a measure of the strength of the wish. What makes the elation pathological is not that there is nothing in the conscious content that would justify it if it were true —there often is, in the form of fleeting grandiose ideas, for example—but that there is nothing in the external circumstances that apparently justifies the elation. The reason for the elation lies outside of consciousness, although often very close to it, breaking through sometimes in the fragmentary utterances of the flight of ideas. What happens is that from some very strong wish that has been repressed into unconsciousness, the repression is at least partly removed, and the patient feels and behaves as if the wish had been fulfilled. Sometimes the wish is for some adult gratification, *e.g.* marriage, but more often the wish is one that has developed at the childish stage of mental development and has persisted into adult life, *e.g.* for the death of a disliked parent. Sometimes external circumstances contribute to the wish-fulfilment, and so precipitate a psychosis. For example, the hated relative dies—let us suppose it is the mother of an individual who has from childhood had an abnormally strong liking for her father, and so, as a child, wished her mother out of the way (the 'Electra complex'—the feminine counterpart of the 'Oedipus complex'). This wish was repressed at the time and ever since. Then if the mother dies the wish is fulfilled, and the now adult woman, with the childish fixation of her affection on her father, has the chief obstacle to her exclusive possession of his affection removed. She becomes elated, but the elation appears causeless, *i.e.* pathological, and the fulfilment is poorly formulated in consciousness, if it appears there at all—either because repression continues to operate to some degree, or because the conscious formulation of unconscious wishes is a difficult task. The degree to which conscious expression is attained varies very much. Often the releasing causes of a manic psychosis are entirely within the patient's own mind, consisting in phantasy.

If, on the other hand, there has been a strong feeling of guilt associated with the wish, adult or infantile, its fulfilment, whether in fact or phantasy, is apt to lead to a depression, which again appears pathological, especially because here repression continues to operate much more decisively, since the ideas are altogether unpleasantly coloured, and must be kept completely out of consciousness.

Depressions

In many depressions a precipitating cause is not recognizable. In others, the depression results from disappointment or deprivation. In a third group, the precipitant is the reanimation, often by some external event, of an unconscious trend ('wish') which, if allowed to reach consciousness, would ultimately destroy the personality. Hence a gigantic effort is made at repression (inhibition), and the inhibition becomes generalized, so that all thinking is interfered with. The trend may have a strong feeling of guilt attached to it, because something antisocial is the object of the trend, *e.g.* the death of a near relative. As in the manic, such trends may be either infantile or adult in origin. In any case, repression of the guilty trend having occurred, depression appears as the conscious correlate of the now unconscious guilt-feeling. The depressive ideas which appear in consciousness are largely rationalizations, but may have also some disguised relation to the repressed wish.

The psychoanalytic view of the psychopathology of the depressive phase is that the following factors are involved:

1. A constitutional factor in the form of inherited accentuation of oral erotism.
2. A special fixation of the libido at the oral level, that is the patient's erotic

interests have lingered round the mouth zone when they should on the contrary have developed to the genital zone with complete object love. The fixation is considered to be at the second oral stage when ambivalence first becomes possible (biting is an aggressive act, not co-existent with suckling).

3. A severe injury to infantile narcissism brought about by early disappointments in love, especially love of the mother.

4. The occurrence of the first disappointment in love before the Oedipus wishes have been overcome.

5. The repetition of the primary disappointment in later life as the exciting cause of the depression. But for a detailed understanding of this theory it is necessary to refer to Abraham's paper (1927) on the development of the libido.

SYMPTOMATOLOGY

Manic Phase

We have become accustomed to describe four main varieties of mania, termed respectively: 1. hypomania; 2. acute mania; 3. delirious mania; and 4. chronic mania. The cases which we include in the group of chronic mania run a course so different from the cases in the other groups that it will be best to consider the chronic manias together under a separate heading. All of these varieties, however, are characterized by three main symptoms, which vary in duration and in intensity in each case. These three symptoms are (a) elated though unstable mood, (b) flight of ideas, (c) increased psychomotor activity. These basic symptoms, although present in every case, are to be considered as a background or setting for the development of other symptoms. In some cases the elated mood may predominate clinically, whereas in other cases it may be the restlessness or the over-talkativeness. Other features may complicate the picture, and irritability, cantankerousness, suspicion, a clouding of consciousness, with delusions, hallucinations, disorientation and lack of insight, may all appear. Such symptoms as suspicion, hallucinations, etc., are usually transitory, occurring at the height of the illness, and are not of the same ominous significance as they would be if they occurred in a setting of clear consciousness.

Another important general point which should always be kept clearly in mind is the fact that practically in all cases the attacks are acute in onset, the history dating back only for a few days or a few weeks.

While such conditions as hypomania, acute mania and delirious mania can readily be recognized, we wish to point out that the differentiation of these states is not by any means clean cut, and that many cases pass through such stages without any definite gradation; some may never pass beyond the hypomanic stage, while others may from the very beginning be either acutely excited or delirious.

MANIC STATES

Hypomania

Hypomania is the mildest variety, and although it is characterized by the individual symptoms previously mentioned, e.g. elation, over-activity, flight of ideas, these are not greatly developed. The patient continues to have a keen realization of his position and environment, and does not exhibit such extreme disorder of conduct as to bring him into conflict with his fellows. For a time he is merely considered a 'live wire', witty, a man with ideas and aggressiveness, a social success; and it is only in the further course of the illness when he becomes interfering, irritable, domineering, and has too many schemes on hand, that his friends suspect that something is wrong. He tends to monopolize conversation, expresses his views dogmatically, drifts from one topic to another and shows a flight of ideas. His schemes, though feasible, are never thoroughly worked out. He is inconsistent and changeable; yet he feels more fit than ever before. When reasoned with, he is intolerant of criticism, becomes sarcastic or rude, changes the subject, thinks that the person who does not see eye to eye with him is a fool and does not hesitate to say so. He is lacking in moral control, and may indulge to excess both sexually and in regard to drink. It is frequently on the basis of such disordered conduct that he comes under hospital treatment or is apprehended by the police and taken to prison; *e.g.* a man with a very distinguished record was apprehended for buying motor cars with worthless cheques, and it was not until he recovered that he became fully conscious of the significance and serious-ness of his action. Under hospital conditions such a patient is most difficult to manage. He resents restraint, wants to better the ward arrangements, is arrogant towards officials, staff and other patients, and constantly lodges com-plaints, writing long letters to the Board of Management of the hospital, the Home Secretary, Members of Parliament and others. In his conversation, all manner of trivial details are introduced, but the talk never develops into incoherence; whatever he says can be followed and understood, but the patient rarely completes any topic. His memory is excellently preserved. Although many incidents may be distorted, ready explanations are given (*folie raisonnante*). Perhaps the most striking symptom of all is the extreme restlessness; such a patient must be doing something all the time; he feels that he can do everything better than anyone else, writes long letters, takes part in all manner of games, is never still and yet does not seem to experience an ordinary sense of fatigue. There is no clouding of consciousness; his orientation for time, for place and for person is correct; and there is no evidence of hallucinations or delusions. As a general rule, he does not realize that he is seriously ill, his judgement being impaired.

CASE NO. 18

An enterprising successful man almost continuously ill for the past sixteen years with alternating attacks of depression and elation; now in a state of hypomanic excitement; over-active, talking continually and writing numerous letters; both talk and writing show-ing obvious flight of ideas and play upon words (rhyming and punning); his mood elated, but changing rapidly to irritability when he is crossed; and the content of his utterances showing a strong erotic trend.

P. S., 50 years old; a professional man. He has been ill more or less continuously for 14 years, with alternating attacks of depression and excitement. One sister was stated to have been in a mental hospital, and another was described as a 'nervous wreck'.

P

The patient himself had been an extraordinarily capable man, who had taken a high place in examinations, and had reached a position of great distinction. He was always of an aggressive type, very much a leader, described by some as too independent, by others as an agitator and, by his son, as one who could not brook opposition.

He has been treated in various mental hospitals. In his first excited attack in 1919 he was so exalted that it was suspected he might be a case of general paralysis. At that time he said that he was very wealthy, that he was the deputy of Lord Kitchener. He was taken to prison because of insulting behaviour towards a Jew, whom he accused of being a German spy.

The state which he has shown since he has been under our care has been essentially a hypomania.

He had been admitted to a mental hospital but was transferred to a private home. His condition there was described as follows:

After arrival he stated that it seemed as if he had entered Paradise after escaping from Hell, but he immediately wished to alter the domestic arrangements to meet his own whims. He woke early, and passed the time whistling in opposition to the black-birds and thrushes. When asked by the nurse not to disturb the others, he abused and cursed her. At breakfast he talked incessantly, and made offensive personal remarks. He pointed out that one of the Matrons did not look well—that no doubt she had 'spent the night on the tiles'. During the day he wandered about, acting in the most unconventional and irresponsible way. He called on the local lawyer, and wasted his time, telling him of all the actions he intended to bring. He troubled the doctor, who in consequence tried to avoid him, but this could not be done, as the patient stood beside his car until the doctor was forced to appear and listen to his rambling talk. He threatened to get the banker into serious trouble, so that the latter complained. He disturbed the postmistress, and abused her loudly before the public, so that she also was compelled to lodge a complaint. He called on strangers, who were relatives of the staff, and demanded tea. He hinted by innuendoes, by winks and gestures, that one of the Matrons drank, and that he was going to keep his eye on her. At table, in the presence of others, he was disrespectful to her. He suggested that gross immoralities were going on, and he thought this must be so because there were 'one male attendant and twelve beautiful nurses'. He himself would go to the kitchen quarters to talk to the maids, and when reproved by the Matron, flew into a temper and went to bed. He made a formal proposal of marriage to one of the nurses, and decided to divorce his wife for desertion. He told all his intimate affairs to complete strangers, such as his coming marriage, his intended divorce and so on. At table his conversation was most objection-able, as he discoursed among the ladies about public conveniences. He asserted that he himself was a lady-killer, and provided details. He was in communication with many lawyers, requesting actions to be brought and demanding money. On one occasion he forged the name of the lady in whose house he was staying, and sent a telegram to his wife demanding £25, which was forwarded immediately.

A good example of his condition is obtained from the following letter, in which he makes his proposal of marriage:

'My dearest G.—Y'day, I fondly believe, was as happy a day as I ever spent in this weary world of Drink, Work, & Sin. All on A/c. of you "Matey".

'Do you not believe in love at first sight? I do most emphatically assert that *the moment I met you at N. station my fate was sealed*. I am not an old Turk, or even Mahommedan, but I believe in *FATE*. And if I have your "promise true" ("which ne'er forgot shall be" mind) then "*I* am yours, and *YOU* are mine"—(For ever and Beyond) as the grand old Hymn phrases it. "And *ye* sall walk in silk" (real—not celanese) "attire an' siller hae tae spare"—bonnie sang that, a' aboot *LOVE*?

"And we shall all the beauties prove,
        Of Hills and Valleys, Seas and Towns, etc., etc., etc."

'When I give my promise I make good. With St. Paul it is a case of "What I have said, I *have* said" always.

'But perhaps you will rejoin: "You have a wife?" Yes, but after many years' treacherous thieving, lying, failure to do that which she vowed, viz.: "Love, *Honour* & Obey", instead of putting me into vicious Asylums, I am not risking her company again. So, as I *know* she won't (*and cannot even if she would*) resist my Divorce Action for her Desertion of me in 1921, you must wait until Autumn for Ct. of Session Judge's decision. The cost is small for undefended actions nowadays under the 1922 Act, which allows "desertion" as a reason for granting Divorce. (It used to be that Adultery must also be proved, but that was amended.)

'So you are not taking an adulterous *lunatic* (?) If you'll have me, of course I'll settle a big sum on you for your own use, and make over my insurance and estate by Will in your favour, less one or two legacies for Charitable Institutions.

'Meantime you are my nurse—I am your Guide, Philosopher, Humble Servitor, and Lover. I could not sleep after 5 A.M. for thinking of you—and my songs were all of thee, my ideal woman, for face and figure and grace, and gracious womanly sympathy for a man without friendly relations when he is in "these places", but whose relations were proud of him when his income was large. "Telle est la Vie", m'amie fidèle.

'"I fear no foe with thee at hand to bless", as Toplady wrote together, in his immortal Hymn, "Rock of Ages".

'Tout à vous.'

The above letter, with its underscored passages (here printed in italics), interpolations, brackets and flight of ideas, yet at the same time coherent, is completely characteristic of a hypomanic state.

Since his arrival under our care his condition has been very much as already outlined. He is diffuse and circumstantial in his conversation, his statements are apparently quite accurate, and dates in his career are given rapidly and without confusion, and are remembered in minute detail, even to the hour and the day when certain things happened. He talks so continuously that it is almost impossible to get in a question, but he usually answers correctly and to the point; a few seconds later, without any break in the continuity of his flow, he is talking about something totally different. Yet after a long digression he is capable of coming back to the main point at issue—usually, however, only to leave it again. His mood is one of constant elation. At times he is definitely euphoric, and his list of wrongs, which is very long, he recites in a whimsical, jovial way; but every now and again, especially when interfered with, or when his wishes are not immediately conceded, he becomes very irritable, often obscene, and always scurrilous and threatening. There has, however, not been any evidence of hallucinations, nor does there seem to be the slightest impairment of his intellectual faculties, except, of course, that he has no realization of his condition, and therein shows defective judgement.

He spends a great deal of his time writing letters to various members of the staff, to the Sheriff of the County, to other high officials and to his own relatives and friends.

A letter, addressed to the Matron, is typical:

'Matron B.—Do you want to get hung at the Yard Arm as Pirates used to get hung for Piracy on the High Seas?

'If not, better come to terms with P. before the Directors are apprised of *your* piratical ways at G.

'And that may be sooner than you dream.

'Do your duty first—attend to your own private down-town pleasures when off duty here. Otherwise the consequences may send you into retirement without a pension, and with only a bad character from your last place. P.'

So long as this patient's threats are not taken too seriously, he is quite pleasant to get on with, but he has to be handled with a considerable amount of rope. He is able, however, to conform to regulations to a wonderful extent; he has now had the privilege of parole for a good many months, and has not in any way misused it.

The case is a good example of the constitutional reaction-type—repeated attacks, with no sufficient precipitating causes to be found.

In the following case there is a clear indication in the content of the patient's utterances of the factors leading to his illness:

CASE NO. 19

A brief mild hypomanic excitement in a hitherto quiet, docile youth, following upon a transitory mild depression. The hypomanic elation showed the usual characteristics— over-activity (with erotic tendencies coming to the fore), an infectious and excessive gaiety, over-talkativeness with some punning and rhyming and lack of sustained attention. The flight of ideas and the general over-activity are not so marked as in the previous case and the whole condition was comparatively short-lived—features which are probably related to the essentially shy, quiet type of personality in whom the illness developed.

L. M., 24 years; male; single; farmer. The patient had been a very quiet, sensitive, docile youth, who was not fond of company, avoiding the society of girls especially. He had been clever at school, and had just missed obtaining a medal in his last year. Since leaving school he had worked on his father's farm. He had seemed to think that having done well at school he was too clever for farm work. Nevertheless, he worked hard on the farm, except when suffering from 'stomach' troubles—he had headaches, and had to go to bed sometimes after food. During the War he showed no anxiety to join the Army, but afterwards he expressed regret at not having done so. In the early months of the year he was mildly depressed, but nothing remarkable was observed till April, when he began to behave oddly and was removed to a nursing home. There he was mildly elated, talked diffusely and circumstantially, rhyming and playing on words, and was distractible. He was restless and sleepless, and in the latter part of May he had brief influenzal symptoms, his sputum being blood-stained and watery, and containing pneumococci and pneumobacilli, *Micrococcus catarrhalis* and diphtheroid bacilli. On admission to hospital in June from the nursing home he showed all the above mental symptoms to a mild degree. He walked about aimlessly, smiling and laughing. Anything presented to him distracted his attention. He was mischievous, and tried to caress the nurses.

The following is a sample of his speech in response to questions: (Do you want to do some work?) 'Yes, I want to get out and practise music for a while.' (Do you want to earn a living?) 'Yes, I got a gold disc with a lion in the centre, with a wild cat down below and a tree above, from the King.' (Why?) 'For bravery, service to my country— and writing letters to my friends.' (Have you always been happy at home?) 'No, at times I was very angry—had wanted a shift—had seen these things too long—got into arguments.' (When you were young what did you do?) 'Well, that was a long time ago. I may have felt queer—I hurt my chest climbing trees—my lungs grew, but my stomach was too small—I could have gone without food for a long time.' (Do you sleep well?) 'I don't care to sleep—I've so much energy.' (Do you dream?) 'I dreamt I was flying— and if that doesn't prove that your spirit roams at night when you're in bed—electricity in your backbone which attracts eyes.' (What else?) 'I'd like to be married—hadn't money—I was shy—there's a change in me—I was kind of entranced—lifted clean out of myself.'

In addition he mentioned that he felt that his stomach would have to be very different before he could get married, and that he had read many sentimental books, and 'thought it might be very nice sometimes—buying rings and then taking a tiff'.

His memory was good, except for events of the very recent past, which had not been attended to and therefore were not well retained. Orientation was slightly interfered with for the same reason. Insight was lacking for the nature of his illness—'I was supposed to be in consumption.'

Within ten days he became less restless, his elation gave place to uneasiness and his talk became more connected and relevant. Within two weeks of admission he had returned to his normal state, *i.e.* a docile, quiet and agreeable fellow, rather self-conscious in manner.

Several trends were obvious in the content—the compensatory phantasy of the award of a medal (which he had missed at school), which also served to compensate his lack of war service; the remark indicating dissatisfaction with his employment on the farm—'he wanted a shift'; his erotic preoccupations and overt tenderness (caressing nurses); and his references to his bodily ill-health. The conditions which these trends indicate combined to produce a mild degree of depression, followed by an elation, in which his failings were compensated in phantasy, and in which his personality underwent a change of which he was conscious—'I was shy—now there's a change in me.'

Acute Mania

There is no sharp distinguishing line between hypomania and mania—the one grades into the other. There are cases in which a state of acute excitement develops at once without any previous hypomanic stage. Acute excitement may be preceded by a short period of sleeplessness and irritability. In this stage the elation, flight of ideas and over-activity are all more intense, and, in addition, there may be a certain clouding of consciousness with disorientation and great impulsiveness. The patient affirms he 'never felt better in his life'; he has an air of utter superiority, he orders everyone about, and his conversation and conduct are so disordered that residence in a mental hospital is imperative. The mood is merry, gay, infectious, but periods of irritability and anger are frequent. At such times his conversation becomes obscene, and his conduct unrestrained. Violent assaults are made on the officials and nurses, the furniture and bedclothing are broken and torn, the walls may be smeared with excreta, but just as suddenly there may be a return to a state of good humour, and apology may even be expressed for the previous conduct. The speech shows a typical flight of ideas, and this may proceed to incoherence. He is extremely distractible, and his attention can be held only momentarily, because whatever he sees or hears he comments on. Such a patient is 'on the go' night and day. He may not be quite clear in regard to time or environment; he tends to misidentify people, and to greet perfect strangers as old friends.

Hallucinations are occasionally present, but they are transitory. The delusions expressed are of a wish-fulfilling kind, and are in harmony with the patient's excited mood.

It is impossible to carry out an accurate examination of the memory and intellectual functions, but there is nothing to indicate that they are disordered *per se*. The insight and judgement are very poor, as a secondary result of the disorders of affect and attention.

The following case illustrates the more acute type of manic excitement, and shows the rapid transition which occurs from one stage to another:

CASE NO. 20

Rapid onset of an acute manic excitement in a healthy young woman of energetic happy disposition; extreme restlessness; excessive talkativeness with continuous screaming at times; elation reaching at intervals a pitch of ecstasy; distractibility so great that comprehension was vastly impaired and the patient disoriented in consequence; shamelessly erotic behaviour along with a pronounced religious trend in her talk; gradual subsidence with occasional exacerbations of destructiveness; complete recovery with insight.

A. L. A young lady, 32 years old, single, a school-teacher, had been ill for four days previous to her admission to hospital. She had come from a healthy stock, and had developed quite normally. She was a bright, happy, cheerful girl, who at school took many prizes in English, arithmetic and French, and after leaving became a pupil teacher. She was fond of fancy sewing, played the piano, sang in a choir, liked dancing and company, mixed with boys as freely as with girls and was a general favourite. She may have been somewhat over-sensitive, and is stated sometimes to have imagined slights where none were intended. On the whole, however, her personality was that of a very steady, normal, efficient girl. For about one year previous to her breakdown she had been teaching a special class of physically defective children. A few days previous to the onset of her illness she was noticed to be more 'on the go'—at the pictures, at a dance, and attending a meeting in church. She showed an unstable emotional state, burst into tears without provocation and next moment would be laughing and saying that she was all right, 'just needing a rest', 'just tired'. Soon she became more talkative and restless; she took little food, she did not sleep, except under the influence of a drug; she tended to recall the past, and to talk about former imaginary slights. Subsequently, she expressed peculiar ideas, declaring that her mother was dead, and when reassured about this, that her friend upstairs was dead. She declared that she was acting under God's orders, that she had spoken to God, and a good deal of her conversation consisted in her repeating what she said God was telling her.

At the time of her admission she asked the doctor to kiss her, and because he refused she said she could not trust him. She talked incessantly, accused the doctor of having been drinking and then immediately began to talk about God, and about how God meant her to suffer. 'I have got a pain here', pointing over her heart. 'It is me that is going to have the baby; God has made me say it now that I am going to have a baby; it was my fault—his fault—he was selfish; it is that that has nearly driven me out of my mind.' She explained how God meant everybody to be happy—God had told her to have a baby, and, at the same time, she felt sure that she was going to die. This idea of death constantly recurred throughout her conversation. At times she refused any nourishment—she would not even take fluids. She screamed at the pitch of her voice, saying that the doctor was to 'die, die, die', shrieking it till her face was livid, the veins congested almost to bursting, and her pulse racing at about 160 per minute. On account of her great excitement she had to be tube-fed, and had to be given paraldehyde to help her to rest. The intense excitement was accompanied by great motor restlessness. She was distractible, commented on things around her, misidentified people and was disoriented both in regard to time and place. Her conduct at times suggested that she was seeing visions. Her condition approached a state of ecstasy, when she would sing, 'How blessed are the messengers that preach the Gospel of Peace', and then would continue the air in a kind of recitative, interspersed with questions and conversation. She maintained that she still heard God's voice talking to her, believed herself to be God's spokesman and frequently identified herself with God. In contrast, she was foolishly erotic in her behaviour, made attempts to embrace the medical officers, exposed herself and was quite shameless.

In the course of a few weeks improvement began to take place, but at intervals she had very excited periods, when she smashed the crockery, tore her bedclothes, smashed the glass panels in her room and flung the fragments at the other patients. These periods gradually became fewer and briefer, and finally she reached a stage where she was able to discuss her illness, and gained complete insight for the fact that she had been mentally ill.

Here, then, was the history of an acute illness of rapid onset, rapidly passing through the various stages of the manic reaction and terminating in an excellent recovery. The condition seemed to be partly explained by exogenous causes, *e.g.* the strain of teaching, and the fact that she was the main support of her home. Her psychosis exposed erotic trends, and the fulfilment of her wishes, at the expense of sane thinking.

Delirious Mania

This is the extreme stage. It may spring from a hypomania, and then pass through a stage of acute mania, or may develop at once without the other stages having preceded.

The individual is totally disoriented for time, place and person. Conversation is incoherent, and the patient is so excited that he can be restrained only by a powerful hypnotic. He is never at rest; he tosses and rolls about, is in a ferment of activity bodily and mentally, and unless this is controlled by means of drugs or otherwise he rapidly exhausts himself. Auditory and visual illusions and hallucinations, and suspicions and delusions, develop. Such patients behave in the most shameless way; they not only do not take any pride in their personal appearance, but they are careless in all their habits. They have no realization at all of the serious nature of their illness, and do not therefore co-operate in treatment.

Such cases were first described by Luther Bell in 1849 and were known as Bell's mania. From their acute nature and high death-rate they were also named typhomania, delirium grave, or collapse delirium. If recovery occurs, the condition, when arising *de novo*, does not usually recur, or at least there is a long interval between attacks. Kraines (1934) gave an excellent review, and suggests that they should continue to be known as Bell's mania.

The following case illustrates the delirious type of excitement:

CASE NO. 21

Extreme manic excitement of rapid onset in a young woman of an enterprising, hardworking disposition. Continuous wild excitement, regardless of physical needs of any kind; talkativeness so incessant and disconnected as to amount to incoherence; great elation; attention given to nothing for more than a second or two; intercurrent infection; gradual subsidence with playful happiness in the meantime; ultimate complete recovery with insight, but amnesia for the period of extreme excitement.

M. A. An unmarried woman, 26 years old, was admitted to hospital in a state of great excitement. She would not co-operate in an examination, answered questions at random, talked in a fragmentary, almost incoherent way and had no appreciation of time or place, or people around her. She tore her clothes, refused her food, jumped in and out of bed, spat on the bedclothes and often would run up and down the ward in an aimless way. It was impossible to gain her attention. Her excitement was so intense and her co-operation so poor, that it was necessary to tube-feed her. Her mouth was in a foul condition, her tongue was thickly coated, she was careless and inattentive to bladder and bowels and she had bruises on her arms and legs. There was no evidence of any organic disease, but physical examination on account of her great restlessness was very difficult. Her weight was 6 st. 3 lb. After a few days her mouth became much cleaner, she looked better, but she was sleeping very poorly at night, was still very restless, tended to be flighty and flippant in her talk and was tremendously elated. She talked in a low, hoarse voice, and was very difficult to follow. During any examination she would shift about in her bed, attempt to get out, play with her hair, tuck the sheets round her arms and so on. When asked how she was, she said, 'Just daft, dearie. Knife and fork—no, they would not do it.' She paid very little attention to questions, and answered more or less at random. She said she wanted 'One, two, three sugars: Aunty Jinty filled her pockets—dickey birds—it's the highest—you can roll round as much as you like.'

Six weeks after admission she was still restless and inaccessible, and her temperature now rose in the evenings often as high as 103° F. Two weeks later it was found that she had a swelling of her left leg, which seemed to be caused by a thrombophlebitis, which reacted to treatment. This condition was accompanied by an irregular but gradually declining temperature. At this time she was constantly wetting, and a catheter specimen of her urine showed a considerable bacilluria. Gradually she became less restless, her temperature came down to normal, she began to take her food well and slept for from seven to eight hours every night. She still was flippant in her answers, and when asked what place this was, she replied, 'I suppose it is a blooming hospital.' What is my name? 'Walter.' What is my business? 'Nothing at all.' She then laughed uproariously, and said, 'Excuse me for laughing.' When asked what had caused her illness, she said, 'An explosion in San Francisco', and enjoyed this reply very much. Her whole attitude was still one of great elation; her laughter was of a merry, infectious character, and there was a great deal of restless energy about her conduct.

After a period of two and a half months she was able to give a comprehensive account of the onset and development of her illness. She stated that she had no recollection of having been excessively energetic or excited. She remembered having been taken to a nursing home, but of events following this she had no remembrance until several weeks after her admission to this hospital. She also recalled that when her family doctor had come to see her she had misidentified him.

This young lady's father had died from a shock: her mother was stated to have had epileptic fits, and to have lost all memory before her death, at the age of 45.

The patient herself had been a delicate child, who had suffered from the ordinary childish ailments, but in addition had had two separate attacks of chorea, from which she had made good recoveries. Her personality was of the leader type, a steady worker, perhaps rather older than her years, but inclined to be very active in whatever she took up.

Her illness had a very rapid onset, during which she became over-energetic, over-talkative, sleepless and did not take her food; her friends explained it on the basis of excess of work. She had been helping in the work of the Crippled Children's League, which necessitated a great deal of strenuous activity, including such things as office work, teaching a class of boys, helping them to finish off their toys, visiting in their homes and helping to arrange outings in their summer time.

During her period of convalescence she rapidly put on weight, and at the time of her discharge she had come up to her usual level of 7 st. 7 lb.

This case was one with a rapid onset, which quickly passed through a stage of acute excitement, until at the time she came to the hospital she was delirious, and had no memory of what happened during a period of six weeks. The type of reaction was characteristic of the manic-depressive psychosis. The thrombophlebitis which developed during the course of her illness was purely incidental.

Depression

Depression exhibits three main grades of severity, termed respectively simple or mild depression, acute depression and depressive stupor.

We again recognize a triad of symptoms which is present in all of the above grades, namely, difficulty in thinking, depression and psychomotor retardation. Many other symptoms may be superadded—delusions, hypochondriacal, self-accusatory or persecutory; hallucinations, irritability, etc. The mood change gives the impression of being the fundamental feature. The depression is not infrequently accompanied by anxiety. The other features are such as might be expected to go with a depressed mood: for example, difficulty in thinking and a small output of talk. Sometimes there is considerable talk with much reiteration, while instead of reduction in activity there may be motor agitation [see under 'Mixed States'].

The most important feature of depression in general, from the point of view of care and treatment, is the danger of suicide. Suicide is not necessarily an indication that a person is mentally ill; but a large proportion of those who commit suicide have been so affected. East, in an analysis of a thousand consecutive cases of attempted suicide, estimated that about one-fifth were psychotic. Gaupp, without attempting to make a distinction between certifiable and non-certifiable, found that among 124 cases 44 were definitely insane, while one person was considered to be mentally sound; the others were described as psychopathic and as showing poor mental equipment and balance. A study by Sievers and Davidoff (1942–43) showed that of 150 cases of attempted suicide referred to a general hospital only eleven had been seen previously by a psychiatrist. This corresponds to our experience. We have been impressed by the large proportion of cases of attempted suicide admitted to the Royal Infirmary, Edinburgh, and Guy's Hospital, London, who have never previously seemed to require psychiatric guidance or control. The rapidity with which recovery may occur is also a factor to be noted and is in striking contrast to the prolonged treatment of the average case of depression.

We have also been struck by the trivial nature of the precipitating factors in some cases; for example, in a husband requested by his wife to sleep for the time being in an attic to make room for a guest; in a girl who had been 'walking-out' with a soldier of whom her father disapproved, so that being afraid to return home she walked into the Thames, near London Bridge, instead. Such people are no doubt in some ways psychopathic, but not always to an extent which brings them to notice before the suicidal attempt itself. Sometimes spite enters as a basis for the suicidal gesture, but it is a gesture which is sometimes carried to the point of successful self-destruction. The type of mental disorder most likely to be associated with suicide is depression of the anxious, agitated type characterized by hypochondriacal bodily delusions and the futility of existence. The mental and executive retardation of the depressions of the manic-depressive group may not infrequently act as a safeguard but cannot be relied upon.

Simple Depression. This type is characterized by depression and by a general slowing, both mental and physical. The bearing of the man is altered. He has a sad, careworn expression, his brow is wrinkled, his eye is dull, and he looks older than his years. He describes himself as a failure, or hopeless, or a disgrace. Thinking is difficult and slow. The slowness may not be apparent, and the only evidence of retardation may be the complaint of difficulty in thinking. He is unable to take an interest in what goes on around him, and thinks of himself as a man apart, and that it would be better if he were dead. His answers are usually monosyllabic: he speaks in a low voice, in typical cases with a delayed reaction-time. Sometimes questions have to be repeated before an answer is obtained. What he does say, however, is relevant. He blames himself for trivial mis-demeanours in his past, makes mountains out of mole-hills. In the psychomotor field the retardation is also conspicuous. The patient sits idly in one place, gazing at the ground, and when asked to do anything there is usually a delay of a minute or two, and then the action is carried out in a slow, deliberate way, as if his limbs were weighted. He has to be assisted with his dressing, his food, and often has to be urged to attend to the calls of nature. The patient understands everything that goes on in his environment. There is no clouding of consciousness, there is no disorientation, no defect of memory or intellect. The patient himself recognizes the need for specialized treatment, and may come to the out-patient department of a general hospital, or apply voluntarily for admission to a mental hospital.

Milder forms of depression occur, which often masquerade under some other guise. Patients will consult the doctor in general practice, or come as out-patients, complaining sometimes of mild depression, but more often of anything but depression. They have vague or emphatic complaints of headache, often of an ill-defined and ill-localized type and very persistent, of dyspepsia of various kinds, including lack of appetite, feelings of weight in the abdomen, a bad taste in the mouth, constipation, blurring of vision, irritability, especially to noises, lassitude, general weakness and (what is very common) fatigue or actual exhaus-tion. When thoroughly examined physically, they present nothing that will satis-factorily account for their symptoms. They are probably continuing at their work, but finding it very difficult, and on closer inquiry it will be found that although their difficulty is at first attributed to the complaints just enumerated or to the exacting nature of their work, as a matter of fact they cannot concen-trate, and it is an effort for them to keep to the task in hand. Reading may be easy enough, but when it comes to writing, it is difficult for them to do it, words and phrases come with difficulty, and if the latter requires any invention it takes a very long time. Sleep is frequently, but not always, disturbed, with early waken-ing and it is always unrefreshing. It is especially difficult to get started in the mornings. It may be impossible to get a clear statement of mood disorder from these patients; they may even deny that they are sad or depressed in any way. But when a patient presents a number of the above symptoms and when no adequate physical lesion can be found, and especially if the condition has per-sisted more or less unchanged for some months, and if there has been a previous similar attack perhaps some years before, it is probable that one is dealing with what is primarily a mental disorder—in these cases a mild depression. If, further, it is found that the patient has been of an anxious, gloomy, foreboding disposi-tion, or, on the other hand, of an habitually or even unusually cheerful turn of mind with perhaps very transient episodes of depression of spirits (the 'cyclo-thymic' temperament), the conclusion is strengthened. A family tendency to affective disorders is also of confirmatory value.

Such patients as these do not usually enter a mental hospital. They can be treated outside, and are sometimes better so treated. After a time, usually months, they recover gradually or suddenly, and the particular method of treat-ment they were undergoing at the time gets the credit of their cure; but that is fallacious; they recover often in spite, rather than because, of the physical treatment meted out to them. In a few instances there is not this happy result. We have known cases, almost monosymptomatic in character—perhaps only a persistent headache, without physical signs, but with a good deal of concern about it—who committed suicide.

CASE NO. 22

A second attack of simple retarded depression of acute onset in a quiet, shy girl, with a suicidal attempt early in the illness. Inactive, hopeless, slow and brief in her replies, with ideas of unworthiness, but some insight. Recovery in two months with insight, probably hastened by stimulation of interest in simple occupations.

A. B., 18 years old, is a good example of a simple retarded depression. She had had a former attack one year previously, which had lasted only for about one week, and from which she made, apparently, a good recovery. The family history indicated suicidal tendencies, because a paternal grandmother had taken her life when she was 62 years old, and a maternal uncle had committed suicide at the age of 45. This family history seemed to have a definite bearing on the case.

She had always been a strong, healthy child. She was not nervous, but was quiet, shy, reserved and not inclined to make friends easily.

She did quite well at school, but was described as being more practical than intel-lectual, and was especially interested in housewifery tasks. It was while she was attend-ing a course of instruction at a School of Domestic Science that she broke down. The illness developed acutely, and three days before her admission she suddenly told her parents that she had drunk a bottle of eye lotion that had been in the house. On the night following this she got out of bed, and attempted to leave the house. It is of interest that preceding the onset of her previous attack she had overheard talk about suicide. This reminded her of similar incidents in her own family, and she was depressed for about a week afterwards.

At the time of her admission she was in a dull, depressed state, feeling hopeless and that she had not been learning and concentrating as she should have done. She feared in consequence that she would become a burden on her friends. Suicide had therefore seemed the simplest solution of her difficulties. She was slow in answering questions, replied for the most part in monosyllables, readily admitted that she was melancholy and that her mind was not at peace, but was occupied with morbid feelings and thoughts. As a result she had not been sleeping well. She said, 'I seem just to have been slipping along, and not doing my duty. I feel as if I had got everybody into a mess. I thought I was not so efficient as others, and that I could not hold my own with them.' Her answers to questions were always quite coherent and relevant. She denied ever having suffered from ideas of reference, from hallucinations or delusions. Her memory, her grasp on school knowledge and her intellectual faculties generally were not im-paired. She realized that she was ill and in need of treatment in a mental hospital, so much so that she came as a voluntary patient. Her general physical state showed that she was in good condition, and there was no evidence of physical disease. She had an erosion of her lower lip, due to the eye lotion which she had swallowed.

After a short period in bed she was allowed up, an attempt was made to cultivate her interest in the occupational department and this she readily took to. She found that she was able to do certain simple pieces of work comparatively well, and in consequence her self-confidence rapidly returned, and in the course of two months she made a good recovery. She put on weight, her sleep improved, she realized more clearly than heretofore what her actual difficulties had been and was able to return home.

A case such as the above illustrates very clearly a simple, depressed, retarded state, occurring in a somewhat shy, sensitive girl. There is no reason to suppose that she will not be able to carry on satisfactorily in the future.

Most cases of depression belonging to the group of affective reaction-types correspond closely to Kraepelin's classical description as given above. In some of these cases retardation is not to be detected, at least by the ordinary clinical methods; yet the depression may be profound. In others, instead of depression, there is a total loss of feeling—the patient complaining bitterly of the lack of any emotion whatsoever, including a loss of affective response to those whom he formerly loved. As our appreciation of reality depends so much on our ability to 'feel ourselves into' the activities of other people (or more technically to project our feelings as well as our perceptions), patients suffering from emotional deficit of this kind frequently complain that everything seems unreal to them. (This is probably not the only basis of such feelings; they may arise also, as Lewis (1934) points out, in association with disturbed states of consciousness such as perplexity and dream-like states.) This *feeling of unreality* may be distressing in itself and may even be the chief complaint.

The following is an example of the so-called 'reasoning' type of depression, where retardation was not in evidence:

CASE NO. 23

An unretarded depression in a single woman who had had a previous attack of mental illness. Definite precipitating factor. Extreme depression, without slowing, but with carelessness in dress and comparative inactivity at first. Insight fairly complete during illness and utilized in an attempt to help herself. Several suicidal attempts, ultimately successful.

G. H. She was a single woman, 32 years old, a native of Ireland. This patient came to the hospital of her own accord, saying that she wished to be admitted as a voluntary patient.

She had been born in Ireland, but came to Scotland when about 16 and learned typing and shorthand. After a number of years she returned to Ireland, where she had a long attack of mental illness of approximately three years' duration. Four months before her admission to this hospital she left Ireland and returned to this country, where she took a temporary position as a typist, but within the course of two or three weeks she became depressed.

At the time of her admission to the hospital she said frankly that she would prefer to die, but she feared that death might not end her misery. She insisted that she was not insane, but that she had become introspective, and on this account that her sufferings were terrible. She described it as a perversion of her personality, with an atrophy of her affections. She was enveloped by her own misery, buried her face in her hands and had frequent outbursts of crying. She was unable to employ herself, and paid little attention to her personal appearance. Her extreme introspection is well shown by the type of expression she used: 'This pain is with me always. I cannot get away from my conscious self. I keep comparing states of feeling.'

An attempt was made to investigate the actual factors responsible for her breakdown, and she frankly enough told a story of unrequited love. She had returned to Scotland to renew acquaintance with a friend who had professed great affection for her. She told him of her previous mental illness, and discovered that under these circumstances he was not prepared to consider marriage. She strove bravely against this great disappointment, but eventually the strain became too much, as all her hopes had been centred on him. 'Now', she says, 'life is dead for me: my universe is shattered.' It was for this reason that she had no wish to live, and was sorry to find that she was so healthy, because had she not been so well physically she might have found a more easy way out of her wretchedness. She had refrained from suicide only because she believed that such an act was wrong.

Physically, she was a large-framed, well-developed woman, who presented no signs of any bodily illness.

Following her admission, she declared that she was 'trying to batter back her fearful tendency to introspection', and at times she thought that she might win what she described as her 'terrible battle'. To this end she attempted to interest herself in various ways, took her food well, slept well and tried to make herself helpful to some of the younger and less able patients. For a number of weeks her condition was very variable; there were times when she was rather better, when she felt that she was getting the upper hand, but there followed periods when she felt that her struggle was overcoming and mastering her, and that her life was simply 'a large pretence'. She selected Foster Fraser's book called *Red Russia* from the library, and in talking about this, said that she had got some consolation from it, because she learned that other people besides herself (in Siberia) have to lead a life without hope.

Three weeks after she had been admitted she was found one evening with a strip of bed-sheeting tied tightly round her neck. After this had been removed she had a severe emotional outburst, during which she cried convulsively and trembled all over. Following this episode she again improved, but a few days later it was found that she had again tried to strangle herself with a piece of cord which she had surreptitiously obtained from another patient. The following morning she snatched some methylated spirits from one of the nurses and drank a quantity of it, but the only result was that she became sick. During the course of the next few days she made two further attempts to strangle herself. On account of these repeated attempts to injure herself, she was discharged as a voluntary patient, and certified. She told the medical examiners that she wished that they had come to kill her, that her life was her own, that she had a right to take it if she wished to do so, and that she would have actually accomplished her object unless the nurses had been very vigilant.

Eventually, four months after admission, she had made so much improvement, and was so anxious to be discharged, that she was taken to the house of friends, who said that they would be responsible for her until arrangements could be made for her to return to Ireland. The evening after she had gone, when she had retired for the night, a noise was heard in her room. When her friends went to see what was wrong, they found that she had swallowed a considerable quantity of Lysol. Prompt measures were taken to wash out her stomach, and she was immediately recertified and returned to the hospital. Her friends stated that on the night she had arrived home she had seemed bright and happy, and had spent a very pleasant evening. Such an act was not anticipated by them. Her friends asserted that they never kept Lysol in the house, and that the patient must have bought the Lysol one day when she was out, and kept it for the first suitable occasion. When she had recovered sufficiently from the effects of the attempt, she stated quite emphatically that the deed had been long premeditated, and all the time she had been in hospital (even although she had improved) her feelings and her outlook had remained quite unchanged. She cried bitterly throughout the conversation, and seemed in the uttermost depth of depression and complete hopelessness. Several months later she again created great anxiety, as she smashed a thick glass skylight window, and then pulled herself up on to the roof, clad only in her nightdress. Her escape was soon noticed. A nurse went up after her, and was successful in bringing her down. She said afterwards that once she got to the roof she realized that if she did take her life it would mean great trouble for others, and therefore she had not acted at once; if she had thought only of herself, she would have jumped immediately.

About this period she willingly reviewed her illness, and described the period of depression she had suffered from while in Ireland. Her condition then she described as being similar to what it was now. She said, 'I was perfectly sane, but the mental pain was so intense that I wanted to end it all.' At that time she attempted to commit suicide by drowning, and for this reason she was certified. She had become careless in her appearance, and had taken her food in a ravenous way. 'I know that that means that the animal part came uppermost.' At no time did she have hallucinations. Her recovery was described as being a complete one: life seemed worth living again, she took an interest in everything social and felt that she had a broader outlook on life than she ever had before. It was very much in this spirit that she returned to Scotland, and met with her great disappointment.

This patient was eventually transferred to another hospital, and after being discharged from it she accomplished her end by committing suicide by drowning. The interesting points about this patient, besides the suicidal determination she exhibited, were her clear insight, the absence of any retardation, and the success with which at one time she concealed the depth of her depression and her suicidal intentions.

Acute Depression. In this stage the retardation is more marked. The patient may never make any spontaneous remark; he is asocial, sits apart, refuses to mix with his neighbours in any way. The whole attitude is one of great misery and dejection. The patient accuses himself of the most heinous wrongdoing, of having committed the unpardonable sin and of bringing misfortune on others. There is nothing for it, he says, except to go to prison to expiate all his misdeeds. Hypochondriacal ideas are frequently expressed; the patient may believe that he has ruined his health because of early sex practices, that his body is wasting away, and that he will never be able to apply himself again. His bowels, he believes, are stopped, and his brain is wasting. The patient is thoroughly convinced that no one ever suffered as he does, that he is doomed, that it is hopeless to think of the possibility of getting well. Sometimes he feels that his whole personality is changed, that he is altogether different from what he was before. The environment seems unreal to him. Occasionally hallucinations, illusions and delusions occur, and orientation may not be quite correct (from inattention), but the memory and the intellectual faculties are well preserved. The patient realizes that he is ill, and needs careful looking after. Bleuler has stated that the depressive delusions of such patients usually concern themselves with conscience, as delusions of sin; with health, as delusions of disease; with fortune, as delusions of poverty. He draws a distinction between such depressive delusions and the katathymic hypochondriacal delusions expressed by the schizophrenic. 'Usually the difference consists in the fact that the depressive delusion of disease postpones the worst for the future, while the katathymic hypochondriacal worries about the present. The depressive patient believes he suffers from closure of the intestines and will perish in a particularly disgusting way, while the hypochondriac asserts that he actually suffers from intestinal inactivity, and demands, and expects, relief.'

Depressive Stupor. This condition may be defined as a state of intense psychic inhibition during which regression may occur to an infantile, if not more primitive level. The patient, usually, is confined to bed, is mute, inactive and uncooperative. His bodily needs require attention in every way; he has to be fed, washed and bathed. Precautions have to be taken to prevent the retention of faeces, urine and saliva. In some cases all attempts at movement are strongly resisted. In other cases the muscles are more flaccid, and the body and limbs can be moulded into any position. On the surface it may seem as if there was a total absence of feeling or emotion, but that is often more apparent than real, for, after recovery, many patients give a vivid account of the distress which they have experienced. The idea of death is believed by some to be almost universal in stupor reactions, and may be regarded as a form of expiation for the wickedness for which they hold themselves responsible. Some patients may have a clear appreciation of their position and surroundings throughout the whole period of the stupor, but in the majority a considerable dulling of consciousness occurs.

During all these stages of depression the *physical health* suffers greatly. The patient becomes weak, loses weight, has a poor appetite, a coated tongue, and constipation. The peripheral circulation is reduced, and there may be cyanosis, especially of the extremities.

CASE NO. 24
Depression with hypochondriacal ideas of a somewhat grotesque kind in a previously healthy but somewhat anxious man of 52, following influenza and business worries; extreme taciturnity, refusal of food, retention of urine and general resistiveness—in short, the manifestations of a type of negativism; clear orientation; fairly rapid improvement with general care and encouragement; interest in occupational pursuits followed by recovery.

B. W. A severe grade of disturbance occurred in a married man, 52 years old, who for about one year previous to admission had been experiencing a good deal of business worry.

About six months before admission to hospital he had suffered from an attack of influenza, and was in bed for a period of about ten days. He gradually made some improvement, but two months prior to his admission he seemed to change completely. He expressed the idea that he might have cancer, then that he had syphilis; he did not wish his wife or children to come near him in case they should get infected. He feared to go to the lavatory lest it would become choked, and infection would spread all over the house. This condition was followed by a period during which he would talk only in monosyllables. It was difficult to get him to take his nourishment; he tended to retain his urine, and on account of the difficulties of management he was sent to the hospital. He would not speak or answer questions when spoken to. He became restless, moaned and cried, and said, 'I cannot, I cannot.' He refused to take his food, and resisted being touched; and it was with the greatest difficulty that a physical examination could be made.

This man had come from a healthy stock. He had developed normally, and was described as a 'wild youngster, with lots of go'. He did well at school, and after leaving became a successful business man. He had been married for ten years, had two children and had a happy married life. He was always even-tempered and good-natured. He took life seriously, was rather inclined to worry, but was generous to his friends, devoted to his family and considerate to everyone. He had many outside interests, including art, drawing and latterly photography. His principal hobby had been his garden.

At the time of his admission he was in a miserable physical state, greatly emaciated, with small abrasions over the back of the left scapula and over both shins. His bladder was distended, and he had to be catheterized immediately. There was no evidence of any gross organic disease. For the most part he lay in a dull, depressed state. He answered one or two questions in monosyllables, but usually he refused to reply to questions. There was no evidence of any hallucinatory or delusional formation. He was able to tell the month correctly, but refused to reply to questions as to the day or the year. He seemed to realize quite clearly that he was in a mental hospital. He had to be tube-fed, and had to be catheterized. His condition, in short, was one of stupor. Even five weeks after admission he was more or less unchanged, except that artificial feeding had improved his general health. Gradually improvement was effected, so that he began to show more initiative, shaved himself, went out walking, spoke a little more and started to take his food better. Gradually it was possible to interest him in the occupational division, where he soon began to do satisfactory work, and after a residence of several weeks at a convalescent home at the seaside he made a complete recovery, returned home and resumed his work.

This case is therefore a rather more pronounced type than the case previously recorded. It is true that the history of influenza several months previous to his actual breakdown may have had an important bearing on the development of his illness, but at no time was his condition accompanied by any actual toxic state. It seems therefore that although his influenza was an important aetiological factor, it acted more by lowering his general resistance than in any specific way.

Alternating States. Some patients alternate continuously for years between states of depression and states of elation, with little or no interval of normality.

CASE No. 25

Alternating depression and elation over a period of thirty-five years with brief intervals of apparent normality, but later without normal intervals. At first, chiefly mild depression and subjective uncertainty, with slight restlessness; gradual increase in signs of depression (e.g. diminution in activity) in subsequent episodes; then exaggerated self-satisfaction (mild elation) over successful work. Then depression again, of greater duration, followed by elation, completely spontaneous this time. Similar alternations continuing over a long period of years, but with the passing of time a gradually increasing lack of emotional restraint (considerable exaltation or deep depression) with corresponding deterioration in judgement (grandiose ideas, grossly exaggerated opinion of his own abilities). Elated periods characterized by aggressiveness, frequent irritability and pronounced erotic tendencies. Some hallucinated episodes. Intense depression with suicidal attempt, preceding death.

D. P. A good example of a persistent alternating state is afforded by the history of a patient who was first admitted to hospital in 1889, when he was 26 years old, and who for the next thirty-five years, until his death, suffered persistently from recurring attacks of excitement and depression. At the time of his first admission he expressed the feeling that his brain was failing, and spoke about a strong hereditary predisposition, which had made him afraid. From thinking about this he had become excitable and nervous, felt that he could not stand the strain of business and decided on that account to put himself under observation. He did not express any delusions, and a note was made in his history to the effect that it would be difficult to detect any abnormality. During the period of his first admission he gradually gained control over himself, and after a period of four months he was discharged as recovered.

He was readmitted in December 1889, as a voluntary patient. He stated that after leaving in August he had resumed his occupation, but in the course of a few weeks found himself unequal to it, and had placed himself under care in another mental hospital. He stayed there for a period of three months, and then, on his return home, felt himself still unable to take up his work, and decided to put himself under treatment again. At the time of his admission he talked intelligently and rationally, but he showed a striking lack of confidence in himself, was depressed, unstable and rather restless. In a short time, however, he rapidly gained control, and in February 1890 he was discharged as recovered.

In November 1893 he was admitted for the third time, but previous to this admission he had been a patient in still another mental hospital. He showed the same symptoms as previously. He talked quietly in a low voice, and complained of nervousness and inability to stand the strain of business. He was depressed, dull, unable to rouse himself, to shake off his doubts and fears. Gradually he improved, and in the course of five months was discharged as recovered.

His fourth admission was in February 1895, when he stated that he would like to stay about the place, as he felt the need of protection. He was discharged on June 3, 1895, but readmitted on June 26, 1895. After leaving he had gone to a farm, but while there he became so depressed that he started to write letters urgently entreating to be allowed to return. He felt incapable of exerting himself or of doing anything at all with his mind. At this time he was encouraged to interest himself in the steward's office, and for a period during the steward's illness he carried on the duties of the steward. As a result of this—no doubt as a reaction to it—he became too pleased with himself; he felt that he was indispensable, and was fussy and excitable. This condition was in great contrast to his previous behaviour.

He was readmitted in March 1899, having been discharged previously in December 1896, but in the meantime he had been a patient in another mental hospital. On this admission he was depressed, frightened lest he should become insane and said that he frequently felt stupid and inadequate.

Gradually, in the latter part of 1901, he began to mix with the other patients, and finally became so excited that he had to be removed to another ward. He was very nasty to the staff, and excited many of the other patients. Gradually these symptoms passed away, and he developed a hypomanic state. He was exalted, was perhaps too active and energetic, played golf, danced, mixed a great deal with the other patients, both men and women, and showed a certain lack of common sense. At this time he acted as editor of the hospital *Gazette*.

During subsequent years his condition constantly varied from one of mild depression to one of mild excitement. The variation was not great, but the alternations in his mood were definite.

In July 1907 he became very exalted and irritable. He struck an attendant, had exaggerated ideas of his own abilities, thought that his poetry was better than that of anyone in the land (it was very bad); declared that he was going to marry a lady with £40,000, and 'be upsides with the medical officer'. He wore his watch chain as a bangle, rode in a wheeled chair and said it was a car, shouted and imitated an officer drilling soldiers.

On May 20, 1912, he was allowed to go out for a walk, but took the opportunity to escape. While absent from the hospital he raised some money by pawning his belongings and took the train to London. On his journey to London he threw his gold watch and chain out of the carriage window, and then started to take off his clothes, much to the alarm of the other passengers in his carriage, who fled. After he had divested himself of everything, he paraded the corridor, and eventually was taken in charge by the guard, and was handed over to the police when the train arrived in London. He was taken to one of the London County Council mental hospitals, and was transferred to his former hospital on February 21, 1913. The medical certificates on which he was brought

Q

back stated that he was alternately angry and suspicious, plausible and friendly. He wrote stating charges of immoral conduct against various persons, which he was unable to substantiate. He was impatient of contradiction, believed harm was meant when no such intention was entertained, and wrote amorous letters to certain ladies.

His subsequent history consisted of alternating attacks of depression (during which he would retire to bed and complain of all sorts of bodily symptoms), and periods of excitement when he would behave in a very self-confident, egotistical way. Latterly he tended to develop hallucinatory states, and one afternoon while the other patients were at dinner he upset the fire buckets in his ward, and clipped off part of his beard, stating in explanation that he was being tormented by devils, and that they could not cross a running stream. On one occasion, when allowed out with an attendant to visit his tailor, he walked the attendant round by a circuitous route, and left him standing out-side, while he himself went to call on a lady with whom he had previously been friendly. Much to this lady's astonishment, he proposed immediate marriage to her, and asked her to go to the registrar for the ceremony to be performed, so that he could go home with her and take up his position as her husband. The lady was so frightened and startled by his visit that she called at the hospital the following day and asked to be protected from any such further episode.

During the latter months of this patient's life he became tremendously depressed. He blamed himself for his conduct in the past, and became intensely suicidal, so much so that on one occasion after having asked permission to write a letter, and after having been given his eye-glasses, he suddenly took off his glasses—while the nurse was stand-ing beside him—placed them in his mouth and swallowed them; but fortunately the X-ray photograph showed that they had stuck at the cardiac end of his oesophagus, and they were successfully removed. He made other determined attempts to injure himself, but eventually passed peacefully away.

MIXED STATES

Kraepelin described 'mixed states', which he formed by a combination of the cardinal symptoms of the manic and depressive states. He differentiated six principal types as follow:

    1. Maniacal stupor.
    2. Agitated depression.
    3. Unproductive mania.
    4. Depressive mania.
    5. Depression, with flight of ideas.
    6. Akinetic mania.

These conditions, according to Kraepelin, not only occur singly in the course either of an acute excitement or an acute depression, but as transition stages during the change from excitement to depression.

In our experience mixed states, other than agitated depression, are not un-common and are often misdiagnosed as schizophrenia. They show an admixture of manic and depressive symptoms, rapid fluctuations of mood are commonly noted, and perplexity may be a prominent feature. Such mixed states tend to run a rather more prolonged course than the average case of manic-depressive psychosis. Briefer mixed states also occur as transition phases, and the condition known as maniacal stupor is usually a transition stage between a depressive stupor and a manic attack.

The following is an example:

Case No. 26

A shy, timid Italian girl of 18 who became mute and incontinent, but retained certain simple responses to her environment; then passed into a typical manic attack; recovered incompletely and without insight; became seclusive, expressed some religious ideas and relapsed into her former condition of mutism, etc., from which again she passed into an infectious elation, but this time with curious inhibitions in her flow of talk; once more recovery, again without insight.

A young Italian girl, 18 years old, who had always been shy and timid, was admitted to the hospital in a state of mutism. There was no evidence of infective-exhaustive factors, or of hallucinations, so that the diagnosis seemed to lie between a katatonic and a manic-depressive condition. The expression of the patient was impassive, but not unobservant. She obeyed commands promptly and quickly, her movements were free and graceful, and when given a pad and pencil she would cover pages with scribbles. She was incontinent both as to bladder and bowels, and on several occasions she smeared herself with excreta. She reacted very slightly to pin pricks. There were no assumption of fixed attitudes, no stereotyped movements, no catalepsy; on the other hand, there was no evidence of depression. Retardation or blocking or negativism could be inferred from the mutism.

This girl had had a previous attack, which lasted for a period of eight months. Before her first attack she had complained of some headache, and one day while in church said that it was full of cats. On admission to hospital she presented features similar to those seen in the condition above described, but later she exhibited a playful mood, free, graceful movements, some distractibility, flight of ideas and sound associations—a typical manic state.

She recovered from this attack, but at the time of her discharge she had very little real insight into her condition, and was rather careless and indifferent.

For five months she was able to remain at home. At first she did a certain amount of housework, but gradually she lost interest, became seclusive, sat in a room by herself and could hardly be got to leave the house. On one occasion she expressed the wish to become a nun, complained of seeing devils at night-time and seemed afraid.

During her second attack the patient gradually developed a condition of elation, becoming talkative and restless. Her talkativeness was peculiar in that there was no steady flow of words, as is usual in the frank manic, but rather an abrupt, inhibited mode of speech, a short sample of which is as follows:

'You know I'd love—you know—let me have a pencil—you know, you know—you know sometimes when—we didn't have any—we didn't have any news—you know sometimes (hums a tune)—I love the Italian band. You know sometimes we——' The content of her remarks was not specially odd or peculiar. She was extremely alert, and was much more in touch with the situation than her conduct seemed to indicate. She laughed excessively, but her laughter was gay and infectious. She was distractible, and showed occasionally clang associations.

She made a good recovery from this attack, but again without any real insight.

The essential part of the picture had been her elated mood, with restlessness, alertness and talkativeness. Apart from her make-up, there was little that could be considered ominous. At the beginning of the attack the association of mutism with a slightly happy, smiling mood and free movements constituted a fairly typical example of the mixed phase of the manic-depressive psychosis. A similar mixture was shown later by the association of inhibited talkativeness with bright, happy, alert behaviour and increased psychomotor activity.

Physical Symptoms. There are no outstanding physical symptoms characteristic

of affective states. The chief physical changes are disorder of sleep and emaciation. These two symptoms are more difficult to control in the manic than in the
depressed case. A history of sleeplessness or loss of appetite, or both, is often
said to have been the first indication of the patient's being out of sorts, but a
careful analysis of the case history usually shows that these symptoms were
dependent on some already existing mental change. Control of these two factors
is a keystone of treatment, particularly in the acute phases. It can be said that
practically every case of acute or delirious excitement, and every case of acute
depression, suffers from sleeplessness and from a disorder of appetite; the manic
patient, on the one hand, is so restless, so distractible and so busy that he has no
time either to sleep or to eat; whereas the depressed patient may be so tormented by depressive ideas, and feel so unworthy, that he does not consider
himself entitled to any food that is offered him, and either refuses it altogether
or states that he has no appetite for it. In consequence the body weight diminishes, often to an alarming degree. One of the first signs of beginning improvement is an increase in the bodily weight, usually with a relish for food, and
improved sleep.

Particularly in depressed patients there is a sluggishness of the whole
gastro-intestinal tract, and constipation is a very common complaint. Rarely the
depressed patient gains weight due to the retention of body water, and disturbances of sodium and potassium metabolism have been recorded.

The menstrual function tends to be disturbed or to disappear at the onset of
any mental illness, and it frequently remains absent during its whole course.
Return of the menstrual function is sometimes an early sign of improvement.

These are the main physical symptoms. None of them are in any way pathognomonic of the manic-depressive state, and all of them have to be looked upon
merely as incidental to the acute mental disturbance from which the patient is
suffering, and as having no specific aetiological relation to it.

INVOLUTIONAL MELANCHOLIA

The involutional period is a physiological epoch common to men and women,
bringing in its train certain mental and bodily changes. The mental faculties in
general become less acute. There is a tendency to bewail the past, and to feel that
the future has nothing in store. The mind is occupied with the 'might-have-beens',
and in consequence doubt, indecision, fear and anxiety readily show themselves.
The glands of internal secretion begin to fail in their functioning, and the bodily
health is lowered.

It is impossible to state definitely when the involutional period begins and
when it ends, but, roughly, it ranges from 40 to 55 years in women, and from
50 to 65 years in men.

When Kraepelin made his broad differentiation between the manic-depressive
psychosis and schizophrenia, he kept cases of depression occurring at the involutional period apart, and termed them melancholia. Some years later Dreyfus

reviewed the material on which Kraepelin had based his findings, and concluded that the great majority of 'melancholias' should be included in the manic-depressive group, that cases of involutional melancholia corresponded to mixed states of manic depression, and that there was no such entity as involutional melancholia. Altogether, Dreyfus investigated 81 cases, and of these 34 were personally examined, 8 were not personally examined, and 39 died. He considered that 2 cases should be left undiagnosed, that 4 were doubtful, and that all the rest were cases of the manic-depressive psychosis. Of these cases 66 per cent. recovered, 8 per cent. developed arteriosclerotic symptoms, and 25 per cent. died either of some intercurrent disease, or as a result of suicide. Kraepelin accepted and concurred with the conclusions of Dreyfus. Kirby, in commenting on the work of Dreyfus, made the significant statement: 'In a number of cases the manic-depressive symptoms were plainly in evidence, the cases having been improperly placed with the melancholias. In a considerable number of other cases the author's conclusions that manic-depressive symptoms were present is based on extremely meagre data.' We agree with this conclusion of Kirby, and are not willing to accept the Dreyfus–Kraepelin findings. We believe that there is a group of cases which we can term involutional melancholia distinct from manic-depressive states. In Scotland cases of involutional melancholia used to be very common. If we take the figures at the Glasgow Royal Mental Hospital for a period of five years—from January 1, 1915, to December 31, 1919—we find that 299 patients (160 women and 139 men) were admitted between the ages of forty and seventy years. Of these 65 women and 32 men showed anxiety states characteristic of the involutional period. The great majority of these patients had never previously suffered from any attack of mental illness, and cases in which there was a definite history of previous attacks were grouped not as involutional melancholias, but with the manic-depressives. In the county mental hospitals (*e.g.* Inverness) the figures for such states of melancholia were much greater than those here recorded. We believe that involutional melancholia, though less common now than formerly, has certain features of its own. These features are *depression without retardation, anxiety, a feeling of unreality and hypochondriacal or nihilistic delusions*, the last being in the allo-, somato- and auto-psychic fields.

The above definition is merely a tentative formulation, and certain reservations must be made. There is no one of the above-mentioned symptoms which is peculiar to the involutional period, but their occurrence together is unusually common at that time of life. A very similar syndrome may occur at an earlier age, in the twenties and thirties in women, and before the fifth decade in men. A series of 80 cases of agitated depression of various types has been carefully examined by us, and there were at least four, not at the involutional period, who were not easy to distinguish clinically from many cases of involutional melancholia. We mention this matter as one for further study and observation.

The general plan which we have adopted is to reserve the term involutional melancholia for those cases who have never previously suffered from any form of mental illness. There is no known reason why a person should not suffer from manic-depressive symptoms during the earlier period of life, and then at the involutional period exhibit an agitated state. When such is the case, it is considered better to keep it in the manic-depressive group. The term involutional melancholia is a convenient label for a certain group of cases occurring at the involutional period, because cases exhibiting the characteristics given in the above definition are particularly common at that epoch.

The most characteristic involutional qualities lie in the content of the psychosis, especially in the apprehension, hypochondriasis and nihilism, and these qualities are the result of the psychological changes associated with advancing years.

AETIOLOGY

In certain cases the involutional period itself seems to be the most important factor. This is possibly more true in women than in men, because the physical concomitants of the menopause are well recognized. The mere fact, however, that many people reach the involutional period without having previously shown signs of mental disorder is an indication that those who develop this type of disorder have stouter mental and physical qualities than those who break down from the more purely constitutional disorders, such as manic-depressive and schizophrenic psychoses. Nevertheless it is stated that schizophrenic psychoses are unusually frequent both in the ascendants and descendants of these patients. There is often a history of exciting factors, either psychic, physical or a combination of the two.

But the underlying type of personality in many of them has certain characteristics which can bear emphasis. They have a record of hard work behind them. They are sensitive, meticulous, over-conscientious, over-scrupulous, busy, active people who take a pride in their work and have a high sense of duty towards others. Titley has described them as showing 'a narrow range of interests, poor facility for readjustment, asocial trends, inability to maintain friendships, intolerance and poor adult sexual adjustment, also a pronounced and rigid ethical code and a proclivity to reticence and sensitiveness'. It will be readily appreciated that such a type of pre-psychotic disposition has little or no relationship to the manic-depressive constitution.

Naturally the theory has been advanced that in women, at least, such conditions are due to hormonal alterations associated with the menopause; but treatment with oestrogens (e.g ethinyl oestradiol, 0·05 mg. daily orally), though it may relieve the troublesome vasomotor symptoms of which many menopausal women complain, will not cure an affective psychosis.

In the group of material which we examined in the Glasgow Royal Mental Hospital, we found that 57 per cent. of the women and 70 per cent. of the men broke down as the result of psychic factors, whereas physical factors were of importance only in 21 per cent. of the women and 6 per cent. of the men. The psychic factors which are usually stressed are the death of near relatives, financial and business worries, unfortunate home conditions, and the breaking-up of the home. These figures are in agreement with those of William Mabon, who found that in his involutional cases 47 per cent. were of psychic origin, 34 per cent. of physical origin, and 17 per cent. were due to a combination of these. We have already pointed out that in country districts the percentage of such cases is higher than in cities, and the fact of environment as a predisposing cause should be kept in mind.

SYMPTOMATOLOGY

It has been indicated by the definition given above that the symptoms centre round a state of anxiety and agitation, accompanied by delusions of a depressive nature, frequently hypochondriacal or nihilistic. This state, although common to the great majority of cases, shows all kinds and shades of variation, so that no two cases are ever exactly the same. Kirby attempted to differentiate four main types:

1. Cases showing a simple form of anxiety or general uneasiness, apprehensive anticipations, with or without ideas of sin.
2. A severer form, showing anxiety, with fear, perplexity, and allo-psychic concepts.
3. Cases presenting a sensory somatic complex: abnormal bodily sensations, hypochondriacal trends and feelings of unreality.
4. Cases developing with arteriosclerosis.

These types may be recognized, but they could very well be increased to as many more. Their differentiation in this way does not make matters clearer, for any patient during the course of the illness may show all the grades described by Kirby. Furthermore, it seems wrong to complicate the picture by emphasizing the occurrence of such states with arteriosclerosis. There are bound to be cases of this type, where the occurrence of arteriosclerosis complicates the picture. But the arteriosclerosis need not exert any specific action unless it is so marked as to give rise to definite arteriosclerotic symptoms, when the case would much better be grouped with the arteriosclerotics than with the involutional melancholias. We have mentioned this here because we wish to emphasize that the real involutional cases seldom show any involvement of the intellectual faculties. Considering the depth of distress which they exhibit, their intellectual clearness always stands out prominently. Farrar described three main forms, which he termed, first, 'melancholia vera', which is characterized by a self-accusatory state, with clear consciousness. The patient may also express some somatopsychic delusions, and a slight degree of anxiety is present. The second type he termed 'anxietas presenilis', in which there is an extreme anxiety and feeling that things in the world outside are unreal. These cases of the second type were supposed to be complicated to a greater degree by arteriosclerosis, and the prognosis was considered less favourable than in the other types. The third group he termed 'depressio apathetica', in which there is simply a state of apathy, without the expression of much affect, and in which the prognosis is considered to be relatively good.

MacCurdy (1925) has also described four main groups:

1. Ridiculous delusions, insufficient emotional reaction, anti-social conduct, indulgence in infantile sexuality. This is probably a schizophrenic reaction-type.

2. Hoch's organic insufficiency, characterized by lack of interest, apathy, mild hypochondriacal ideas and mild restlessness.

3. Cases that are really simply another recurrence of a manic-depressive state.

4. Cases with fears of impending death, of poverty and of bodily disease.

This last group he termed true involutional melancholia.

These again are arbitrary subdivisions which do not by any means always hold.

In short, we must not attempt to group cases too closely along any of these lines, but as with other mental states we must recognize that the psychotic picture is largely determined by the character traits present in the individual in his normal, healthy state, and that the mental picture may vary just as one individual does from another.

The outstanding feature in all this group of cases is the anxious depression, and this has often been preceded by a stage during which the patient has complained of tiredness, of feelings of inadequacy, of being easily fatigued and of sleeplessness. They may also have physical symptoms, such as feelings of pressure in the head, difficulty of thinking, flushing, vertigo and irritability. The appearance and the attitude of such patients is one of great misery; they feel frightened, are restless, wring their hands, moan and groan, tend to rake over their past, the slightest faults becoming the most terrible crimes. They feel that there is no hope for them, and fear that they are to be thrown out, that they will be taken to prison, and that they will be tried and put to death. Such patients in their misery may attempt to mutilate themselves, and the danger of suicide is great. In addition, they are very resistive to care and treatment, refusing food because they feel they are not entitled to it, or because they are suspicious lest it be poisoned; and, besides blaming themselves, they hold themselves responsible for the condition of the others with whom they are associated.

There is, as a rule, very little clouding of consciousness; they are correctly oriented, the memory is good, and the individual realizes to a certain extent that he is ill.

In the most acute types of disorder, hallucinations of a terrifying nature may occur, and a certain amount of disorientation is present.

Any physical change which occurs apart from accidental intercurrent disease is secondary to the mental state. The most impressive sign is the rapid loss of weight, due in part to the intense agitation, and in part also to the refusal of food. Many of these patients complain of inability to take their food, of a loss of appetite, and of a feeling of weight and pressure after meals, and their bowels are apt to be constipated. There may be a transitory glycosuria. There are frequently vasomotor disturbances, with complaints of flushing, sometimes excessive perspiration, and other indications of involvement of the sympathetic nervous system.

PSYCHOPATHOLOGY

MacCurdy made a consistent attempt to explain the type of mental content common in involutional melancholia. There is an increasing egoism equivalent to a progressive restriction of external interests, one of the results of which is a preoccupation with death, because pure egoism finds no satisfaction in this life. The idea of death is an epitome of the all-round loss of interest. But egoism implies in itself resistance to the idea of death, so that at one and the same time there is a revulsion from death and a wish for it. The presence of the two tendencies is shown by the presence together of apparently contradictory tendencies in the form of apprehension and of delusions of impending death, or of apprehension of death together with suicidal attempts. Sleep being a symbol for death, insomnia is accounted for by supposing that these patients are afraid of sleep because it has this (unconscious) symbolic meaning. Delusions of poverty are mild forms of delusions of death, money being the chief symbol of social value— a value which the patient feels he has lost. If the loss of interest in the world is projected, nihilistic delusions appear—the very existence is denied of that which is no longer interesting. Irritability and negativism are likewise attempts to exclude reality. Hypochondriacal trends are supposed to be compounded of self-centredness and auto-erotism.

Involutional melancholia can be summed up as a regression to the 'primary subjective phase' of the minimum of mental effort (= death) and auto-erotism (= hypochondria). Anxiety is the natural reaction to ideas of murder, torture, etc., which are symbolizations of the unconscious desire for death and derive their intense motive power from the latter.

The most striking aspects of the following case were the interrelations of the content of the delusions, the day-dreams of her childhood and her unsatisfactory married life. Evidently her revolt from her husband's coarseness had caused her to return to her early dreams, but with the realization that they could now never be fulfilled—hence everything she had dreamed of was gone—'all buried; . . . under the earth'. The precipitating factor was evidently the birth of her third child.

CASE No. 27

Onset in fifth week of normal puerperium in cultured woman of 38, with a family history of suicide and an unsatisfactory married life. Mild anxiety and self-consciousness, followed by complaints of fatigue, then by depression accompanied by nihilistic delusions and later by suicidal attempts. On admission, depressed, mildly agitated, with nihilistic delusions and ideas of transformation of her personality, but with a certain amount of insight; finally suicide. Probable relationship of content of delusions to phantasies compensatory for the disappointments of her married life.

A. B., a cultured, married lady, 38 years old, became mentally ill five weeks after the birth of her third child. The symptoms first were those of a 'neurasthenic' state, during which she complained that things had been too heavy for her, and that she was easily tired both mentally and physically. An attempt was made to treat her in a nursing home, but while there she became gloomy, depressed and began to express delusional ideas, believing that she had no money and no children, and saying that her husband and her children were dead. For a time she seemed to improve, and gained in weight, but suicidal tendencies appeared, and on one occasion she jumped out of the window and fractured her collar-bone.

This patient had a family history of suicide, as both her grandfather and a maternal uncle had taken their own lives. Her father had died just before her third child was born, and this also had been a great shock to her. As she did not make progress, she was brought to a mental hospital.

A letter from her own doctor stated that her confinement had been perfectly normal, and had not been accompanied by any rise of temperature. During the fourth or fifth week after her pregnancy, she seemed to become self-conscious, concerned herself about trifles, a spot on the face and the like. The doctor also stressed the fact that her married life had probably not been entirely satisfactory to her. He described the patient as refined, cultured and religious, and her husband as coarse, godless and with no interest in life beyond hogs and his own gratification.

At the time of her admission to the hospital, she is described as believing that the world had entirely changed—that formerly there had been no sin or unhappiness, but now everything was horrible and dirty. She stated that the food was beastly, and that there was no necessity to take food, because she could live eternally without it. On another occasion she stated that the Golden Age was past, that everything was now dirty and unclean.

Physically, she was a tall, squarely built woman, who had the appearance of good health. Her hair was almost grey; she looked older than her years. The thyroid gland was visible and considerably enlarged, the increase affecting each lobe as well as the isthmus. The swelling was of medium and uniform consistence, and no pulsation was palpable. There was no exophthalmos. Her facial expression was one of depression and anxiety, and she showed her agitation in pacing to and fro, and in occasional wringing of her hands. She was willing enough to answer questions, and gave the impression of making an effort at keeping herself under control. She understood clearly why she was in the hospital. She constantly referred to her delusions with much display of feeling. She believed that the world had changed, and compared the brightness, beauty and purity of what she calls 'the golden days' of her earlier life with the ugliness, squalor and sinfulness of the present. Everything is different—sun, moon and stars are not as they were, 'the beauty of the earth and the glory of the sky' do not now exist; the seasons are not as the seasons of yesteryear; the flowers, the trees, the birds are not arrayed in the glory of old times; people display only repulsiveness, deceit and all forms of wickedness. Even the children are innocent and of good report in name only. 'All, all is gone, those days of bygone splendour, and things can never be as I once knew them.' She herself has been completely changed; body, soul and spirit have been altered, until she has become but a weariness to herself. There is nothing to live for, no joy, no hope. She wishes everything were at an end. But she did not say she would end her own life. She had no wish to discuss things apart from these colossal changes, but when subjects among her old interests (art, literature, etc.) were touched on, she would talk with momentary animation and freedom, only to come back sharply and soon to 'the things that really matter'. Her intellectual faculties were very well preserved, her memory was good and she had a realization of her own disordered state. Occasionally she showed little impulsive acts, during which she would strike a nurse, and then immediately afterwards would express great regret. A few months after her admission her condition was more or less unchanged. She was quiet, composed, polite, but she was still possessed by a marked feeling of unreality, and continued to express the belief that things were different from what they used to be. Many determined attempts were made to organize her activities, and she took an interest in physical exercises, in reading to a number of the ladies and in doing pieces of work.

A careful investigation of her personality was made, in order to obtain some light on the onset and development of her illness, and it was striking to see the close relationship between her original disposition and the psychosis. Intellectually, she had always been much above the average, heading her class in German, and being particularly gifted at languages. She had always read a great deal, used to tell fairy stories to herself and was imaginative. In her day-dreams she used to want to become great and happy, and to be a great authoress, 'people to be fond of me, and everything to be beautiful around me'. All this would come to her mind, thoughts of a beautiful home, of a husband, children and happiness. Later in life she had become a successful authoress, her books being closely modelled on her own life. It was evident that there had been considerable conflict, because she had dreamed of a rather spiritual, artistic type of existence, which her husband's nature rendered entirely impossible. In consequence her life had undoubtedly not come up to her expectations. She talked at this time as follows: 'The beautiful furniture, the beautiful needlework—all the excellent trams in X—— (the most perfect in the world), such clean and beautiful people in them, clergymen, professors, county gentlemen, officers—think of them all, all buried: these things are literally under the earth. All the lovely scents, the lovely, lovely clothes that everybody had—the beautiful industries. I used to sell beautiful crochet, and beautiful baby-clothes of beautiful Irish work, always on St. Patrick's Day in London. That is all over—all these beautiful ladies have gone, there is none of that now—all is gone—absolutely, and here am I. We are now at a standstill, all the wonderful inventors and their things are buried, the wonderful telescopes and phonographs are buried. I wish I had never seen the world, and how I have ruined it.'

About a year after her admission she was discharged to the care of her friends, in a slightly improved condition. Later she committed suicide.

CASE No. 28

Gradual onset of depressed, anxious, apprehensive state in a man of 65; ushered in by apprehension over financial losses, followed by depression, loss of interest, irritability, insomnia and headache; stereotyped anxious queries and stereotyped expressions of distress; increasing automaticity of actions and emotional expression; noisy, gluttonous and careless of his appearance; but ultimate recovery in two years.

E. F., male, 65 years old, was admitted to the hospital in a very restless, depressed, excited state. He threw his arms and legs about, knocked his head against the wall, pulled at his hair and cheeks and frequently made strange noises. This condition had been of about six months' duration.

He had been a strong, healthy man, successful in business, and had been married for a period of about thirty-eight years. He had always been reserved and silent but kindly, and had very few interests outside his business. Three years before his admission he had been able to retire, but during the war years his investments began to depreciate, and he worried greatly about his financial state, and exaggerated his losses. He began to fear that his income would be insufficient, though his family asserted that he had no grounds whatsoever for such an assumption. His habitual reticence gradually gave place to a deepening depression; he brooded about himself, took no interest in the daily papers and continually accused his eldest son—on whose advice he had acted in regard to his investments—as the cause of his ruin. He was sleepless, suffered from headache and complained that his head felt as if it was in a vice. He was irritable over the smallest things, and was totally unable to rest. For a minute or two he would sit down but then would be up, jerking his legs, pulling at his hair or his face. A holiday at a farmhouse had been tried, but while there his excitement increased, and as he seemed to be getting rapidly worse he was brought to hospital.

The patient's condition was one of great depression and anxiety. He said that he had always been a nervous man, and that he could not seem to control his movements or what he wanted to do. He answered all questions on general topics without any hesitation or confusion, and his memory for remote and recent events was good. His knowledge of current events had been gained by hearsay, as he had not been able to sit down and read a newspaper for many months. He knew exactly where he was, and expressed deep regret at the worry that he was causing his wife and family.

Physically his condition was satisfactory. There was no evidence of any organic disease. His hair was rubbed bare in patches over the temples.

Following his admission, he slept very badly, and he frequently had to get medicine to help him. He was always in a state of panic about himself, was constantly demanding an explanation of his condition and wanted to know the prognosis. He was treated by prolonged baths and as much nourishment as possible, but his excitement and restlessness continued undiminished. Whenever spoken to he was quiet, but when left alone he would continue to pace up and down the ward, shouting out some stereotyped phrase such as 'Oh, my God', at constant intervals. He never could give any explanation of why he shouted—whether he was impelled to do it, or whether he derived any special relief from it. His stereotyped attitude was also seen by his daily queries. 'Do you think I will ever get better?' 'Is there anything wrong with my brain?' 'Am I insane?' 'If I could stop the shouting would I get home?' 'What is it that makes me shout?' 'Could I live as I am just now in a tenement?' These questions, or similar ones, were repeated day after day. Attempts were made to interest him in various kinds of work both in the garden and in the house, but he never could be made to apply himself to anything.

Five months after his admission, his excitement and his manifestations of grief became more and more automatic, and were often continued, though with diminished vehemence, even when conversing. At this time his weight was persistently falling. He never passed a night without more or less frequent outbursts of shouting. It sometimes happened that he did not sleep at all; he would then jump in and out of bed, and pace the floor of his room shouting, 'Oh, my God', or meaningless and inarticulate sounds. He stopped before the mirror, where he examined his reflection, and increased the din by striking the chest of drawers with his fist or the back of his hair-brush. When in this highly excited condition he would pull at his nose, or pull his too closely cropped hair. During the daytime he was even more noisy, and attempts to keep him in check were unavailing. Later his appetite became capricious, and gluttony alternated with abstemiousness. His sons usually brought him cakes and other 'tit-bits'. These he would put away in a drawer in his room, and at odd times in the day he would bolt various articles of food either in the way of fruit, fancy cakes or confections. While he was still a patient he was left a certain amount of money, which completely made up for all the money which he had lost as a result of his investments, but in spite of this his state of anxiety and depression continued. He continued to express abhorrence of his own conduct, and constantly asked 'Why do I make this noise? Can I not help it? Will you not give me something to keep me quiet?' Gradually a certain amount of improvement was effected in his condition, and after a period of two years he was able to be discharged.

During the whole of his illness his intellectual faculties remained perfectly clear. A certain continuity of personality and subsequent psychosis is clear in this case. His financial losses were the precipitating cause, but were not in themselves by any means sufficient to account for such an illness; and their redemption led to no immediate improvement. The fact that his chief topic in his illness was his health suggests strongly that his financial losses merely served to bring to the surface the general concerns of advancing years. The stereotypy of his utterances ('Oh, my God', etc.) and his deterioration in personal habits, both of which would have seemed prognostically ominous, are interesting in view of the fact that he ultimately recovered.

CHRONIC MANIA

At one time chronic mania was regarded as the aftermath of an attack of acute mania which had persisted for a period of twelve months or longer. A time limit, however, did not prove a very reliable guide, as in the absence of the specific methods of treatment which have in recent years proved so successful in manic-depressive states, many cases did eventually make good recoveries even after several years. This led Schott, in 1904, and a number of other workers of whom we may mention Von Hösslin in 1909, Nitsche in 1910, and Laignel-Lavastine and Vinchian in 1921 all quoted by Wertham (1929), to consider whether chronic mania had a symptomatology which was peculiar to it, or any other factors which differentiated it from the manic-depressive psychosis. The four cases which Schott reported exhibited a manic state which had persisted for thirty, twenty-five, twenty-one and seventeen years respectively. All of them had had previous manic attacks of a similar nature to the final persistent one. All of the above-mentioned psychiatrists were impressed by the long duration of the final attack, by its intensity, and by the astonishing integrity of the intellectual functions even after a period of many years.

In our original investigations of such cases, published in 1927, we suggested that chronic mania was the counterpart of involutional melancholia, that it started comparatively late in life, and might be maintained for many years at a persistently high level. We further suggested that the diagnosis should be reserved for those cases in which the first manic attack had occurred after the age of 40 years. Under such circumstances the condition was likely to be intractable. The absence of emotional fluctuations or periodicity seemed to justify its separation from the much more familiar and recoverable manic-depressive psychosis. In 1929 Wertham's review of a group of 'prolonged manic excitements' which had persisted for periods of from five to eleven years was extremely valuable. He reported seven cases, in three of whom, aged 58, 52 and 60 years respectively there was no history of previous attacks. He was impressed by what he terms 'the psychobiological rigidity' of his patients in conjunction with a manic constitution.

We do not wish to over-elaborate the position, but as examples of the clinical states which were not uncommon, previous to the introduction of electric convulsion therapy, we submit the following.

CASE No. 29

Chronic mania. An excited, noisy, elated state with over-talkativeness and distractibility. Frequent angry episodes. Paucity of ideation, but a caustic wit. Hallucinatory and delusional trends. Ten years' duration.

A single woman, 49 years old, was admitted to hospital in an excited, elated, hyperactive state. Her conversation was imperious, domineering and abusive. Her language was obscene. Her mood fluctuated so that she had phases of irritability which might give place to the expression of grandiose ideas, or else she lapsed into a happy, humorous, witty stage, in which she cracked *risqué* jokes, and laughed heartily at the ensuing consternation. She was destructive of her clothing, or dressed grotesquely in a red dressing-gown adorned with gaudy bows. An example of her pressure of speech is as follows: 'You are not able to write. Give me a clean page. You are not a doctor—if I had a son like you I would drown myself, but first I would shoot the man—I see a vision—very fine—you are insane—I never met anyone worse—these bloody men—I loathe men.'

Throughout her illness her memory and general intellectual faculties remained intact, and she showed that she had considerable insight into her disordered state.

CASE No. 30

Chronic mania. Sudden onset of an elated, over-active, talkative state in a widower, 44 years old. Condition continued unchanged for five years.

A farmer went to a neighbouring estate where he liberated all the horses from their stables. He rapidly became so excited and irrational that his admission to hospital became a matter of urgency. He addressed the doctor as King Edward, King George, the Pope or as plain Geordie Boyle. He said he had been to Windsor Castle and had let the horses out to grass.

In hospital he was restless, excitable and noisy. He was constantly 'on the go', never stopped talking and showed a typical flight of ideas with clang associations: *e.g.* 'They were all stolen from me—King of Spain, Queen of Spain, twins, Heavenly twins, Esau —he sold his soul for a mess of pottage. Shah, Shaw of Persia I suppose you are.' When he was asked to explain his behaviour he replied: 'Mad, sir. Mad as a mad dog sir.'

The intense pitch of his excitement continued unabated for five years. There was no evidence of hallucinations or delusions; his memory and intellectual faculties remained intact.

Course and Prognosis

Affective states have, almost invariably, a comparatively rapid course with a good prognosis. That is true, particularly, when the attacks are of an isolated nature or of the intermittent type which occur so frequently in young people. In Rennie's investigation and analysis of 200 cases 93 per cent. of the patients recovered from the first attack but, unfortunately, 79 per cent. had recurrences. If the mania or depressive episodes are of a mild or simple nature they may resolve quickly under home care, but if there are frequent repetitions the duration of the episodes is inclined to be more prolonged, the care and treatment of the patient becomes more hazardous, and it may be imperative to arrange for the patient's admission to a mental hospital. Irrespective of that fact, and often in virtue of it, ultimate recovery can be expected even although it may be impossible to foretell with accuracy the duration and course of the illness. It is, however, often a matter of extreme urgency, for family, business and economic reasons, to be able to give an approximate forecast. With the modern methods of treatment which are now in everyday use we can usually assure the patient and his relatives that recovery from the episode will probably occur in from one to three months. Naturally enough, depending on a variety of circumstances, some cases may tend to persist much longer. In those cases in which the aetiological factors precipitating the cyclothymic reaction are of an exogenous nature the prognosis is better, and there is less tendency to recurrence than in those cases of an endogenous or constitutional nature determined by an hereditary predisposition. The individual with well balanced, wide interests can usually be helped through his periods of stress without too much difficulty.

When the psychotic episodes continue to recur, periodically, in persons who are over 40 years of age, or, even more significantly, if they appear for the first time after that age, then the prognosis must be more guarded owing to the possibility that the patient may be more vulnerable to incidental factors such as arteriosclerotic or other organic changes. We have already emphasized the persistence of attacks of excitement of the chronic manic type. In the few cases of affective disturbance which fail to recover there is an emotional deterioration characterized by a loss of interest, diminution of affect, and a state of chronicity which may persist indefinitely. It has been asserted that when hallucinations have complicated the clinical picture the prognosis has been rendered more unfavourable. That suggestion, however, has never been adequately substantiated. In our experience hallucinatory phenomena occurring in affective states are of a transitory nature determined by the acuteness of the psychotic process.

Previous to the introduction of electric convulsion therapy the depressive states associated with the involutional period of life constituted a great problem. The illness was usually of intense severity, caused great distress of mind and body, and might be prolonged over many years. Usually the intellectual faculties remained intact, and so long as the affect was maintained, and there was no organic cerebral involvement, we felt justified in maintaining an optimistic outlook. Now, we know, that with electric convulsion therapy at our command, we can usually give a good prognosis.

Hoch and MacCurdy (1922) made a comprehensive survey of this group of cases in the hope of making a symptomatic differentiation between the recoverable and irrecoverable. In the recoverable cases they found intense emotional reactions which found expression in anxiety, restlessness and agitation, and prominent delusions of death and poverty. In the irrecoverable they drew attention to the narrowing of interest, severe hypochondria and restriction of affect. While, as has been stated above, electric convulsion therapy has transformed the course and prognosis of involutional depressive states yet the clinical acumen of Hoch and MacCurdy deserves to be recognized. Their findings are closely analagous to 'the psychobiological rigidity' of chronic mania which makes that condition so resistant to successful treatment.

Diagnosis

In the majority of cases the personality of the patient, the relatively acute onset and the unequivocal nature of the mood changes are typical of the affective reaction types.

There are, however, a number of cases in which the clinical picture may be complicated by extraneous symptoms such as hallucinations, or by conduct disorder which points to a high degree of regression to a more primitive and instinctive level, e.g. exhibitionism, incontinence of urine and faeces, smearing the walls and floor, and so on. Superficially it might seem as if such features were more indicative of a schizophrenic rather than an affective reaction but they serve to teach us not to divorce symptoms from the setting in which they occur. So long as the mood, thought and conduct of the individual are in harmony we can remain assured of the correctness of our diagnosis. It is true that affective states may show schizophrenic features and vice versa, but in diagnosis it is safer to pay more attention to the acuteness of onset and the personality structure rather than be side-tracked by the symptoms which are subject to so much variation. The mood of the manic patient is a gay, happy, jolly, infectious one—you want to laugh with him because of the warmth of his personality. The excitement of the schizophrenic is a blind, confused, impulsive, episodic state, during which the conduct is bizarre and determined by the hallucinations and delusions which are so predominant.

The depressive stupor state may appear to be identical to the katatonic stupor of schizophrenia, and again it is safer to be guided, for differentiation purposes, by rapidity of onset and personality type. On the whole, however, the depressive stupor is not so persistent as a katatonic one, and is not punctuated by episodes of wild excitement as the latter is.

Careless observers are apt to mistake the manic phase for the onset of an organic illness such as general paralysis. There is no excuse for this, because the physical signs and the serological tests should be conclusive. Affective states may be complicated by syphilitic disease, and a positive blood Wassermann may be present, but the absence of clinical symptoms pointing to an organic type of reaction, along with negative findings in the cerebrospinal fluid are sufficient to rule out the diagnosis of general paralysis.

Those cases of affective disturbance occurring at the involutional period may occasionally present a certain amount of difficulty in differentiation from paranoid states, but in the latter the heightening of affect is only related to certain specified paranoid ideas, and differs in quality and type from that of affective disorders; in the involutional states the affect dominates the entire clinical picture.

Differentiation from cases of arteriosclerotic brain disease may present certain problems. The fact that a marked degree of peripheral arteriosclerosis may accompany involutional states should not deceive us. That is exactly what might be expected, but provided there is no history of headache, dizziness, convulsive attacks, failure of memory and concentration, we can remain confident of our diagnosis.

Treatment

The affective psychoses are, for the most part, constitutionally determined, and may occur and resolve spontaneously. In other cases trivial or more serious precipitating exogenous factors may be required to trigger off the psychotic cycle which we must attempt to control. Our treatment is directed in a threefold direction: 1. to allay the acuteness of the symptoms; 2. to modify or alter the patient's environment; and 3. to assist the patient to a better understanding of his own personality so that he may learn to live amicably with his disability. No hard and fast rules can be laid down, each case differs in its psychological, physical and environmental components, and must be treated on its individual merits.

The rhythmic swings of mood so characteristic of the affective state may never over-step normal limits, and be very transitory. In consequence, domestic, social and business activities need not be seriously interfered with. Perhaps temporarily the patient may have to modify the pace of his life, to take things easier, to get

more sleep, to maintain his physical strength. A few words of sympathetic encouragement plus a mild sedative to combat sleeplessness may be sufficient to
enable the personality to resume a better balanced tempo. In other cases the
mood swings may be of a higher and deeper intensity, are episodic, prolonged,
alternating in nature, and occur with dramatic suddenness. Even so the tendency
is always towards a spontaneous readjustment irrespective of the number of
recurrences. To facilitate recovery and to allay the mental distress and excitement it is advisable, without delay, to utilize all the modern methods of treatment
which are now at our command.

Before any programme of treatment is instituted, a decision as to where it most
appropriately can be undertaken should be come to. The social, economic and
business circumstances of the patient may be some of the important deciding
factors, but the patient's ability to co-operate is paramount. If he has good
insight into his condition, if his relatives are able to undertake the responsibility,
if a special nurse can be provided, his own home may be eminently suitable.
Otherwise the advantages of a nursing home, a special psychiatric department of
a general hospital, or a mental hospital, have to be carefully considered. Any of
the above arrangements may prove successful; they have become more feasible
because of the rapidity with which electric convulsion therapy and tranquillizing
and sedative drugs can control excitement, noise, depression and restlessness.
Under special circumstances a compromise can be effected whereby treatment
on an out-patient basis can be arranged. In-patient treatment, however, gives a
greater sense of security both to patient and to doctor.

Acutely disturbed, non-co-operative patients are more suitable for mental
hospital care, especially if the illness is likely to be prolonged. Such a hospital
gives a greater sense of freedom, recreational and social activities are available,
and the association with other patients can hasten the rehabilitation process.
At the same time depressed patients obsessed with suicidal thoughts can be
under constant observation, while manic patients have sufficient scope in which
to dissipate their superabundant energy. In coping with the above issues a
serious responsibility is involved but doctors and nurses must remain understanding, flexible, calm and tactful even under the most trying and aggravating
circumstances. Too great rigidity, the inability to take a reasonable risk may
lead to unfortunate consequences by creating antagonism between patient and
doctor. Careful 'timing' of such decisions should be exercised. Supervision
should always be carried out in as unobtrusive a way as possible. No one likes to
feel 'policed'—it may create a sense of mistrust, irritation and frustration. In
case of any untoward accident our conscience may remain at peace provided all
reasonable care has been exercised.

On admission to hospital or nursing home these patients are invariably in
need of bed treatment and careful nursing which should be continued until the
patient has become completely rested mentally and bodily. Some prefer a single
room, others a small dormitory where they may have the companionship of others.
These procedures ensure that the doctors and nurses in attendance become
quickly familiar with the character, conduct and habits of the patient. The

R

problems of insomnia, suicide, undernourishment and so on are kept under constant review. The human interest and attention given to the patient is not only a comfort, but also reassures relatives and friends that everything possible will be done to facilitate recovery.

The vast majority of depressed patients are dominated by guilt feelings, regard themselves as moral cowards rather than as estimable persons who are merely sick in mind and body. The only mistake they have made with their problem has been to struggle unaided, usually for far too long, and to have added bodily exhaustion to their other troublesome symptoms. They feel that they are lacking in will power, that their character has deteriorated, that they should make some superhuman effort to free themselves from all those tormenting thoughts which seem to control and bind them. Their suffering may be intensified by well-meaning, naïvely optimistic friends—and even family doctors—who prescribe cheering up methods, social activities, amusements, sea trips or other dangerous experiments which the patient is unable to accept.

The more sensible plan is to reduce life's activities to as simple a level as possible. The patient should be advised, as a general rule, to have a period of sick leave, to conserve his resources, and to avoid activities which might increase his sense of failure. Anything he undertakes should carry with it a reasonable chance of success. He should be reassured and informed that his illness is not an uncommon one, that it is as real as appendicitis or any other bodily involvement, that there is nothing to be ashamed of, that it is not a punishment for sin, and that the future can be anticipated with equanimity. It is by no means easy for the patient to accept such reassurances, but constant repetition eventually brings conviction.

Insomnia and the dangers of suicide, which are often closely linked, are the most troublesome symptoms to deal with. It is this combination which so often necessitates hospital treatment, and indeed may be a matter of extreme urgency. In the event of a suicidal attempt everything possible must be done to conserve the patient's life by administering first-aid for the injuries sustained, and by arranging for additional psychological care and treatment (Batchelor, 1955). It is surprising, in many cases, how admirably the patient responds; only a day or two may be required for relief. It is as if things had to reach a climax, as if the mounting tension could only be broken by a huge mental explosion. The ensuing peace and calmness in the security of a hospital atmosphere provides the best opportunity to discuss the many problems which seemed impossible to solve. Their revelation constitutes a blessed relief. Perhaps those who are most difficult to help are the so-called sexual neurasthenics. It has been said: 'No woman suffering from amenorrhoea and melancholia is free from danger, and no man who believes he is suffering from impotence, spermatorrhoea or syphilophobia is trustworthy.' We can never afford to be cynical, even although it has been recorded that Esquirol, in talking to a lady who was always threatening suicide, said: 'Very well, it is nothing to me, and your husband will be rid of a great torment.' She made an instantaneous recovery.

The Church and various lay organizations are less heroic and more helpful in their attitudes. London's Anti-Suicide Bureau, the Save-a-Life League in the U.S.A., Vienna's Advisory Centre for those weary of life, Zürich's Anti-Suicide League, and Berlin's Suicide's Aid Society have all accomplished a great purpose. The Salvation Army, the Samaritans Association and the increasing development of psychiatric out-patient clinics are most essential prophylactic agencies (Henderson, 1937). The risk of such a catastrophe occurring is greatest in the early stages of the illness or during convalescence. It is at those times that the conflict between the fear of life and the wish for death is most acute. A familial tendency, and a particular locality may increase the suggestive effect. It is, however, an act which need never be repeated.

Insomnia may also prove most difficult to deal with. The unconsciousness which characterizes sleep and death are closely akin, and it is often the fear of death, of sinking into unconsciousness which prevents sleep. Tolstoy expressed it in this way: 'One must not be afraid of falling asleep if one wishes to avoid sleeplessness.' That is the underlying reason why so many patients refuse sedatives, fight against an anaesthetic or waken up suddenly once they have gone off to sleep. It is because of such doubts and fears that it is so important to establish a good *rapport*. It is only then that hypnotics will operate to the best advantage. If hypnotics, even in large doses, are failing to produce the desired effect it is often advisable to discard them altogether and rely on other methods. In any case, some patients are allergic to certain drugs and respond admirably to others. It may take time to decide the preparation which will prove most suitable. Paraldehyde has the particular merit of being safe, rapid in action and rarely leads to addiction. It is prescribed in from 60 min. to 180 min. doses, each 60 min. with an ounce of water and syrup of orange as a flavouring agent. Chloral hydrate is another safe, quick acting and effective hypnotic: it is prescribed usually in solution in doses of 20 gr. Many barbiturates can be most efficacious. We suggest pentobarbitone sodium, B.P. (*Nembutal*), 1½ to 3 gr.; barbitone sodium, B.P. (*Medinal*), 5 to 10 gr.; cyclobarbitone, B.P., 3 to 6 gr.; quinalbarbitone, B.P. (*Seconal Sodium*), 1½ to 3 gr. For elderly patients a combination of chloral hydrate, B.P., 15 to 30 gr. and nepenthe, 15 min., may prove most helpful. When the excitement is intense and it is imperative to prevent exhaustion, a hypodermic injection of morphine, ¼ to ½ gr. with hyoscine, 1/100 to 1/75 gr., or chlorpromazine injection, B.P., 50 mg. intramuscularly, will usually act successfully.

To allay tension, depression or excitement during the day many thymoleptic and tranquillizing drugs have proved most efficacious. For instance, in depressive states we have found imipramine hydrochloride (*Tofranil*) valuable. It should be prescribed in doses of 25 to 50 mg. three or four times daily; a higher dose is seldom required. In certain instances it has replaced the use of electric convulsion therapy. Troublesome side effects, *e.g.* a manic reaction, dryness of the mouth, tachycardia, disturbance of accommodation, sweating, giddiness, faintness and falling, should be treated by reducing dosage or discontinuing the drug. As a substitute, phenelzine (*Nardil*) 15 mg. three times a day, or one of the other amineoxidase inhibitors, may prove of considerable value.

In manic states chlorpromazine hydrochloride (*Largactil*) reduces the excitement and restlessness, and allows the patient to become more co-operative. The usual dosage is 25 to 100 mg. three or four times daily but when the patient is in hospital larger doses may be given. The side effects which may be encountered are dryness of the mouth, agranulocytosis, postural hypotension, photosensitivity, jaundice, Parkinsonism and dermatitis. Alternatively reserpine may be used [see p. 352].

We have every reason to hope that further psychopharmacological research into the treatment of distressing emotional disturbances will lead to even greater therapeutic accuracy.

It is the use of such drugs plus electric convulsion therapy which has almost transformed the treatment of affective states. As a result hydrotherapy in its various forms has been discarded, and tube feeding is rarely necessary. If, however, the patient's general health has been severely undermined by refusal of nourishment then an easily digested meal of milk, eggs, sugar, grated vegetables, meat juices and other ingredients can be given by nasal or stomach tube.

Occupational therapy is an indispensable adjunct. It can be utilized, in one form or another, throughout the whole course of the illness, and even after the patient has returned home. It should be prescribed in consultation with the occupational therapist, and should be varied according to the particular interest or 'bent' of the patient. The essential point is to create co-operation, a sense of accomplishment, an ability to concentrate, and to persist in whatever is undertaken. It is not merely a matter of learning a new skill or handicraft, but it may be that greater satisfaction will be derived from work in the garden, the kitchen, workshop, laundry or other department. Others with literary and artistic interests are also catered for not only through the Occupational Therapy Department but also by the generous voluntary assistance of the British Red Cross Society and other organizations, some of whose peace-time activities are directed to increasing the amenity of life in a mental hospital. They provide an excellent library service, and choose appropriate works of art with which to decorate the hospital wards. The recreational and social side of hospital life is also incorporated, to a large extent, in the Occupational Therapy Department. Remedial exercises, dances and other types of entertainment, *e.g.* tennis parties, hockey, cricket, do much to build up a sense of well-being and good bodily health and fitness. The ready co-operation of the medical and nursing staff in all the above interests and activities adds enormously to the development of a therapeutic community.

Our main task in treatment, however, is to attempt to give the patient a better understanding of his personality than he has ever had previously. To cure his symptoms is one thing, but a much higher achievement is to increase the patient's subjective sense of strength, confidence and well-being so that he can look forward to the future in a spirit of greater optimism. Our psychotherapeutic interviews are therefore based on good history taking and on an investigation of all the relevant data. It is never wise to minimize the periodicity of this type of illness or its seriousness, but at the same time ways and means can be suggested whereby stress, fatigue and other untoward precipitants can be avoided.

Furthermore, the assurance can be given that the disturbance of mood is a temporary disability, that the intellectual faculties will remain intact, that recovery from the attack will occur but that the length of time can not be predicted. In order to avoid undue suffering the patient should be encouraged to seek expert help at the first indication of oncoming symptoms. Prolonged psychoanalytic treatment is not recommended for the cyclothymic states we have described, but general psychoanalytic principles can be utilized.

The above suggestions regarding treatment apply equally to the affective disorders occurring at the involutional period, *e.g.* involutional melancholia and chronic mania. But these latter forms are not nearly so recurrent as the manic-depressive states, and chronic mania may remain intractable.

During the process of convalescence everything possible should be done by tonics, nutritious diet, holidays, etc., to build up a state of mental, moral and physical fitness. It is only when the patient has returned home and has resumed his former occupation that his complete confidence becomes re-established. A return to work, therefore, should not be too long delayed. (For details regarding physical methods of treatment and occupational therapy, see Chapters 14 and 20.)

REFERENCES

Abraham, K. (1927) *Selected Papers on Psycho-analysis*, London.
Batchelor, I. R. C. (1955), *Brit. med. J.*, **1**, 595.
Henderson, D. K. (1937) *Social and Individual Prophylaxis of Suicide*, 2nd International Congress of Mental Hygiene, Paris.
Hoch, A., and MacCurdy, J. T. (1922) *Arch. Neurol. Psychiat. (Chicago)*, **7**, 1.
Kallmann, F. J. (1953) *Heredity in Health and Mental Disorder*, New York.
Kraines, S. H. (1934) *Amer. J. Psychiat.*, **91**, 29.
Lewis, A. J. (1934) *J. ment. Sci.*, **80**, 277.
MacCurdy, J. T. (1925) *Psychology of Emotion*, London.
Rosanoff, A. J., Handy, L. M., and Plesset, I. R. (1935) *Amer. J. Psychiat.*, **91**, 725.
Sievers, A., and Davidoff, E. (1942) *J. nerv. ment. Dis.*, **95**, 427.
Sievers, A., and Davidoff, E. (1943) *Psychiat. Quart.*, **17**, 520.
Wertham, F. I. (1929) *Amer. J. Psychiat.*, **9**, 17.

11

SCHIZOPHRENIC REACTION-TYPES

Schizophrenia, in its most typical form, consists in a slow deterioration of the entire personality, which often manifests itself at the period of adolescence. It involves a great part of the mental life, and expresses itself in disorder of feeling, of conduct, and of thought, and in an increasing withdrawal of interest from the environment.

We believe that the term schizophrenia is more applicable than the term dementia praecox to the group of cases now to be described. In 1896 Kraepelin first made his differentiation between manic-depressive psychosis and 'dementia praecox'. The differentiation was of great importance, but the name given to the reaction-type was unfortunate. Many of these patients did not show a permanent dementia, and many became ill outside the adolescent period. The term dementia praecox furthermore implied usually a rather hopeless prognosis, and encouraged therapeutic nihilism.

In 1911 Bleuler introduced the term 'schizophrenia' for these dementia praecox cases and for others which he considered to be allied—paranoid states, hallucinoses and prison psychoses; and in doing so stressed the importance of splitting of the different psychic functions. Bleuler's was a wider conception than Kraepelin's: 'We designate a group of psychoses whose course is at times chronic, at times marked by intermittent attacks, and which can stop or retrograde at any stage, but does not permit a full restitutio ad integrum'. He used the term schizophrenia in the singular, but was in no doubt that he was dealing with a group of several diseases. The symptoms of schizophrenia he divided into two classes, the fundamental and the accessory or secondary. The fundamental symptoms Bleuler considered to be disturbances of association and affectivity, a predilection for phantasy as against reality, and a tendency to divorce from reality (autism). Hallucinations, delusions, illusions and katatonic symptoms he called secondary, while conceding that these were the symptoms which often made manifest the psychosis and caused the patient to be hospitalized.

There has been little advance in the classification of this reaction-type since Kraepelin and Bleuler, and their descriptive work has not been superseded. Both Kraepelin and Bleuler believed that schizophrenia was the outcome of a pathological, anatomical or chemical disturbance of the brain.

The point of view adopted by Adolf Meyer and his pupils differs considerably from that held by the purely pathological and anatomical investigators. Meyer did not by any means disregard the latter, but rather sought to include, in a general biological formulation of schizophrenia, whatever is of established value in the field of physical pathology. The essence of his view was that schizophrenia is the outcome of progressive maladaptation of the individual to his environment. Schizophrenia is not a 'disease', but a congeries of individual types of reaction having certain general similarities. 'We must consider mental illness, not in terms of clean-cut groups, but of reaction-types.' The individual may be loaded in various ways—by inheritance, by physical defects of an endocrine disorder or some grosser kind, by intellectual deficiency, or what not—but none of them is in itself a sufficient cause of schizophrenia. It is only when the subject, whether handicapped or not, has to face the usual concrete problems in his journey through life that reactions can appear which cumulatively lead to one of the numerous conditions which have been included under the designation of 'dementia praecox' or 'schizophrenia'. It was from a careful study of patients, and especially of their history before any breakdown was recognized by friends or relatives—a line of investigation commonly neglected—that Meyer concluded that 'schizophrenia' is the end result of an accumulation of faulty habits of reaction.

The healthy attitude to life's difficulties and problems is a direct, aggressive, matter-of-fact one, designed to overcome the difficulty once and for all, with the result that the individual feels satisfied, and can proceed confidently to his next problem. On the other hand, the individual may shrink from facing the situation directly, and may temporize in the hope that something will turn up, or that the matter will be decided for him. In other instances he may evade the necessity for definite action by indulging in some substitute, which is never satisfactory; for example, if unsuccessful in work, he may indulge in day-dreams of wealth; or if unable to face the responsibilities of marriage, he may take to sex ruminations or to auto-erotic habits. A sense of failure is no longer combated by renewed efforts, but by brooding over troubles and by blaming others. Such reactions, occurring only occasionally, are within normal limits; but if they become so frequent as to be habitual, they lead to total inefficiency and social maladaptation, so that the individual exhibiting them comes to be regarded as abnormal. Certain kinds of faulty reaction are especially pernicious, such as hypochondriacal trends—blaming one's health for one's failures—ideas of suspicion or actual fault-finding, phantastic religious motives and persistent brooding and seclusiveness. Reactions which are not morbid when used sparingly and in certain circumstances may become diffused over the whole conduct, and are increasingly used because, being habitual, they are easier than anything else. Negativism, for example, is healthy enough as mere stubbornness in certain directions; but when it extends to every activity as an 'uncontrollable blocking factor' it becomes pathological, and constitutes what has hitherto been called a mental 'disease'.

Since the Second World War, particularly in the U.S.A., the concept of schizophrenia has been enlarged; in our opinion, without sufficient justification. Hoch and Polatin (1949), in an influential paper, introduced the term 'pseudo-neurotic' schizophrenia, describing a condition of persistent tension with multiple and changing neurotic symptoms, which is characterized further by a proneness to develop transient psychotic episodes and which may pass later into unequivocal schizophrenia. Other terms have been used for apparently the same kind of case: for example, 'borderline states', 'abortive' and 'latent' schizophrenia. Usually the presence of a thought disorder is considered to be a necessary criterion for the diagnosis: but the nature of this thought disorder is by some authors left vague and is variously described by many others. Egocentricity, coldness of feeling, inability to develop normal personal relationships, poor work record, and a failure to respond to psychotherapy, are frequently described: these features are said to be persistent, and a progressive and lasting deterioration unusual. This description suggests that many of these cases would be more correctly described as suffering from psychopathic states. Their close relationship to schizophrenia has not been established. It is of course common experience that many cases of schizophrenia, particularly those of insidious onset, begin with the development of neurotic symptoms: but these do not form a distinct group and need not be given a special label.

Langfeldt (1952), from the University Clinic of Oslo, has been prominent amongst those who have deplored any widening of the classical concept of schizophrenia. Langfeldt accepts the Kraepelinian sub-groups of schizophrenia; while noting that the paranoid cases seem to be of mixed aetiology, multiform symptomatology and very variable course. He proposes in addition that cases which seem to fall into the category of schizophrenia should initially be divided into two other sub-groups, according to whether they appear to be typical or atypical: one group he calls typical, genuine schizophrenias, the other schizo-phreniform psychoses. The former, nuclear group shows pre-illness personality deviation and the schizophrenia develops mainly endogenously with dominant feelings of depersonalization (feelings of influence and passivity) and derealiza-tion: these symptoms, with massive primary ideas of persecution and katatonic stuporous features, he calls 'process' symptoms. Such cases mostly carry a poor prognosis and are prone to dement early. The atypical, schizophreniform group, on the other hand, is said to be heterogeneous: the pre-illness personality is not schizoid, exogenous factors are often prominent, and the symptomatology is mixed, with clouding or strong affective features and without process symptoms. This group carries a better prognosis on the whole, though some cases in the group turn out to be dementing schizophrenics: others prove to be cases of affective psychosis or neurotic or organic reactions.

Langfeldt's call for greater discrimination in diagnosis is to be welcomed, and research would be more profitable if it were heeded: but it is doubtful if his clinical designation of a specific schizophreniform group brings any advantage. That many of his schizophreniform cases reveal themselves later as definitely schizophrenic, seems to demonstrate that his concept of the typical group is too narrow: while if the category were generally accepted, many cases would no doubt find their way into this schizophreniform group not so much because of their near resemblance to schizophrenia but because diagnostic acumen is often lacking. For example, there would be little to be said in favour of calling a case of mixed affective psychosis schizophreniform on the grounds that the individual is hallucinated, perplexed and his affect variable; except that to do so would be better than calling it schizophrenia.

The term 'schizo-affective psychosis' has probably created more diagnostic difficulties than it has resolved. Certainly in many cases of schizophrenia there are prominent affective symptoms: particularly depression, in the illnesses of more acute onset. A mixture of manic and schizophrenic symptoms is much rarer. In some of these cases of mixed symptomatology the patient appears to have developed at the same time a schizophrenic and an affective psychosis; in others, where the affective symptoms colour the clinical picture but are not so prominent, one can find a sufficient explanation for them in that they can be linked with the traits of the pre-morbid personality or understood as psychogenic reactions to other distressing or alarming symptoms of the disease. In a small number of cases a schizo-affective psychosis appears to be a clinical entity showing a familial distribution, is inherited as a Mendelian dominant and is probably distinct from schizophrenia (Leonhard, 1939). Much more often the term schizo-affective psychosis is a misnomer, applied to cases of mixed affective psychosis in which the admixture of depressive and manic symptoms has given rise to some apparent incongruity of affect; and the perplexity and difficulty of thinking have been wrongly diagnosed as evidence of schizophrenic thought disorder with blocking. These mixed affective psychoses are not rare, and are much more often misdiagnosed as schizophrenia than is schizophrenia mistaken for an affective psychosis.

Research into the many problems posed by schizophrenia has been frustrated by doubts and uncertainties about the heterogeneity of the clinical material being studied. Possibly the majority of observers now think that schizophrenia is not a clinical entity but a group of syndromes, of different aetiologies though with similarities in their clinical features: yet research has usually proceeded on the assumption that a biological entity was being investigated. The varieties of schizophrenia shortly to be described are clinical groupings of symptoms, they have no known pathological basis: but it might well now be more profitable to select for biochemical research these clinical subdivisions rather than schizophrenia as a whole, and particularly the most typical cases of hebephrenia and katatonia.

AETIOLOGY

Heredity

The evidence from genetic studies is that hereditary factors are of predominant importance in the majority of cases of schizophrenia. Some psychiatrists already hold it to be established that schizophrenia is a hereditary disease or group of diseases, and probably a biochemical disorder determined by a gene-specific type of enzyme deficiency. Major contributions to the genetic study of schizophrenia have been made by Luxenburger, Rosanoff, Essen-Möller, Kallmann and Slater.

Kallmann (1953) stated that his very large clinical material showed clearly that the chance of developing a schizophrenic psychosis increases in direct proportion to the degree of blood relationship to a schizophrenic individual. From an analysis of nearly one thousand twin index families he reported that the total expectancy of schizophrenia varies from 7·1 per cent. for half-sibs, through 14 per cent. for full sibs and two-egg co-twins, to 86·2 per cent. for one-egg twin partners. The expectancy rate for schizophrenia in the normal population is 0·85 per cent. For the children of one schizophrenic parent the expectancy is 16·4 per cent.; of two schizophrenic parents, 68·1 per cent.—that is, the children of two schizophrenic parents have the second highest expectancy of the disease, next to one-egg co-twins. These expectancy rates, which Kallmann recorded for the blood relatives of schizophrenics, cannot, he believed, be explained in terms of increasing similarity of environment. 'About one-quarter of one-egg pairs have been found to develop schizophrenic psychoses in the absence of similar environments, while close to one-half of two-egg pairs remain discordant despite similar environments.'

With regard to the mode of hereditary transmission, Kallmann holds to the hypothesis of recessive inheritance. He does so mainly on the grounds that the distribution of schizophrenia in affected families shows that schizophrenia is transmitted in the collateral rather than in the direct line of descent, and that there is an excess of consanguineous marriages among the parents of schizophrenics: he reports that in the U.S.A. approximately 5 per cent. of schizophrenics are the offspring of consanguineous marriages. Kallmann notes that the children of schizophrenics have a higher expectancy of schizophrenia than the sibs, and that this is not what one would expect if the disease is recessive. He suggests that this apparent discrepancy may be due to a selective process of 'negative mate selection—the unlikelihood of actual or potential schizophrenics having a normal chance to select their mates'.

Kallmann believes that in some homozygotes the genotype is completely inhibited, so that the individual is normal: some schizoid personalities are probably inhibited homozygotes also, while others may be heterozygotes. Kallmann also suggests that the apparently wide differences in the penetrance and expressivity of the schizophrenic genotype may be interpreted as being controlled by genetically non-specific constitutional defence mechanisms, which possibly are related to the effect of certain mesodermal tissue elements.

The hypothesis of simple recessive inheritance of schizophrenia has been criticized by a number of other authorities, mainly because if the condition is recessively inherited the frequency of schizophrenia should be greater among the sibs than among their children. But no other genetic hypothesis fits all the facts better. That the mode of inheritance is not more obvious may be due to the fact that a heterogeneous clinical material has been investigated—the schizophrenias, that is, rather than schizophrenia.

Slater (1953) critically reviewed the literature of twin studies in schizophrenia and reported on a large series of twins personally investigated: of 297 pairs the propositus was schizophrenic in 158 cases. He found a concordance rate for schizophrenia of 76 per cent. in uniovular twins, and of 14 per cent. in binovular twins. While there were wide differences in the severity of the illness within concordant uniovular pairs, taking all pairs of affected relatives together there was a significant degree of resemblance in the course of their illness and the type of onset: but not in the outcome. The facts suggest, Slater commented, 'that genetical causes provide a potentiality for schizophrenia, perhaps an essential one, though environmental factors play a substantial rôle, which may be decisive in the individual case. Those environmental factors which affect personality and constitution appear to be the most important.'

Environmental Factors

The rate of concordance for schizophrenia in uniovular twins has been estimated to lie between 66·6 and 86·2 per cent. It is not 100 per cent. The genetic studies quoted above therefore indicate that inherited determinants are not all important: and there is evidence that social factors, in the family and in the *milieu* of an urban civilization, may play some part in the aetiology.

The Family Environment. Psychotherapists who were treating schizophrenics analytically became interested naturally in the early relationships of their patients to their mothers: and by the late 1940's the concept of a 'schizophrenogenic mother' had gained wide currency in the United States. The typical mother of a schizophrenic was held to be severely rejecting, and the subsequent distortion of the mother-child relationship was believed to have much aetiological significance. Tietze (1949), for example, found the mothers of schizophrenics dominating, over-anxious and obsessive, covertly rejecting and often frigid. Much of this work was, however, based only on clinical impressions. At the same time maternal rejection was commonly believed to produce types of deviation other than schizophrenia.

This interest in the mothers of schizophrenics subsequently widened into several important researches into the nature of the total family environment in which schizophrenic breakdowns develop. The investigations by Lidz and his colleagues (1949, 1956, 1957) at Yale have been amongst the most careful of these studies. They reported initially on a group of 50 young schizophrenics. Only 5 of these patients were considered to have been raised in homes which seemed reasonably favourable and which contained two stable and compatible parents until the patient was 18 years of age. Broken homes, unstable parents and an unusual pattern of child rearing appeared to be almost the rule. Later, investigating more intensively in 16 middle-class families the intra-familiar environment in which schizophrenia had developed, Lidz and his colleagues reached the conclusion that 'serious pathology of the family environment is the most consistent finding pertaining to the aetiology of schizophrenia'. These researchers have found abnormalities wherever they have looked in the schizophrenic's family. The marital relationship of the parents is reported to be seriously disturbed, in one of two ways: either there is chronic disequilibrium, with derogation and undercutting of the marital partner and threats of separation ('marital discord'); or one spouse is dominant and imposes his or her psychopathology on the masochistic partner, who achieves some marital peace by submission ('marital skew'). The schizophrenic's father, they report, tends either to be a passive nonentity; or to sabotage his wife in her rôle as a mother, being himself motivated by jealousy of a son or by a wish to mould a daughter after his own arbitrary fashion.

These researches by Lidz and his colleagues cannot be said to be definitive. The work has lacked controls and suffers from the weaknesses inherent in all retrospective studies. It has stressed effects of environment in the explanation of facts which might be better explained in terms of inheritance. But it has been of considerable value in placing the schizophrenic in his home setting, in raising questions about the mental normality of the heterozygous parents, and in stressing the importance of the complex personal interactions which take place in the schizophrenic's family whether as causes or effects of his illness. It has drawn attention to an aspect which is too often neglected in the investigation and treatment of schizophrenic patients; namely their families, from whom we can always glean a great deal of relevant information, whose co-operation we must enlist if our plans for management are not to miscarry, and to whom, good or bad, stable or unstable, our patients will in most instances return.

The Wider Social Environment. There is a disproportionate number of cases of schizophrenia amongst those of low socio-economic status both in Britain and in the U.S.A., but there is as yet no evidence pointing unequivocally to specific injurious social factors outside the family which may cause schizophrenia. Elements of the urban social environment and social stresses may contribute to schizophrenic breakdowns, may act as precipitants of such breakdowns in predisposed individuals, and may complicate the ascertainment, treatment of, and recovery from the illness; but our present evidence suggests that the rôle of such factors is usually of secondary importance in the aetiology.

In Chapter 4 attention has been drawn to the work of Faris and Dunham, Gerard and Houston, and Hare on the influence of neighbourhood on schizophrenic breakdowns. Here the important researches of Hollingshead and Redlich (1958) must get further mention. Schizophrenia was the most common mental illness in their New Haven, Connecticut, population, at all class levels: schizophrenics comprised 59 per cent. of the psychotic patients. The rate of schizophrenia per 100,000 of this urban population was for social classes I–II, 111; for class III, 168; for class IV, 300; and for social class V, 895. Hollingshead and Redlich state that their data support the conclusion that 'neither geographic transiency nor downward social mobility can account for the sharp differences in the distribution of schizophrenic patients from one class to another'. 91 per cent. of their schizophrenic patients were in the same social class as their families: only 1·3 per cent. were in a lower class, 4·4 per cent. were in a higher class. 89 per cent. of the class V patients came from class V families: and they had lived in the slums all their lives. Neither was there any linkage between schizophrenia and international migration (immigration was the largest geographical movement in this population). Hollingshead and Redlich therefore support the conclusion of Faris and Dunham that schizophrenic patients committed to mental hospitals from slum areas have not drifted there as an effect of their illness.

In a detailed study of family and class dynamics in 50 cases which formed part of the New Haven research, Myers and Roberts (1959) have produced some evidence that certain conditions of life in social class V may be conducive to the development of schizophrenia, by causing isolation and withdrawal. They do not suggest that social class position is a direct cause of schizophrenia, but only that life at a certain social level may expose the potential patient to certain potent stresses. They found that the developing individual in social class V is more exposed than people in other social classes both to adverse economic conditions and to social isolation from community institutions. They found also that he tends to be reared in a family environment where there is little affection, protection and stability: and they link this with the proneness of the adult in this social class to feel 'neglected, rejected, exploited and trapped by unfortunate circumstances'. Furthermore, they report that both intra-familial and community stresses bear more heavily on schizophrenic than on neurotic patients, both in class III and in class V. Myers and Roberts are cautious in their formulations, emphasizing the exploratory nature of their studies and suggesting that their results should be regarded as hypotheses for future research.

In the U.S.A. schizophrenia has been reported to be nearly ten times as frequent in social class V as in the upper two social classes. A similar great social class difference in the incidence of schizophrenia has been found in Britain, where schizophrenia preponderates amongst the unskilled young men of the lowest social class and is concentrated in two occupational groups, kitchen hands and labourers: Brooke (1959) reporting these facts, comments that in both these occupations we should expect to find a high proportion of casual labour and they might prove suitable temporary occupations for the unstable. The Registrar General for England and Wales's figures for first admission rates by social class to mental hospitals, for schizophrenia in males aged 20 years and over were (1956) per 100,000: for social class I, 11; for class II, 8; for class III, 16; for class IV, 17; and for social class V, 45. The ratio of class V to class I rates for schizophrenia were 4·2 for first admissions and 6·7 for other admissions (Brooke). In contrast with the U.S.A., in England and Wales a drop in social status from father to schizophrenic son has been reported by Morrison (1959), who has studied male schizophrenics aged 25–34 first admitted to mental hospitals in 1956. The fathers of these schizophrenic patients had the same social class distribution as the population as a whole. These results are very different from Hollingshead and Redlich's, and further investigations are being made by the Social Medicine Research Unit of the Medical Research Council.

Precipitating Factors

Exciting factors in the sense of immediate precipitants of the illness are often apparently absent; but a certain proportion of cases begin in association with such stresses as toxic-infectious illness, pregnancy and (more often) the puerperium, domestic unhappiness, love affairs and financial difficulties. During both World Wars, schizophrenic cases of acute onset were encountered which appeared to have been definitely precipitated by war stresses, and which were both of a simpler form and had a better prognosis than the average.

Model Psychoses

There have been various attempts to elucidate the obscure aetiology of this disease by inducing what have been called 'model psychoses' in normal subjects.

Some of these experiments have produced psychological data of much importance, but they have thrown little direct light on the genesis of schizophrenia. So-called model psychoses have been produced in two ways: by administering hallucinogenic drugs, and by sensory deprivation.

The hallucinogenic (or psychotomimetic) drugs most often employed have been mescaline and lysergic acid (LSD 25). The effects of lysergic acid, an ergot derivative, have been particularly interesting because they are produced by minute quantities of the drug. These drugs, given to the normal subject, cause changes in attention and affect, as well as hallucinations. Typically, the individual's attention is abnormally arrested by his immediate environment; he becomes anxious, depressed or euphoric; and he has visual hallucinations, which may be coloured or monochrome, take mosaic or graticule forms or consist of human or landscape content. Synaesthesiae may be reported. These phenomena occur in a setting of clear or nearly clear consciousness: insight is retained and behaviour is usually not disturbed. Perhaps the individual under the influence of a hallucinogenic drug has some experience like a schizophrenic's: but the 'model psychosis' which is produced by this means belongs to the classical organic reaction-type, since, if the dose of the drug is increased, the subject becomes delirious.

Sensory deprivation may be produced experimentally by shutting the individual into a cubicle (Heron et al., 1953), where he lies on a couch with frosted goggles over his eyes, sponge-rubber pads over his ears, his arms splinted and his extremities swaddled; or by immersing him in a tank of water at body temperature (Lilly, 1956). These experiences proved more unpleasant than they sound and became intolerable after 24–72 hours. The subjects reported a craving for stimulation, became abnormally restless, and later developed visual hallucinations, alterations in body image and, occasionally, fleeting paranoid delusions. The resemblance to schizophrenia of the symptoms produced by sensory deprivation may be closer than the effects produced by drugs, though they are somewhat similar to the latter: but there is no real evidence that sensory deprivation phenomena are a paradigm of schizophrenia. These experiments seem in fact to have thrown some light on the mechanisms of schizophrenia in a direction opposite to what was originally intended, since Harris (1959) has found that a small group of schizophrenics were more tolerant than normal of sensory deprivation for short periods in a soundproof cubicle: it seemed to reduce the intensity of their hallucinations and to render these less troublesome.

The psychological aspects of phantasticants and the relationship between experimental and social isolation have been discussed by Mowbray (1958).

In summary of this section, we can say that the aetiology of schizophrenia challengingly remains to be fully elucidated. It appears to be a disease or group of diseases, mainly caused by unknown abnormal organic processes which are genetically determined. We are still wholly ignorant of the mode of action of the pathological gene or genes which we suppose are responsible for its diverse symptomatology and its often malignant course.

CLINICAL FEATURES

Schizophrenia affects particularly adolescents and young adults. It has been estimated that two-thirds of the cases occur between the 15th and 30th year, and the maximum incidence is reached about the 25th year. Few cases begin after the age of 40. The incidence in the general population is 0·85 per cent. Schizophrenia is the diagnosis of about three-quarters of the long-term patients in mental hospitals in this country, and it appears to have a world-wide distribution. It constitutes one of the most serious disease problems of western civilization.

Mode of Onset and Previous Personality

In a small number of cases, particularly those showing katatonic features, the onset of the illness may be comparatively acute. More usually, and in contrast to the affective psychoses, schizophrenia develops slowly and insidiously over a long period of months or years. In the vast majority of cases a close analysis of the history shows that the patient has exhibited peculiarities and oddities which perhaps did not seem to have any special significance until the grosser symptoms presented themselves. We believe, therefore, that close attention should be paid to obtaining very complete records of the development of the patient, and that the idiosyncrasies and perversities of childhood should be carefully scanned, because by so doing we may be able to determine traits which are likely to be followed by more serious symptoms. We would particularly emphasize the importance of noting such traits as day-dreaming, fears, solitariness, undue sensitivity, and bashfulness.

It is often difficult to fix a time of onset of the psychosis. It seems to develop more or less from the habits of reaction cultivated by the patient on his way through life. These habits make up in great part the 'personality' of the patient as it was before they were sufficiently developed to constitute a socially recognizable illness. Meyer and Hoch emphasized the frequency with which this psychosis develops in certain types of handicapped personality, especially in the 'shut-in', shy, seclusive type. The same general type of personality has been described by other authors by other names; for example, by Bleuler as 'schizoid', in contrast with the 'syntonic' or 'cycloid' personality in which, if mental illness develops, it tends to be of the manic-depressive kind. Farrar distinguished five main types of 'shut-in' personality: 1. the 'backward' type, lacking ambition, absent-minded, often playing truant; 2. the 'precocious' type, the bookish, serious, prudish, 'model' child; 3. the 'neurotic' variety, selfish and deceitful, with headaches and other minor ailments, and temper-tantrums; 4. the 'asocial'—seclusive and day-dreaming; and 5. the 'juvenile' type, which never seems to grow up.

In at least half the cases there is this special type of schizoid personality, probably partly inborn and partly acquired, out of which the psychosis develops. The morbidly sensitive individual may, for example, become worried about masturbation or a homosexual experience, and go on for years ruminating about it till his feelings of guilt, no longer bearable, come to be projected, first as ideas of reference and later as delusions and hallucinations. The guilty feeling may be treated in other ways—the patient goes into an ecstasy in which he feels himself forgiven, or (rarely) attempts expiation by castrating himself.

A clinical example or two will help to illustrate the gradual development of a schizophrenic illness as an accumulation of mental reactions.

CASE NO. 31

Q. M., who was admitted to the Glasgow Royal Mental Hospital at the age of 26, was reported to have been always 'nervous'. He had stuttered at the age of 15, and as the consequence of a fright, when he had been left alone in a schoolroom, he was kept away from school for a year. He was easily led by companions, and very obedient to his parents. Once at school his teacher had drawn his face on the board and said it was 'like the moon'. He remembered this bitterly, and his personal appearance became an increasingly sensitive point. Partly as the result of this, he was shy, and felt 'like a kind of clown' in company. When he left school at 16, he was apprenticed as an engineer, but as he developed Raynaud's symptoms his over-solicitous parents considered the work unsuitable. Aged 18 he enlisted, and was discharged three years later, but he saw no active service, having spent most of his time in hospital on account of a supposed heart lesion. On his discharge he had an operation for cervical adenitis. He became increasingly preoccupied about his health, so that if he read a book in which a disease was mentioned he at once imagined that he had that disease. At 22 he courted a girl, but 'I felt if I kept it up I'd go wrong in my head'. He ceased seeing the girl, concentrated on his work and felt better for a time. This failure only increased his general sense of insufficiency. 'I never felt I was just a man. I wasn't taking my right place. I was going about things apologetic. I could never talk right clear. I could never take the place I should have taken according to my age. . . . I never let myself go—for fighting or anything like that or taking up with a girl.' After discharge from the Army he had worked for his father, but his anxious preoccupation about his health, his sensitiveness about his appearance and his general feeling of dissatisfaction with himself interfered so much with his concentration that his head 'buzzed', and he had done no work for ten months before admission to hospital. After leaving off work, his preoccupation increased, he became more and more depressed about himself, and more and more secretive, so that he did not wish to see any one, thought everyone was looking at him, and hinted at suicide. When admitted to hospital he was quiet and co-operative, but very jerky in speech and movements, hesitating in the middle of sentences as if his thoughts had been interrupted. Soon he began to express definite persecutory ideas. He was 'being made an example of', and to 'appear the biggest fool in the world'. Finally, there was 'a system being worked' against him. His conduct became impulsive —he escaped over the garden wall, and returned voluntarily, saying he thought 'a race might do him good'. Within four months of admission hallucinations appeared, and at times mutism, verbigeration and flexibilitas cerea. Physically, there was no evidence of organic disease.

This patient shows very well how faulty habits of reaction—shyness, sensitiveness, plastic obedience to others, extreme consciousness of inferiority (based on his physical appearance, his clumsiness of address and of speech and the remarks of others) and hypochondriacal preoccupation—can lead to invalidism and then to inactivity, depression and ideas of reference, and finally to delusions, hallucinations, impulsiveness, automatic obedience, mutism and verbigeration. These, in fact, are the 'symptoms' of the so-called 'katatonic' form of schizophrenia.

The extent to which phantasy can console someone who cuts himself off from the more solid satisfaction of social intercourse and material achievements, and can ultimately replace these entirely to constitute a 'psychosis', is shown by the following case:

CASE NO. 32

A shy, sensitive, seclusive young man who showed increasing incapacity for social adaptation as he grew older; fanciful preoccupation with a girl whom he had never met; misinterpretation of the remarks of others in the light of his phantasies and in accordance with his wishes; gradual loss of appreciation of reality, so that his phantasies became delusions (e.g. engagement-phantasy) in which he lived—hence bizarre conduct and increasing seclusiveness, with correspondingly increased sensitiveness and a feeling of guilt (for phantasied actions), leading to ideas of reference and self-accusations of an extravagant kind.

A young man, M. R., who was admitted to the Glasgow Royal Mental Hospital at the age of 22. He had been an excellent student at school, but when he began work in an office at the age of 14 he was very 'nervous', starting violently even when the house-bell rang, thinking it was a telephone call he had to answer. He tried several occupations in turn, with little success. He was very sensitive and had very few friends, and was increasingly lonelier as he grew older. Masturbation was frequent. His chief recreation was music, and for some years before admission to hospital he had been taking violin lessons. A girl whom he had never met attended the same teacher, who told one pupil about the other. A friend of the patient informed him that the girl liked him, which 'harassed' him, as he 'did not know any way of getting an introduction'. For two years subsequently he ceased taking lessons 'because they occupied too much of his time', but he was induced to return 'by thoughts of the young lady'. He tried to arrange for the girl and himself to play at the same concert, but their teacher refused, and this he thought queer. The patient understood his music-teacher to say on one occasion, 'There is a child which is unwelcome in the world', and he considered that the girl and himself might marry and adopt this child. He 'thought a lot of stuff' about the girl, and five weeks before admission he began to believe that he was engaged to her, although he had never spoken to her. About this time he would say to his dog, 'I'll tell you a nice story', and laugh foolishly. Soon he began to accuse himself of a murder, with a sexual setting, recorded in the newspapers, and of causing a shipping disaster which had just taken place. He began to feel that people were 'talking about him and laughing at him', and that the girl was trying to hypnotize him. He became mildly depressed and tearful, and during the three weeks he was under observation he did not improve.

TYPES OF SCHIZOPHRENIA

Kraepelin first differentiated three principal types, which he termed hebephrenic, katatonic and paranoid; later he added a fourth, termed simplex. In the last edition of his textbook he added numerous other forms, *e.g.* simple depressive, delusional, circular and agitated. No useful purpose is served by a multiplication of such sub-groups. The main groups are reasonably distinctive, but even these are not clear cut, there are admixtures and transitions, and one could if one wished form almost as many groups as there are affected individuals.

Paranoid symptoms may be present in any type of schizophrenia, in the same way that they may be found as secondary features in many other reaction-types, in delirium for example, or in a depressive psychosis or in senile dementia. The

S

term paranoid schizophrenia is no more required to designate such cases than the term paranoid delirium is required for a delirium in which the patient is suspicious. On the other hand, paranoid symptoms may dominate the clinical picture of an apparently schizophreniform psychosis. Where they do, the reaction is in most cases in our opinion much more closely allied to other paranoid psychotic reaction (paranoia, paraphrenia) and should be considered and classified with the latter. We therefore make a clear distinction between schizophrenic psychoses and paranoid psychoses, while recognizing that paranoid symptoms may occur in the former and that there may be cases which are difficult to classify neatly in one group or the other. Our reasons for making the above suggestion may be summarized as follows: paranoid psychoses—

1. develop later in life than schizophrenia, *e.g.* at 35 years, or over;
2. are symptomatically more homogeneous and do not show the same mutual transitions and admixtures as other types of schizophrenia do;
3. have a strong affective component, often of a transitory or cyclical nature, which may be responsive to treatment;
4. rarely exhibit the gross intellectual and emotional deterioration which is so characteristic of schizophrenia.

We suggest therefore that the sub-types of schizophrenia should be limited to the simple, hebephrenic and katatonic forms.

SYMPTOMATOLOGY

The detailed symptomatology is extraordinarily varied, but there are certain groups of symptoms which stand out more prominently than the others, and are common to all the varieties. A most prominent symptom is the failure of affect, or emotional blunting, showing itself in apathy and indifference. This description applies more definitely to cases of some duration. In the early stages the affect may be lively enough, and even in advanced cases there are sometimes more evidences pointing to affective activity than would, on the surface, be suspected. The emotional deterioration leads to a state of mental facility, in which the patient is, up to a point, easily suggestible, and his conduct is more easily affected by those in contact with him. On the surface one gets the impression of a certain mild depression and feeling of failure. The patient does not seem to appreciate joy or sorrow or fear, but his attitude is rather one of indifference to his condition, and 'I don't care' or 'I don't know' is a frequently repeated phrase. Associated with this is a certain dreaminess and a lack of touch with reality; the patient lives a life with which his relatives and his doctor cannot get in touch. The apathy and lack of interest are usually so marked that active attention to any specific problem is fleeting. On the other hand, passive attention is remarkably good, so that he may remember long afterwards events of which he had seemed to take no notice. Such patients may be induced to do some purely mechanical type of work, something which they can pursue without interfering unduly with their ruminations. Another impressive feature is the disharmony between the mood and the thought. It is this more than anything else that distinguishes schizophrenia from other types of mental disorder. Schizophrenic patients may express, without any show of emotion, ideas which in the ordinary person would produce remorse, or pity, or profound depression. Situations in which they find themselves, which would normally have a profound emotional value—as, for example, being placed in a mental hospital—are by them met with indifference. Frequently there are sudden, causeless outbursts of laughter, and a stereotyped, silly, smiling attitude, in which there is no real mirth or hilarity.

The disharmony revealed in these ways between mood and thought is not the only indication of a deep-seated psychic change. There is a general disintegration of all the mental functions, resulting in the appearance of queerness and oddity which is so striking to the ordinary observer.

The result of the mental disintegration is a widespread change in the patient's personality, which vividly impresses itself on his friends. The patient loses his pride in his personal appearance, gradually becomes untidy and slovenly and needs constant attention.

Ideas of reference, illusions, hallucinations and delusions constitute another group of symptoms which are present at one time or another during the course of the illness. Ideas of reference are probably more common than the others. They arise from the patient's attitude, which is one of increased sensitiveness and suspiciousness, in consequence of which he believes that he is being spoken about, and that articles in the daily press have special reference to him and his affairs. He interprets the most commonplace occurrences as having some special reference to himself. Such a patient may feel that the whole world centres round him, and that he is marked out either for persecution or for some great honour. Hallucinations of hearing are particularly common. For a time they may not exercise much influence, but often they dominate the patient so that the hallucinatory suggestions may be acted upon. It is frequently in response to such commands that impulsive and violent acts are perpetrated. Visual hallucinations, hallucinations of smell and taste, are also frequent, but not so common as those of hearing. The striking feature about the delusional ideas is their changeable and transitory nature. Ideas of influence are very important. They take the form of a belief that the patient's thoughts are being read, or stolen from him, or that he is being influenced by wireless or by electrical machines.

The symptoms which have been described are all the more significant in that they occur in a setting of relative clearness, so that the patient recognizes clearly time and place and the people around him, i.e. there is no disorientation or clouding of consciousness. In addition, the patient has a good memory both for things of long ago and for more recent events. The general intellectual faculties are unimpaired, and the remembrance and grasp of school knowledge are not interfered with. Any apparent intellectual deterioration arises from lack of attention and concentration.

The judgement of these patients is, however, greatly interfered with, and they have no proper appreciation of the serious nature of their illness. Gradually the thought-content becomes more and more involved, so that a formal disorder occurs, and incoherence of speech, which may go to the extent of becoming a 'word salad', is not uncommon.

Schizophrenic Thinking and General Behaviour

Some general account of the factors which contribute to the strangely disordered appearance of the schizophrenic's mind is perhaps desirable. The peculiar qualities of schizophrenic thinking and behaviour generally seem dependent principally on four conditions: 1. the schizophrenic turns away from reality (introversion); 2. his thinking is dominated by his complexes (topics with a strong affective colouring) to an extent not seen in the normal; 3. he regresses to a childish or infantile or archaic (as it is variously called) mode of thought; and 4. his personality undergoes a progressive disintegration. These are not separate and distinct conditions, but different aspects of one and the same thing. Different writers lay different stress on the various aspects.

It has been pointed out elsewhere ['General Psychopathology', p. 116] that the individual's personality is the product of the interaction of his instinctive forces and his environment. His personality is not simply the sum of the qualities so produced. It is their combination into a new dynamic whole, in which some of the component forces are allowed direct or indirect expression and some are inhibited. Now if such a personality for some reason (*e.g.* persistent instinctual frustration) ceases to keep in contact with reality (introversion) the necessity for inhibition is removed. Modes of expression which are, from the social point of view, primitive and not permissible, can then come into action. In other words, regression can occur, and tendencies hitherto unconscious, because inhibited, receive conscious expression. But a personality in which such expression is permitted is *ipso facto* no longer the same personality; it is socially a deteriorated one. Moreover, since there is no longer the necessity for conforming to the real environment, which demands a consistent purposive adaptation, all the modes of instinctive fulfilment can be used in a go-as-you-please, haphazard way; now this and now that complex may receive some sort of conscious expression; and the personality not only deteriorates, but becomes disintegrated as well.

This concept of the schizophrenic's personality, with its introversion, dominance by numerous loosely connected complex-derived affects, and its regression to 'archaic' modes of expression, provides a key to a general understanding of the clinical manifestations of schizophrenia. It should, however, be understood that the disintegration seldom is complete. Fragments, so to speak, of the old personality remain with the corresponding conflicts and inhibitions.

The vagueness of the schizophrenic's thought may be attributed largely to his introversion. The schizophrenic patient no longer seeks to commune with his fellows, but lives instead in a world of his own. There is then no need for clear definition in thinking, and the very lack of clearness itself helps to make possible another of the conditions mentioned—that as much as possible in his introverted world may be as his wishes dictate. The lack of necessity for communication with others makes possible such 'telegrammatic' and metaphorical thinking as that described by Jung in the case of a dressmaker who fell ill in her thirty-ninth year. She said, for example, 'I am Socrates'. This delusional statement proved to be an ellipsis for the thought that, like Socrates, she had been extremely able and accomplished and had been falsely accused and placed in prison (the hospital) where she would have to die. That the vagueness and disconnection of thought which reaches its extreme development in the complete incoherence of some cases may be largely dependent on the factors of introversion and dominance by affects, and that it does not necessarily depend on organic cerebral changes, is well illustrated by an occurrence that is not very uncommon; namely, that a patient whose utterances have long been unintelligible may talk coherently and entirely naturally for a time if he is overtaken by some severe physical illness which brings him up against reality with a shock, so to speak. A woman of 60, admitted thirty years previously as suffering from 'dementia praecox' and who had remained in hospital ever since in an apparently demented condition, began during an attack of influenza to ask intelligently for the relatives and friends who had been dead to her those thirty years. Between the thought-processes in schizophrenics and the type of thinking found in primitive man there are certain similarities, but some writers on the subject have tended to go too far in their identification of primitive and schizophrenic thinking. Some schizophrenic utterances are superficially reminiscent of the 'sympathetic magic' of savages. For example, a male patient, 30 years of age, was observed to carry always dead leaves next to the left side of his chest. Closer inquiry revealed that his mother, to whom he had been specially attached, had died in the autumn some years before, and that at the funeral he had seen the withered leaves strewn on her coffin. He believed that his heart was weak, and that autumn leaves placed over it would have a curative effect, because they had been associated with his mother.

Ideas of death and rebirth, such as are common in primeval myths and in religious writings, are frequently found in schizophrenic patients, who tend, moreover, to act according to such ideas and to give dramatic representations of them. For instance, the stupor of some katatonics seems to be a dramatization of the idea of death, and some states of ecstasy have as their corresponding mental content the idea of being born again. Such conditions, however, are not peculiar to schizophrenia. Religious trends in schizophrenics are sometimes of a type that would perhaps have been permissible in persons still claiming to be normal in the Middle Ages, but now bear the stamp of grotesqueness. One young man, for example, hears a voice saying, 'Yea, we shall relish thee', while at prayer, sees a picture of the Last Supper scintillate and sparkle six times in one afternoon, finds that his room is illuminated with a bright unearthly light, and observes that a bottle of medicine momentarily assumes the shape of an angel. His personality being disintegrated, and working inco-ordinately, instead of as a harmonious whole, it has been said of the schizophrenic that he is at the mercy of his complexes.

Whereas in the manic, as in the depressive, there is one prevailing affect, in the schizophrenic numerous affects, associated with as many complexes, are at work and at war with one another in the disintegrated personality. This affective disorderliness probably contributes to producing the curiously chaotic appearance of the schizophrenic's mind. In the minds of normal people all things are possible—a feeling of love, or its opposite, or apparent indifference, may be entertained towards the same person; what determines the choice is external circumstance and the individual mind as a whole—that feeling comes uppermost which is most in harmony with the rest of the mental experience, conscious and unconscious, of the individual concerned. But in the fully developed and therefore mind-disintegrated schizophrenic this decisive solution is impossible. He hesitates between one feeling and the other, so that he may waver between strong like and dislike, between wanting and not wanting something—rejecting and accepting almost at the same time. This is the so-called 'ambivalence'. Hence, something rejected, which the schizophrenic still succeeds in inhibiting from full conscious expression, does not remain totally inhibited, but, because it is still keenly wished for, crops up in an indirect way as a projection, *i.e.* as a delusion or a hallucination. Thus, a young married woman consulted a physician, whose voice she soon afterwards began to hear following wherever she went. She wrote letters to him and to the hospital authorities, protesting vigorously against this persecution. Persuaded, however, to interview the physician again, she smiled a great deal, especially when reference was made to the voice, and said that it 'spoke of love'. Further, at the same time as she complained of the physician's persecution, she proclaimed her engagement to him. It is not surprising that such an ambivalent affective attitude which follows from the disintegration of the personality also contributes to it. Bleuler supposed that a similar 'ambivalent' tendency is at the root of schizophrenic negativism, a stimulus evoking with equal readiness the appropriate (normal) psychological reaction and its opposite. But negativism is probably fundamentally an expression of the desire to shut out reality (introversion). In Bleuler's opinion, ambivalence is simply one aspect of the not-yet-fully-understood disorder of association which he supposed to be the fundamental defect in schizophrenic thinking.

The combination of loss of contact with reality and domination of thinking entirely by the emotions centred round certain complexes makes all kinds of fantastic delusions possible. The patient in phantasy has anything he wants. For example, a young medical student talked of his will-power, and said that he had a motor-car, a house of his own, and that he was a doctor, having qualified at the age of 21, and was going to marry the girl of his heart. This is a mild example.

Guilt complexes, *e.g.* remorse for masturbation, also lead to compensating phantasies, at the same time as there exist delusions of reference (that everyone can see his guilt, *e.g.* in his eyes). In such an instance the phantasy may be translated into acts of expiation. One young man, for example, mutilated himself by sawing with a safety razor blade round his penis just behind the corona, in an attempt at castration and 'purification'.

These are among the commoner instances of the very numerous types of 'autistic' (introverted) and 'katathymic'[1] thinking and consequent action found

[1] Katathymic thinking = thinking along the lines determined by some complex.

in schizophrenics. Other examples will be found in the case-records included in this chapter.

PHYSICAL ASPECTS

The pathogenesis of schizophrenia is unknown, though many physical abnormalities have been reported. A few of those reported are now fairly widely accepted by critical opinion to be significant, but none of them, with the possible exception of the biochemical changes described by Gjessing, go near to providing a comprehensible physical explanation of the mental symptoms. From the genetic findings we might expect schizophrenia to have a specific physical pathology, but a great many research workers over the past fifty years have failed to find it; though several of them indeed have thought that they had succeeded. Some of what appear to be the most important findings will be described briefly here. A full review and references can be found in the book on the somatic aspects of schizophrenia edited by Richter (1957).

Central Nervous System

There is no unequivocal histological evidence that schizophrenia is a disease of the brain. There are no gross changes in the brain, and though many microscopical abnormalities have been reported, none of these is yet accepted by the majority of expert investigators to be both constant and significant.

The position here has in fact changed little since Dunlap, an American pathologist of great discrimination and technical ability, reported in 1924. Dunlap formulated certain conditions which should be fulfilled in studying *post mortem* the brains of schizophrenics. The clinical diagnosis must be so clearly established as to be acceptable to the most critical; the age of the patients should not be over 40 years; and death should be caused by some acute disease and not by a wasting condition such as tuberculosis. The post-mortem examination should be performed immediately after death.

Dunlap examined eight cases, contrasting his results with control material, and found very much the same nerve-cell changes present in the control brains as in the schizophrenic ones. He concluded that schizophrenia is a condition lacking in any fundamental or constant alteration of nerve cells, and that any nerve cell alterations which have been found in schizophrenia have probably been reactions to various other bodily conditions, post-mortem changes and the result of technical factors (that is, artifacts).

The various microscopical changes which have been reported by other workers include loss of nerve cells, mainly in the cortex, and cell changes of many kinds—amoeboid, shrinkage, sclerosis, vacuolization, lipoid infiltration, and the presence of inclusion bodies. Glial changes described have been microglial proliferation, macroglial hyperplasia, and swelling of oligodendroglia. It is a ragbag of a catalogue.

The Vogts and their co-workers (1948) directed attention to pathological changes in the thalamus in schizophrenia, particularly in the nucleus medialis dorsalis of young katatonic patients. They reported two special changes: 1. the presence of a large number of dwarf cells (schwundzellen), these being clusters of cells which show dissolution and disappearance of the cytoplasm with unaffected nuclei; and 2. alveolar degeneration, in which the cytoplasm has become vacuolized and the nucleus distorted. These investigations have been critically and painstakingly conducted; and they seem sufficiently promising to be worth pursuing in other laboratories.

It may be that insufficient attention has been paid in the past to the thalamus and hypothalamus in seeking the neuropathology of schizophrenia. New and more refined techniques are also now being developed (Meyer, 1960), which may be used to discover abnormalities not revealed by earlier methods of examination. We would emphasize the importance of correlating good clinical records with the pathological investigations.

Hill (1957) has reported on the encephalogram in schizophrenia. There is no specific pattern or constant type of abnormality. Some schizophrenics have abnormal E.E.G.s, particularly katatonics. 'Subcortical type discharges, similar to those found in some epileptics, occur particularly in young katatonic schizophrenics': but Hill does not think that these discharges are evidence for the organic-pathological process theory of the aetiology of schizophrenia.

Nitrogen Metabolism

In katatonics following a periodic course, who are said to form only 2 or 3 per cent. of schizophrenics, Gjessing (1938), as the result of painstaking intensive studies continued over many years, of the metabolic exchanges in patients of this type, described certain disturbances of nitrogen metabolism which appear to run parallel to the periodic clinical alterations. Such illnesses are described as occurring usually before the age of 20, the onset being sudden with a state of confusion and excitement or in other cases of stupor, which clears up after days, weeks or, rarely, months, and repeats itself at varying intervals of longer duration, and are characterized by apathy, lack of insight and gain in weight. Ultimately there is a permanent state of mental deterioration which made Kraepelin change his opinion and place the condition among the dementia praecox group instead of among the manic depressives.

Gjessing distinguished two types: 1. the 'syntonic' type, so called because the metabolic changes synchronize with the changes in mental phase and with one another; these patients enter the excited or stuporose phase suddenly and emerge into comparative clearness; and 2. the asynchronous group, in whom the change of phase is gradual and the intervals characterized by apathy and lack of initiative, and where the metabolic alterations are chaotic.

Gjessing's results are important because they were the first record of uniformly recurring metabolic changes running parallel with clinical alterations, the correction of which by chemical means is followed by disappearance of the episodic clinical disturbances.

He began by eliminating focal infection, and gauged its elimination by the subsequent stabilization of the blood picture, pulse and temperature.

The main methodological principle of the research was the simultaneous recording of many of the physical functions of the organism, over a considerable period of the illness, covering a number of phasic recurrences and intervals in the same patient. The patient served as his own control.

Gjessing described the changes in periodic katatonia, as follows. In type (1) the metabolic changes are the same whether the phase is one of excitement or of stupor, but the course of the changes shows two sub-types. In sub-type A at the beginning of the phase (of excitement or stupor as the case may be) there is evidence of generalized sympathetic stimulation. It is of special interest that, even in the stuporose phase although the patient is kept motionless, the O_2 consumption rises. The excretion of total N_2 is also increased whatever the kind of phase, compared with the more or less quiet intervals. In these intervals there is an N_2 retention and therefore a positive N balance, and N_2 goes on being accumulated until it reaches a threshold characteristic of the individual patient (between 15 and 28 g. N_2) and then at the point of maximum N_2 accumulation, stupor or excitement, as the case may be, sets in. It is not the excitement that causes the excessive excretion to begin, as the latter may begin a day or two beforehand. Similarly in the excited or stuporose phase retention begins again before the end of the phase.

What characterizes this group is that excitement or stupor sets in shortly after N_2 retention has reached its maximum. In the sub-type C stupor or excitement sets in just before the lowest level of N_2 accumulation. The stuporose or excited phase coincides with a phase of N_2 retention and the quiet intervals begin when the N_2 store has reached the maximum.

Gjessing early suggested that at the time of the change of phase in the N_2 balance, a toxic substance, derived through a disturbance of protein metabolism, might act through the blood stream on the diencephalon: later he thought that the diencephalic autonomic functions might be influenced by periodic alterations in thyroid activity. With the object of emptying the N_2 store he used thyroxin in large doses (as much as 44 mg. in 8 days—intramuscularly, 1 mg., increasing by 1 to 2 mg. each day) and later dried thyroid so that the N_2 consumption was stabilized at 10 to 15 per cent. above normal. In this way he found it possible to stop the periodic katatonic disturbance. He recommended immediate discontinuance of thyroid if the pulse becomes irregular, and continuing with it when the pulse has fallen to 80 or 90. In type A he recommended that thyroid should be given during the last 8 or 10 days before stupor or excitement begins, and in type C shortly before the patient becomes quiet and stupor free.

Gjessing's reports of nitrogen retention in periodic katatonia and the response to treatment with thyroid have been generally confirmed by other workers (Stokes, Danziger, Rowntree and Kay); but the causal relationships between the biochemical and mental changes, and questions of where and how the biochemical changes originate, have not yet been elucidated. More research is required along these lines, and it might well be profitable to bring cases of periodic katatonia, which are not common, to one or more general hospital psychiatric units for further intensive metabolic study.

Cardiovascular System

Lewis (1923) was the first to record hypoplasia of the circulatory system in the majority of schizophrenics. The abnormalities consisted in a small heart, weighing usually less than 300 g. and on the average 254 g.; an abnormally thin aorta; and a reduced lumen of other major vessels.

Olkon (1939) reported a reduction in capillary density, and abnormalities of capillary size, shape and blood flow, in the finger webs of schizophrenics.

Shattock (1950) has made a detailed study of the vascular disturbances which schizophrenic patients, particularly katatonics, may exhibit and which are well known to all doctors working in mental hospitals. Peripheral vasoconstriction of the hands and feet may be severe, with cyanosis, oedema, atrophy and thickening of the skin and superficial ulceration. The nose and ears may also be cyanotic. The cyanosis is not always related to inactivity. Extreme constriction may be found of the brachial, radial and dorsalis pedis arteries; also of the retinal arteries: and vasoconstriction is relieved as the patient improves mentally. These vascular changes in schizophrenics resemble those seen in normal and cold-sensitive subjects exposed to cold, but they are elicited at room temperatures, and are unusually intense and lasting. Shattock is commendably cautious and critical in drawing conclusions: 'some of the abnormalities of behaviour observed in refractory patients may be related to a relatively inadequate cerebral circulation.'

It is unlikely that cardiovascular changes play more than an adjuvant part in the production of schizophrenic symptoms. The cerebral blood flow has been reported to be normal by Kety (1948).

Physique

Kretschmer (1925) linked leptosomatic (asthenic), athletic and dysplastic physiques with schizophrenia [see p. 80]. By dysplastic physical types he denoted those approximating to the results of endocrine disease, and he found 34 patients of this kind of physical constitution among 175 schizophrenics, and none of this type in 85 manic-depressives. Bleuler (1948) reported an association found in Switzerland between schizophrenia and an acromegaloid physique.

Rees (1943) confirmed Kretschmer's theories in part. He found schizophrenics more leptosomatic than normal controls and manic-depressives: but there was also a considerable overlapping in the distribution of physical types between manic-depressive and schizophrenic groups of his subjects. He reported that the schizophrenic group gave statistically highly significant smaller measurements than the normals in stature, chest circumference and expansion, hip circumference and biacromial diameter.

Endocrine Aspects

Schizophrenia is not associated constantly with any known abnormalities in any endocrine gland. There have been numerous investigations, tending to link schizophrenia with disordered action of the endocrine system and in particular of the sex glands, since Mott in 1919 first reported a regressive atrophy of the cells of the testicular tubules in schizophrenia. And most of the reported findings have gone through a cycle of affirmation and denial similar to the fate of Mott's. Mott's work was most damagingly criticized by Morse, on grounds which included his failure to take into account the effects on the testes of physical disease and malnutrition. Later Hemphill and Reiss (1944) reported testicular changes in schizophrenia resembling those seen after partial hypophysectomy: there was said to be marked degeneration of the testicular elements. Blair and his colleagues (1952) could find nothing in the testes outside the limits of the normal. Apart from the paucity of securely established positive findings, the clinical features of schizophrenia give no hint that the clue to its aetiology will be found in the endocrine system.

Other Investigations

Osmond and Hoffer (1952–59) have developed a hypothesis that schizophrenia may be caused by a defect in adrenaline metabolism, and have reported evidence that adrenochrome and adrenolutin (adrenaline metabolites) may both occur in the human body and be psychotomimetic. Recently they have found differences between adrenochrome metabolism in normals and schizophrenics. They reject the view that the effects of mescalin, LSD 25 and adrenochrome more closely resemble toxic-confusional than schizophrenic illnesses. The theories of these Saskatchewan workers have aroused a good deal of interest but their findings have not been confirmed.

Other workers have investigated carbonic anhydrase and serotonin metabolism, liver function and the excretion of indoles in schizophrenia, all alike inconclusively. Again and again the schizophrenic is reported to show an unusual biological variability, but within normal limits.

PSYCHOPATHOLOGY

Various psychopathological concepts have been employed above in describing the symptoms of schizophrenia and in trying to get a working grasp of their significance. Here we will refer more specifically but briefly to a few of the many detailed psychopathological theories which have been formulated in attempts to comprehend schizophrenia in psychodynamic terms. The pursuit of a unitary psychopathology of schizophrenia is probably as illusory and doomed to failure as is the search for a single physical pathology common to all cases: but whether or not the cause of schizophrenia is found ultimately to be physical, psychological interpretation of the clinical phenomena will remain a necessary aspect of our understanding of the total pathology of the disease.

Prior to 1907 Bleuler and Jung of the Zürich School of Psychiatry had become interested in Freud's psychoanalysis in relation to the psychoses. Developing Wundt's experiments in association by interpreting the findings in psychoanalytical terms, they made a bridge between experimental psychology and psychoanalysis. Freud (1914) acknowledged the importance of their work: '(Bleuler) showed that light could be thrown on a large number of purely psychiatric cases by adducing the same processes as have been recognized through psychoanalysis to obtain in dreams and neuroses; and Jung successfully applied the analytic method of interpretation to the most alien and obscure phenomena of dementia praecox (schizophrenia), so that their sources in the life-history and interests of the patient came clearly to light. . . . As early as in 1897 I had published the analysis of a case of schizophrenia, which however was of a paranoid character, so that the solution of it could not take away from the impression made by Jung's analyses. But to me the important point had been, not so much the possibility of interpreting the symptoms, as the psychical mechanism of the disease, and above all the agreement of this mechanism with that of hysteria, which had already been discovered. At that time no light had yet been thrown on the differences between the two mechanisms. For I was then aiming at a libido theory of the neuroses, which was to explain all neurotic and psychotic phenomena as proceeding from abnormal vicissitudes of the libido. . . .'

Jung wrote his *Psychology of Dementia Praecox* in 1907. The thought disorder in schizophrenia he considered to be due to the operation of unconscious complexes of ideas and feelings. The inner tensions and conflicts produced by these complexes precipitate states of panic, and the complexes themselves become split off from the ego in autonomous activity: in the schizophrenic patient's conscious mind they come to replace the normal traffic with reality. These complexes also cause resistances, which are revealed by negativism. As a technique of investigation he made much use of word-association tests, in which a line of stimulus-words is read off to the subject and he is asked to respond to each word with the first idea that comes into his mind. Different types of response are noted, according to the length of time that elapses between the giving of the stimulus-word and the reply, and according to the nature of the reply itself. By this means Jung obtained clues to the unconscious mental content, especially to the complexes. The method is, however, not generally of much value clinically. Jung thought schizophrenia to be psychogenic in its origin, but suggested that there might develop secondarily a biochemical disorder with toxic effects. Later he came to interpret the mental content of the schizophrenic, much of which appeared to him to be archaic and archetypal, in terms of a phylogenetic collective unconscious common to all men, a deposit of primordial and primitive experience. Bleuler adopted many of Jung's earlier ideas. Jung's later esoteric preoccupation with religion and mythology has had little impact on clinical psychiatry. His papers on schizophrenia have recently been republished (1960).

In Freud's view (summarized by Fenichel (1946)) the central process in schizophrenia is a profound unconscious mental regression and turning inwards, with the withdrawal of libido from reality, its objects and relationships. This regression may be precipitated by emotional traumata or conflicts of various kinds, and is particularly apt to occur at critical periods of biological development: it is facilitated by some earlier trauma in the development and organization of the ego, which has caused a fixation at a more immature level of auto-erotism or narcissism. Contacts with reality are progressively lost as the illness develops, and the ego, reinvested with its libido, becomes again egocentric and narcissistic. The abandonment of relations with reality and the withdrawal of libido from objects lead to the development of feelings of depersonalization and derealization, and to such delusions as those of the death of relatives or of world destruction. The increased narcissism and inflation of the ego result in hypochondriacal preoccupation and delusions, and infantile feelings of omnipotence. Other symptoms are interpreted along similar lines: regression is revealed in behaviour also, in oral and auto-erotic activities, in incontinence and smearing, in echolalia and echopraxia. In addition to these regressive symptoms, breaking with reality, Freud identified restitutional symptoms which indicate efforts on the part of the sick individual to regain reality. Delusional ideas of saving mankind are adduced as examples of this trend: hallucinations are interpreted as creating a substitute reality in place of the perceptions which have been lost, and certain katatonic symptoms, stereotypies and mannerisms, are seen as attempts to regain lost object relationships. Freud pointed to the particularly close resemblance between visual hallucinations and dreams, and stated that in the disordered language of the schizophrenic words are subject to the 'primary' process which produces dream images out of dream thoughts.

Federn (1952), whose views have been recently influential, interpreted schizophrenia in terms of an ego psychology which he personally elaborated and for which he provided a special terminology. The ego he described as having a fluctuating boundary, which delimits the self from the environment. The ego is driven (cathected) by libido. Ego feeling, conscious and unconscious, floods the area of the self and is sensitively involved with reality at its frontiers. In Federn's view schizophrenia is a disorder of the ego: the ego is weak, because its cathexis is weak. The ego boundary disintegrates, with the result that ego and environment, thought and feeling and their objects, become confused, and reality is falsified. The production of delusions and hallucinations then leads to a withdrawal from reality, and the ego regresses to states of childhood functioning, with the appearance in consciousness of previously unconscious mental material.

Freeman, Cameron and McGhie (1958) follow Federn in regarding a disturbance of the development and maintenance of adequate ego boundaries between the self and the not-self, and a deficiency in ego feeling, as the central features of the schizophrenic disease process. 'The illness of the ego results in an impairment of the functions usually associated with it, namely the loss of adaptive capacities, perceptual disturbances, changes in the memory function, alterations in the relationship with reality, disorders of the motor apparatus, and varying degrees of loss of personal identity.' They emphasize that the ego is never completely lost even in the most demented patient. Their theoretical framework is used to develop a therapeutic programme which is, in its earlier stages, essentially non-verbal, and is dependent on the formation of durable nurse-patient relationships: treatment is orientated specifically towards the restoration of ego functions. These workers, like many others with a psychoanalytic orientation, are careful to state that their views do not have any fundamental aetiological implications: the causation of the dissolution of the ego is left an open question.

Psychologists have also made important contributions. N. Cameron has made an experimental analysis of schizophrenic language (1938) and thinking (1944). Weckowicz (1959, 1960) has studied the relationship between constancy of perception and concept formation, and disturbances of body image in schizophrenia: the latter, which are reported to include a tendency to underestimate the size of the distal parts of the body, it is suggested may be due to a breakdown of size constancy and distortions in the perception of space. This sort of objective approach to the clinical phenomena should be cultivated. Both Kraepelin and Bleuler concluded that there are no perceptual changes in schizophrenia, and it now seems probable that they were wrong. Disorders of perception and attention in schizophrenia are the subject of a number of current researches in Britain and North America.

Schizophrenia Simplex

In this type there is an absence of any definite trend. There is simply a general falling away of interest. Kraepelin described it as consisting of an 'impoverishment and devastation of the whole psychic life, which is accomplished quite imperceptibly'. The change in the personality may be so insidious that it is not recognized as being due to any definite type of mental disorder, but such individuals seem to lack ambition, and are content to lead idle, shiftless lives, constantly changing their employment, being never satisfied with what they have. People who suffer from this type of disorder fill the ranks of the unemployed, the vagrants and delinquents. They are able in mild cases to carry on a coherent conversation, and give an appearance of normality which is not borne out on further acquaintance.

Such conditions frequently have their beginning in early adolescence. At school the potential schizophrenic is content to slip along. Afterwards he never reaches a position of any special responsibility, because he is apt to be dreamy, to be lacking in attention and concentration, and is content usually with routine tasks. Such a person may do good work, but always in a subordinate capacity.

As time goes on, a certain change may occur in his temperament, so that he becomes irritable, moody, distinctly asocial, and rarely takes part in the pleasures of his comrades. Even from his own family he becomes estranged. Inability to sustain a conversation is noticed, and the thinking becomes disorganized, even to the extent of incoherence; but it is rare for such a patient to have ideas of reference, hallucinations or delusions. The memory is well retained, and the chief feature is the extreme apathy or emotional dulling. We are all familiar with this type of individual. These are people who at one time have looked as if they might develop into something much better. They are quiet, pleasant individuals who gradually sink more and more into themselves, and who never fulfil the promise of their earlier days.

CASE NO. 33

Simple schizophrenic deterioration. A quiet well-behaved patient with little initiative but performing simple routine tasks satisfactorily; shallow in his affective responses—a facile

*empty laugh, a lack of resentment at detention in hospital or of desire to leave it; absence
of significant thought-content and complete want of insight.*

A good example of this type is that of a single man (D. R.), 32 years old, who had
served for a period during the war years.

He had a history of having been ill for about two years. At the time of his admission
to hospital he was quiet, looked a little dull, but smiled pleasantly, and answered
readily and agreeably. His memory was good, and there was no evidence of hallucinations or delusions.

Following his admission he has been employed at various jobs about the hospital,
and has always led a contented and happy life, quite satisfied with his surroundings,
and never asking to be allowed away. A good idea of his condition may be obtained
from the following questions and answers:

He said that he had nothing special to complain of, that he was quite happy.

'Do you think it strange being here so long?' 'Yes, that's true.'

'How do you account for it?' 'I feel very well. I feel all right.'

'Is your head right?' 'My head feels quite clear.'

'No strange thoughts?' 'No.'

When these questions were asked, the patient often laughed or smiled, in a simple,
foolish way. His laugh did not have the 'infectiousness' of manic cases. There was
always an element of silliness in it. He stated that he felt just as well now as he had
ever done, and denied hallucinations and strange ideas of any kind. His answers were
given quickly and to the point. The impressive features were contentment and apathy;
and yet he had been long resident under hospital conditions. He was able to tell the
day, the month, the year quite correctly, and he was able to give a history of his life.
He told when he was born, where he was born, mentioned the different members of his
family, what he had done at school.

'Did you get on all right at school?' 'Oh, yes.'

'Were you clever?' Patient laughed, and said that he could always get through his
lessons.

'Were you top boy in the class?' The patient laughed loudly, said that he was not,
but that he had never been 'kept back'. He was able to do simple calculations correctly,
and he had a good grasp on general information, but no appreciation of the serious
nature of his disorder.

The picture, therefore, is a very good example of the so-called 'simplex' type.
The patient had suffered from a general slumping of his interest, to reach a state
of apathy and contentment, in which he calmly accepted his detention in a
mental hospital. He is protected by the hospital, and has no fears; but neither
has he any ambition of any kind, nor any great capacity for enjoyment. His war
service had probably little or nothing to do with precipitating such a reaction.

Hebephrenia

This type may be difficult to differentiate, because often in it there are some
symptoms pointing more to a katatonic reaction. Hebephrenia, however, seems
to occur usually at an earlier age than the katatonic varieties, and it is especially
characterized by great incoherence in the train of thought, marked emotional
disturbance, periods of excitement alternating with periods of tearfulness and
depression, and frequently by illusions and hallucinations.

The people who develop a hebephrenic disorder have in their earlier days
shown an unstable emotional condition; they may give a history of tantrums,

and have often been of the over-pious, ultra-conscientious type, apt to be too idealistic, and to brood on obscure topics. Their acquaintances generally have looked upon them as queer. In such people the emotional response is shallow, and they laugh and weep without very adequate cause, or have sudden violent outbursts of anger, explosive in character and rapidly passing away.

Hallucinations of sight and hearing are particularly common in hebephrenics, and are usually in the nature of symbolic interpretations. They come and go during the course of the disorder. It is the vivid hallucinations which especially dominate the picture. Kraepelin particularly remarked on the changeable, phantastic, bizarre nature of their delusions, and he gave certain examples: they 'have no brain any longer', their 'back is broken in two', their 'blood has been taken from them'.

The hebephrenic patient often suffers greatly from ideas of reference; he feels that he is being watched and made fun of. Feelings of influence are common.

The most prominent symptoms are the incoherence in the train of thought, the strange, impulsive, senseless conduct and the vivid hallucinations.

The following is an illustrative case of the hebephrenic kind. The very rapid deterioration to a condition of silly, impulsive activity, with inadequate and inappropriate emotional manifestations, great incoherence of speech and thought, hallucinations and apparently absurd ideas, e.g. of influence—in other words, the 'molecular disintegration' of the personality—is very well shown.

CASE NO. 34

P. R., a girl, 20 years old, who had been employed as a nurse, was admitted in a restless, agitated state, but a few minutes later she was smiling and happy. These phases rapidly alternated, even in the course of a few minutes. It was difficult to get her to co-operate in a satisfactory examination; she spoke in a simple, childish way, said that she wished someone would do an operation on her head and make her better. She told how she had worked in various hospitals, but had not been able to continue steadily at her job, because she 'seemed always to be working in a maze'. Perhaps the question and answer method brings out certain points better than a mere description.

'You were at a fever hospital?' 'Yes, just a few weeks.'

'Why did you leave?' 'I am not sure.'

'Do you hear voices?' 'No—yes—very seldom. I seem to be going sort of dead.'

Later she admitted that she did hear voices, and that they terrified her dreadfully.

She was able to do simple calculations correctly, and answered some questions on general information correctly, but her diffuseness and inconsequent talk can be gathered from the following:

'Who discovered America?' 'Well, I think it was a Murray. I had an old Aunt Sally who died and an old brother went to Hudson Bay.'

She behaved in a disturbed, excitable way, and made such a noise that she had to be removed to a room by herself. While there she promptly smashed several panes of glass. Her impulsive, violent conduct continued at intervals. She refused food, so that for a time it was necessary to tube-feed her. Still later she deliberately poked her fingers into her eyes and caused conjunctival haemorrhage.

During her residence in the hospital she continued to be hallucinated, and talked freely about her experiences. She said that voices told her things had been done to her during the night. During the day also she hallucinated, and often sat gazing at the ceiling in an ecstatic way.

Gradually her impulsiveness subsided; she began to look after her appearance, to help the nurses in the ward, but often she would have outbursts of weeping without any apparent cause. She was asked about this time why it was that she frequently sat with her eyes tightly shut, and would only open them for a moment or two at a time. She explained that when her eyes were wide open the doctor, or the sister in charge of the ward, or the nurses, saw what she was seeing, and that they were therefore seeing through her eyes, and to prevent this she shut her eyes. She also explained that she had two voices; the one which was speaking she called her 'top voice', and what she said with the 'top voice' was true; but there was a second voice, an 'under-voice', which she apparently believed or felt was what her auditors at times heard, replacing the true 'top voice'. Consequently we were getting false ideas by believing this second voice. She also expressed the idea that the doctors and nurses used her as a 'medium' to affect others. She held up the three middle fingers of her hand to illustrate the idea clearly to us; pointed out the first outside finger as representing the number 'six', the finger in the middle was herself, and the other outside finger represented 'the others'.

Her condition became gradually worse. She wandered about in a restless, aimless way, and when the physician visited the ward she clutched him by the arm, and could only be detached with difficulty. Her thought-processes were blocked and her speech was incoherent, her sentences being composed of detached words and phrases which had no relationship to each other, except for an occasional superficial association. An example is as follows:

'Losh, I don't know what it is. You see—she says—I don't know, I'm sure. There's Cinderella. There is a much better play than that. "I don't know," I said. He is an awful idiot. O dear God, I'm so stupid. That's putting two and two together—saying I really don't know—saying Cathie, and so I observe and—flowers. An orange, and shoe laces. A gaberdine skirt. Pettigrew's and the jazz band, with cream cakes. She says no. They like my hair bobbed, but I'm so stupid. Contrary Mary. Statues at Copland and Lye's. "Oh," I said, "yes, yes, yes." I'd go off to sleep immediately afterwards. I said, "I know quite well." "Nothing," I said. I forget all that I saw next. The next thing was —eh? The poor man's mad. They'll be chopping off our heads next, and—calendars tied with blue ribbons. Oh, dear God. Contrary Mary again. What period—that's right. I don't like acting the goat at all. A cream-sponge sandwich. My memory is so slow, that all I'm sure. It was caramels then and fruit cakes. Well, well, I said, I can't help it— I don't want to help it, and well, I don't care. Contrary Mary again, and says—Nurse Grant—dogs barking. What's the matter with me anyway? I'm so terribly stupid. I'm fed up with this place—that's all. Sago pudding. She looks pale and tired often, but not —I know that. Sings "Take me over there, drop me anywhere, Manchester, Birmingham, Leeds, Well I don't care. I should like to see my best girl"—Mrs. Patrick, she says—"though 'tis time for parting, that's it, Jean, and my tears are starting". I've got the Kruschen feeling.—Blue belts and medals—three eggs for tea. No, that won't do. Oh, dear God, I'm so stupid. I won't see my way—white rabbits. "Back home in Tennessee"—that the way it's spelt. Oh, I don't know what I am going to do now. It's all wrong. Dear God, I'm so silly. It's killing, isn't it? Cream cakes, French cakes and meringues. Flies, fleas, butterflies,' and so on.

She had the idea that she was changed, and sometimes remarked, 'My face is changed.'

The course of her illness had already been of five years' duration, and she was steadily going downhill.

A sample of her letter-writing shows very well the incoherence and the tendency to repetition.

T

DEAR SIR,

I have just had dinner. I ate my dinner the monkey and I feel better. change I. Nurse is always making the tea. Betsy's nurse.

> Wearing for a cup of
tea.
> > Bathing patient.
> > (Ogalvie).
> > > Your—
> > > > I   j   g   u.
> > > > gins Druce,
> > > > > Yours
> > > > > > sincerely,
> > > > > > > P. R.

DEAR DR. HIND,

I am just that watea ahe bring me som gin snap & I u—a lobster — — — 1 a. the water's hot what a monkey goes with.

> > Y   I am
> > > s incere.
> > > Nurse Bruce
> > > > gave
> > > > > me two
> > > > > snaps.

> > > > > > > Thursday.

Caristic.
> Soc.
> > Sit up latest
Ruby was away with it—Shorthand. So that I don't get a bath.

Katatonia

The katatonic type of reaction is more easily differentiated than the other types of schizophrenia. This katatonic condition was first described by Hecker and by Kahlbaum as a variety of mental disturbance *sui generis*, with symptoms and a course peculiar to itself. Kraepelin, however, recognized that the great majority of cases of this sort ultimately ended in a state of considerable dementia, and therefore he included these katatonic cases in his dementia praecox group.

Katatonia is usually described as an alternating state characterized by a stage of depression, a stage of excitement and a stage of stupor. We would reserve the name katatonia, as Kraepelin did, for these cases in which one sees the conjunction of peculiar excitement with katatonic stupor.

There is no doubt that this type of schizophrenic reaction develops much more acutely than the other types. Kraepelin himself said that 41 per cent. of such cases tend to develop acutely, 31 per cent. insidiously and the others subacutely.

There is no group of symptoms which can be looked upon as in any way premonitory. The usual history is a more or less general statement that there has been a general falling off in interest, an apathy, a lack of concentration, a dreaminess and often episodes of an odd nature. Then a state of dull stupor develops, with mutism, refusal of food, and with such a diminution of all activities that the patient may sit idly in one position, with the hands stretched out on the knees, and the head bowed between the shoulders, the whole aspect being that of a mummy. The facial expression is vacant, and no apparent interest is taken in the environment or in the people around. The muscles of the mouth may become pursed up into the so-called 'schnauzkrampf'. Patients in this condition have to be dressed and undressed, and have to be moved in bed: they may have to be tube-fed. Urine and faeces are often retained, or there is incontinence. Mannerisms are common. Perseveration may reach an extreme degree; for example, a patient who took his meals in a singularly mechanical way, shovelling his food into his mouth with his fork and then with his knife, used to go through the same motions long after he had finished the food before him. The saliva may be retained, so that the cheeks become bulged out with it, or drooling occurs from the mouth. These patients are so insensitive that they may not react to painful stimuli, such as pin-pricks, nor even close their eyelids when told that a pin is going to be put into one of their eyes. They understand perfectly clearly everything that is going on around them, but their apathy is so great that they take no part in it. Not infrequently they are intensely negativistic, and an attempt to do anything for the patient is resisted with every ounce of his strength. On the other hand, he may obey everything automatically. There are also stereotypies of thought and action; the patients ask the same questions over and over again, write words or letters in a stereotyped way, or walk in a peculiar fashion, perhaps always stopping for an instant after so many steps; or they assume strange attitudes, which are maintained unchanged for long periods of time. Flexibilitas cerea is common; they will allow their bodies and their limbs to be placed in awkward positions, which are maintained indefinitely. Other symptoms commonly present are echolalia and echopraxia.

Suddenly, without any warning, the picture may change at any time, so that the patient begins to speak, answer questions and often gives a detailed account of everything that has occurred. A state of extreme frenzy may alternate with the period of stupor, during which the patient behaves with extraordinary impulsiveness and assaults whoever comes into contact with him. During this stage he may not only be homicidal, but impulsively suicidal. Such episodes of excitement usually come from a clear sky, and there are no premonitory symptoms. For instance, one of our patients, who had been going about as usual, and had actually been in town with his mother, and had seemed rather better, suddenly got up early one morning and made a dive through a window two storeys high. The frames were of iron, so that he was not successful in precipitating himself, but the violence of the attack was so great that he broke his collar-bone and had numerous cuts about his face and arms. Following this attempt he tried to mutilate himself. Another patient used to prop herself against the wall, then stand on her head and attempt to screw her neck. She also repeatedly tried to smother herself in the bedclothes, and several times dived from her bed on to the floor. These episodes of violence are usually associated with hallucinations, but they are not necessarily so. Often at these times the patients express delusions;

they feel that they are not only commanded to do such things, but that they are all-powerful, or that they are being persecuted. Sometimes they believe that it is the voice of God that they hear, and that it is God who has commanded them to destroy themselves. The duration of these paroxysms is usually short-lived, not lasting more than a few hours or days or weeks. It is in this type of schizophrenia that the vasomotor symptoms already mentioned are prominent.

The following is a typical katatonic state:

CASE No. 35

Katatonic schizophrenia. Onset of a dull, listless state, with vague ideas of reference and feelings of influence. Later, auditory and visual hallucinations, unsystematized paranoid delusions, refusal of food and incontinence. Alternating periods of stupor and excitement, with progressive dementia. No response to treatment.

There was no family history of mental illness in the case of F. C. He had been an average scholar but introspective and solitary at school, with no liking for games and no hobbies. He became a mill-worker at the age of 15 and was 'more a boy for home, never keen on girls'. He served in the Army during the Second World War and had some sort of transient mental breakdown, of which no records are available. After demobilization he was idle for six months: he appeared depressed and mixed up, seemed to take no interest in things around him and did not even respond to questioning. Then he had a job for six months, but was dismissed and again hung around the house, making no attempt to seek further employment. Thereafter he became even more dull and apathetic, looked vacant and faraway, refused to get out of bed or take food. He declared that people were trying to take a rise out of him, that some unknown individual was 'making him think about things', and that he himself was a 'riddle of bones'. In the year following his demobilization from the Army he was admitted to a mental hospital, aged 23 years.

In hospital at first he lay in bed with an occasional vacant smile, and refused food. He was correctly oriented and could give his history with reasonable accuracy, but he had little insight, saying that he had been sent to hospital on account of fits of bad temper. He was both auditorily and visually hallucinated: he complained of hearing buzzing noises, sounds like someone squealing and voices which he could sometimes understand but whose messages he could not remember, and he described flashes of light and shadows in the middle of the room. He expressed the belief that the doctors and nurses could manipulate their shadows, and that there was another person in his bed. Later he complained of tasting soap in his mouth and of receiving poison from the post beside his bed.

Treated initially with E.C.T. and then with reserpine, he remained withdrawn and apathetic, often could not be engaged in conversation, sat vacantly by the hour and had both to be taken to his meals and pressed to eat. At times he was incontinent, chewed the end of his tie and hoarded rubbish. For weeks on end he would be in a state of stupor or near to it, showing catalepsy and flexibilitas cerea. Then a period of excitement would intervene, when for days or weeks on end he would be hyperactive and talk a great deal in a disjointed and usually incoherent way. At these times he would strike out impulsively at the nursing staff. On occasion he clowned in a crude way and would walk on his hands.

Repeated courses of E.C.T., various tranquillizing drugs, and treatment in occupational and social groups, have had no effect, and he has become grossly demented.

DIAGNOSIS

Probably mistakes in the diagnosis of schizophrenia are made most often because undue attention has been paid to single symptoms and the clinician has failed to view these in perspective. Certain symptoms in a young person, feelings of influence and passivity, for example, and hypochondriacal complaints of a wholly unexpected, unjustified or bizarre kind, will quite strongly suggest the diagnosis of schizophrenia: but the diagnosis cannot safely be allowed to rest on isolated symptoms. Later, when the illness is obviously a psychotic one, the persistent presence of auditory and visual hallucinations occurring when there is no excitement, and when there is no toxic basis, are very much more in favour of schizophrenia than of anything else.

Much help is to be got from a detailed history. Schizophrenia is usually an illness of slow, insidious onset, developing over years; whereas a manic-depressive psychosis develops, if not very acutely, at any rate over a period of weeks or months. The patient's relatives may report strange, odd, inappropriate behaviour. One should find out always if there has been progressive deterioration in the level of performance, at work and socially: school reports, examination results at university or college, and the employment record will provide objective and usually reliable indices of intellectual performance, its maintenance or decline.

Adolescent turmoil of feeling and behaviour, and neurotic symptoms, usually of an anxious or hysterical kind, in a young adult may for long mask the true diagnosis. Usually external precipitants are suspiciously slight or hard to define, the response to psychotherapy is disappointing, there is a deficiency in rapport and the illness drags on. The clinical picture is often gradually recognized to be becoming more atypical. There tends to be a diffuseness and vagueness in thought and expression, one cannot follow the patient's thought processes without strain, his thoughts may become blocked, or an unexpected emotional reaction may jar the sympathetic observer into recognizing the patient's deeper disorder.

The young schizophrenic may become profoundly depressed, and he may come into medical care after a suicidal attempt. His schizophrenia may be revealed only after his depression has been treated, in residual symptoms. Whether or not the patient is acutely emotionally disturbed, schizophrenia in the adult has in fact most often to be differentiated from a manic-depressive psychosis. Superficially the apathy, listlessness and even stupor which occur in schizophrenic cases are apt to be confounded with a state of depression. One or two questions may be sufficient to elicit the fact that the listless schizophrenic does not have any subjective feeling of sadness, but, on the other hand, often feels contented and prefers to be left alone. In the depressed phase of the manic-depressive psychosis, the individual not only looks sad, but feels miserable, and his thoughts are despondent. In general, the schizophrenic, as contrasted with the manic-depressive, is full of discrepancies between his mood and his thought, so that ideas of persecution or disaster leave him comparatively unmoved; and between his thoughts and his actions, so that he does little to fulfil his day-dreams or to stop his persecution. There are also discrepancies in his thought-content itself, clear contradictions going uncorrected.

The type of excitement which one sees particularly in katatonic cases is sometimes very difficult to distinguish from an episode of manic excitement, but here again there are certain points which help to differentiate the two states. The excitement of the schizophrenic is much more episodic; it may occur quite suddenly following a period of stupor, and it is usually characterized by a blind impulsiveness, during which the patient may be dangerous to others and himself. There is a poverty of ideas as compared with the free production of the manic: there may indeed be something in the nature of a flight of ideas, but it is stilted, and poorly sustained. On the other hand, the manic excitement runs a much more prolonged course, the mood is typically one of great happiness, flight of ideas and distractibility are prominent features and there is commonly a joy and an infectious hilarity about the patient which are very easily observed.

Close attention should be paid always to the nature of the previous personality and to the adequacy of the previous social adjustment: and one should ask oneself, under stress what kind of reaction would be expected from a personality so constituted or limited.

The difficulties of diagnosis are best illustrated by the report of two cases: the first, one in which the schizophrenic symptoms predominated, but which ended in complete recovery; the second, one in which for a time the manic-depressive features were preponderant, but which went on to considerable deterioration.

CASE No. 36

A young unmarried woman, 28 years old, had shown mental symptoms for one month previous to her admission to the Glasgow Royal Mental Hospital. There had been an initial period of depression lasting for a few days, which was followed by the expression of strange ideas. She announced that she had cast a spell over the family, that neither she herself nor any member of the family had any sense of taste, that she had no blood in her body, that she could feel nothing. She tried to leave the house dressed only in her night clothes. Her language became obscene, a thing quite foreign to her. On admission to hospital she was in a state of stupor, which was punctuated by impulsive episodes. She would suddenly leap out of bed and destroy the ward furniture. On one occasion she struck her brother violently, tore her bedclothes with her teeth and in doing so broke one of her teeth. She constantly rubbed the top of her head, or picked her skin. She hung over the edge of her bed, spitting out large quantities of saliva, and she became very filthy in her personal habits, smearing herself with excreta. Thirteen months after admission she was still most difficult to manage, and her mood was one of angry resentment. The only explanation vouchsafed for her conduct was that she was 'in love with some other fellow', and that 'he was an actor'. When asked about her picking habits she explained, 'I have been shedding my life-blood for you.' Twenty months after admission she began to show signs of betterment, which went on rapidly to recovery. She co-operated in a review of her illness, and showed good insight. She stated that at the onset of her illness she had the idea that she might have become pregnant, and worried over the disgrace which this would mean both to herself and to her family. A study of her personality showed that she had been a bright, happy, jolly girl, and a great favourite at school, where she had done well.

CASE No. 37

A young married woman, 24 years old, had shown mental symptoms for one year previous to admission. She exhibited a variable emotional state, having periods of excitement, talkativeness and restlessness, followed by periods when she was depressed, dull, 'lifeless' and lacking in interest. During her excited periods she talked of seeing lights and hearing bells, was erotic in her conduct, exposed herself and used filthy language. She gave the impression, however, of great happiness, showed a flight of ideas, was distractible and misidentified those around her. For a time her conversation was incoherent and obscene, but her mood was always one of elation. In the course of six months she had made a satisfactory adjustment, and was discharged. Fifteen months later she was readmitted. Her condition was now one of apathy and lack of interest. She grimaced, showed flexibilitas cerea, had periods of mirthless laughter, had to be spoon-fed and was careless in her personal habits. During the next four years her mental health showed a steady decline. There were times when she had periods of excitement, which superficially simulated a manic state, but these periods were poorly sustained, her conversation was incoherent and irrelevant, she hallucinated, was foolish in her conduct and utterly lacking in appreciation of her disordered mental state. An investigation of her personality showed that she had been vain, reserved, hypersensitive and had peculiar tastes.

In the first of these two cases the behaviour sank to a very low level. Yet the patient made an excellent readjustment, with considerable insight, and there seems no reason to suppose that she will have a further attack.

In the second case at the time of the first admission the picture resembled a manic excitement. In estimating the prognosis at that time, more weight should have been placed on the long prodromal period of one year previous to her admission, and on the vain, reserved type of personality.

PROGNOSIS

It is now generally recognized that although schizophrenia has in general a most serious prognosis, there are a considerable number of cases which can, and do, readjust themselves satisfactorily. There are a larger number who make a social rather than a complete recovery, and there are still others who reach a quiescent stage so that they can be cared for at home. The majority gradually show a state of mental deterioration, which particularly involves the emotional field and habits, and such patients are best cared for under mental hospital conditions. It is uncertain how far current methods of treatment have improved the prognosis in schizophrenia: their efficacy must be measured against the percentage of remissions reported previously. Three groups of workers gave the following percentage of total remissions in cases followed up prior to the Second World War: Stalker (1939), 12 per cent., and Guttmann, Mayer-Gross and Slater (1939), 21·5 per cent., both in Britain; and Rennie (1939), 24·6 per cent. in the U.S.A. Norris (1959), in a survey of mental illness in London, has reported that still about one-third of those admitted to hospital are not likely to recover sufficiently ever to leave hospital, while of those who are discharged, over one-third are admitted at least once again in the ensuing four years. She states, however, more hopefully: 'There is reason to believe that the prognosis is less gloomy now than fifteen years or more ago, since the outcome for the unselected schizophrenics included in this study was almost as good as that for a group specially selected in 1933–34 for its favourable prognosis.' In every case we should attempt to come to a comprehensive understanding of the individual aetiology and should try to discover what factors can be modified: the over-all seriousness of the prognosis has too often discouraged therapeutic efforts.

The specific symptoms developed are of very little help in estimating whether the outcome of the illness is likely to be favourable or unfavourable. One must look at the total clinical picture, its setting and evolution. A long history of insidiously developing withdrawal of interests and progressive inefficiency is very ominous. Cases of acute onset—in particular, the katatonic group—have generally a better prognosis than those developing insidiously, but although this holds true for the majority it is no absolute criterion. We have seen cases of very acute onset who, far from showing signs of improvement, exhibit a gradual deterioration. Those who have been ill for less than a year before admission to hospital have a better prognosis than those who have been ill for longer.

Emphasis should be placed on an attempt to estimate how the individual met his difficulties in his pre-psychotic period. If he handled them for the most part in a satisfactory way, and if his general interests have been well maintained, then he has a much better chance of readjusting himself than the shut-in, introverted individual. The preservation of more or less adequate affective responses and rapport during the illness is a hopeful sign.

Illnesses precipitated by obvious exogenous factors, physical and psychical, tend to be more favourable: but there is no hard-and-fast rule. In certain cases the exogenous factors seem even to release latent pernicious trends which can never again be thoroughly held in check. If the exogenous factors have been heavy, and are transient or reversible, the conditions for recovery are obviously made easier.

It has been claimed that cases which have a family history of affective psychoses, those which present with some clouding of consciousness and those which are in other ways atypical, have a better prognosis. This is hard to gauge. Undoubtedly some or many of these are cases of manic-depressive psychosis, not of schizophrenia. Langfelt has stated the situation succinctly in these terms: 'Schizoid character, leptosome body, insidious onset, lack of precipitating factors and initial symptoms such as massive influence and derealization phenomena as a rule indicate an unfavourable prognosis; cyclothymic temperament, pyknic body build, acute onset, demonstrable exogenic factors and a non-typical schizophreniform symptomatology on the other hand indicate a favourable prognosis.'

The prognosis depends also on how soon, how vigorously and how persistently the illness is treated. In treatment what matters most is perhaps the individual attention given to the patient; and even although the methods used are not in any way specific, the fact that doctors and nurses are constantly stimulating the patient along one or other line is helpful. After the patient's discharge from hospital much will depend on the understanding and support of relatives, on the tolerance of neighbours and on whether or not the patient can be found suitable employment. There is nearly always a certain falling away from the pre-illness level of adjustment. Recoveries seldom occur with complete insight, and the patient who becomes re-employable is seldom able to return to his own job, something simpler being required.

TREATMENT

We have no specific and effective treatment for schizophrenia. Our attitude has to be melioristic: but much can and should be done which is helpful. In a considerable proportion of cases the treatment given determines the prognosis, at least in part. We can probably assist in arresting the disease process, we can certainly often limit the degree of deterioration, and we can sustain and develop the patient's undamaged assets.

Neither is there any sure way of preventing schizophrenia. Even if it were legally permissible, sterilization would not be a useful measure, since schizophrenia is inherited probably as a recessive and the parents are in most cases outwardly fairly normal individuals. We cannot for certain identify the carrier state, though we suppose that the schizoid individual may be heterozygous for the abnormal gene or genes. Fortunately, some biological circumstances tend to limit the spread of the disease. Schizophrenics have low marriage rates and low fertility rates, and few children are born to schizophrenics after the onset of their illnesses. If medical opinion is sought, one should usually advise a person who has had a schizophrenic breakdown not to marry: it is true that an understanding spouse might greatly help such a sensitive and predisposed individual, but childbearing and child-rearing would be liable to bring stresses which would prove insupportable.

A more promising field for mental hygiene lies in the special care and understanding which can be given to the child who is recognized to be shy and withdrawn and to have schizoid trends. We have as yet no proof that such special care of the schizoid individual at an early age can prevent the onset of schizophrenia, but it seems both humane and realistic to take deliberate precautions. We must encourage, stimulate, explain and try to 'exteriorize' those who tend to day-dream and to lead asocial seclusive lives. If there are difficulties in any part of the instinctual life, these difficulties must as far as possible be resolved; the shy and nervous and sensitive individuals who suffer from such difficulties must be encouraged to talk them over more freely, and must be urged to meet their problems face to face instead of dodging them. Consideration must be given to habit formation and character training, so that the child does not come to suffer from the kind of dangerous accumulation of faulty reactions to which Adolf Meyer drew particular attention. We may have to choose the sensitive child's school with care, and later by vocational guidance try to make sure that he enters the most suitable type of occupation or further training. These are tasks for parents, teachers, ministers of religion and family doctors: and, in the case of the more disturbed child, for the child guidance and specialized child psychiatric services. Every endeavour must be made to identify the child who is labouring with problems of adjustment, and to bring help at an early stage.

When the illness has been diagnosed or suspected, admission to hospital is in most cases advisable even if the patient's disturbed conduct does not make it imperative. The young schizophrenic patient is unpredictable and at home he imposes great strains on his family. The orderliness and discipline of a hospital regime, and the understanding attitudes of the staff, have a calming effect, the patient's mental condition can be more thoroughly assessed in hospital, and the effects of various methods of treatment can be more certainly ascertained. The co-operation of the patient's relatives must be secured from the outset by explaining to them something of the nature of the patient's illness, the objectives of treatment and the lines of management which are proposed; and the relatives should be encouraged to visit the patient regularly and frequently in hospital. The therapist should never imitate the patient in ignoring the claims of the world outside the hospital: and if the patient's home circumstances are reasonably good, the objective should be to return him home as soon as his more acute and disabling symptoms have been controlled. In considering discharge from hospital one has to weigh up both the patient's need for rehabilitation in a more normal environment and the ability of his relatives to sustain any residual mental disabilities which the patient may show. To discharge a patient prematurely is perhaps usually less of a mistake than to keep him in hospital too long, but it may lead to losing the ground gained therapeutically and may so antagonize relatives and the public that after re-admission to hospital the patient's next discharge may be very difficult to effect.

It has often been stated, erroneously, that the schizophrenic is incapable of rapport. In a state of stupor or acute turmoil he may be, and lack of rapport is a feature of advanced schizophrenic dementia. But most schizophrenic patients are accessible and capable of developing emotional bonds; and these bonds may be intense and ambivalent. The therapist first gains the patient's trust by himself taking his history in detail and listening attentively to his symptoms. Probing and interpretations of an analytic type are usually unwise, since they may easily result in the patient becoming more confused and disturbed. The therapist must not only seek to understand the symptoms of the illness, but also intimately the personality of the individual who has become ill, his defects and assets and the environmental pressures which have moulded him. He should orientate his treatment in much the same way as one does for a brain-injured individual, building upon what is uninjured or relatively intact in the personality, re-educating, encouraging, advising, praising, rewarding; directing the patient persistently towards normal ways of thinking and acting. This sort of supportive psychotherapy is relevant in every case. The therapist must be optimistic and not give up easily, since it is often a long haul until the patient can be discharged from hospital relieved. Analytic psychotherapy should be considered an experimental form of treatment in schizophrenia, to be undertaken usually only in hospital and only by most experienced psychotherapists. Modified analytic techniques for treating schizophrenics have been developed by Fromm-Reichmann, Federn, Powdermaker, Frank and other American workers (Brody and Redlich, 1952).

Individual interest in the patient is of prime importance. To be most effective, the doctor must leave his consulting room and the interview situation, to join the patient in the other business of hospital life. He must make contact with his patient at social functions, at games, dances and religious services, at the canteen and in the occupational therapy department. In short, the therapist must never limit himself to formal verbal exchanges with the patient. The nursing staff, more constantly with the patients and participating with them in many small activities and purposes, have commonly an even more important and potentially effective therapeutic rôle than the doctor. Nurses must be educated and encouraged to see that all their contacts with patients are potentially therapeutic, and not just those which have been conventionally described as nursing duties. All the time the patient must be brought sympathetically into contact with reality and helped to climb a ladder of social readjustment. Aggressiveness should be met with calm handling and explanation, as well as being diminished by the prescription of drugs. It is of the greatest importance to insist on good personal hygiene and posture, cleanliness, clean shaving, tidiness of dress, acceptable eating habits. The patient should be helped to take an interest in his clothes, to select new ones and to take an active pride in his appearance: anonymous clothing of the institutional type depresses morale. Exercises and games will help to restore the patient's physical tone and sense of well-being. All this gives the schizophrenic patient needed self-confidence. As well as being given individual attention, he should of course participate in group activities, and never be left to stand or lie about in lonely self-absorption. Group psychotherapy may be even more helpful to the long-term patient than individual psychotherapy.

The patient's general physical health must be cared for, his nutrition attended to and any concurrent physical illness actively treated. Though not in any way specific in their effects, other physical methods of treatment directed towards amelioration of the schizophrenic process itself play an important part in the total therapeutic programme. E.C.T. is often of value in alleviating depressive symptoms and in disrupting acute hallucinatory states. Tranquillizing drugs, in particular chlorpromazine and trifluoperazine, are useful in allaying turmoil and tension and in allowing the patient to become more accessible to other therapeutic influences: and these drugs apparently sometimes have a distinct effect in diminishing the strength and persistence of delusions and hallucinations. Chlorpromazine is prescribed usually in doses of 150 to 400 mg. daily by mouth, and as much as 800 mg. daily has been given; the dose of trifluoperazine is 5 to 25 mg. daily: both drugs produce Parkinsonian symptoms as their main neurological side-effects. A tranquillizing drug should probably be persisted in for 1 to 3 months, to give it a fair trial, and patients who respond to a particular drug may have to continue to take it regularly for many months or even years. We give our reasons on page 347 for abandoning insulin coma treatment. Leucotomy is very rarely indicated, it being so apt to increase deterioration. Physical methods of treatment have also psychotherapeutic effects, and there is some evidence that the contacts of physical nursing may help the schizophrenic patient to reconstitute the disturbed boundaries of his ego.

Occupational therapy assists the patient to regain his interests and to develop manual skills. When thus busy he is distracted from his delusional and hallucinatory preoccupations; but distraction is only a step on the way to his rehabilitation.

Occupational therapy must be followed by therapeutic occupation; first, in the grounds of the hospital or on a hospital farm, or in one of the indoor departments of the hospital, the kitchen or joiner's shop or elsewhere. There every attempt should be made to train and fortify the patient to become fit to take a job outside hospital.

When the patient is discharged from hospital, he must not be allowed to fall into a social void. It is seldom of any use to return him to a lonely life in lodgings: if he has no home, boarding out with a suitable family should be considered. His return home must have been prepared by encouraging visits to him in hospital, by giving him increasing parole and later by allowing him home for short trial periods. The patient's relatives too must be prepared by an understanding of his illness, his needs and his limitations. A psychiatric social worker is often very helpful in smoothing the way for a patient's discharge by visiting the home and discussing with his relatives in that more intimate setting the problems and challenge the patient's return home may bring. If the patient can be discharged to a job, so much the better: he must certainly not be allowed to return to a life of slippered indolence around the house. His relatives must often continue at home the work which has been done in hospital by nurses, and the patient's family doctor must attend to his medical needs, which include taking the drugs upon which his being able to live outside hospital may depend. Continuing visits by a health visitor or social worker may support both doctor and relatives in their efforts to keep the patient at a socially acceptable level in the community. Membership of a social club may draw the patient further out of his loneliness and diffidence.

The more enthusiasm and staying power we bring to the treatment of schizophrenia, the better are likely to be our results: but complete success cannot often be claimed for treatment. All our treatments are empirical and limited in their effects: we are frustrated by our very slight knowledge of the aetiology of the illness. Schizophrenia still accounts for about two-thirds of those who require long-term care in our mental hospitals, and is thus one of the major unsolved problems in the whole field of medicine.

REFERENCES

Blair, J. H. (1952) *J. ment. Sci.*, **98**, 464.
Bleuler, M. (1948) *Arch. Psychiat. Nervenkr.*, **118**, 271.
Bleuler, E. (1950) *Dementia Praecox or The Group of Schizophrenias*, New York.
Brody, E. B., and Redlich, F. C. (1952) *Psychotherapy with Schizophrenics*, New York.
Brooke, E. M. (1959) *J. ment. Sci.*, **105**, 893.
Cameron, N. (1938) *Psychol. Monogr.*, No. 221.
Cameron, N. (1944) in *Language and Thought in Schizophrenia*, ed. Kasanin, J. S., Berkeley, California.
Dunlap, C. B. (1924) *Amer. J. Psychiat.*, **3**, 403.
Federn, P. (1952) *Ego Psychology and the Psychoses*, New York.
Fenichel, O. (1946) *The Psychoanalytic Theory of Neurosis*, London.
Freeman, T., Cameron, J. L., and McGhie, A. (1958) *Chronic Schizophrenia*, London.
Freud, S. (1914) *The Standard Edition of the Complete Psychological Works* (1953), London.
Gjessing, R. (1938) *J. ment. Sci.*, **84**, 608.

Harris, A. (1959) *J. ment. Sci.*, **105**, 235.

Heron, W., Bexton, W. H., and Hebb, D. O. (1953) *Amer. J. Psychol.*, **8**, 366.

Hill, D. (1957) in *Schizophrenia, Somatic Aspects*, ed. Richter, D., London.

Hoch, D., and Polatin, P. (1949) *Psychiat. Quart.*, **23**, 248.

Hollingshead, A. B., and Redlich, F. C. (1958) *Social Class and Mental Illness*, New York.

Jung, C. G. (1960) *The Psychogenesis of Mental Disease*, London.

Kallmann, F. J. (1953) *Heredity in Health and Mental Disorder*, New York.

Kraepelin, E. (1913) *Lehrbuch der Psychiatrie*, 8th ed., Leipzig.

Kretschmer, E. (1925) *Physique and Character*, London.

Langfeldt, G. (1952) *Proceedings of First World Congress of Psychiatry*, Vol. 2, 237.

Leonhard, K. (1939) *Allg. Z. Psychiat.*, **112**, 391.

Lewis, N. D. C. (1923) *Nervous and Mental Diseases Monographs*, No. 35, Washington.

Lidz, R. W., and Lidz, T. (1949) *Amer. J. Psychiat.*, **106**, 332.

Lidz, T. (1956) *Amer. J. Psychiat.*, **113**, 126.

Lidz, T. (1957) *Amer. J. Psychiat.*, **114**, 241.

Lilly, J. C. (1956) *Psychiat. Res. Rep. Amer. Psychiat. Ass.*, No. 5.

Meyer, A. (1951) *The Collected Papers*, Vol. 2, Baltimore.

Meyer, A. (1960) *J. ment. Sci.*, **106**, 1181.

Morrison, S. L. (1959) *J. ment. Sci.*, **105**, 999.

Mowbray, R. M. (1958) in *Topics In Psychiatry*, ed. Rodger, T. F., Chap. 2, London.

Myers, J. K., and Roberts, B. H. (1959) *Family and Class Dynamics in Mental Illness*, London.

Norris, V. (1959) *Mental Illness in London*, London.

Olkon, D. M. Z. (1939) *Arch. Neurol. Psychiat. (Chicago)*, **42**, 652.

Osmond, H., and Hoffer, A. (1959) *J. ment. Sci.*, **105**, 653.

Rees, L. (1943) Physical Constitution in Relation to Effort Syndrome, Neurotic and Psychotic Types, M.D. Thesis, University of Wales.

Richter, D. (1957) *Schizophrenia, Somatic Aspects*, London.

Shattock, F. M. (1950) *J. ment. Sci.*, **96**, 32.

Slater, E. (1953) *Psychotic and Neurotic Illnesses in Twins*, London, H.M.S.O.

Tietze, T. (1949) *Psychiatry*, **12**, 55.

Vogt, C., and Vogt, O. (1948) see Richter, D. (*op. cit.*) The Pathological Anatomy of the Schizophrenias.

Weckowicz, T. E., and Blewett, D. B. (1959) *J. ment. Sci.*, **105**, 909.

Weckowicz, T. E., and Sommer, R. (1960) *J. ment. Sci.*, **106**, 17.

12

PARANOID REACTION-TYPES

The history of paranoia and paranoid states as we know them to-day may be said to date from 1818 when Heinroth described them as disorders of the intellect under the term *Verrücktheit*. In 1845 Griesinger described similar conditions, but he regarded the intellectual disorder which was present as secondary to an affective disturbance either of a manic or depressive nature. The above contradictory opinions have never been completely resolved or co-ordinated. The matter is one of considerable academic and clinical interest and is worthy of further study and investigation.

Kahlbaum, in 1863, was the first to use the term paranoia, and later it was accepted by Westphal, Krafft-Ebing, Mendel, Snell, Sander and Cramer, all of whom supported the view that paranoia was a disorder of the intellect. For instance, Krafft-Ebing defined it as 'a chronic mental disease, occurring exclusively in tainted individuals, frequently developing out of the constitutional neuroses, and having as its principal symptoms delusions'. These delusions were believed to arise independently of any disorder of affect. They were bound together systematically, and by reasoned judgement and inference were welded into a formal delusional system. This disease was slow in its course, was subject to a certain degree of remission, but showed neither a complete recovery nor complete mental deterioration. Particular attention was directed to a study of the personality prone to develop such a disorder, and it seemed remarkable how often shy, solitary and suspicious persons expressed persecutory delusions; the excitable and egotistic were grandiose; the over-conscientious and eccentric showed a predilection for religious topics. Krafft-Ebing postulated two main types: 1. original paranoia, developing at or before puberty, and always attributable to hereditary predisposition; 2. acquired paranoia, a form which developed late in life, particularly at the involutional period.

Meantime, Magnan in France was making a determined effort to give an even more systematic account of this disease which he described under the general term of *délire chronique à évolution systématique*.

He described four main stages:

1. A hypochondriacal stage, or stage of subjective analysis.
2. A stage of persecution.
3. A transformation of the personality, characterized by the expression of delusions of grandeur.
4. Occasionally a stage of mental deterioration.

During the primary stage the patient becomes self-centred, believes that remarks he overhears, or things he sees, or items he reads in the newspapers have some special significance, and are directed to him personally. Naturally he resents such happenings, he worries about them, sees meanings in them which were never intended, becomes resentful, avoids his friends and colleagues and shows an inability to concentrate on his work as he had done formerly. In the second stage, the morbid introspection which has been described is replaced by the development of delusions of persecution which dominate his life and conduct. All his suspicions are transformed into beliefs so that he may seek the help of the police, or may employ all manner of devices to protect himself from his supposed persecutors. He may even change his home and his employment, but wherever he goes he seems to be followed and feels that he is the victim of a huge organization which is determined to ruin him and to make his life unbearable. Occasionally he may turn on his persecutors and attempt to right his supposed wrongs by criminal action. Such delusional states are not infrequently complicated by an hallucinosis which may affect any of the special senses but is, predominantly, auditory. In the third stage it appears almost as if a complete transformation of the personality had occurred. The persecuted man becomes the grandiose man, and he does so in his attempt to find an explanation or compensation for all the trials to which he has been subjected. He appears to argue that because so many people seem to be interested in him that therefore there must be something which calls for special consideration and in consequence he may identify himself with God, or at least with some very distinguished person. During the passage of years a certain degree of mental deterioration may occur, but it is surprising that the memory and general intellectual faculties remain remarkably intact.

Kraepelin, in 1893, in his effort to obtain a clearer clinical differentiation suggested a nosological grouping which he termed respectively paranoia, paraphrenia and paranoid schizophrenia. We have found such a grouping cumbersome and we have already stated our reasons [see p. 262] for rejecting the concept of paranoid schizophrenia. We would, likewise, in the interest of clarity and to effect a better classification, suggest that the term paraphrenia should be discarded, as it does not serve any useful purpose. Paranoia and paranoid states should be grouped together rather than differentiated. They are merely individual instances of the rigid, biased, sensitive, suspicious personalities who, under certain circumstances, are liable to develop a delusional system which may or may not be highly systematized. Furthermore, while paranoid symptoms may build themselves into a specific and distinctive grouping, yet that does not imply that they may not occur in schizophrenia, just as they may involve or complicate a manic-depressive state, or an organic psychosis; under such circumstances they are secondary phenomena which need not influence the course of the illness.

The term paranoia was reserved by Kraepelin for cases showing a prolonged course, unfavourable prospects of recovery, and fixed delusions. He laid particular stress on the insidious development of a permanent and unshakable delusional system, resulting from endogenous causes, and accompanied by preservation of clear and orderly thinking, willing and acting; there is no real or genuine hallucinosis. The underlying personality type is usually consistent with the clinical state. They are apt to be violent, excitable persons, self-willed, distrustful people with 'a chip on their shoulder'. Homosexual tendencies may play a significant part in their make-up; this will be mentioned later in relation to the psychopathology.

But apart from the full-fledged paranoia there are lesser states which have been described, notably by Gierlich and Friedmann (1908), as 'abortive forms and formes frustes'. Their cases had recurrent tendencies which were precipitated by certain situations or circumstances. 'These are patients who present the picture of paranoia, who develop systematized, persecutory delusions, with great irascibility, with happy or sad affective states which last for several weeks, without sensory impairment, and who rather rapidly recover, with perfect insight into their condition, with a tendency to a periodic recurrence.' In analysing their case material both Gierlich and Friedmann had comments to make which are of significance in helping us to understand the mechanism of such cases. For instance, Gierlich concluded that a compelling emotion, anxiety, expectancy, envy, might lead to a delusional formation, provided it had sufficient strength and duration. Friedmann's views were very similar. While he emphasized the sensitive, obstinate, egotistical nature of his patients, yet in addition many of them had been struggling with complex emotional forces. It was usually a disturbing experience which had created uneasiness or mistrust and remained the sole topic of the abnormal trend of ideas. Such happenings give rise to shame and guilt feelings, to uncertainty in relation to others, and ultimately to delusions. Friedmann believed that the experience preceding the development of the disorder corresponded very closely to Wernicke's conception of 'overvalued' ideas, and that the entire condition rests upon congenital traits, particularly of character. In our experience delusional states of a transitory nature, with or without hallucinations, are among the commonest of psychotic reactions occurring in the wards of a general hospital. The types we have in mind arise acutely after operations, child-birth, and debilitating illness of all kinds, especially if associated with a transfer to a novel environment, e.g. to hospital. The condition usually subsides almost as quickly as it arose. The content of the delusions and hallucinations is usually self-accusatory and may be accompanied by fear, and even clouding of consciousness. The mood is depressed, and for that reason these cases might be classed with the depressions (on an infective-exhaustion basis) rather than with the paranoid reactions, but clinically the prominent features are the ideas of reference and the delusions.

While the above description gives the basic features of paranoia and paranoid states, yet we must take notice of the contributions which have been made by Bleuler, Adolf Meyer and Freud.

Bleuler was critical of the symptomatological differentiations of Kraepelin, and was much more liberal in his interpretation of paranoia and paranoid states. Bleuler (1912) also took issue with Specht and sought to prove that paranoid states were not related to manic-depressive psychoses (as Specht had claimed) and that they were not dependent on the 'pathological affect of suspiciousness'. Bleuler maintained that suspiciousness was not an affect, that it was not a mixture of pleasure and displeasure, and that therefore paranoia could not be regarded as an 'affect psychosis'. On the contrary, Bleuler argued that suspicion and mistrust were the result of faulty perception and interpretation and were dependent on intellectual processes. 'Suspicion simply means that one cannot definitely foretell, and in consequence the affect may be either positive or negative, the former being what we term hope.' He analysed the position further when he pointed out that the manic-depressive state is the typical affect psychosis because of the variability of mood, whereas in paranoia the affect remains stable. Furthermore, in the affective psychoses any delusional formation which is present is secondary to the mood change, whereas in paranoia and paranoid states delusions are the predominant feature, and any change of affect is based thereon. If, for instance, the patient's attention is shifted from his delusions, his affect is similar to what it is in sane people. Furthermore, paranoia can actually exist without the feeling of suspicion, as it does, for instance, when the delusions of persecution are replaced by those of grandeur. Surprisingly enough Bleuler's experience led him to believe that many paranoid patients never become dangerous. Our experience is that the majority are, potentially, dangerous. And our view seems to gain support from Bleuler's formulation of the development of a 'katathymic state'. It appears to arise in consequence of a complex of ideas (usually of a delusional nature) associated with intense emotion which may show itself in some form of criminal conduct. It is of some significance to note that Bleuler found evidence of lack of sexual power almost invariably in his paranoid cases, and no doubt it was this failure which led so often to the expression of delusions of jealousy and infidelity. His general summing-up was as follows: ' The constitutional predisposition will explain why these people and not others suffer from paranoia (and paranoid states) and Freud's complexes will tell us why the critical events have brought out the paranoia and, eventually, why the developed paranoia immediately connects itself with the events.'

Meyer (1951) regarded all paranoid states as transformations of the personality, in which reason appears preserved, but side-tracked, and no longer fitting into the natural and real work of the world or of the individual, but still active along set lines. It is the type of personality which is continually ready to see a biased meaning in things, to be suspicious and asocial. They are always wondering what others think, and attribute deliberate intention to casual and indifferent actions. Such paranoid tendencies, for a time at least, may be compatible with formally correct conduct, but there is a certain inability to adapt the personal trend of thought and elaboration and attitude to the actual facts. He suggested that certain grades or stages might be recognized in the development of a paranoid reaction:

1. Uneasy, brooding, sensitive type, with an inability to correct notions and to make concessions;
2. Appearance of dominant notions, suspicions, or ill-balanced aims;
3. False interpretations with self-reference, and a tendency to systematization;
4. Retrospective or hallucinatory falsifications;
5. Megalomanic developments or deterioration, or intercurrent acute episodes;

U

6. At any period anti-social and dangerous reactions may result from lack of adaptability and excessive assertion of the aberrant personality.

Freud (1911) and his co-workers and pupils have, however, been much more bold in their formulation, and have not hesitated to propound an explanation for the origin and psychopathology of paranoid states which is most ingenious, and in certain instances seems to be borne out.

They state that paranoia and paranoid states are dependent upon homosexual fixation which is repressed, but when a failure of repression occurs the paranoid symptoms develop as projection phenomena. Freud's views stemmed from his analysis of the case of Dr. Schreber. He showed that in the genesis of delusions of persecution the persecutor is the one who, before the illness, had a great influence on the emotional life of the patient, or was an easily recognizable substitute for that person. The person who, on account of his supposed persecutory activities, is hated and feared, is the one who was formerly loved and revered. Schreber, for instance, had had at one time a great trust in and affection for his physician, Flechsig, but during his illness he called Flechsig a 'soul murderer', and also exhibited a feminine wish fantasy (passive homosexuality) which had taken Flechsig for its object. The person longed for had become the persecutor. Eventually Flechsig became replaced by God, and this seemed to afford a way of escape from the unbearable homosexual wish fantasy. Flechsig and God both probably symbolized the father. Freud then came to believe that all the recognized forms of paranoia could be represented as contradictions of the proposition 'I (a man) love him (a man).'

(a) *Delusions of persecution.*—The contradiction in this case is 'I do not love him, I hate him', but such a familiar principle cannot become conscious, the mechanism of projection comes into play and instead of saying 'I hate him' a transformation occurs into 'He hates me which justifies me in hating him.' Then the contradiction really becomes 'I do not love him, I hate him because he persecutes me.' The persecutor is always the former beloved one or a recognized substitute.

(b) *Erotomania.*—The contradiction is 'I do not love him, I love her.' Then the mechanism of projection causes the following change. 'I notice that she loves me. I do not love him. I love her because she loves me.'

(c) *Delusions of jealousy, e.g. alcoholic.*—A man disappointed in a woman may take to alcohol, which means that he may go to a public-house where he may meet other men. The contradiction then becomes, not 'I love a man', but 'She loves him', and in consequence he suspects the woman in relation to all the men whom he himself is tempted to love.

Analogous to this is the jealous paranoia of women: not 'I love the women.' 'He loves them.' The jealous woman therefore suspects the man towards all the women who please her.

(d) A fourth kind of contradiction is possible, 'I love nothing and no one', which is equivalent to saying 'I love only myself.' This is at the basis of delusions of grandeur, and may be regarded as a sexual overvaluation of the ego.

One of Freud's most distinguished pupils, Ferenczi, went even further than his master. He drew a contrast between the neurotic who frees himself from what is unacceptable by the process of conversion, transference, or substitution, with the demented person who withdraws his interest from the object to the ego, and also with the paranoid person who succeeds only in part in his withdrawal—a greater or less part of the interest cannot be set free from its original object, nor turned back to the ego, and so out of a feeling of love arises the feeling of its opposite. According to Ferenczi, repressed or distorted homosexuality is the explanation of paranoia.

We believe that the best method of illustrating the difficult problems which such cases present is to submit a series of case histories which have been carefully chosen.

CASE NO. 38

In the timidity, shyness, sensitiveness and lack of application of his boyhood, he early exhibited a tendency to be out of touch with reality and with his fellows—a very common foundation for feelings of dissatisfaction and actual antagonism, and one which would readily be strengthened by the occurrence of such incidents as the homosexual adventures he met with. Homosexual incidents, being covertly focussed upon, readily act as a basis for sensitiveness towards the 'herd', as the patient rather significantly called his fellows.

Lack of application to his work led to inefficient performance and failure, and a definite feeling of social inferiority from another direction. Masturbation seems also to have contributed to his many-sided sense of unworthiness. His attempt at compensating his inferiority, not unhealthy in itself, soon reached unhealthy dimensions. His compensating feeling of superiority went far beyond the bounds of reasonable possibility, and produced the grandiose ideas of his psychosis, of which the muddled, high-flown mystical trends were an example. His exhibitionist tendencies (Müller's exercises in full view of the public) were, of course, related to his other sexual trends. His overweening sense of general superiority and his exhibitionism are different aspects of what McDougall would have called his self-regarding sentiment, what the Freudians would call 'narcissism' and what others have called the paranoic 'hypertrophy of the ego'.

The course of the symptoms is clear enough as far as the sexual trends are concerned— rumination over homosexual episodes, with the stirring up of homosexual desires; repudiation of them at first, and projection of them on the environment; but finally, increasing acknowledgement of their subjective origin.

The fact of transition from an attitude of inferiority to one of superiority is also sufficiently clear; but in this patient the ideas of superiority are certainly not a matter of logical deduction from delusional premises, but of something deeper—a craving for the satisfaction which life has denied him.

Symptomatically the clear thinking on other topics, the absence of hallucinations and the attacks of impulsive violence are all noteworthy.

The patient was described as a shy, sensitive, timid person, who did not interest himself in his school work, and was inclined to resent any criticism. His apparent backwardness at school was due much more to lack of application than to any intellectual defect. If teased or cuffed by any of his comrades he did not retaliate but went home and wept to his mother. He was unable to pass the university entrance examination, and went into an office in the city. He soon changed his occupation, and, after being in several positions, he set out on a voyage to South America, but, behaving in a strange, excitable way, he was put ashore at the Canary Islands, and eventually brought back to the British Isles. We have no description of what happened on board the ship. Prior to his voyage, however, it had been noted that his behaviour was strange, in that he had left his positions without adequate reason, but always on account of some imagined slight. Following this, he went to Canada, and stayed there for a period of seven months. On his return home he obtained a position in a laboratory, but after changing from one to another he decided that he was being persecuted. In consequence he entirely gave up his employment, and for twelve years previous to his admission he had not done any work. Gradually he began to express his ideas of persecution more constantly. Everything that went on around him seemed to have some special reference to himself, and everyone with whom he came into association seemed to be conspiring against him. The war preyed on his mind. He was much against it, gave the usual high-flown pseudo-philosophic reasons of war's insanity and uselessness and refused to do anything for his country. He began to state that the police were shouting in at his bedroom window at night-time, making insulting and obscene remarks, that people were pointing at him in the streets and that he was surrounded by a host of watchers. His suspicions became more and more diffuse, and every sound made, every action that was done, was interpreted by him as a sexual symbol. A night or two previous to his admission he rushed into the room where his sisters were and threatened either to rape them or kill them. At this time he was talking in a very grandiose way, stated that he had revolted from organized society, that he objected to vote as 'the herd' did and that law and government and social organizations were 'all nonsense'.

At the time of his admission the patient adapted himself pleasantly enough, but he resented having been brought to hospital, said that the whole procedure was quite illegal and that there was no necessity whatsoever to admit him on an emergency certificate. Without being urged, however, he began to tell the medical officer how the police had been shouting in at his bedroom window. He spoke in an affectedly humble way of his knowledge of philosophy, and how few people understood it. He answered questions readily and correctly, but in his answers he was apt to become diffuse, and frequently dragged in some ideas connected with his delusions. He stated that he had known that sooner or later 'the herd' would 'get him down' and have him put in hospital, and he expressed the idea that the herd was always against those who had enough brains to think for themselves. He related an incident when he was 10 years old when a ticket-of-leave man from Perth prison had attempted improper practices with himself and a friend. No actual relation occurred, but the episode frightened him, and, looking back on it, he is certain that this man was a police spy. He could give no reason for this assumption save the light of his subsequent experiences. When he was about 14 years old, the same thing happened, he said, with a man who purported to be a night-watchman, but the patient then added, 'As he went home to bed at night, and did not appear to watch anything, I think I am justified in saying he was also a police spy'. At that time, and for some years following, he was greatly troubled with nocturnal emissions, and he now regards these as having been manifestations of some malign influence.

In reference to his beginning work in an office at 16, he said, 'I will not say I was persecuted, but I was just made to feel—as always—that I did not belong, that I was different and regarded with suspicion'. On this account he left the office and entered another one, but left for a similar reason and tried to enter the university. He is certain, however, that the Registrar was not sympathetic towards him, and told him that without his Leaving Certificates he could not enter. The Registrar seemed to be making much of two young men, and was saying to them, 'I see that you were at a public school. We are always very glad to get public school boys here', and while saying this he gave the patient a scornful glance, as much as to say, 'That is you washed out'.

The patient described how a system of spying and persecution had been going on for the past twenty years. Always his remarks were coloured by an artificially humble attitude about his own abilities. 'You can see, I expect, that perhaps I'm not just exactly below the average. I am not altogether shallow-minded.' He spoke a great deal about the interrelation of philosophy and science, how one could not have, or even think of, the one, without, or in terms of, the other, explaining that that was where

Haeckel failed. 'A good sound man, unimaginative perhaps, but sound, and yet no-where, because he had no science. Now that is where I want to begin.' He related how when he had been working in a certain laboratory his urine had been examined, and that afterwards his teachers seemed to twit him rather unkindly about the presence of mucus and vaginal epithelial cells. He believes that this was part of the plot on the part of society to make him 'cave in'. Eventually he left there on account of 'petty attentions which I did not mind very much really'. He then told how he had fitted up a small laboratory at home, but when he mentioned this to a friend it seemed to be construed into an allusion to tender passages with some girl. It was about this time, he said, ten or twelve years previous to admission, that the police began to pay special attention to him. Insulting remarks were frequently shouted in to him through his open bedroom window while he was asleep. This was done by a policeman whom he knew quite well, who had no personal enmity to him, but was obeying orders. The police, he feels sure, were told to do this by the Chief Constable, because 'the herd' were outraged by the patient doing Müller's exercises before an open window, and had complained to the City Fathers. Having described this episode, he gave a diatribe on the theme, 'To the pure all things are pure'. He then related what he called his 'Blank Experiment'. It seemed to him that people might try to annoy him by jingling money in their pockets. He waited for a year, and never heard anyone doing it. This struck him as significant, and he wrote down, in a notebook he used for jottings, that people might, to annoy him, jingle money in their pockets. From that day onwards, more and more, he heard people jingle coins as they passed him. This proved that 'there must be a plot' against him, and also that his notes were being systematically perused by others. He related an endless number of such incidents—how beggars on the street made strange gestures as he passed, how people looked out of the window at him, how blinds were pulled half-way down on his approach, as a signal to those farther up the street, how bags were opened in the theatre as a special signal.

His memory, both for recent and remote events, was unimpaired; his grasp of general school knowledge was excellent, and he had a clear realization of his position, but had no real insight into his condition.

Physically he was in excellent general health. He was a tall, well-built man.

His blood pressure was 135/80: there was no evidence of any disease of the internal organs, and there were no neurological symptoms.

Following his admission, he took up the position that he was misunderstood, that his detention was part of the plot of society against him, that it was quite unjustified, that it was a criminal proceeding, that the superintendent and all associated with him would be made to pay dearly for it. His attitude at all times was one of superiority and condescension; he always felt that he was on a higher intellectual plane than anyone else. For example, he stated that his coming here had interrupted a small job that he was on. He explained that he had been writing a piece of music on the subject of a chapter in *Travels with a Donkey*. When asked if this was for the piano, he said, 'No, for a small orchestra of about forty performers', adding, 'it was as easy as falling off a fence—to me at any rate'. The most insignificant, trivial happenings in the ward were interpreted as being done with the sole purpose of annoying him. He stated that he experienced pains in his abdomen, due to the movements of the mouth of the sister in charge, which he looked upon as a sex symbol. At night-time he did not sleep well, and he alleged that he was purposely prevented from sleeping. He constantly spoke about 'the herd', whom he described as 'haters of bravery and individuality', and then arrived (as he invariably did) at the sex aspect of the situation, and said, 'What they always do is to grab the unfortunate man by the genitals who dares to think for himself, and keep ragging at him until he gives in and lies down to it. It is just all part of the plot.'

A few days after his admission he rushed out of his bedroom at seven o'clock in the morning and attacked the attendant in charge. The assault was a violent one, and two other attendants had to come to the rescue before the patient could be controlled. He did not give any explanation for this assault, except to say that the attendant had annoyed him by walking up and down the ward, that there was no necessity for him to do such a thing and that it was done with the purpose of raising sex ideas. He said, 'It is the same old system of punishment for self-abuse. There can be no such thing as self-abuse; it is a contradiction in terms. I refuse to take orders from a man like you.' The explanation for this idea was obtained later, when he said that he supposed that one of the methods of treatment in an institution such as this was to nauseate him with the thing that was supposed to trouble him. A similar outburst occurred the following day. He rushed out of his room in the middle of the night and assaulted one of the attendants, who, he claimed, had been making a peculiar noise with his mouth with intent to annoy him. He declared that the attendant's conduct was 'equivalent to striking him in his privates'. He demanded to be set free at once, and used the most abusive language to all the members of the staff, accusing the superintendent particularly of instructing his nurses in such methods of persecution. On one occasion he admitted that when he was in the presence of other men he felt what he called 'a wild sexual urge', which seemed to dominate him. He also said that he had dreams, usually accompanied by nocturnal emissions. In the usual type of dream, which the patient said is 'quite free from any element of sex', and which is accompanied by a feeling of pleasure, he is plodding along a road, through a beautiful countryside. In this dream he is always alone. Once, however, he had a dream in which he saw himself walking outside his room along with one of the other patients. The other patient was striking him on the side of the neck with a newspaper at every step.

Six months after admission he was given parole of the grounds and was allowed occasionally to go into the city, accompanied by a male nurse. For a time he enjoyed these outings very much and appreciated the privileges, but he continued to suffer from impulsive outbursts. On one occasion he got into conflict with one of the other patients, and before they could be separated our patient had been put forcibly on the ground, and sustained a severe bruise on his left eye, a cut on the lip and a cut on the right ear. His attitude towards this was remarkable. He pretended to treat the matter very lightly, said that he had no recollection of what had happened, that he must have been in a phantasy and that it was the first time that he had ever been so affected.

Seven months after admission he again made a violent assault on one of the night attendants. He caught him by the throat, threatened to strike him and only after a severe struggle was he overpowered. When asked for an explanation he refused to furnish one, but demanded that he should be allowed into town to see his lawyer. Later in the morning he attempted to leave the ward without permission. He stated that he wished to be allowed out into the grounds to pass urine, because he was quite unable to perform the act in the lavatory. On this occasion, while the physician was talking to him, the latter happened to rattle some money in his pocket. This was immediately seized on by the patient as a form of annoyance, done with the object of inciting him to attack the physician. He made many wild accusations against the officials in the institution, saying that it was their object to 'down' him and to persecute him in every way.

In contrast to his delusional formation, and to his persecutory ideas, it was found that on ordinary topics he talked clearly and intelligently, showing no affective disturbance and behaving like an ordinary individual. If conversation with him was continued over any period of time, however, his persecutory ideas always came to the surface. He believed, for instance, that certain lady patients had been deliberately set to follow him by the medical superintendent, and that the object of this was to stimulate him sexually so that he would misbehave himself and therefore be subjected to some form of punishment.

His delusional system is unchanged. He refers frequently to his persecution by the police, who are under orders to annoy him by making 'disgusting sexual signs'. He continues to have a very high opinion of his scientific knowledge, and says, for example, that he has no difficulty in understanding Einstein's theory. On one occasion he resented being given lettuce to eat: 'Fancy giving a bachelor lettuce; that is an insult; lettuce contains vitamin E, the reproductive vitamin'.

CASE NO. 39

This case is of interest as the symptoms seemed to be the direct outcome of a 'complex' (a feeling of guilt for a venereal sore) which had existed for twenty years without producing psychotic effects, but which finally led to a psychosis. The reason why symptoms at last appeared depended probably in part on his age, but the immediate precipitating cause was a visit from a policeman on entirely indifferent business (Voters' Roll). The persecutory ideas which ensued centred very obviously round his feeling of sexual guilt, and were associated with some compensatory phantasies, which were also projected as delusions (e.g. a woman was to take care of him, and marry him when he had recovered from his venereal disease). A passive homosexual trend latterly received very frank expression, and it seems reasonable to suppose that part of the strength of his guilt-feeling about venereal disease was derived from his original resistance to acknowledging his homosexuality. His alcoholism is also of interest since it is supposed to be sometimes a symptom of underlying homosexual trends, and a means of substitute satisfaction of them, since alcoholism usually involves the close companionship of other men.

It is very unfortunate that the nature of his previous breakdown at 26 is unknown. It was evidently serious, since he did odd jobs only for five or six years. It may have been one of those transitory paranoid episodes, the existence of which Kraepelin is unwilling to admit, except as manifestations of 'latent' paranoia.

The lack of any noteworthy predisposing trait in the personality is also of interest.

For about five months previous to his admission to hospital at the age of 50 the patient had been on holiday, but eventually he decided to return home, as he said that everyone was spreading the report that he was 'mad and poxed'. He stated that his brother was at the root of it, that it was a conspiracy, that records were taken of everything that he was doing and thinking and that reports were spread abroad to do him harm.

On admission to the hospital he adapted himself well, was pleasant and frank and said that he looked forward hopefully to getting better. There was no disorder in his train of thought, and he was able to give a complete account of the onset and development of his illness. He complained of persecution by an unlimited number of people, who had formed a great conspiracy against him. He stated that he had contracted a venereal sore about twenty years ago, and that ever since he had been bothered with its constantly breaking down. This had worried him, and gradually he had become convinced that outside people knew of it. He related how a man was sent to his room to spy on him, and how this man had hidden underneath his bed. He asserted that the manager of his firm had sent detectives after him to spy on him and to tell everybody about him. The spies, he thought, had tampered with his lunch. He is convinced that they thought he was using the lavatory too frequently, and knew that he had a sore. If his manager 'had asked him in a straightforward way to explain things' everything would have been cleared up, as he 'could never understand what motive was behind it all'. He thought that all his friends were in league against him, that they were notifying the manager about his movements and spreading the same reports as formerly. He was thoroughly convinced that he was not suffering from delusions of persecution, declaring that everything he had related was true.

Physically he was in excellent health.

At a later date he stated that his mind felt more settled, and that he had no complaints. He added that 'the outside organization' had not interfered with him while he had been in hospital, and he was convinced that he was just as capable a man as he had ever been. He felt that he could devote his mind to anything that he cared to take up, and said spontaneously, 'When a fellow loses interest he loses life, and I don't want to part with that without a struggle'. His nights at this time were undisturbed. He slept well, and he worked regularly in the garden every day. He described himself as always having been a strong, healthy man. Always full of life, fond of company, of play and nonsense, he played games, liked rambling and walking and being with others. He was not shy or bashful and preferred mixed company. If he felt convinced in his own mind that his opinion was the right one he did not bother about what people thought, but asserted that he was not egotistical or argumentative, or pig-headed, but tolerant. 'If a man proves to me that I am wrong then I will give in to him at once.' He was not superstitious, but liked to get at the truth and at facts. He always was inclined to be optimistic. He was broad-minded and catholic in his views, but liked a man to have some kind of religion.

When about 26 years old he had had a breakdown in health, which he attributed to overwork. It was ushered in by a faint. The doctor told him that he would need a long rest, and on this advice he returned home, remaining there for a period of about five or six years, during which he did odd jobs. According to his friends he had been drinking very heavily previous to this breakdown. Questioned about his drinking habits, he admitted often having drunk to excess, and he also spoke about the venereal sore which he had contracted twenty years ago. One day his landlady told him that a policeman had called to ask his name, his age and his occupation. His landlady explained to him that the Voters' Roll was being made out, but this did not satisfy him. He noticed that the policeman seemed to come back and forward to the house, and that people watched him while he was at his work. On the night of September 27–28 the forenoon timekeeper at his place of employment, he said, spent the night underneath his bed, and he came to the conclusion that he must have been sent by the manager. The patient did not speak to him, but he maintains that he saw him. His landlady told him that he was suffering from a delusion, whereupon he concluded that his landlady must have been in collusion with the man, and that the whole thing was done so that the landlord might get a better position. He complained of his eyes feeling peculiar, of strange pains in his chest and he accused the night-attendant of having drugged his cocoa. In addition, he asserted that one of the other patients constantly came into his room both during the day and at night, and he was certain that the night-attendant and this patient were in the employment of his firm, and had been sent here specially to watch him. When explaining this he became tense, excited, emotional, showed a great deal of tremor and twitching of his facial muscles, said that he wished he had a bolt on the inside of his bedroom door and that he would like to go away where no one knew him.

Following the above conversation, the patient withdrew himself from the society of others, and refused to discuss his illness or his ideas. If the matter was approached he usually became emotional, asserted that the physician knew all about it and that it was not worth while discussing it. He complained of a pain over the region of his bladder and requested that 'the pump' which was being used on him should be stopped. He asserted also that the previous night his supper had been drugged, that he had been put into a 'corpse-like' state so that the pump might be worked on him. He was so tense and worried that he described himself as 'shaking from head to foot'. Because of the persecution which he felt he was being subjected to, he gave notice that he wished to leave the hospital, since he was a voluntary patient and could go when he desired. On account of his attitude, two outside physicians had to be asked to examine him, and they certified him as being of unsound mind. One of the medical certificates was to the effect that 'he stated that someone paid several men to spread a report that he had venereal disease, that he had overheard a woman in the train talking about it to a man, that everyone spoke about it (there are good reasons to know these are delusions). He stated that someone in hospital made a hypodermic injection into his penis while he slept.' An attendant stated that the patient had extraordinary sexual delusions: that two nights ago during the night a patient from upstairs had relations with him, and injected seed into his flesh. The other medical certificate said 'he believes he is being spied upon, watched and followed, and his present condition published abroad on account of the disease he contracted some time ago. He tells one that when he last travelled north he was followed by nurses, who told everyone in the train about his state, and that these nurses were engaged to do so by his employers, with whom he had had a difference concerning a patent, of the benefits of which they wished to deprive him.' He blamed the physician for this, stating that he had not behaved like an honourable man, and that it was unjust to receive him as a voluntary patient and then to detain him against his will. In addition, he had all sorts and kinds of delusions, principally of a sexual nature. He felt that the physician and some of the patients and nurses were in the employment of his firm, and that their sole purpose was to pump his body up so as to make him feel as if he was having sexual relations. He accused the physician of coming to his room in the middle of the night so as to accomplish this purpose. Apart from his delusions, his memory and his general intellectual functions were intact. He stated that he had only one complaint, namely, the annoyance that was caused him by letting people into his bedroom at night, and then he added, 'Of course you deny this'. He described it as sinful for the physician to go on like this, but when asked if he was getting sound sleep, he admitted that he was getting plenty of sleep, but that it was always a disturbed sleep. He stated that every night his bed was prepared in some peculiar way, that three or four times during the night he was gassed and that, in addition, pumps were used on him. It always seems to him that it was the physician who was doing this, 'or that man you put on to me as a chum'. He said, 'I don't know what you have done to other people, but you have tried me as much as any man could. All that I say is as true as I am sitting on this chair.' Reports of his treatment were spread by the physician throughout the house, and he heard attendants and other patients constantly saying that 'a pump will be used', and so on. Letters which he wrote were at once made known to all the other patients, and the information contained therein was spread by the physician. This was done to annoy him. He stated also that two fellow-employees were in the hospital at night to annoy him, that the physician had been responsible for letting them in and that they must be friends of the latter. While they were present they talked about business and patents, and other things, in order to annoy him. He 'would swear to it on oath before God that these things that he says are true'. Mentally he felt that he was just as right then as he was when he left school. 'If I were as sure of going to Heaven as of swearing to the truth of these statements, I would be a happy man to-day.' 'You are the most awful man I have ever met in my life, the most thorough-paced scoundrel that I have ever known'—this to the physician. He stated that he had pleaded to be given an easier time and that no attention was paid to him, and he described himself as being 'the daftest man that ever was to have come into such an institution as this'. In going over his previous history he corroborated the statements which he made on admission, and gave a history of sleep-walking when a child. He confirmed his previous allegations about the persecution to which his employers subjected him, and he again asserted that it was all done in order to deprive him of a patent. They 'wished to chase him away, and to give him such a facer that he would never come back again'. When he got into the north train the two women came into the compartment after him, and there was also in the compartment another woman with a child. In the next compartment were four or five men, who were spying and drugging him. One of the women in the carriage was tall, slim and fair, about 35 years old: the other was stout and dark, and seemed very strong. Just as soon as the journey started these two women began to talk about him—the whole thing was schemed. The stout one said that he had had a venereal sore, that she was going to his home to nurse him and that afterwards she was going to marry him. On one occasion she held out her hand, saying that she had never done any hard work, meaning that she would have to be very comfortably looked after.

His ideas of reference and pseudo-memories continued unabated, but, eventually, he was discharged in a slightly relieved condition.

CASE No. 40

This patient came from a family described as 'neurotic'. His personality was in many respects a good one, but he was at the same time unusually sensitive and prudish.

In this case the important factors were endogenous ones, of which the personality traits mentioned were manifestations. Homosexual trends became evident in the course of the psychosis, suggesting that they formed a considerable part of the 'endogenous' element. Symptomatically there was a gradual deterioration, with hallucinations, feelings of influence, and incoherence and crudity of ideas, facts of some interest in view of the slow onset, and in which the psychosis is distinguishable from a 'paranoia' in Kraepelin's sense.

A man, 38 years, single, was admitted to hospital in September 1920.

The medical certificates stated that he believed he was subject to continuous persecution by some unknown persons, who interrupted him at his work, in sleep and at recreation. For instance, while reading Scripture from the pulpit a foul thought is slung at him: at golf he slices and loses balls through their agency. A friend, a fellow-clergyman, stated that on one occasion he had identified one of these persons who persecuted him as his niece, and threatened to injure her, and also threatened her mother when she criticized him.

His friend described the whole family as being somewhat neurotic.

The patient was described as having been a strong, healthy, active man. A good student, he took honours in his classes, and was an excellent athlete, taking a prominent part in football. His friend described him as 'one of the best men I have ever met'. In his conduct and behaviour he was always very chaste. He was not alcoholic. He is said to have had a frank, open personality, sociable and making friends easily, although somewhat shy. He was not argumentative, but was most exact in the expression of his thought. He was not at all egotistical, but rather modest and humble. Once, abroad, when a woman appeared on the stage indecently clad, the patient left the theatre. A good preacher, he always gave of his best. His inclinations were philosophical, and latterly he was a professor in a colonial college.

His friend dated the beginning of his illness to the period when he was 22 years old, when he had a breakdown while studying for his degree. He was advised to take a rest and to give up study. After a few weeks he seemed better. The exact nature of the above attack is unknown. He told his friend, however, that ten years ago he was subject to little disturbances to which at first he did not pay much heed. If he were reading a book a blank would seem to come over him, which would quickly pass away. In 1916 he was sent back from his colonial post, undoubtedly on account of his mental condition. His friend met him again in 1918, and at that time he was speaking in a strange way, talked about 'striking out' at someone, and on being questioned he said that he might possibly strike the wrong person. He was so sensible on other topics that little attention was paid to this. One year previous to admission it was more evident that something serious was wrong, as it became impossible to follow his reasoning. He would say such things as 'they will never leave me alone', but he would never specify who 'they' were. He began to say that he was being worked on in various ways, that profit was being made out of the use to which his body was put, that the medical profession, for instance, had tapped his body, and several doctors through using him gained the D.S.O. and the M.C. So long as his body was used for healing purposes—particularly during the war—all this was quite agreeable to him, but he now wanted to know why he was not demobilized when others were. He mentioned two persons in particular as his persecutors, one a man and the other a woman. He could not give their addresses. He has seen only the man in the flesh, and that but once, and he cannot describe him. These persons were earning their livelihood through him, the man about £5 a week and the woman £4. They were now 'giving the secret away', and 'even children are in the know'. On one occasion, just previous to admission, the patient accused his niece (a little girl about 12 years old) of being in the affair, and spoke to her in a threatening way. When his sister found fault with him he replied, 'What would you say if I gripped you'. The patient believed implicitly that he was watched and followed, and at times he seemed to have difficulty in restraining himself, and said to his friend, 'I might lose my temper with you'.

On admission the patient adapted himself quietly, but on the following day he became domineering, demanded his clothes and said that he wanted to leave. He complained about being interfered with, and threatened to 'make it hot' for the whole medical profession. The following day he had calmed down, co-operated in an examination and gave an account of the development of his illness. When asked to state his complaint in a few simple words, he described it as 'an interference with my ordinary ways of life', and gave as an instance that, when reading, his thoughts were constantly interrupted and interfered with. He felt that whatever was occurring must be of some advantage to someone. He related how when 21 or 22 years old he had had a short spell of what he described as 'strangeness', and he did not get the advantage out of a course of summer study that he should have done. At that time he was working on a thesis. He gave a description of this which was circumstantial, detailed and difficult to follow. It was in 1912 (aet. 30) that he first began to experience definite feelings of influence and a feeling of fogginess which never entirely passed away. He told an involved, confused story of his work and experiences abroad, of how eventually he was examined by two doctors, and somehow or other he was given 'sealed orders' and was told that 'it was a wash-out with Russell'. He felt that these doctors might have had 'something in their minds which I did not know'. He was puzzled to know why he should have been sent home from abroad, but he accepted it pleasantly. After returning he obtained an assistantship at X——, and there things seemed to happen all the time. His thoughts were read, and strange, disgusting, obsessive ideas would suddenly come into his head. He declared that on the day of admission to hospital a muscle had suddenly twitched in his arm, and asked, 'What is that going to lead to?' He argued that the same forces which operate on the voluntary muscles might also operate on his involuntary muscles, and if that is so then one can be 'interrupted in all sorts of ways'. He said that on the previous night he awoke at 3 a.m. and found that certain people were giving him what he called 'consciousnesses', thoughts 'articulate or inarticulate', and apt to be unclean. 'These people must be paid for doing this.' Regarding the episode with his niece, he explained that he only spoke to her as a warning. He demanded that steps should be immediately taken to stop the interference to which he was being subjected. At times he said he heard a long harangue, 'a consciousness like a human voice'. He went on to say how medical men had used him to write books, and of how during the push on the Marne he nearly died from sleeplessness. (He was in this country.) His body was being used for 'certain purposes'. His orientation, memory and general intellectual faculties were unimpaired, but he had no realization of his serious mental condition.

Physically he was in excellent general health.

A few days later he stated that he was contented, that he had been free for the most part from interference, that he had been able to read more, and expressed himself to the effect that 'it has not been outrageously bad; a little discomfort, that is all'. During a conversation he seemed suspicious and evasive, not wanting to say anything which might be used to his disadvantage. At other times, however, he would speak in rather a threatening way, saying the time might come when he would have to take things into his own hands, and that if things got much worse he might even have to sever his connection with the Church. He said, 'People may be paying to keep certain ones tormenting me'. Occasionally he hallucinated—one day whilst in conversation with the physician he answered a 'voice', which he said was that of a woman.

On May 18, 1921, he requested a special interview and handed three letters to the physician, one to the town-clerk, one to a lawyer and one to a leading divine. All these letters were to the effect that he wished steps taken to rid him of his persecutors. He refused to discuss his illness directly, but simply hinted at things. In reference to his resigning the post at X——, he said he did so on the understanding that something good would follow, but instead he had done practically no work since. During the past five years he had earned only about £350. 'The persecution has now reached such a length that it must be stopped. It will be a sore knock if I gather the information that is possible, for all this must stop. If it cannot be stopped, then I go to another place. A man could not be incarcerated for eight months for nothing, nor will the people causing it get off; if eight months has not been long enough to rouse their latent virtue, then the next step may be of a different nature.' Even if this meant his resignation from the Church he would not mind. He suspected that jealousy was at the back of it all, but there was one thing that he would like to investigate further: it is a trifle that happened when he was a boy. Occasionally during this interview he would stop for a minute or two, look away, smile, and there was no doubt that he was hallucinating. His legs began to shake and tremble, and this he explained as being due to outside influences. If he played golf badly, if he had a restless night, or anything happened to him whatsoever, all such phenomena were due to interference by his persecutors. Perhaps some day, he said, he would be able to name them.

On November 1, 1921, he said that during the war he had thought of charging certain people, that he simply came here so that he might get into touch with the medical men, talk over things and have things stopped. He stated that what had happened was that he was now fixed in a certain place, and that if he had been in the physician's place he could have beaten 'the thing I refer to'. People, for instance, knew where he slept, his habits regarding meals, golf, reading the newspapers, etc., so that in every way he was fixed and made a target. He was not going to allow anyone to examine his body. 'If I am here I am not going to have things stolen from me; that is the only basis I can put it on, the basis of theft. During the war I used to think that it was a matter of honour', but he felt now that it may come to a matter of killing. He was going to demand some return for these years which he had spent since his return from India, and then added again, 'Theft it is, accompanied by something one might term assault'.— 'I would not mind a man like you handling my body, rather than some rough tyke.' He referred to the days when he was an assistant in X——, how he applied for a parish at W——, but was not considered owing to the fact that he was not married. Then he was asked to take charge of a parish church for a year, but they refused to allow him. 'If one could only state things in a Church Court or in a Law Court one could see how preposterous it is. Suppose one does find that he has been played with, suppose some suggestion of sex is made, here is a thing which can be thieved, and then what is going to happen.' He described it all as 'a matter of having been abused, having been played with and having been abducted'. 'Am I going to stay here and be stolen from any longer?' He then asked 'whether the psychic thing is in his clothes, it can't come from the skin'.—'Suppose a part of my body is to be watched—they may affect my breathing if that is so—they may get thoughts from me, original suggestions from me; these are things which can be stolen, that is what I mean by theft, by assault.' He then referred to his being in hospital for over thirteen months, put forward the supposition that a man was doing the work and said, 'I don't want it on me, and if that blighter can work in your stomach what are things coming to', etc., etc.

In December 1921 an almost verbatim account was given of his conversation. He had stated that he wished to explain things, and to make things clear to the medical staff. He explained how he was being kept awake at night-time, and said, 'It's another thing to have one's body abused while it may also be used. It took place at midnight, violently. The thing must come to its legitimate close. I repeat, it is one thing to have one's body abused while it may also be used. Last night again I was awakened. I think it is time we got to grips. Here am I for a year and a half, a person with a fairly sufficient training. I get reading the papers with difficulty. I cannot read a book of any weight but have got to go back and pick up the thread.'

At another point he stated that 'the things that were subconscious were being taken from him', but he evaded giving an explanation of what he meant. He said, 'This cannot continue without theft. I am not going to stay here like an animated wooden thing.' He then gave other instances of how he was interfered with, and said, 'I am reading, say, about Matthew Arnold. Immediately there comes to my mind a thought, and then—close. As if that were all I had in connection with Arnold. Suppose someone were watching this—he would have thought it was a stop, but some other things come, you see.' When he was questioned about his body being abused, he hedged, and suggested that these were matters not to be talked about. Then he said, 'Take a simple instance—I get a slight twitching in my left arm when lying down, and then a little after in my heart, and if I had been delicate it would have finished me'.

'What other parts?'—'Various parts—the private parts.'

Asked whether it was a man or a woman who interfered with him, he said, 'There used to be'.

'Is it always men?'—'Not always.'

'If these things are so,' he asked, 'do you think it right that the patients should be allowed to do things of that sort? Is it a good thing for the asylum that these practices can be carried on so readily? It is certainly a bad thing for me.' He then explained how every hour of the day 'they' knew where he was, and on what particular chair he was sitting. He admitted that the same interference would probably occur in a home of his own, and he told how while he had been outside he had consulted a lawyer, because he thought someone should be put in jail. In February 1922 he again announced that matters must come to a finish, and that if in a month's time this interference did not cease he would make a decided effort to bring things to a termination. At this interview he reiterated his ideas about his body and brain being used to enrich others, and dwelt upon the disadvantage of being confined in an institution for one and a half years, because such confinement enabled his persecutors to 'centralize' their efforts. His talks were apparently designed in order that those who were taking advantage of him might hear him and take warning.

He maintained his general health very well indeed, but he was not so tidy in his habits as previously. He developed the habit of spitting on the floor, and then rubbing the carpet with his foot. When the sister in charge spoke to him about this, he became extremely angry, and told her that she was dismissed. When the doctor spoke to him he was also very angry, marched into the lavatory, spat on the floor and asked the doctor what he was going to do about it. He then repeated that he would not have any of the patients using his body, and told the physician that he was fined £1000, and that he would refuse to recognize him as a doctor henceforth. He took offence very easily, and any simple incident was apparently looked upon as an attempt to persecute him; for instance, when playing in a cricket match, in which he had been bowling, he was given a rest after a few overs, and showed his displeasure by immediately leaving the field. It was very difficult to get him to discuss the position; he maintained the attitude that he was being unlawfully detained, and he was inclined to threaten various penalties which would befall if he was not liberated at once.

In 1935 his intellectual level was noted as being well preserved. He was an ardent student of philosophy, with a particular interest in searching for a rational explanation of supernatural phenomena. This was, probably, motivated by his desire to find an explanation for the forces which he believed were stealing his thoughts, using his knowledge and implanting evil into his mind. He had periodic outbursts, with very little accompanying affect, in which he protested against this interference.

CASE No. 41

This patient had been to all appearances a very normal woman, with wide interests, but in one direction there was a very important suggestion of abnormality—she delayed marriage as long as possible, there were no children and her attitude to men was betrayed in the remark about 'beastliness'. Furthermore, she had a very strong attachment to her sister. It is not therefore without significance that her psychosis followed soon after the death of her husband in tragic circumstances, and that the first evidences of a change in her mental condition were in the nature of over-compensations for her failings in married life, in the special form of morbidly exaggerated regard for the views of her dead husband. Her delusional trends seem to point much more to a projection of heterosexual tendencies (which she consciously abhorred) than of homosexual ones. Her early antagonism to her father is of interest, but no direct light was cast upon it.

A widow, 39 years, was admitted to hospital in 1925.

There was no history of nervous or mental disease in her family. At the time of her birth there was some difficulty, and instruments were used, but she walked and talked at the ordinary age, and developed normally. As a child she took a violent dislike to her father, and the family butler was the only person who could do much with her. The dislike of her father passed as she grew older, but from time to time she has brought up reminiscences of her antagonism to him, saying, for example, 'You remember when I was 3, I was able to cope with my father'. She received a good education and was very intelligent. Learning was easy to her, and she took prizes in literature, history and painting. She was an excellent sportswoman, played cricket and hockey, rode and was in every way interested in outside things. Among her associates she was most popular, and of the 'leader' type.

In 1915 she married, but her husband died in 1920 from a haemorrhage from the lungs. He died very suddenly; his end was rather a terrible one. She was greatly upset by it and did not resume her ordinary activities for about a year. She gradually readjusted herself, and returned to live with her mother and her sister, but the memory of her husband was kept always very much in the forefront. Everything she did was 'what he would want', and she brought his name into everything.

Her sister described her as having 'a very angelic nature, with not a selfish drop in her body. She would do anything for anybody, and always was most generous.' The patient and her sister did things together, and they were always happiest when the other was about. The patient was extremely capable in household matters, and had varied interests, meeting people, attending sports meetings, hunting, dancing and so on. She had many male admirers, and 'could have married half a dozen times if she had liked', but marriage did not appeal to her. She had known her husband for about fifteen years, and for about ten years there had been some sort of understanding, but she could not bring herself to marry. She never looked at any other man. Probably the actual facts of marriage were abhorrent to her, and she used the expression 'men are horrible'. It is doubtful whether marital relations were satisfactory; certainly there were no children.

About two years before her admission she began to change very definitely. One incident was as follows: Her sister had arranged to play golf on a certain day with a friend, and told the patient so, but added that she would put the match off if the patient cared. The patient would not hear of this, said that if her sister did put it off that she would not play anyway. Later, however, she said that her sister had arranged this other match deliberately so that she could not play with her. This was the first abnormal incident, but after this she began to state that people seemed to be either too interested in her, or were avoiding her. A number of incidents referred to a certain gentleman in the county, whom she sometimes referred to as 'the toad', and sometimes 'the comedian'. She seemed to believe that this man wanted to marry her. The patient also declared that this man was instigating people, and influencing them to do all sorts of annoying things to her deliberately, so as to make her 'give in'. At first it seemed to be people outside the family, but her mother and her sister did not agree with her ideas, so she turned against them, and stated that they also were in league with this man. She reviled them for thinking that she would ever deign to marry such a man. Her own husband had been extraordinarily handsome: this man was not, and in addition, he sang comic songs—hence the name 'the comedian'. She began to declare that all sorts of things were done to annoy her, e.g. her car suddenly stopped with a stuck valve—this was done deliberately. She also imagined that she was being followed. When she went to a hotel where her husband and herself had been in the habit of staying, she declared that her sister knew the room she was in and tampered with it. Whenever she went to the bank, her sister seemed to know of it. Her pullets, which she had ordered from England, were changed on the journey. She had a severe attack of illness, with vomiting and diarrhoea, and she declared that either her sister or the butler had tried to poison her.

There was no evidence of any hallucinations at any time. About six months previous to her admission she began to display another sort of trend. She stated that she had been asked to help a woman in the village who was pregnant, and ventilated the idea that there were several women in the same condition, and that the man who was responsible for annoying her was also chiefly responsible for the condition of these women. Even her own niece was implicated in this. On one occasion she found her niece reading from the Bible, 'Unto thee a child will be born', and the patient asked, in a sarcastic tone, how the niece was getting on, and why her niece did not marry this man.

It was so difficult to deal with her under home conditions that she was certified.

The medical certificates described her as talkative and domineering and suffering from delusions of persecution, stating that 'a comedian' who lived in the neighbourhood influenced her mother, sister, servants and everyone against her; that in churches the clergy preached their sermons in reference to her, and the newspapers wrote articles concerning her. She also believed that her mother and her sister were plotting against her, and were thwarting her in all her actions. She believed that people turned to look at her and laugh at her in the streets, and on several occasions she actually accused her mother and her sister of giving her poisoned food.

At the time of her admission to hospital she was extremely resentful. She stated that there was no cause whatsoever for her having been brought, that the incidents which had been annoying her had actually happened, that she would have been insane if she had not spoken about them and that she believed that they had been done deliberately at the instance of some person or persons. She stated that her being brought to hospital was a good indication of the criminal intentions of her mother and sister. She stated that she did not care what happened now, that she was prepared to remain until Doomsday and that it was not the smallest use attempting to discuss matters. She spoke rapidly and diffusely, showing an extraordinarily well-preserved memory for all sorts of small happenings, which she told with great circumstantiality. There were times during the interview when she became emotional, but, under the circumstances, her affect was not unnatural, and was in keeping with the painful topics she was discussing, particularly the matter of her husband's death. She began by stating that everything connected with the death of her husband was 'sanctified', an expression which she used several times throughout the interview. She related that after his death she had received certain extraordinary letters, and mentioned two—one which she received about ten days after her husband's death, in which she was called by her Christian name. The other contained an 'extraordinary' remark or word which struck her as being most indelicate and inappropriate, and that letter she burned. (Her husband had taken ill very suddenly, and he had been laughing and joking a few minutes before his death, and died practically in the arms of the patient within a few minutes.)

Regarding the golf episode mentioned by the informant, she explained that the course was specially sacred to her because of her husband's memory. After the golf episode, she said, the same sort of thing happened constantly. No one seemed to ask her to join with them in their activities, whereas formerly she had always been asked to everything. If the patient chanced to ask them to play, they would always give ridiculous reasons for not doing so. On one occasion she asked a lady to play in a certain match, but in return the lady lost her head and wrote an extraordinary letter saying why she could not do so. The patient said that people used to laugh when she went about in her black clothes. She referred to the arrival of a new butler, who behaved 'in the most strange way'. On one occasion particularly, he put red paint over the pantry floor, and paint seemed also to be sticking to his clothes. This incident was related somehow to her husband's death. The butler sat down in front of the fire deliberately when she came into the dining-room, and at another time he sat down also in her presence. She considered that these acts were done specially to annoy her. Her car, too, was interfered with. Such incidents took place more frequently when her mother and sister were away from home, so that she grew to expect trouble whenever they left, and the annoyances occurred particularly on anniversaries and special days—Saturdays (the day of her husband's death), the date of her marriage and so on. These happenings were not confined to her home. On one occasion when she went to a neighbouring city, she had hardly arrived when an extraordinary old woman came up to her and seemed to follow her around, and tried to talk. When the patient returned home, she found that a new housemaid had been installed, and either the new housemaid was the old lady herself or a very near relative, because 'they were the image of each other'. While she had been away, she was quite certain that articles in her room were tampered with, so that she had to lock the door. On another occasion when she had gone to a servants' registry, which she had used for many years, she was treated quite differently from former occasions. She wanted a housemaid, but, instead of being given the names of housemaids, she was given the names of children's nurses, and was actually asked whether she wanted a maternity nurse. 'There was much talk of perambulators and babies, and one woman was carrying a baby.' She could not believe that such incidents as these were accidental.

In contrast to these delusional ideas, her memory and her general intellectual functions were well retained.

Physically she was in very good general health.

After her admission her condition continued unchanged. To the staff generally she was very pleasant, but maintained the attitude that she had been declared to be insane, that she had been put in an asylum and that she would remain there for the rest of her days. Under this surface equanimity there was a very bitter resentment against the whole situation. An idea of her bitterness and sarcasm may be obtained from a letter which she wrote to her mother, in which she says—'Of course I am not writing *you* as you deserve. I shall not do that just yet. I suppose you all realize that you belong to a *criminal* organization, which in the list of crimes is only about two removed from murder. How long is this abnormal pantomime and criminal act going on for? I shall stay here till I die, and never change my opinions; but it only makes it all so easy for me just now, and shows how right I was in my opinions, which are consolidated in every way by everyone.' She related various other episodes, and particularly mentioned an incident when, in a moment of irritability, she had thrown her shoe at a door behind which her sister was. She stated that her sister accused her of trying to shoot her with a revolver. A few days after this incident a policeman's revolver was found in the garage, and then on the following Sunday there was a sermon which had some reference to these episodes. She felt sure that, instead of her mind being abnormal, there must have been an abnormal mind that was ordering these things to be done—for instance, having the wheels of the car turned the wrong way in the garage, her relatives not replying to a gift of chickens and the doctor not making any remarks when he won a prize which the patient had presented at a charity sale.

After entering hospital also, she expressed very definite ideas of reference. One day, while she was having a bath, the plumber came to the ward to do certain repairs. The nurse went to the bathroom door with him. The nurse opened the door to see whether it was possible for the plumber to go in, but when she saw the patient there she immediately shut the door and went away. The patient, however, got a glimpse of the plumber, although the plumber did not see her, and she immediately thought that this incident was on a par with the incidents which had happened at home, and that it was done deliberately to annoy her. She also believed that the other patients knew all about her affairs, and that they had been instructed by the Medical Superintendent to make things difficult for her. When visited by her mother and sister, she at first refused to see them. When she did see them she accused them of having been responsible for her present position, and said that she would not do anything unless they gave her a complete and full apology, and explained to her why all these abnormal actions had taken place.

A further attempt was made to get a more detailed description from her, but she was evasive and averse to discussing her illness.

She related how her persecution had seemed to start about six months after her husband's death, how she had received certain letters which she had resented and how the person termed 'the toad' and 'the comedian' was probably responsible for this. She said, 'Who murdered the Rhode Island cock? Who prevented my sister from playing golf with me? Why did I have a period of sickness, with perspiration and diarrhoea? Why did the butler sit on the sofa when the daughter of the house went into the room? I am a person who cannot be upset unless I am given frightfully strong medicine.' She recalled events in regard to the maids, said that the servants had been perfectly appalling, that they had all been put into the house for certain purposes, that the matter had been arranged from the very beginning and that the family were suggesting things. 'Why was the big bacon slicer covered with red paint? It was only done to frighten me. Why was it that they all said that the old gardener was going off his head? It was only an indirect hit at me.'

CASE No. 42

This patient was originally regarded as a paranoid schizophrenic, but since deterioration has progressed little or not at all, he is now classed among the paranoiacs. Kraepelin would probably have regarded him as a paraphrenic (especially in view of the hallucinations).

He was of the quiet, dreamy, intellectual type, but very capable nevertheless in practical matters.

The onset of the psychosis followed a combination of severe infections. The loss of his government post was probably the result of the psychotic development (although details are lacking), but it certainly contributed to his persecuted attitude, since he had no insight for his condition, and regarded his dismissal as an injustice. At first his paranoid trends were comparatively localized, and referred chiefly to his wife's identity, and to the injustice of his dismissal; but they have gradually diffused themselves, partly as a means of rationalizing his position. Although his attitude to his wife was one of repudiation, he showed strong heterosexual interests during his illness, so strong that his parole had to be withdrawn. Some ruminations on sodomy were evident, but their significance is doubtful.

X

The dilapidation of his reasoning in some directions is in striking contrast to its pre-servation in others, and to his very intellectual activities (dictionary making).

An official in the Civil Service, 47 years old, he was admitted in 1920.

His family history was described as negative.

The patient had been a healthy child; he had developed normally, was always a very keen student, quiet, dreamy, clever, never much of a mixer. He had a career of great distinction at both his universities and in his profession. He married when 32 years old, and there was one child.

In 1909, while abroad, he had nephritis, malaria and typhoid, and was delirious. He was given six months' leave of absence, and the news was broken to him that he must retire. He did not see the necessity for this, consulted lawyers, entered into litigation and spent a great deal of money in trying to reinstate himself. He developed the idea that his wife was antagonistic to him. All this resulted in his being committed to a local mental hospital in 1917.

In 1919 he was sent home, and on account of his mental symptoms was certified and sent to hospital. At the time of his admission he was quiet, agreeable and co-operative. He said that he had no particular complaint and that he felt perfectly fit. He was correctly orientated for time and place: his memory was excellent in every way. All questions were answered clearly and relevantly, and he was able to give a fair account of the onset and development of his illness. He stated that he did not know why he had been taken to a mental hospital, and that he had been retired from a position of high responsibility without any definite reason being assigned. After he had been retired, he constantly wrote to the government asking them for their reasons. In con-sequence of this the government got 'ratty' and ordered the doctors to put him in the asylum. He said that the doctors declared he was suffering from hallucinations and delusions of persecution, but he denied that he had ever suffered in any such way, and said that the government had simply become tired of his persistence and had him incarcerated. He felt, too, that someone must have spread a story about the poor state of his physical health.

In 1920 he left his brother and took rooms in Glasgow. After he had been a few days in residence his landlady asked him to leave, but this he refused to do without receiving a week's notice. His landlady then asked him if he had heard a noise during the night. He admitted that he had, that he had got out of bed and had gone to his sitting-room, as he thought he had heard someone saying, 'I bought a ham at Cooper's'. It was suspected that he was suffering from a mental illness, doctors were called in and he was certified as being of unsound mind.

The striking feature was that he accepted the situation in which he found himself with a certain amount of apathy, showing a lack of aggressiveness. He was in good general physical health, and there was no evidence of any organic lesion.

Following his admission, he adapted himself well, but he readily expressed delusional ideas. He stated, for instance, that his wife was not the woman to whom he had been engaged, and he was certain that his wife must have taken this other girl's name and have substituted her. This idea gradually became more and more elaborate, so that he now maintained that his wife had not merely been substituted, but that she was dead, and that the girl who said she was his daughter was not so. He kept himself well em-ployed, spent a great deal of his time translating foreign works and in compiling an Arabic dictionary. Every now and again he complained about his incarceration, failed to see that he should be kept any longer in the institution and asked for his discharge.

In September 1921 a detailed examination was made. He asserted that his incarcera-tion in the hospital was illegal, and to support his claim he produced the Lunacy (English) Act of 1857, and pointed to the definition of a lunatic, saying that the 'or's' in it, as in all legal documents, were not disjunctive, but introduced simply limiting clauses. He supported this by reference to his will, where a list of possessions was given without any intervening conjunctions, and said that in this case the terms could be construed as equivalent. The view was also advocated by him that in the law of England a person could be detained in an asylum only if he were dangerous or wandering at large. He explained how, when he had acted as a magistrate himself, and when the patient brought before him was unable to give his name, he classified him as being insane, and therewith committed him; but if he gave his name correctly, then he said, 'The man is sane; I cannot grant a warrant'. This type of reasoning seemed to indicate a state of mental deterioration, but he was clear and correct in his general contention that there are certain types of mental disorder, amounting to actual insanity, which cannot legally be detained in a mental hospital. He believed that his own case was in this category. He stated also that a reference had been made to the specific gravity of his urine, and he wished to know the meaning of the word 'specific'. He seemed to think it related to syphilis, and that there were pathognomonic changes in the urine in syphilis.

For a long time it was possible to give him parole, but on several occasions it had to be stopped, owing to his paying particular attention to one of the female patients. When spoken to about this, on one occasion he stated that he had proposed marriage to her, and at another time that he was married to her. He further alleged that the lady was not whom she purported to be. This difficulty recurred from time to time, but the patient's delusional system increased, so that he stated that he was in hospital to investigate conditions in the institution. He rationalized his talking to the other patients by saying that it was his business to talk to them, and to straighten out any difficulties they may have had, and that it was his duty to investigate the mental state of the patients in the institution. He explained, furthermore, that no one could be kept in an institution unless a crime had been committed. He believed that all the patients had committed crimes of various natures. One patient, he said, had stolen his yacht; others were guilty of murder, and he was sure some were forgers. He also declared that patients were sent from mental hospitals to the colonies, and that Southern Nigeria acted as an outlet for certain of the parochial institutions. When his own illness was discussed with him, he said that he had been in an institution abroad and had been accused of sodomy with native boys, but he entered a total denial of this crime, saying that he had been confined without a proper trial. In further explanation, he said that a high official had been accused of sodomy with English boys, and this matter had been reported to the patient, but he had not had time to inquire into it. In order to shield himself, this high official had therefore ordered that the patient should be accused of the crime, and should be confined in a mental hospital. Various magistrates had been 'substituted' at his trial.

He did not believe that such things as auditory hallucinations existed; a person could not hear a voice without the organ of hearing being stimulated. When told that patients did complain at times of hearing voices, the patient immediately remarked, 'Oh, that's dementia praecox. The person is confessing to the doctor that he is suffering from dementia praecox, and that he should be confined in an asylum.'

This patient is still in many respects very well preserved. He is perfectly polite, careful in regard to his dress and in regard to his general cleanliness. He now believes that his being in hospital is probably a result of misidentification. He elaborates the idea of his wife's death (which is a delusion), and states that she died on his estate in a certain county in England, and that his estate is at present being managed for him.

His general physical health is very good.

CASE No. 43

In another patient there was no evidence of inherent predisposition, either in the family history or in the personal make-up. A 'complex' of very long standing seemed to be the underlying cause—the memory of her husband's unfaithfulness, and the hurt he had done her many years before, had been accompanied (judging from the content of her psychosis) by a good deal of vengeful rumination, in which she had fancied herself unfaithful in her turn. Her illness began at a period of life when repressions are apt to fail, and the repressed material blossoms forth more or less indirectly as symptoms. Not all the paranoid developments occurring at this age are as completely elaborated as this one was.

Symptomatically, the following case shows some common symbolizations of sex feelings —'electricity' and feelings of influence of various kinds. The paranoid trends are to be considered largely as projections of illegitimate heterosexual fancies.

This patient was 52 years old, and was admitted in 1923. There was no history of nervous or mental disease in her family. The patient married when she was 18.

She was supposed to have been a very healthy child, and to have developed normally. She had five children. The second was still-born, the remaining four were alive and well.

Her husband stated that she had been a most capable woman. He always considered her 'a bit better than himself', and she was the leader of the household, though never domineering. Her interests were centred in her home and in her family. She was sociable, a good hostess, even-tempered and met her difficulties courageously. She was well read, and interested in affairs generally.

Her present illness was stated to have begun six years previous to her admission. At that time, while on holiday, a room in the house in which they were staying was kept locked. The patient complained that she thought there was someone in the room who came out when they had left the house and examined their property. At the same time she told her husband that she was certain that some man was following her. Her husband investigated this, and found that there was no foundation for her belief. She stated that she could not stay in the house any longer, and returned home after a fortnight, having intended to stay one month. On her arrival home she at once complained that the house was in a filthy condition. This was not true. She began to accuse her husband of allowing people to come into the house 'to show off the dirt', and so induce people to believe that she was not doing her duty. She also stated that she was certain that her husband had men in the attic of the house who influenced her by X-rays in order to prove her immoral. About the same time a young woman visited the house as a collector for a bazaar. When her husband returned home the same evening he was challenged with keeping company with this woman, whom he had never seen. She was told that her ideas were imaginary, that she was suffering from delusions, but in reply she stated that her husband was trying to make her out a lunatic, and when the law of divorcement for lunatics was introduced, that he would then marry this girl. She refused to allow her husband to leave the house in the evenings; she accused him of making signs to his agents, the X-ray operators, to influence her. She changed in her disposition, became irritable and in fits of temper she struck several members of her family. A doctor was called in to see her, but he was informed that he was an agent employed by her husband to make her do things in order that her husband might get rid of her. She complained of the noise of the traffic, and said that the noise was made at her husband's desire, to annoy her.

At the time of her admission she denounced her husband for having brought her to such a place, saying that he would never be forgiven, and that there was no justification for it. Later she said that it had been a great shock to her, that her husband had exaggerated her illness in order to get rid of her and that he would live to regret it. She said that she had been annoyed and worried because electric sensations had been entering her body, and that she had seemed to see twinkling lights and shades in her own house, and also in the doctor's house, which was not far away. These phenomena were all produced by agents, unknown to her, but probably employed by her husband or by the church. The motive was to make her do and say things in order to make people believe that she had delusions, so that she could be put away by her husband. She stated that two years previous to her admission, she had had a quarrel with her husband, during which she had told him that he should give up his eldership in the church, as he was not good enough to hold it. He agreed to do this. Later on, in the same year, she had gone to stay with friends, and while there a gentleman in the house told her about a woman whom the patient identified with herself. This woman had had suspicions of her husband, and the description of her family and her household surroundings corresponded so closely with those of the patient that the patient became convinced that she was the woman referred to, and that this gentleman must have got all his information from her church people. She began to notice now that people in the street seemed to know about her domestic affairs and were talking about her; her husband, she thought, must be spreading tales broadcast. Later she was convinced that an agency was formed to influence her, in order to make her appear to be suffering from delusions, so that her husband could get a divorce and marry again; he exaggerated her illness to such an extent that there could be no other motive. She also became convinced that the family doctor was in her husband's employment. She spoke quite clearly and connectedly, and had an excellent appreciation of time and place and those around her. Her memory, both for recent and remote events, was excellent, and her power of retention, her grasp of general information and her memory for school events were all very well maintained.

Physically she was a stout woman, in good general health.

Following her admission, she requested an interview with the physician, and stated that she had neglected to tell him that when she was pregnant with her second child she suffered from venereal disease, for which she blamed her husband at the time. There was no evidence of hallucinosis at the time of her admission, and she denied that she had ever heard voices. She described her condition somewhat as follows: 'At times it seems as if words were being put into my head, as if I was being the mouthpiece of somebody else. I will tell you the sort of feelings I have had. I have had different experiences: I have had the feeling of being almost benumbed—like catching the handle of a galvanic battery—I have had other experiences of something that makes my pulse beat faster. Perhaps I would be in the middle of something, when suddenly there was something like a stop put into my head, and things forgotten would come back, songs perhaps, or even conveying some message to me.'

When asked if she had ever heard anything that sounded like a voice, she said, 'No, I have never heard a voice at all; but I gave utterance to things; in regard to the church —I have been the friend of the church, and I have been religiously inclined all my life, and yet I have spoken and said terrible things about the church while that particular thing was on me. I acted under influence. I have no tendency now to swear as I did before, a thing that used to make me shudder. Once or twice the electric forces worked on me since I came, but nothing like to the same extent.'

During her residence in the hospital her condition showed considerable progress. She was very well preserved in her general mentality, but she was now constantly dominated by auditory hallucinations. Often she could be heard talking and shouting in her room, in response to them. She would not go out into the grounds by herself because she felt that everybody was talking about her and making remarks about her, and she continued to believe that she was being persecuted by X-rays. In addition, she felt that she was being watched at all times, even when she was in her own room. She felt that it may be all on the basis of jealousy. She had been so tormented that on occasions she had refused to sleep in her room, and for a time refused to go to bed. She was certain that if she did so she would be interfered with when she was asleep. A sample of her talk is as follows:

'There is going to be no insane certificate for me. It is M——, N—— and Company who are doing this. I am only claiming my legal rights to leave the institution. My husband has been paying for me, but N—— puts it all in his pocket. It is thousands of pounds they are swindling. I would not have a medical man made a criminal to save me. I should have been home long ago. M—— and N—— have called me a forger, a prostitute, and I am a highly respectable lady. Please sign my letter of clearance from the institution. Would you believe what N—— had the audacity to say to me, "Would you, for a piece of money, allow M—— to commit adultery with you?" I would never sell my honour to anyone.'

Her condition showed no improvement.

Case No. 44

In this patient the paranoid development occurred late in life (at age 58). The significant points are the patient's personality—ambitious, sensitive and suspicious; and the origin of the condition in a very definite event—the failure of a cherished ambition. This case furnishes a very apt illustration of the psychogenesis of certain paranoid psychoses, as described by Bleuler.

G. H., a married woman, 58 years old, was admitted to hospital in 1921.

Both her father and mother were stated to have been alcoholic.

The patient had six brothers and sisters.

Her early life was a somewhat hard one, because her parents neglected her. She received a good schooling, however, and after leaving school worked as a dressmaker. She married comparatively late in life, when she was about 40 years old. There were no children. Her husband described her as being naturally ambitious, anxious to climb socially, of rather a suspicious cast of mind, 'apt to put two and two together very quickly', and to read meanings into things. She was sensitive, and apt to apply remarks to herself which were not intended for her.

She was stated to have been well until about six months previous to her admission. Two years before her admission she had suffered a serious disappointment, having failed to inherit from a millionaire relative a large sum of money which she had expected. In 1921 her brother, who was a trustee of the estate, told her quite definitely that nothing had been left to her. She felt that a gross injustice had been done her, and began to speak of taking legal action. A few months later she became definitely suspicious. She began to think that someone must have been slandering her reputation, so that she was kept out of the estate on the plea that she would be unable to manage it. She gradually elaborated this idea. First she became suspicious of her brother-in-law, then of her relatives in general and finally of her husband. She began to pour out her troubles to various friends, and even to the clergyman. She imagined that people would come in the night and take her away. She accused her husband of throwing dirty linen out of the house to expose her, so as to damage her reputation, and of spreading stories that she was addicted to drink. Her husband stated that she had not been in the habit of taking alcohol at all. Three weeks previous to her admission she began to believe that another millionaire had left her a large sum of money, and she called on various people to see what could be done about it.

At the time of her admission to hospital she was in excellent physical health, and there was no suspicion of any organic disease. She stated that she had been in a highly nervous state, that she was in need of a rest and had decided to come voluntarily. She spoke about her ideas quite freely, stating that she was certain that her husband and others had been working against her, that she had been left a large sum of money and an estate, that the money had actually been deposited in a certain bank, but that for some reason or other she was denied access to it. She declared that her husband was spreading tales about her to the effect that she was dissolute and immoral, that he was hand and glove with a man called Brown, a publican, and that these stories were spread with the idea of damaging her reputation, so that she would not be considered fit to receive the money left to her. When she was in Edinburgh, and walked in the Gardens there, she saw a woman talking to one of the gardeners. The woman lifted her elbow as the patient passed. The latter interpreted this act as an indication that the woman was signalling that she (the patient) drank.

After a month's residence she stated that she did not feel that she could stay any longer, and she was discharged.

Four months later she was readmitted under medical certificates. After she left the hospital, she stayed quietly at home for a fortnight; then she engaged a room in a hydropathic establishment, and remained there for a period of five weeks. She then went back to her own home, arriving late one night, and for some time after she behaved in a most extravagant way. She ran up bills with tradespeople and for motorcars, and began to express ideas of grandeur, saying that she was the laird of a vast estate, that her husband was bound to give her £5000 a year and that she would see that she got justice.

When she was brought to the hospital she was in an angry mood, saying that there was no reason why such an action should have been taken, that it was gross injustice and that she protested very strongly against it.

During this second admission her ideas of grandeur became even more marked, and were freely expressed. She maintained that she had estates, that she was a millionairess and that she was being kept out of her money and her estates by certain financial trusts. She claimed Mary Queen of Scots and King David of Scotland among her relatives.

A good idea of her condition may be obtained from one of her letters:

'I claim the privilege of a private citizen. After two years of annoyance, my house open to ladies and gentlemen, everything inspected by them, drawers opened, letters read, garments displayed, fun made of them, the most private relations of home life, I have been tracked both outside, and watched in my home, by land and sea. Men have been engaged to traduce my kith and kin, because of the inheritance which is the dowry belonging to the heirs of Queen Mary and King David, grandson of Robert the Bruce. Everything has been done to disgrace me. I was brought here by force, and am kept until the inheritance is divided.'

Her personality was well maintained. She was always most careful about her appearance. Her antagonism to her detention was undiminished, and her grandiose ideas went on increasing steadily. When she began to talk about them she became slightly incoherent, but her ordinary conversation did not show this.

AETIOLOGY

It is probable that the causation of paranoid conditions is due to a constellation of factors of a constitutional and environmental nature. Very similar symptoms, all with the general stamp of a paranoid psychosis, are capable of arising on the basis of factors which differ greatly in their relative importance in individual instances. The personality-type is one of the most potent predisposing elements. The sensitive, suspicious, jealous, ambitious person; the shy, prudish, dreamy and impractical; and the selfish, vain type were all represented in our case material. It must, however, be recognized that in some cases no suggestive personality traits can be disclosed. Another significant feature is the frequency of a 'complex' with a very strong affective component, e.g. a history of venereal infection accompanied by shame, guilt and self-consciousness. When a person is so involved then the effect of some innocent and trifling incident may be profound. Memories and former associations are re-lighted, e.g. the routine visit of a policeman to a man who had long cherished in secret his shame of venereal infection. Conversely, in cases dating from such an incident it is nearly always possible to trace a particular predisposition, either of the total personality, or in the form of some more localized 'complex'. We do not believe that homo-sexuality, in the aetiology of a paranoid psychosis, is so widespread or so specific as the psychoanalytic school would have us believe. It seemed, however, to be predominant in four out of a group of eleven cases. The remainder were prepon-derantly heterosexual, judged both by their ordinary lives and by the content of their delusions. Homosexuality appears to act largely as other causes of social difficulty or ostracism do—by producing feelings of inferiority or actual guilt; it can however act, in the manner Freud described, by being repressed and projected on individuals in the immediate environment. Feelings of influence may represent equally the projection either of homosexual or heterosexual feelings.

In the genesis of paranoid states the rôle of inferiority feelings, on whatever ground, is considerable. This sense of inferiority may be the result of disap-pointment in inflated ambition, or it may be associated with guilt feelings, auto-, hetero-, or homosexual in origin. In any case, the resulting paranoid develop-ment consists first in ideas of reference, and then delusions of persecution. A sense of superiority, or at least a striving for it, may exist concurrently, and leads eventually to grandiose delusions. Not less important than feelings of inferiority, guilt and superiority are wishes which may or may not have been repressed. These wishes are either sexual or social—for wealth and position. The sexual desires being of a forbidden kind (heterosexual in woman, and usually homosexual in men) have been repressed, but are now projected as delusions of persecution, or as phantastic delusions of marriage to important personages. The persecutory types of sexual delusion seem to be more common in men (homo-sexual), and the frank, wish-fulfilling type more common in women. Projected heterosexual trends were plainly evident in four out of five female paranoid states, two of them wish-fulfilling in nature.

The sources of secondary elaboration of the delusion, especially the develop-ment of grandiose trends concurrently with or after persecutory ones, are mul-tiple—the affect of the original complex continues to operate; more or less logical influence is brought to bear on phenomena observed under the influence of the first factor; and the compensatory superiority feelings sometimes present in great force produce flattering rationalizations. The sequence, delusions of persecution and delusions of grandeur, in that order, is usual. One does not see the reverse order, although sometimes the development of the two delusional trends seems to be concurrent.

Amphetamine intoxication may be responsible for precipitating an acute paranoid reaction, which can be quickly diagnosed by the methyl-orange test [see page 369].

PROGNOSIS

The prognosis of well-established systematized delusional states is extremely serious. It is very seldom that such cases ever make an adequate, or satisfactory, adjustment irrespective of any form of treatment which may be employed. A person so affected believes that he is right, that he is justified in his beliefs, and that anyone who opposes his point of view is behaving maliciously or at least non-understandingly towards him.

There are, however, lesser states, conditions where the delusional ideas are not so firmly established, and where the affective element is powerful. A considerable number of such cases are transitory in nature, are developed often in reference to certain specific situations and subside when such situations are no longer present. These cases are of more acute onset, are more environmentally than constitutionally conditioned, and in consequence we expect a fair number of them to make a reasonable recovery. A number need never be admitted to a mental hospital because they will co-operate very well on an out-patient basis. It is impossible to lay down any hard-and-fast statement as to how long recovery may take; it depends on the insight and understanding of the patient, and on the skill of the therapist.

TREATMENT

The desirability of arranging for admission to a mental hospital is determined not only by the degree to which their delusional beliefs lead them into conduct producing discomfort and loss to themselves or into antisocial activities, whether these be in the nature of homicidal attempts or simply of annoyances to others by accusations, petty litigation or what not. They almost invariably refuse to go to hospital voluntarily, and to effect compulsory admission is not easy. But circumstances arise when mental hospital treatment becomes imperative, and indeed may be the only way in which some form of treatment may be carried out. As a preliminary it is essential to have a detailed and thorough study of the patient's life-history, as this may establish a basis of co-operation, and may win the patient's confidence. The skilful preparation of the ground may enable the physician to enter into explanation, persuasion and analysis with some hope of a result sufficient to enable the patient to be a useful, if still not at all a normal, member of society. The cases, however, which are completely established are not susceptible of therapeutic success, and can only be regarded as extremely disappointing. This is greatly to be regretted because, apart from the delusional formation, the general intellectual and emotional faculties remain intact. In the less firmly systematized cases, with a strong affective component, readjustment can be effected; the use of chlorpromazine and electric convulsion therapy may prove to be valuable aids.

REFERENCES

Bleuler, E. (1912) *Affectivity, Suggestibility, and Paranoia, State Hosp. Bull.*, New York.
Ferenczi, S. (1916) *Contributions to Psychoanalysis*, Boston.
Freud, S. (1911) *Collected Papers*, Vol. 3, 287, London.
Gierlich, N., and Friedmann, M. (1908) Studies in Paranoia, *Nervous and Mental Disease Monograph Series*, No. 2, New York.
Meyer, A. (1951) *The Collected Papers*, Vol. 2, 523, Baltimore.

13

PSYCHOPATHIC STATES

In Chapter 21 it will be noted that the Mental Health (England and Wales) Act, 1959, has differentiated four groups of mentally disordered persons. Psychopathic states form one of those groups. The official definition describes them as 'persistent disorders of mind (whether or not accompanied by subnormality of intelligence) which result in abnormally aggressive or seriously irresponsible conduct on the part of the patients, and require or are susceptible to medical treatment'. That definition may not prove acceptable to everyone, but it has the merit of providing a useful working basis whereby a large number of mentally abnormal persons can become more clearly delineated. It is to be deplored that the Mental Health (Scotland) Act, 1960, has, in the meantime, not accorded it statutory recognition.

We include under the above title persons who have been from childhood or early youth habitually abnormal in their emotional reactions and conduct, but who do not reach, except episodically, a degree of abnormality requiring compulsory detention; they show no intellectual defect, as measured by the usual intelligence tests, and therefore cannot legally be classified as subnormal (mentally defective); and they do not benefit under prison treatment. They are not sufficiently well-balanced mentally to be at large, nor yet are they sufficiently involved as to be suitable for mental hospital care. They have never seemed to be the particular province of anyone, and in consequence they have often been knocked about from pillar to post with no satisfaction to those looking after them and with no benefit to themselves. And yet they are desperately in need of help, of guidance, of encouragement, and the psychiatrist should be better qualified to assist them than anyone else. It is in their homes, in their schools, their factories and workshops that they should be studied and dealt with rather than under hospital conditions. To deal with them successfully requires the co-operation of all persons interested in the problem of human betterment.

Let us attempt a further description: They constitute a rebellious, individualistic group who fail to fit in to their social *milieu*, and whose emotional instability is largely determined by a state of psychological immaturity which prevents them from adapting to reality and profiting from experience. They may be adult in years, but emotionally they are so slow and backward and uncontrolled that they behave like dangerous children. They lack judgement, foresight and ordinary prudence. It is the sheer stupidity of their conduct which is so appalling. 'The judicial, deciding, selecting processes described as intelligence, and the energizing, emotivating, driving powers called character' do not work in harmony. They are the misfits of society, the despair of parents, doctors, ministers, lawyers and social workers. It is probably social workers more than any others who are impressed by the complexities of such cases, and by the difficulty in placing them in satisfactory employment. It is hoped, however, now that so much more attention has been directed to them that they will receive more skilful attention and understanding. They constitute a challenge to preventive medicine, and make us aware, not only of the necessity of ensuring that children will be born healthy but also of doing everything possible to improve the environmental conditions, so that the stability of family life can be ensured.

In 1835 J. C. Prichard, a Bristol physician, under the title of 'moral insanity' and 'moral imbecility' described a series of cases which may be taken as the prototypes of the psychopathic state as we know it to-day. The term 'moral imbecility' was incorporated and defined in the Mental Deficiency Act, 1913, but we consider it advisable to remove it from that classification altogether, and to make a clear distinction between states of intellectual and so-called moral defect. Prichard made the position abundantly clear when he wrote: 'There are many people suffering from a form of mental derangement in whom the moral and active principles of the mind are strongly perverted or depraved; the power of self-government is lost or greatly impaired, and the individual is found incapable, not of talking or reasoning on any subject proposed to him, but of conducting himself with decency and propriety in the business of life.' While Prichard was the first person to give a systematic description of those so-called moral disorders, yet others before him, notably Pinel, Esquirol, Georget and Rush, had drawn attention to their existence, and had appreciated their significance. Then later came interesting contributions from Morel and Magnan in France; from Lombroso, Bianchi and Tanzi in Italy; and from Krafft-Ebing and Ziehen in Germany.

In 1888 Koch introduced the term psychopathic inferiority, and suggested that certain hysterical and obsessional states might be so regarded, or at least had a certain psychopathic component which might influence prognosis adversely. This conception was widened and elaborated by Kraepelin, who drew attention to the fact that a vast variety of syndromes occurred which could be described in terms of the most obvious presenting symptom, e.g. excitable, impulsive, eccentric, liars and swindlers, antisocial and quarrelsome. He further suggested that closer clinical analysis might show that the psychopathic element formed a constituent part of certain neurotic and psychotic states. During the present century the contributions of Healy, Kahn and Partridge in America, and of Birnbaum in Germany, each from their individual viewpoints, have been outstanding. While Healy and Kahn have attempted a more accurate clinical analysis and differentiation, Partridge and Birnbaum have drawn attention to the sociological implications of the group, and have suggested that the term sociopath might be more appropriate. This is not altogether a happy term, since society does not always suffer as a result of their instability; some, as will be seen, even benefit the society in which they live. For such a diverse group it is difficult to devise a satisfactory nomenclature. We feel that it is better to describe samples of the group under convenient but admittedly somewhat arbitrary headings, so as to give a foundation upon which experience may provisionally be based. It has never been easy to differentiate those cases from many of those who constitute

the prison population. It is probable that Prichard had this difficulty in mind
when he postulated 'that there is a state of mental derangement'. It may be
suggested that the disordered conduct of the psychopath is determined at a subconscious or instinctive level, in contrast to the reason and intention and free-
will which governs the conduct of the criminal. This is a matter worthy of much
more detailed consideration. In order to illustrate the general complexity of the
group the following case may be submitted:

CASE NO. 45

M. B., 24 years old, single, was a young lady of attractive appearance and address,
who came from a neurotic stock. For a long number of years this patient had been
creating a great deal of difficulty in the home, so that her brothers and sisters felt that
their mother's life was not safe. It was stated: 'Her vindictiveness is so extreme that she
is capable of anything, while, at the same time, she is so plausible and cunning that she
is able to impress all strangers that she is a persecuted saint condemned to live in a
family of criminals and savages.' A few instances of her conduct are sufficient to
describe the case. One of her brothers arrived home on leave from France to visit his
father, who was dying. She refused to sit by her father when he was ill, to prepare food
for him or to relieve those who had been constantly with him night and day. On the
contrary, she jeered at the constant 'morbid atmosphere' of the sick-room. The family
tried to induce their mother to have a nurse in the house, but she refused to do this lest
a stranger should talk outside about her daughter's conduct. She terrorized the home
for years, and drove more than one of her sisters away from home by her threats and
her violence. On another occasion when her brother came from France she did not
speak to him during the whole time he was in the house. She sat at meals with her face
turned away from him, and when he left to return to France he had to search her out
to say good-bye, and his farewell did not meet with any response. Her mother had to
sleep at night with her bedroom door locked for fear of her daughter's violence, and
she had also to lock her door by day in order to guard against thefts. The patient for
weeks on end would not speak to any member of the family, except to demand money
or clothing. It was also stated that one of her brothers, who was an apprentice engineer,
had to stand over the water which he had heated to have his wash, because if he relaxed
his vigilance the patient would take the warm water and pour it down the sink. One
day in mid-winter she threw a bucket of cold water and deluged his hens, which were
his hobby, 'just to see what he would do'. Frequently she told her mother that she
'would make her suffer'. On one occasion she walked through the house and crumbled
every gas mantle into dust. She lit all the gas jets of the gas stove, and put over them
every pot, pan and kettle the stove would hold, and then slipped quietly out of the
house. Her habit was to rise any time from 11.30 to 2 P.M. to cook a meal for herself,
and then to leave the house without a word to anyone. 'What she does, where she goes,
and who her friends are, none of us are quite sure.' Indian ornaments, sent home by
a sister, disappeared, and some Greek metal-ware which was also in the house disappeared and was discovered hidden in the commode in the patient's bedroom, awaiting
a chance to be smuggled out of the house. A brother came home unexpectedly, and
found his sister arguing with a rag-woman for the sale of his boots—his second-best
pair.

On account of the difficulties of management, she was certified as being of unsound
mind, and was admitted to hospital. During her stay in hospital she was unreliable
in every way. There were times when she was better controlled and better behaved,
but sooner or later she got into difficulty again. When found fault with, or criticized,
or restrained in any way, she had outbursts of great passion, during which it was
almost impossible to control her. She was sullen, sulky, spiteful and destructive, making

life difficult for the other patients, and even striking those who were most helpless. At other times she could be most attractive and charming, and seemed almost out of place as a patient in a mental hospital.

CAUSATION

There is no specific cause, no single traumatic event either of a psychological or physiological nature which need necessarily be present. On the other hand, in every case we require to think of a combination of hereditary and personality factors working in association with a great variety of environmental ones which may have affected the health or social circumstances of the individual. Some persons are much too prone to over-emphasize the predispositional or constitutional factors, while others pin their faith and their treatment on a modification of the obvious and difficult environmental situations. No such division is possible. The whole situation must be considered in the light of all the surrounding circumstances, and if this is done then conduct which has seemed meaningless, foolish, irrational may be capable of being more fully understood. We may then be spared the remarks of the judge who, in dealing with such a case, exclaimed: 'I am asked to show my pity to you on the ground that the documents you produced were nonsensical, that they were incredible, like documents out of *Alice in Wonderland*. I can find no excuse for all this, and I must deal with you severely. The sentence will be one of 4 years' penal servitude.' It seems incredible that the judge could not have been open-minded enough to ask for the help of someone who possibly might have been able to deal with the matter in a less arbitrary and impatient manner. We know that conduct disorder may be in the nature of an over-compensatory reaction for those things which ordinary daily life has been unable to supply, *e.g.* for poverty, broken homes, illegitimacy, etc. We also know, however, that even more intricate mechanisms may be brought into play by a disturbance of the prefrontal hypothalamic connections, by organic disorders such as encephalitis, chorea, idiopathic epilepsy, brain injury, brain tumour, or by the even more subtle metabolic and biochemical functionings associated with an involvement of the autonomic system, and imbalance of the endocrines. In all of the above instances the conduct of the individual may be so affected as to render him unfit for ordinary society owing to the transformation of his personality. He becomes governed and dominated by thoughts and feelings which are uncontrollable. That is why it is always so imperative to insist on a comprehensive medical examination being carried out in those cases where the conduct is incomprehensible, and in complete contrast to the person's real character. It should never be forgotten that intellect and emotion and character do not always go hand in hand; one may not develop any more than the other. In the case of the intellectually defective the situation can be measured and assessed, but so far no yard-stick has been devised to allow us to estimate the emotional factors in a person's make-up. 'We thus have people in our midst, semi-insane or semi-responsible, if you like to use such terms, in every walk of life from the highest social and political offices to the ranks of the unemployed and the delinquent, who not only are unable to conform adequately in their own personal lives, but may even be responsible for some of the greatest social crimes in history.'

From the point of view of psychoanalysis a number of clever, interesting and ingenuous articles have been written arguing in favour of an Oedipus situation—the endless seeking after his mother and the extermination of his father. 'He goes to Hell rejecting in a grandiose way any feelings of guilt or atonement. Very frequently he is overtly homosexual but attracts both women and men because they feel and love the child in him.' It is true that in many cases of a psychopathic type such mechanisms can be demonstrated, but the same mechanisms occur in other conditions as well and the psychoanalytic interpretations which are often so glibly suggested must still be accepted with a good deal of reserve.

The more organically minded have turned with eagerness to the investigation of the cerebral rhythm. Electroencephalographic studies have shown that 65 per cent. of aggressive psychopaths, and 32 per cent. of inadequate psychopaths, have abnormal E.E.G.s compared with 15 per cent. of normal controls (Hill and Watterson, 1942). These authors suggest that the abnormality exhibited by the E.E.G.s points to a failure in development in the central nervous system, especially as similar findings are obtained, although not invariably, in 'problem' children of the irritable, hyperactive, moody and aggressive type (Bradley, 1942).

In his more recent work Denis Hill (1952) grouped the E.E.G. patterns into two classes, those found in normal children and sensitive to the age factor, and those not found in normal children, and not sensitive to age. He believes that the first class may be associated with maturation defects in the nervous system, and the second class with processes of homeostatic regulation. In the case of episodic psychopathic or psychotic behaviour no single type of E.E.G. has been found, but in episodic catatonic schizophrenic states he noted paroxysmal patterns characterized by fast spike and wave and grouped spikes. Focal abnormality in the temporal lobes (especially posteriorly) was prominent in personality disorder with antisocial conduct.

It need only be added that E.E.G. changes are so delicately determined that their interpretation demands great skill.

In 75 criminal psychopaths, characterized either by aggressiveness and hostility, or by extreme selfishness, or by inferiority feelings and self-destructiveness, the great majority were found to have either an abnormal E.E.G. or an unsatisfactory early home life, or both (Silverman, 1943). Simons and Diethelm have reported results very similar to those mentioned above, while Brill and Walker have drawn attention to the unusually high incidence of cerebral dysrhythmia in children with severe behaviour disorders, and 'many with aggressive, impulsive, anti-social behaviour were found to have epileptic-like cortical electrical activity in the absence of any convulsive phenomena'. That last statement is important because, not infrequently, the impulsive conduct of the psychopath is closely akin to the trigger-like reaction of the epileptic.

A social factor which stands out pre-eminently in a large number of psychopathic cases is illegitimacy. In a personal study of 34 mothers of illegitimate children we found that 50 per cent. were psychopathic. Binder's analysis of 350 cases of illegitimate pregnancies showed that one-third of the mothers were nor-mal, one-sixth subnormal (mentally defective) and 50 per cent. psychopathic. It was further noted that 113 of the women were under 20 years of age; the love factor had not entered into the pregnancy, and in many cases there was hatred towards the unwanted child. It is easy to see that any inheritance of psychopathy from the mother will be reinforced by a sense of insecurity in the child, with the possible consequence of antisocial behaviour, e.g. stealing in the 'affectionless' thieves, who apparently try to compensate and revenge themselves materially for that of which they have been emotionally deprived. According to the psycho-analysts, stealing is intimately associated with lying, swindling, robbery, murders and suicide, and all such deviations can, it is believed, be explained and under-stood by a displacement of sexual desire into criminal conduct.

It is of considerable interest to draw attention to the fact that according to the criminal law of Scotland special provision and consideration is given to mothers of a psychopathic type who commit infanticide. Such persons, although they cannot be considered completely of unsound mind, are yet so affected in their reason that they are assessed as 'only partly responsible for their actions'. Under such circumstances the charge may be reduced from one of murder to culpable homicide. In the above instance the law is really taking into consideration miti-gating circumstances, and it is urged that in other types of criminal offence, e.g. assault, sexual offences, the same beneficent attitude might be more frequently practised. While the psychopath is not psychotic and not subnormal (mentally defective) in terms of intelligence, yet in many instances he shows a close ap-proximation to both of these categories, and is not so fully responsible as the average man. Under certain conditions of stress and conflict the psychopathic person is no more able to control his conduct than the paranoiac to correct his delusional beliefs.

CLINICAL GROUPS

The line to be drawn between psychopathic states as a medical problem and delinquency as a penal one is sometimes very narrow indeed, and a degree of overlapping is almost bound to take place. On some occasions, when face to face with such problems, it has been thought that the law should take its natural course, but on other occasions, when dealing with the same case, care and treat-ment under mental hospital conditions has been suggested. There are numerous delinquents who have psychopathic personalities but who are best treated and dealt with under prison conditions, and there are many psychopathic persons who may never come into conflict with the law at all. The term psychopathic state, therefore, is not to be applied indiscriminately to every type of delinquency; it should only be employed when it has acquired a degree of specificity which cannot be questioned, and it should never be advanced in a criminal court merely as a plea ad misericordiam.

There are a huge number of persons, unfortunately, who suffer from a psycho-pathic state or constitution which has often been present from their earliest days, and which has remained unaltered irrespective of all the medical and social measures which have been tried. They respond neither to kindness nor to a beating, they remain a law to themselves, show an absence of altruistic feeling and require very special consideration. The varying clinical states exhibited are almost as numerous as the persons involved, but to facilitate classification we suggest three broad groupings:

1. Predominantly aggressive.
2. Predominantly inadequate or passive.
3. Predominantly creative.

Predominantly Aggressive

Those who constitute this group exhibit disorder of conduct which may reach the highest degree of violence either directed towards themselves or others. The characteristic feature is that it is not sustained but occurs in the form of episodes of shorter or longer duration, and is followed by a period of relative calmness, often with considerable insight into the occurrence. The attack, whatever the nature of it, seems to clear the air just as an epileptic fit so frequently does. The principal clinical features of this group may be exhibited in the form of suicide, homicide, alcoholism and drug addiction, epilepsy, and sexual perversion. All of the above conditions may be part and parcel of an accompanying psychosis, but in the present instance we are considering them merely as features or symptoms of the underlying psychopathic state. A detailed investigation of the life-history will show that from an early age, and at intervals throughout their development, whether at home, school or place of employment, their conduct has given cause for alarm owing to its wayward, impulsive, violent and undependable nature. As has been explained already, this conduct may be determined on the basis of a multiplicity of factors, some of which may be entirely obvious, but its intensity and fierceness seem often to be related to feelings of hate and frustration which have their roots in the instinctive life of the individual. There is little or no pre-meditation, the action is almost in the nature of a reflex—a trigger-like reaction giving rise to the 'chance, affect and opportunity' criminals described by Asch-affenburg; there is usually a clouding of consciousness with a varying degree of amnesia. There is a coldness, a hardness, an insensibility to the feelings of others, and an absence of remorse which relates the condition to a primitive level, and exemplifies the catathymic crisis described by Hans Maier and Wertham.

While the above-described features are evident, especially in cases of suicide and homicide, yet it is the same type of impulsive, ill-adapted personality that uses alcohol or drugs, or shows epileptic phenomena or sexual perversion. The drunken bout, the unconsciousness of the epileptic, or the retreat to sex-perversion, are sometimes methods of escape from situations which for the moment have proved intolerable. They are the immature ways in which the personality attempts to evade reality. The persons who constitute this group are, obviously, a very dangerous social class, and the problem is made even more difficult by the inadequate provision for caring for them, and the difference of opinion which exists in regard to them.

CASE No. 46

A young man, 18 years old, was charged with the murder of an elderly woman, 63 years old, who had befriended him. The facts of the case were as follows:

He was an only child, whose father died when he was very young; in consequence he was over-protected and spoiled by his mother, who subsequently married again. He was a big, sturdy, ungainly youth who suffered from a stutter on account of which he had been teased. He was educated at a good school, but a report from his headmaster described him as an unsatisfactory pupil who had no interest in school work, and was probably below normal mental capacity. He left school when 15 years old, obtained work in a factory but was dismissed on account of his lack of interest. When 16 years old he was charged with 'Serious assault, robbery and lewd practices'. At that time he was considered to be strange and lacking in control; he was treated in mental observation wards, was given a course of electro-convulsion therapy and was put on probation. His probation officer eventually reported that he was deceitful, cunning, untruthful and not suitable for probation. He was again put under mental observation, was considered unfit to plead to the charge against him and was certified as of unsound mind. After a period of nine months' treatment an appeal on his behalf for an independent medical examination was granted. Two experienced and distinguished psychiatrists testified to his controlled behaviour and sanity, and in consequence he was discharged. He obtained work on board ship and was away from home for several months. On the day after he returned he committed the crime with which he was charged.

The lady whom he murdered was a friend of one of his relatives and he had known her throughout his life. While in her home he battered in her skull with a poker or other blunt instrument. So far as could be determined there was no ostensible motive for this foolish, unprovoked crime. The prisoner had a clear memory of all the events preceding and following the offence. He denied being prompted by hallucinations or delusions, and yet he acted with great violence. He could offer no explanation of why he had behaved in so impulsive a manner.

During his examination the outstanding feature was his strange, smiling, callous, unconcerned manner, and his complete nonchalance in relation to the dangerous and serious position in which he was placed. On account of this mental attitude, his lack of insight, his disordered judgement and his emotional instability, he was considered to be of unsound mind and was ordered to be detained in a criminal lunatic asylum during His Majesty's Pleasure.

The case illustrates very clearly the difficulties and dangers involved. Here was a youth with a poor school and work record who had been brought up under unsatisfactory home conditions, and who on account of his erratic conduct and unstable disposition had required care and treatment in a mental hospital. Under such conditions he had behaved well, and in the examination carried out by experienced psychiatrists he had so comported himself that he was considered fit to be discharged. His subsequent conduct showed how narrow his margin of control was, and how, without provocation, he again committed a dangerous assault which resulted in the death of the victim. Surely such a case teaches us the necessity of treating all such psychopathic states with the greatest possible care, with greater care than one would bestow on the psychotic patient who has recovered, or even on the so-called sane criminal. We would even go as far as to suggest that the psychopathic person who has committed serious offences of the type described should not be liberated except under the most stringent safeguards, and only after a prolonged period of stable conduct.

Y

It is the occurrence of such cases which brings forward the advisability of introducing an indeterminate sentence into the criminal code.

Such partly affected, emotionally immature persons are far more dangerous than either the sane or insane criminal. The former may readjust, the latter may recover and never commit another crime, but the partially involved very seldom recover sufficiently to be considered as reasonably safe. Their margin of control is too narrow and delicate. Repetition of the offence is seen particularly in the case of sex offenders, and everyone knows how futile it is to sentence such persons to short terms of prison treatment. We appreciate likewise that the majority of such cases are not susceptible to psychological treatment, but at least they should be given an opportunity for readjustment.

Predominantly Inadequate or Passive

This again is an important and numerous group exhibiting symptoms which may not be so dramatic as those already described, but which may be more persistent and with less chance of readjustment. Roughly we see two main types: 1. the petty delinquent class with thieving, lying, swindling propensities; 2. those who develop types of invalidism closely allied to neurotic and psychotic states. The background in each is essentially the same. On the one hand we have placid, suggestible, rather charming persons who readily accommodate themselves to the domination of others, and always follow the path of least resistance; on the other hand we meet cold, frigid, apathetic persons who, irrespective of the fix in which they may find themselves, are utterly detached and individualistic. Under these circumstances and with such ill-balanced personalities it is not at all to be wondered at that a multiplicity of symptoms should on occasion present themselves as reactions to the various situations in which the persons become involved. For instance, we see the so-called kleptomanias and pyromanias, conditions which are more common in children than in adults, due to their greater state of emotional instability and their embryonic state of social development. It has been shown, especially by Healy and Stekel, that the antisocial acts are very frequently the outcome of some conflict produced by ill-understood sexual impulses. Stekel uses the term 'parapathic impulses', representing a craving for repetition, a striving for infantile impressions and pleasure. The criterion of pathological stealing (kleptomania) is similar to that of pathological lying, namely, that the misconduct is not proportionate to any discernible end in view (Healy). Of 'kleptomanias', Godden says that 90 per cent. are women, that most are at the menstrual period, and that a lack of conscious intent is shown by the fact that the stolen goods are commonly returned anonymously. But this is not everyone's experience.

Pathological Liars. These are persons who lie habitually and without external need. The condition seems to involve two processes: 1. falsification of the memory of actual occurrences; and 2. entirely new creations of phantasy. The haziness which normally obscures the details of remembered events is filled in circumstantially, at first perhaps with a feeling of uncertainty, but later, when the true details and the false have become inextricably mixed up, with assurance.

The pathological liar never tires of phantasies, which are usually of the nature of wish-fulfilments (often compensatory for a felt inferiority), and which he recounts to others with apparent belief in their veracity. The condition is the continuance into adult life in an exaggerated form of a tendency not uncommon in children. One lie leads to another, since previous statements have to be sub-stantiated. The usual topics of the phantasies are the possession of wealth and position. The phantasies do not develop, however, into actual delusions—the patient seems privately to realize that they are fabrications.

A patient of ours, for example, recounted how he could indulge in imagina-tions for hours at a time. 'I could go to a dealer's and buy a Rolls-Royce, pay for the car, drive it home, visit my friends and so on', and he could recount such events to any chance acquaintance. But he had full insight, and said he realized he must stop the practice. This attitude of reform and desire to do better is not by any means always present. Some deny that they ever made such statements, and assume the attitude of injured innocence. Emotionally they are usually light-hearted, and have very little sense of responsibility. The patient mentioned above gave up his post as ship's officer, and was entirely unconcerned that there was no prospect of any other occupation for him. This attitude of complacency is usually accompanied in such patients by confidence in their own powers. They make a good impression socially, being gay and talkative, and full of information, which is superficial and, of course, unreliable. Intellectually they are usually equal to the average, and sometimes above it. Healy states that a few ultimately abandon the habit.

The pathological liar develops readily into the *pathological swindler*. In them the phantasies are translated to some extent into reality. The swindler not only says he is the Earl of X., but acts as if he were so—putting up at expensive hotels, running up bills for motoring and clothes. Such cases are frequently reported in the newspapers. East described a good instance of this type:

CASE No. 47

The patient had an intellectual capacity considerably above the average for her station in life. There was no record in her family of mental illness, epilepsy or nervous disease of any kind. She was dismissed from her last school on account of pilfering. She was described as having had a good, but superficial, education, as being a singer and pianist of more than ordinary merit, with attractive conversational powers. At the age of 15 'Jane' became intimate with her mother's lodger, and subsequently married him when she was 17 years old, her baby being born shortly afterwards. Her married life was very unsatisfactory; she was recklessly extravagant, involved her husband in debt and they shifted about from place to place. She neglected her home and children, and led a gay life, on account of which her husband eventually left her. Before they actually parted she posed to a lady as an heiress having a guardian. After leaving her husband she obtained a situation in a hotel as a book-keeper, but was discharged on account of her unsuitability. It was then found that she had obtained goods from local tradespeople, representing that she was the hotel proprietor's wife. She was arrested, and sentenced to a short term of imprisonment. After her discharge from prison she went to a rescue home, from which place she wrote to Mrs. X., the lady to whom she posed previously, representing the home as the mansion of her guardian, Mr. Y., who, she stated, was asking her to marry him. She stated that as her fortune was tied up until she was 23 years of age she felt at his mercy, but was determined to resist his attentions, and she asked Mrs. X. to take her as a paying guest. This plan did not materialize, and J. was recommended to another rescue home, where she made herself popular with the inmates on account of her social talents and engaging personality. She told them that she was about to be married to a young gentleman, who eventually arrived for the ceremony. As soon as he discovered that she was a married woman with children he left her abruptly. Later she stayed in a local hotel at a seaport town. Fire broke out a few days later in one of the bedrooms, and the place was gutted. The next day it was discovered that the cash-box and a sum of money were missing. J., who had left the town, was traced, pled guilty to the theft and received a short sentence of imprisonment. On her release she resided in a leading hotel, posed as a rich ward in Chancery and at this time had plenty of money. She took a situation, succeeded in introducing herself into the manager's home circle, and while there she met a gentleman, Mr. Z., who within a few days proposed marriage and was accepted. Ultimately she married Mr. Z., but her life soon became very unhappy. She involved him in debt with her reckless extravagance; at one time he was paying rent simultaneously for three different houses she had taken in his name. She alleged that she was ill-treated by Mr. Z. She was attended by various doctors, and to one she said that she was the illegitimate daughter of a lady, an admiral's wife, who had erred during the absence of her husband at sea, and that she was under guardianship. This doctor considered her to be morally insane, and informed Mr. Z. that she had already had children. On hearing this Mr. Z. separated from her. Soon after this J. wore her hair in public as a long plait reaching below her knees, but no explanation was given for this conduct. Later she obtained a situation, but was discharged for stealing. Next she was companion to a lady under treatment for inebriety, but J. continued to supply her with intoxicants, and the inebriate lady became so much worse that she had to go to an institution. She then set fire to this lady's bedroom, stole a large quantity of her clothing, saturated some of the other beds with water, lighted a large fire on the kitchen floor and so terrorized the other servants that they all left the house together. She was arrested, charged with theft and sentenced to imprisonment. Following this she carried out various impersonations. She called herself a nurse, and was engaged to take care of a lady who was dying of cancer. A night or two afterwards she was discovered bringing men into the house, and instead of attending the patient she was usually absent from her.

The swindling and lying were the prominent aspects of this case, which would formerly have been classed as one of 'moral imbecility', secondary to inherent emotional instability.

A form of psychopathic behaviour which occurs as a wartime phenomenon—masquerading in uniform—has been emphasized by Stalker (1945). He reported a group of seven cases in whom the underlying motive seemed to concern itself more with personal prestige than with any materialistic purpose. The cases in themselves were of great interest as showing the length to which people will go to attain their ends even although that end may be a source of discomfort and annoyance to themselves, their relatives and every one interested in them. In all Stalker's cases the constitutional element was prominent, but he draws particular attention to the over-compensation mechanisms which were at work, mechanisms which were determined by a state of physical or mental inferiority. One of the most amazing of these cases was that of a young man, the son of wealthy parents, who throughout the whole period of his supposed medical career led a life of make-believe. He eventually returned home saying that he had been the most distinguished student of his year—a story which was accepted by his parents, his family doctor and his friends. Later, when he was arrested for masquerading as a Naval Surgeon-Lieutenant, his life-story was exposed; he accepted the whole position in the most nonchalant manner, stated that he had always craved for adventure, and that he would like to join the R.A.F. as a pilot. Unfortunately their practice lags woefully behind their expectations and they do not succeed any better in the Armed Forces than in any other walk of life.

Pseudo-querulants. The pseudo-querulants are usually described as a separate type. It is really a matter of accentuating a trait that is not uncommon in the emotionally unstable. They are very irritable. Hence they readily come into collision with other people, and regard trifling differences as grave injustices. They are also arrogant, and this combination of irritability and arrogance leads them not only into quarrels but lawsuits. They seek satisfaction from higher and higher courts, if permitted to do so. If frustrated in this direction, they try other methods—making charges of perjury against the witnesses, and indulging in other slanders. This quarrelsomeness never involves them in actual delusions. Their feelings would be legitimate in isolated cases; it is the aggregation and universality of their feelings of grievance, and the manner in which the latter lead them into falsifications and inventions, that mark them out as abnormal. They are further distinguished from the litigious paranoid type by the fact that in the pseudo-querulants the tendency exists from youth up.

Eccentrics. 'They are the only representatives of the constitutional aberrations in whom the affectivity is apparently not preponderatingly disturbed' (Bleuler).

The group is one which does not usually come within the physician's purview. When it does, it is usually difficult to distinguish the symptoms from schizophrenic manifestations.

Numerous other types of constitutional psychopathic inferiority could be described. Thus Schneider (1958) mentions, among others, the 'insecure', characterized by feelings of insufficiency; the 'self-seeking', including the 'hysterical character', so called, which he rightly regards as a misnomer, holding as we do that the 'hysterical character' and 'hysteria' are not at all the same condition; the 'explosive', the 'weak-minded' and the 'asthenic', the latter including those whom we have elsewhere alluded to as the scanty group of 'congenital neurasthenics'.

There is considerable evidence to show that the inadequate, immature, dispositional background of the psychopath may exercise a considerable influence, prognostically, on cases which symptomatically might be classified as neurotic or psychotic. We should pay more attention to this influence, and should not think too exclusively of neurosis, or of what we term schizoid, cycloid and paranoid. The outlook, heretofore, has been too circumscribed.

Predominantly Creative

At first sight it may seem strange to associate creativeness developing to a condition of genius with the aggressive and inadequate groups already described.

Popularly, genius and 'madness' have always been closely associated, but that is an over-statement, and just as the aggressive and inadequate groups do not include madmen (as that term is used generally), neither does the creative group. We find, however, intense individualistic people who carve out a way for themselves irrespective of the obstacles which bestrew their path. Genius in its truest and greatest sense is a multiple quality, it has many facets, and associated with it there must be sufficient energy to accomplish whatever has been conceived. Such persons are not many in number. Kretschmer postulated the interesting idea, while recognizing that 'gifted parents have gifted off-spring', that individual geniuses are more frequently due to cross-breeding, and that this may produce a variety of contrasts and conflicts which, while leading to genius, is also productive of psychopathological conflicts. It is understandable that the sensitive nervous system of the genius is one which might quite well show vagaries in many directions. It is something which crops up in the process of variation. When we study the lives of those who have been famous in many diverse fields we find with singular regularity dispositional traits which are in fairly close conformity to the psychosexual immaturity, and emotional instability, and individuality of others termed psychopathic. Joan of Arc, Napoleon, Lawrence of Arabia, may all be taken as examples of persons with great qualities of leadership and of vision, but yet associated with a certain unevenness in their make-up which differentiated them markedly from their more ordinary companions. There is an uncanniness and an inspiration about them which is far beyond what, ordinarily, may be expected. Their objective is gained by a feeling that their way is right rather than by thoughtful, methodical planning.

It is believed that the clinical groups delineated are of great psychiatric and social interest, and that while they may seem heterogeneous, yet they have a common background in their constitution and their psychobiological development.

PROGNOSIS

It is obvious that the prognosis of such a diversified number of clinical states cannot be discussed in a categorical manner. The prognosis is likely to be more favourable when the patient is young in years, referred early for expert advice, and proves co-operative in treatment. But when the hereditary loading is severe, and personality defects have been intensified by unfortunate environmental circumstances then we are faced with a set of factors which may prove difficult, if not impossible, to modify. In any case the course of the illness or mental disturbance is so prolonged that many months or even years may elapse before the patient's future stability can be regarded as reasonably secure. So many become dogged by a sense of failure and resentment that they feel that every man's hand is turned against them. In consequence, all too often they develop a cynical fatalism which seems to glorify their rebellious, individualistic, selfish conduct rather than to despise it.

On the other hand it has been our experience that a much larger number of cases than might be thought have a genuine desire to obtain help, and are willing to co-operate to the best of their ability. They have their lapses and failures but if the physician continues to exercise individual care combined with great patience a *rapport* can be effected which breeds mutual trust and confidence, and leads to a sense of greater hopefulness. The importance of the ageing factor should never be lost sight of; a state of greater emotional maturity and stability may be delayed until the middle thirties. That fact by itself should encourage us to persevere in our therapeutic efforts. It may be that as our knowledge of personality structure and character formation increases that we will be able to offer a more favourable prognosis than heretofore.

TREATMENT

The successful treatment of psychopathic persons does not rest with the medical profession alone. It is a medico-social problem of great complexity which constitutes a challenge to society in relation to every aspect of social health and welfare. While we are unable to specify definite forms of treatment yet we can formulate some general principles which, in certain instances, may prove of value. We are never likely wholly to prevent the occurrence of psychopathic states, they will continue to appear during the natural process of variation of the species. Just as some persons, from birth or an early age, are handicapped physically and intellectually so there are others who, irrespective of their heritage and education, are lacking in mental stability, emotional maturity and social adaptability. In the former, precise methods of training can deal reasonably well with defects of intelligence and physical incapacity, but in the latter the problem presented is much more complex. For we are then called upon to deal with anomalies of character and personality which prevent the individual's adjustment to his social *milieu*. Every medical and social discipline may require to be called into action. Through our understanding of the psychobiological principles which govern reactive tendencies we should, medically, be able to give a lead as to how treatment might most profitably be directed. This entails the co-operation of parents, schoolmasters, social workers, probation officers and all others concerned with the health and welfare of young people. And this is also the reason why we so strongly support the development of organizations such as the Cubs, Brownies, Girl Guides, Boy Scouts, Boys' Brigades, etc. It is during puberty and adolescence that everything possible requires to be done to inculcate high standards of decent conduct. It is at this preventive level when all deviations of conduct should be examined in their entirety that we are most likely to attain success. Undue delay may spell disaster, and may lead to Juvenile Court proceedings, referral to a Remand Home, and perhaps to indoor treatment in an Approved School or Borstal. We do not gainsay in any way the most valuable work which all the above-named organizations accomplish, but like tends to be attracted to like and the association of groups of psychopathic persons may constitute a dangerous complicating factor in their successful treatment. It is, however, by our intensive study of such case material that we are likely to acquire greater diagnostic skill whereby we can enlarge our concept of mental abnormality. There are shades and degrees of abnormality which do not amount to a psychosis but yet constitute a diminution of responsibility which can lead to disastrous results. We want to avoid such catastrophes. If we are fortunate to deal with such conditions in their incipiency excellent results may be attained by a simple environmental adjustment. A modification in the school curriculum, a change of school or of occupation, a good foster-home, the skilled guidance of a child psychiatrist, an expert social worker or probation officer and above all, kindness, friendship and human understanding may work wonders.

Adult psychopathic persons frequently require indoor treatment over a prolonged period but how and where this can be best carried out has not as yet been definitely decided. Our experience, however, coincides with that of others who believe that the wards of an ordinary mental hospital are not suitable. The psychopath disrupts the lives of the more contented and amenable psychiatric patients. If the mental hospital is used for such patients then a separate department should be built detached from the main hospital. When special security measures are necessary a special department of a prison, where there is an adequate psychiatric service, could be utilized; or else a completely independent organization with its own highly skilled medical, nursing and social service personnel could be set up. A notable example of the latter organization was instituted in 1933 at Herstedvester, Copenhagen, Denmark. It is under the medical direction of G. K. Stürup, and provides accommodation for 180 males and 20 females. Its object is twofold: 1. to effect satisfactory preventive detention; and 2. to treat patients according to their psychical needs so that they may return to a normal life. Detention is regarded as a security measure rather than a punishment. The majority of the patients at Herstedvester are relapsed criminals who have committed serious offences, *e.g.* murder, incendiarism, rape, indecency to boys and girls, and drug addicts. The same court which orders the detention of the patient decides, on the basis of a medical report, when he may with safety be released on parole. The Medical Director is the counsellor to the Ministry of Justice, and the officers of any prison are encouraged to seek guidance from him in regard to the management of difficult cases. An atmosphere of great activity is present throughout the institution. There are workshops with modern machinery, where the detainees work an 8-hour day at a variety of vocational tasks, earning 10 kroner or more per week. A lively, social club life provides an agreeable opportunity for discussion; study circles and correspondence courses are available, and everything possible is done to promote a spirit of hope and encouragement. Stürup maintains that upwards of 50 per cent. are able to resume normal life in the community. Sexual offenders who have been repeatedly convicted are advised to submit, voluntarily, to castration. As an inducement to do so the hope is held out that there may be a remission of sentence and liberation on parole at an earlier date than normally expected. Castration, however, appears to us to be a dubious practice, and is in striking contrast to the other much more constructive methods which are employed.

Maxwell Jones (1952, 1959) at the Belmont Hospital, London, has stressed the value of group therapy and psycho-drama whereby the patients, in co-operation with the medical and nursing staff, work out their life situations and specific problems. An imaginative, elastic technique is used backed up by infinite patience. Frequent staff conferences are held so that grievances—'real or imaginary'—can be talked out. Jones takes a conservative and modest therapeutic outlook and believes that we will require to know much more about personality structure before any fundamental changes can be effected. At present we have to be content with improving social attitudes.

Progress in therapy may be hastened by the use of suitable medicinal agents. As our knowledge of thymoleptic and tranquillizing drugs and hormones increases we may be able to bring disorders of mood and behaviour under more adequate control. At present much discretion requires to be exercised in prescribing them and in controlling the length of time over which they are used.

In conclusion we would emphasize once again that the treatment of the psychopath is a many-sided affair. Our central aim, however, is to maintain a progressive, constructive outlook, to encourage and support the patient so that we can direct his interests and activities into healthy channels. By so doing we may be able to inculcate the art of living harmoniously.

REFERENCES

Bradley, C. (1942) *Conn. St. med. J.*, **6**, 773.
Hill, D. (1952) *Electroenceph. clin. Neurophysiol.* **4**, 419.
Hill, D. and Watterson, D. (1942) *J. Neurol. Psychiat.*, **5**, 47.
Jones, Maxwell (1952) *Social Psychiatry*, London.
Jones, Maxwell (1959) *Lancet*, ii, 1022.
Schneider, K. (1958) *Psychopathic Personalities*, London.
Silverman, D. (1943) *Arch. Neurol. Psychiat. (Chicago)*, **50**, 18.
Stalker, H. (1945) *J. ment. Sci.*, **91**, 383.
Stürup, G. K. (1948) *Danish Psychiatry*, Copenhagen.

14

SPECIAL METHODS OF PHYSICAL TREATMENT

In this chapter a few of the more important techniques will be described in some detail and reference will be made to others, but a comprehensive account of physical methods of treatment in psychiatry will not be attempted.

About 1935 a major advance in psychiatric treatment took place, with the introduction, on the Continent of Europe, of the so-called 'shock therapies'— insulin coma, convulsion therapy and leucotomy. These techniques were then used very widely in treatment of the 'functional' psychoses, and the results obtained were in very many cases remarkable: they constituted indeed a landmark in psychiatric progress. All these three treatments were, however, empirical, and they have remained so. Over recent years electric convulsion therapy has established itself as the most generally effective treatment for the affective psychoses. Leucotomy, on the other hand, holds now only a peripheral position, as a drastic form of treatment for cases of otherwise hopeless prognosis: while insulin coma has lost its *réclame* and has by most workers in mental hospitals been abandoned.

The latest major development in physical therapy has been pharmacological, the production of the tranquillizers (ataractics) and anti-depressant or euphoriant drugs. These new chemical methods of treatment are also empirical. Some of the new drugs are undoubtedly effective in certain cases, but we do not know how they work and their prescription is therefore very often of a hit-or-miss nature. Too many of them are being produced too quickly, and are being used without guidance from properly controlled trials of their efficacy. We are in fact repeating the mistakes made with the 'shock therapies' of the thirties, using these new therapeutic agents too enthusiastically, too indiscriminately and frequently naïvely. Far too often the latest drugs are prescribed before the patient's clinical state has been defined, and far too often he is rendered punch-drunk (as it were) by their cumulative effects. If they are used well, many mentally ill patients are benefited by drugs: and research into their modes of action, both in those cases where they succeed and in those where they are ineffective or harmful, may provide invaluable clues to the aetiology of the psychoses.

The methods which will be described are as follows:

1. Electric convulsion therapy.
2. Leucotomy.
3. Insulin coma therapy.
4. Modified insulin therapy.
5. Continuous narcosis.
6. Various drug treatments: tranquillizers, anti-depressants and narco-analysis.

CONVULSION THERAPY

The treatment of schizophrenic psychoses by induced convulsions was introduced by Dr. von Meduna of Budapest in 1934, on the basis of the dubious observation that epilepsy was rare in schizophrenics, and of the deduction that there might, therefore, exist a biological antagonism between schizophrenia and epilepsy. However that may be, he found that by producing fits in schizophrenics he could influence the recovery rate. The convulsant first used was camphor, injected in oil intramuscularly: later *Cardiazol* (pentamethylenetetrazol) was given intravenously, before Cerletti and Bini introduced in 1937 the present widely used method of inducing convulsions electrically (E.C.T.). It was not long before it was discovered that melancholic patients responded better than schizophrenics to this physical method of treatment.

The *modus operandi* of the treatment is still conjectural. Its effects are almost certainly due more to the bodily changes induced than to the psychological trauma it may be supposed to constitute. It has been suggested that it acts as a threat of death, and in some cases probably this is so, since we know that certain cases of depression get better rapidly after making a suicidal attempt and by atoning thus for the guilt which has overwhelmed them. A more important psychological effect is doubtless the disruption, by the fit and the subsequent period of amnesia, of recently acquired morbid patterns of behaviour and reaction. The physical changes caused by the treatment are often rapid and impressive: appetite and weight are regained, and normal sleep and menstruation re-established. These somatic changes suggest that the treatment affects diencephalic centres in a way beneficial to the whole bodily economy. From electroencephalographic studies also Roth (1952) produced evidence that the primary effects of E.C.T. may be on the diencephalon: his results suggested a cumulative influence of the treatment on some mid-line structure in the brain with access to all cortical areas, though with some special relationship to the frontal lobes.

Method

Since electric convulsion therapy (electroplexy) has almost completely replaced the production of fits by drugs, this method will be described. Suitable patients can be treated successfully in general hospitals, nursing homes or even out-patient departments, although we are not greatly in favour of the latter procedure. There are several convenient types of electro-convulsant apparatus on the market which are small, portable and designed both for A.C. and D.C. mains.

A careful physical examination must always precede treatment. X-rays of chest or spine, electrocardiographic and other specialized investigations may be indicated in cases where the physical state is impaired; and it is often advisable in such cases to obtain the advice of a medical or surgical consultant. Written permission for the treatment should be obtained from the patient or from the nearest relative, to whom the risks attendant upon the treatment should be explained. If the patient has been taking a long-acting sedative at nights, a shorter-acting hypnotic should be substituted—*e.g.* cyclobarbitone, B.P.C., or pentobarbitone sodium, B.P. (*Nembutal*).

Treatment is usually most conveniently given in the morning. If a muscle relaxant is to be used, food should be omitted that morning, since if food were taken there would be a risk of vomiting and regurgitation into the lungs. Half to one hour before treatment the patient is given a subcutaneous injection of atropine sulphate, 0·45 to 0·6 mg., to prevent salivation and vomiting: and the very anxious patient may at this time be given a small dose of amylobarbitone sodium. Immediately before treatment he should empty his bladder and bowels. His clothes must be loosened at neck and waist; dentures, hair-clips, jewellery, etc., are removed.

The patient lies on a padded table or firm couch, which most conveniently is of the same height as the ward trolley, so that heavy patients can be gently slid from one to the other after treatment.

The use of a muscle relaxant to modify the force of the electrically induced convulsion allows us practically to eliminate the risk of fractures and dislocations. A number of relaxants have been used; for example, curare, gallamine triethiodide (*Flaxedil*) and suxamethonium bromide (*Brevidil E*). The latter is very brief in its action, and is outstandingly suitable. Since the onset of paralysis is very frightening to the conscious patient, 0·2 to 0·25 G. thiopentone sodium, B.P., (*Intraval Sodium*) is first injected intravenously, to give light anaesthesia. The needle is left in the vein, and from another syringe suxamethonium bromide is injected in a dose of 30 to 50 mg. according to the patient's weight and muscular development. Its action is signified usually by fibrillation or twitching of the muscles: when these movements have ceased, or at some time between 30 and 60 seconds after the injection of the relaxant, the electrical current should be passed. Prior to the fit the patient is given a few breaths of oxygen through a mask.

In order to pass the electrical current the electrodes, covered by pads wet with saline or sodium bicarbonate, are placed firmly on the temples, and some workers consider it advisable to clean the temples beforehand with ether or cetrimide solution (*Cetavlon*). A mouth gag is inserted, and the current is then switched on by the operator. A typical initial setting of a McPhail-Strauss machine would be 120 volts for 0·3 second: if an Ectron machine is used, which delivers a fixed voltage of electricity, the current should be passed for at least one second and for not more than four seconds. The object is to produce a major fit.

Oxygenation should be continued after the seizure until breathing has restarted, which usually occurs within three to five minutes. Very occasionally prolonged apnoea results, and aeration of the lungs with a pressure bag may have to be carried out for as long as 20 to 30 minutes. No one should undertake to modify E.C.T. with a muscle relaxant who cannot carry out the prolonged oxygenation of an unconscious patient, or who cannot pass an intratracheal tube in an emergency. We prefer therefore always to have an anaesthetist to assist us.

If muscular relaxation has been very complete, it may be difficult to be certain that a major seizure has occurred. Contraction of the frontalis or inversion of the feet and toes may be seen when there is little or no movement visible elsewhere. The passage of the current may in fact not produce a major fit, but only a 'stun' (simple or sub-shock). A 'stun', which is momentary with relaxation again almost immediately, is of no therapeutic value, and tends to cause later headache and confusion: its production is therefore to be avoided, and no more than three 'stuns' should be allowed to occur at any treatment. If a major seizure is not produced by the first setting or timing of the machine, voltage or time or both should be increased and a further shock given.

After treatment the patient is returned to his bed, where he usually sleeps. On regaining consciousness he is often for a period suggestible, and may reveal previously hidden symptoms of his illness.

If for some reason it is not possible to employ a muscle relaxant, and E.C.T. has to be given 'straight', further and extra precautions have to be taken: and despite these, injury may be done to the patient. A small pillow is placed under the patient's back, extending the dorsal spine, and another under his head, and his movements must be controlled manually by a team of nurses. It is the initial jerk and jack-knife flexion of his spine in the fit which constitutes the chief danger to the patient. If only two nurses are available, one should hold the patient's shoulder girdles firmly to the couch by pressure on the clavicles and shoulders transmitted through her own extended arms, the other should similarly control the pelvic girdle by downwards pressure on the iliac crests. If four nurses are available, one should hold the patient's flexed arms to his sides and another keep his extended legs together at the ankles. The doctor giving the treatment should hold up the patient's lower jaw, thus keeping the mouth gag in position and preventing dislocation of the jaw by extreme opening of the mouth. When the gag is in position, the patient is instructed to bite on it and the current is then switched on by the operator. The patient's movements should be carefully controlled throughout the seizure, and at the end of the clonic phase he should be turned into the semi-prone position. If cyanosis is still marked or if breathing has not recommenced satisfactorily, he should be given oxygen from a cylinder through a face mask attached to a pressure bag: usually this is only required for a minute or so. The patient is then returned to bed. He may regain consciousness quickly, and be restless or emotional, or sleep for half an hour or longer.

Treatments are normally given twice a week but preferably they are spaced according to the needs of the individual patient. In those cases which respond satisfactorily, six to eight treatments are usually sufficient to promote recovery: and, in the great majority of instances, if a response to the treatment is going to occur at all, it becomes manifest in the period of the first four treatments. It is doubtful if more than twelve treatments should be given at a single course. Sometimes a patient who has improved during a course of treatment begins to relapse within a fortnight of its completion: in such a case, a further two or three treatments may be required.

Indications for and Results of Treatment

In all forms of nervous and mental disorder we prefer to use conservative measures to start with; we consider it advisable to delay treatment by any of the so-called 'shock' methods provided there is reasonable chance of effecting recovery without them, but on the other hand it is unjustifiable to submit the patient to the prolonged misery of depression with its accompanying risk of suicide, or to a dangerous degree of exhaustion, without resort to E.C.T. Recently imipramine (*Tofranil*) has been used with success in many cases of endogenous depression which would previously have been treated with E.C.T.: but imipramine has not replaced E.C.T., which appears usually to be more effective in the severer illnesses, to act more quickly and to shorten the illness.

The chief indication for convulsion therapy is the treatment of a depressive psychosis. Results are most dramatic in the involutional melancholia group: here about 80 per cent. of the cases respond, the illness is in most instances cut short, suffering is much reduced and management facilitated. Tube feeding is now rarely necessary in these cases. The response of manic-depressive depressions may also be very satisfactory; the attack may be modified, though recurrences are not prevented. One has the impression, however, that in manic-depressive cases treatment is most effective if given when the nadir of the illness has been passed: it may then accelerate recovery, whereas if given very early in the illness a temporary improvement may be followed by a rapid relapse. E.C.T. is usually less effective in those less typical recurrent depressions which, before its introduction, tended to run courses longer than the average; in cases, that is, characterized by hypochondriasis, and in younger people by prominent feelings of unreality or anxiety. E.C.T. may in fact make such patients worse. In general, it is ineffective and not infrequently it is harmful where the depressive reaction is essentially a neurotic response to environmental difficulties.

We have not been impressed by the results in cases of mania; the patient may be quietened, but usually only very transiently so. Some workers have claimed more satisfactory results in mania from E.C.T., given intensively (*i.e.* 1 to 3 times per day initially), but we are inclined to deprecate its use in this way. Where depression is a prominent affect in a schizophrenic or paranoid illness, E.C.T. may be helpful but its effects are seldom lasting.

Old age is not a bar to treatment with E.C.T. Patients in their seventies or even older may be treated successfully, provided that there is no organic deterioration of their mental faculties.

Physically, there are, since the introduction of muscle relaxants, few contraindications to the treatment. Cerebral arteriosclerosis and recent coronary thrombosis debar the treatment; marked hypertension does not necessarily do so. In cases where there is evidence of myocardial damage the strain on the cardiovascular system incurred by prolonged agitation must be weighed against the strain imposed by a modified convulsive seizure. In cases of pulmonary tuberculosis also the risks must be weighed against the advantages, since it appears that E.C.T. might light up a tuberculous lesion. Orthopaedic disabilities frequently call for the use of muscle relaxants but rarely debar treatment.

The ease with which E.C.T. can now be given has unfortunately led to its rather widespread abuse. Too often it is applied in a hasty and routine manner as soon as evidence of a depressive affect has been observed in a patient, and before any adequate investigation and assessment of the illness has been made. It is a method of treatment which should be handled with the greatest consideration and should only be utilized in carefully selected cases.

Risks and Complications

Since E.C.T. evidently produces its effects by altering brain function, and indeed its effects clinically may resemble closely those which follow head injury, the question at once arises whether or not pathological lesions are produced in the brain and, if so, whether these structural changes are reversible. The results of animal experimentation have not given a clear answer: and pathological studies of human brains can rarely be made shortly after treatment. It may be said that there is no evidence that a previously normal brain suffers permanent damage of any consequence from a standard course of E.C.T. Organic sequelae may, however, follow the giving of too prolonged or too intensive treatment: memory gaps of weeks or months may then be produced and these must have a pathological basis. Corsellis and Meyer (1954) reported two cases in which irreversible histological changes in the brain may have been caused by unusually heavy electro-convulsive treatment. The changes, which were mild, consisted mainly of a proliferation of the marginal glia and of the glia of the white matter.

All patients have an amnesia for the fit and for a variable time afterwards extending over the period when they are drowsy or confused; a momentary retrograde amnesia is also usual, but may transiently be much more extensive. During the treatment course and for a week or two subsequently many patients complain of forgetfulness, particularly over dates, names and such details. This memory disturbance, after a normal course of treatment, may be expected to disappear within a month. With more intensive or prolonged treatment, however, memory disturbance may be more severe and permanent impairment may be caused. This complication points to the need for caution especially in the treatment of those whose livelihood depends on their memory and intellectual capabilities.

The main and commonest danger of convulsion therapy used to lie in the production of fractures and dislocations by the intense motor excitation of the fits. The commonest fracture was a compression of the vertebral bodies (more than one might be involved). When *Cardiazol* was used, this complication was recorded in as many as 40 per cent. of the patients treated (Polatin, 1939): with 'straight' E.C.T. an incidence of 23 per cent. has been reported (Lingley and Robbins, 1947). The incidence was highest in muscular men and in cases with osteoporosis. The injury varied from a slight crush in the extreme tip of the body of the vertebra, usually 4th, 5th or 6th thoracic, to a telescoping of the vertebral body. Fortunately many of these fractures were symptomless: in other cases there was complaint of pain in the back for a few weeks, but lasting disability has been exceptional. Dislocations of jaw and shoulder, and more rarely fractures of long bones, also occurred during treatment. With careful manual restraint of the fit the incidence of such physical injuries can be much reduced, and by the use of muscle relaxants they can practically be eliminated. If a fracture has occurred it may still be justifiable to continue the convulsive treatment, but a muscle relaxant must be employed.

We have had experience of manic-depressive patients who, as a result of treatment, have passed from a depressive into a manic phase. This is very uncommon. In such instances the last state, at any rate so far as relatives are concerned, may be considered worse than the first. We once received a letter imploring: 'Please de-electrify my daughter'. More commonly, towards the end of a course of treatment, the patient may show for some days a euphoria which is probably organically determined.

If the patient has been carefully examined beforehand as to his physical fitness to stand the treatment and if the E.C.T. is properly carried out, the risk of death under treatment is negligible.

LEUCOTOMY

In 1935 Egas Moniz, a Portuguese surgeon, introduced this operation which divides the pathways between the frontal lobes and the thalamus. The original method consisted in the injection of small quantities of alcohol into the white matter of the prefrontal region, but this was superseded by the use of a steel leucotome to sever the white matter.

Rationale

The operation was devised on the basis of clinical and experimental observations. In 1848, in Vermont, U.S.A., a man named Phineas Gage had an iron crowbar driven through the frontal region of his skull, but lived for twelve years afterwards. Autopsy showed that only the prefrontal cortex was involved. After his injury Gage was described by Harlow in these terms: 'He is fitful, irreverent, indulging at times in the grossest profanity (which was not previously his custom), manifesting but little deference for his fellows, impatient of restraint or advice when it conflicts with his desires, at times pertinaciously obstinate, yet capricious and vacillating. . . .' Cases such as this showed that widespread and bilateral damage to the frontal lobes could produce a state of disinhibition and euphoria. Later, evidence from animal experiments led to the general conclusion that in monkeys, too, there was a change in temperament as a result of bilateral frontal lobe injury, J. F. Fulton remarking that the animal became like a 'good-natured drunk'. Chimpanzees which had developed an 'experimental neurosis' in that they became irritable over their mistakes in learning, lost all concern over them after leucotomy.

Ritchie Russell (1948) speculated that the beneficial effect of prefrontal leucotomy may be derived in one of three ways: 'Either the operation prevents the relay of the nervous activities engendered by mental conflict to the fronto-thalamic mechanism; or the fire of the mental conflict loses its fuel when no longer stimulated by the mechanism; or most likely the mechanism of mental conflict at a cortical level is highly complex and may be directly interfered with by this operation to such an extent that it can no longer develop the intensity required to stimulate the emotions'. Fulton (1951) suggested that its effects may be due to interference with a visceral afferent system—the so-called 'visceral brain', which is believed to include parts of the temporal lobe, the hippocampus, the amygdaloid nucleus, and nuclei of the thalamus and hypothalamus as well as the cingulate gyrus and posterior orbital cortex; and suggested that these two latter regions may be the optimum target for the operation. But it is impossible to do more than theorize until much more experimental work has been carried out.

Anatomical Considerations

The anatomical basis of leucotomy was discussed in detail by Meyer (1954) who emphasized the interdependence of the frontal region with the thalamus, hypothalamus and—indirectly—with rhinencephalic centres. The principal afferent connections with the frontal region arise in the thalamus: fibres run from the dorsomedial nucleus to areas of granular frontal cortex, and from the anterior nucleus to the cingular region. The thalamic nuclei which project to the medial orbital and cingular regions receive fibres from the hypothalamus. Efferent fibres from the granular frontal cortex run to the dorso-medial nucleus of the thalamus (particularly), and to the hypothalamus and pontine nuclei; while those from the agranular frontal cortex connect with the ventro-medial nucleus of the thalamus (particularly), the corpus striatum, corpus subthalamicum, substantia nigra, red nucleus and pons. The operation severs thalamo-frontal pathways. After it there is retrograde degeneration in the thalamus, most marked in the dorso-medial nucleus, and in the anterior nucleus following involvement of the anterior cingular region. The importance in the operation of damage to the diffuse thalamic projection system is still uncertain.

The Standard Operation

McKissock (1943) advocated the following procedure:

A point 3 cm. behind the lateral margin of the orbit and 5 to 6 cm. above the zygoma is taken as the centre of a 2 cm. to 3 cm. skin incision. A 1 cm. burr-hole is then cut in the line of the coronal suture and a cruciform incision made in the dura. For sectioning the brain substance an ordinary brain needle with a side eyelet, just short of the blunt point, and a close-fitting stylet is used. The needle is directed in front of the anterior horn of the ventricle to a depth sufficient to be just clear of the grey matter of the medial aspect of the frontal lobe. The stylet is withdrawn and the needle made to pivot about the point of the entrance through the dura so that the blunt inner extremity travels upwards towards the superior surface of the frontal lobe. As the point is made to travel upwards the needle is pushed more deeply into the brain so that the line of the section runs parallel with the falx and does not, as it otherwise would, become steadily more distant from it. When the needle has reached sufficiently close to the upper surface of the hemisphere it is withdrawn and reintroduced along the original

z

line in order to deal with those fibres running from the lower part of the frontal pole; on this occasion the point of the needle is made to travel downwards, again parallel with the falx, and is then brought laterally across the anterior fossa roughly in the same vertical plane as the lesser wing of the sphenoid until it reaches a point just short of the lateral aspect of the skull. During this part of the section the needle is progressively withdrawn for fear of damaging the grey matter of the orbital surface of the frontal pole.

Indications for Operation

The general aim of the operation has been to modify the disordered behaviour of psychotic and neurotic patients whose illness has been of a prolonged type, and the tendency is to select patients for treatment more on a symptomatic than on a nosological basis.

Freeman and Watts stated that: 'The individual who is ideally suited to prefrontal leucotomy is one whose emotions are largely concerned with himself. This is the patient who fears heart disease, cancer, syphilis or contamination; who is a prey to ideas of guilt or persecution, who broods over the future and who is confused in the presence of others and obsessed with the idea of death. A less favourable group are those who have drifted away from reality, who are hallucinated and are lacking in emotional tension. If the patient is completely apathetic, then psychosurgery (*sic*) is unlikely to be very helpful. A patient with obsessive compulsive symptoms is supposed to have a better chance than patients persistently hallucinated; an illness which develops in an older person is more hopeful than when a younger is affected.'

Strecker and his co-workers considered that a syndrome composed of fear, anxiety, actual mental suffering and aggressive violence was a better criterion for suitability than a diagnostic label. In involutional melancholias which had failed to respond to electric convulsive treatment, and which had lasted a very long time, leucotomy was justified by its results.

Our experience has been similar. The best results have been obtained in severe involutional melancholic, obsessional and paranoid states, which have been characterized by great subjective suffering. The possibility of serious and permanent damage to the mental functions makes it necessary to reserve the method for cases where all other suitable methods of treatment have been tried and failed, where the illness offers no reasonable hope of spontaneous recovery, and where the patient is disabled more or less completely from useful occupation or from modest enjoyment of his life. In general it can be said that in those cases where tenseness, aggressiveness and gross symptoms of a delusional and hallucinatory nature are present, and when such conditions have not reacted satisfactorily to any of the other methods of treatment which have been employed, then leucotomy may not only be justified but advisable.

Results of Leucotomy

An analysis of the first 100 cases operated on at the Royal Edinburgh Hospital for Nervous and Mental Disorders may be quoted as typical of the results obtained. Thirty-six of these patients made a social recovery so that they returned home; 40 improved; 22 were unchanged; 2 died. We were dealing with patients who were desperately ill mentally, had been in-patients for many years, and had failed to respond to all other methods of treatment. An analysis of the schizo-phrenic patients in whom good results were obtained showed that in the vast majority a strong affective colouring had been maintained, and furthermore exogenous factors had been prominent. Our experience has led us to the view that the constitutionally loaded, apathetic, indifferent schizophrenic patient does not respond well to the operation: and that opinion can be extended to any mentally ill patients who are complacent, immature, lacking in forcefulness and are accepting their illness in a resigned, lifeless manner.

Similar results to the above have been reported from many centres. Ziegler (1943) surveyed the results of bilateral prefrontal leucotomy operations per-formed in 18 clinics in the United States and Canada on patients with a variety of psychiatric reaction-types, schizophrenics predominating. The first operation was performed in 1936: 75 per cent. of the operations had been carried out since 1939. Total number operated upon, 604; died as the result of operation, 11; died subsequent to operation, 18 (2 from suicide); rendered clinically worse after operation, 8; clinically improved, 59; clinically slightly improved, 106; clinically much improved, 188; recovered, psychotic or neurotic symptoms disappeared, 213; recovered, and better than at any previous time in life, 1; number of patients known to be in hospital, some able to work, 266, number known to be outside hospital, unable to work, 59; number known to be outside hospital working part or full time, 250. In 1947, the Board of Control for England and Wales made a comparable survey, analysing 1000 cases, 348 males and 652 females. Of these there were 599 cases which had been diagnosed as schizophrenia. After the operation approximately 5 per cent. died, and 25 per cent. could be discharged from hospital; 36 per cent., while still in hospital, were regarded as improved. There was a small relapse rate amounting to about 4 per cent. of the total material. The groups of patients in whom the best results were obtained were manic-depressive, involutional and obsessional states. Later experience has gener-ally confirmed these earlier reports. Relapses occur most often in the schizo-phrenic group. The significance of the premorbid personality in determining the quality of the results obtained has become apparent, as also has the importance of a stable and understanding home and family to which the patient can return. Careful rehabilitation after operation is essential if the best results are to be obtained.

These, then, are the results in broad outline. It is important to stress that, in giving symptomatic relief, the operation does not produce a cure. In depressives the apprehension and anxiety are relieved or disappear, and obsessional think-ing tends to die out perhaps because it is no longer sustained by its effective component. But hallucinations and delusions may remain, though the patient is no longer so disturbed by them. Apart from this relief of distress and tension, there has been recorded a restoration of energy and interest, increased appetite, a gain in weight, and even, although rarely, an improvement in the pre-psychotic personality. Thus Strecker, Palmer and Grant record of one patient that she exhibited resourcefulness and common sense to a degree which she had never previously possessed. In the violently disturbed patients the gain consists at least of their being made an easier problem of management.

These beneficial effects are won, unfortunately, at the price of some change in the personality, in the direction usually of coarsening and blunting. Symptoms of frontal lobe deficit appear, and may be disabling: euphoria, tactlessness, lack of initiative and laziness have been recorded in many cases. Freeman and Watts state that these defects are mostly temporary, the only one in their experience that tends to persist in the majority being diminution in tactfulness. They relate this diminution to a loss of self-consciousness and to an inclination to be content with an inferior quality of performance socially and intellectually. They emphasize particularly also a diminution in foresight and care for the future. Intelligence tests show usually no measurable loss, but there is probably a tendency for thinking to become more concrete. These unfavourable personality changes are most marked if the cuts have been too extensive or placed too far posteriorly; or if there is involvement of the dorso-lateral white matter, and particularly the cortex of the lateral convexity (Meyer, 1954). Thus in every case the benefits of leucotomy must be weighed carefully against its disadvantages: while there may remain a certain bleaching of affect and a lack of the finer sensibilities, at the same time a peace of mind has often been attained which makes life bearable for the patient, and gives some pleasure to relatives who have often been intensely distressed.

The mortality rate from the operation itself, the result usually of haemorrhage or infection, is about 2 per cent. Of after-results in the physical sphere incontinence is one of the commonest. It is usually temporary. Epilepsy occurs in 10 to 15 per cent. of cases, but can be satisfactorily controlled with anticonvulsants. A morbidly increased appetite may lead to obesity: and, if the cuts are too posterior, marasmus, restlessness, vasomotor and trophic disturbances, and uraemia, may lead to 'delayed death' (Meyer and McLardy, 1948).

Meyer stressed the importance, for clinical improvement after the operation, of the quantitative adequacy of the cuts made: but, according to McLardy and Davies (1949), schizophrenic and affective psychoses can recur after practically complete isolation of the prefrontal cortex from its long fibre connections.

There are evidently three main factors which govern the results obtained: the previous personality of the patient, his reaction-type and the extent and locus of the surgical cuts.

Later Developments. Much research has been directed towards finding out whether the benefits of leucotomy can be gained without causing adverse personality changes, and many attempts have been made to render the operations more precise. In a blind operation such as the standard Freeman-Watts leucotomy, it is difficult for the surgeon to know the exact location of the cuts made either in the antero-posterior or in the transverse planes. Meyer and McLardy, on the basis of 27 cases which had come to post-mortem, commented on the variability of the surgical lesions, and stated that only in a few cases was a bilateral lesion through the whole of the white matter actually effected. Though the clinical results of the standard operation were on the whole remarkably satisfactory, the general tendency in recent years has been to perform this operation only in the most severe, psychotically involved cases; and to prefer a procedure more limited in extent. Freeman and Watts themselves (1950) made cuts in three different planes—rostral (2 cm. anterior to the coronal suture), standard and radical, seeking to suit the severity of the cut (the most radical being most posterior) to the severity of the illness. Freeman (1949) introduced a blind operation, transorbital leucotomy, in which the cuts were made by a stylet driven through the orbital plate on each side, and which was aimed at isolating the orbital parts of the frontal lobes. He claimed results which, except in cases of schizophrenia, compared favourably with those of the standard operation, while complications were said to be fewer and personality changes slighter. But this procedure is open to the objections which may be made against all blind brain operations, and its simplicity lead to its abuse.

Other workers, in the pursuit of surgical selectivity and better clinical results, have performed open operations. Heath and Pool and their colleagues have performed bilateral cortical ablations (topectomy) of Brodmann areas 9, 10, 11; Whitty and Cairns ablation of Brodmann area 24 (cingulectomy); and Greenblatt and Solomon a bimedial lobotomy.

Scoville (1949) introduced undercutting of the orbital area. Personality changes are said to be slight after this operation, and patients suffering from chronic neurotic tension states, with anxiety and depression, which have been unresponsive to psychotherapy, are said to benefit. Knight and Tredgold (1955) reported that 23 out of 52 such cases were markedly better after the operation, and 21 somewhat better. Ström-Olsen and Northfield have also reported favourably (1955).

Of the various developments of leucotomy, orbital undercutting and the bimedial lobotomy introduced by Greenblatt and Solomon (1953) have seemed the most promising. The results obtained correspond also with the deductions which Meyer (1954) made from the pathological study of 102 cases mostly treated by a standard leucotomy. Meyer stressed that this material showed that quantitative adequacy of the cut is a most important factor in the degree of improvement obtained, and that full social recovery may be obtained without involvement of medial orbital and cingular segments. But he concluded: 'While the quantitative factor thus retains its importance, a few facts have emerged which point to some regional localization. The dorsal and, in particular, the dorso-lateral sectors of white matter do not appear to be as significant for improvement as the mid-central, orbital and cingulate sectors.'

With the introduction of surgical procedures which appeared to produce less damage to the personality, there was a widening of the clinical field in which leucotomy was used. Cases of neurosis other than obsessive-compulsive states have been operated upon, and Sargant advocated a modified leucotomy in intractable psychosomatic states, in anxiety hysteria and in anxiety and depressive states in obsessive personalities (1953). Unilateral and bilateral leucotomy has been performed by Freeman and Watts for the relief of unbearable pain in physical illnesses such as carcinoma and causalgia.

Present Position. Undoubtedly much relief of human suffering and important advances in our understanding of frontal lobe anatomy and function were brought about by the operation of leucotomy. But the indications for its use have in the past five years been much reduced with the introduction of new drug therapies. Leucotomy is now rarely carried out in cases of schizophrenia, having been replaced by tranquillizing and allied drugs in the treatment of those whose behaviour is grossly disordered. Some cases of involutional melancholia, resistant to E.C.T., which would previously have been considered suitable for leucotomy, are found to respond to imipramine. Probably the main indication for leucotomy now is for the relief of cases of obsessional neurosis, where there have been many years of suffering and relief cannot be brought in any other way.

INSULIN COMA THERAPY

In 1935, Sakel (1936), while working in Pötzl's Clinic in Vienna, was the first to suggest that insulin might be utilized to produce a hypoglycaemia which might prove valuable in the treatment of schizophrenia. Previously Sakel had used insulin in the treatment of drug addicts and had been impressed by the manner in which insulin tended to control the restlessness and irritability which characterizes such cases. It was not long before insulin came to be used extensively in the treatment of schizophrenia, and results were reported from many quarters which raised hopes that at last a form of treatment had become available which could do much to prevent the slow deterioration which is so common a sequel in schizophrenia.

This method of treatment, the use of which has been practically confined to schizophrenic psychoses, depends on the production of severe hypoglycaemia, usually to the depth of coma, on many successive occasions. It is a method that in insufficiently skilled hands can entail considerable risk to life, but in practised hands the mortality is about one per cent. It is time-consuming and requires as much vigilance as the administration of an anaesthetic. The patients selected have to be free from serious physical disease. It is necessary to have a specially trained nursing staff and experienced doctors, who should have obtained first-hand knowledge under supervision of carrying out the treatment. One doctor can attend six to eight patients, but another should be on call for emergencies.

The treatment is entirely empirical: it has no rational basis in applied knowledge of the aetiology of schizophrenia.

In the last edition of this book the opinion expressed about the effectiveness of insulin coma therapy was as follows. 'Insulin is capable of shortening the course of schizophrenic illness. What is not yet certain is whether it does more than this, whether it cures or improves permanently cases which would otherwise not have been cured or improved. It is conceivable that in those cases in which it is effective, it is effective only in shortening an illness which would in the long run have been recovered from, wholly or in part. The fact that it is more effective the more recent the illness may be construed as meaning either this, or that after, say, the first year a considerable proportion of those cases which would have been helped by insulin have already recovered, so that the percentage of cases remaining improvable by insulin is less. The problem of the effectiveness of insulin or of any form of therapy in schizophrenia is very much complicated by certain difficulties of assessment.' Attention was drawn to problems in diagnosis, in particular the differentiation of schizophrenia from the affective psychoses, and the opinion was expressed that many manic-depressive illnesses had been numbered among those which were reported as having responded to insulin coma. The work of Gottlieb and Houston (1943) was quoted as strengthening 'the suspicion that treatment with insulin, even if it is undertaken early, does not increase the ultimate rate of recovery, whether in acute recent cases or others. The efficacy of insulin shock therapy is still somewhat difficult to estimate. One effect of its introduction has been to emphasize the frequency of recovery or social recovery without insulin.'

Our personal experience since then has confirmed our scepticism. We have ceased to use insulin coma therapy and so have many others, some of whom were previously enthusiasts for the treatment.

Ackner, Harris and Oldham (1957) have published a very important report of a controlled study of the insulin treatment of schizophrenia; which they prefaced with a critical review of previous studies, exposing their frequent fallacies and deficiencies. They allocated 50 young schizophrenics (ill less than one year), by randomization, according to sex and diagnostic subtype, into an insulin treated group and a group treated by narcosis. Every matched pair of patients having insulin or narcosis was treated otherwise in the same therapeutic environment. The insulin treated group were given 35 to 40 insulin comas: the narcosis group were given, on a similar number of occasions, a mixture of sodium amylobarbitone and sodium quinalbarbitone which induced deep sleep or a state of unconsciousness near to coma. The only difference in treatment between the two groups was the method by which unconsciousness was produced.

The results of treatment, assessed by observers who had no knowledge of the kind of treatment which had been given, showed at the end of six months no significant difference between the two groups. The results were in fact better than those reported in any previous series: 40 per cent. were fully recovered at the end of six months. Ackner and his colleagues comment—'No conclusion can be drawn about the therapeutic value of the coma regime, but the results suggest that insulin is not the specific therapeutic agent'.

No published study which has claimed to show that insulin coma treatment is effective, has been as carefully designed to avoid fallacies as the investigation quoted above. We therefore support Ackner in his conclusion that insulin cannot be shown to have a specific effect on schizophrenia, and we are of the opinion that the treatment should be abandoned. Insulin coma therapy brought hope to the schizophrenic, individual attention, therapeutic enthusiasm and a constructive group experience. Many patients were benefited by it. Some interesting physiological and neurological studies derived from its use. Therefore, if insulin coma can now be abandoned as a treatment of schizophrenia, the things that went with it must not be. It probably had its most striking results in units where previously schizophrenic patients had had too little care and attention: and the history of its transient success and reputation indicates some of the ways in which the schizophrenic will continue to need understanding, nursing attention and therapeutic stimulus.

Modified Insulin Therapy [1]

This method derives from Weir Mitchell's treatment of neuroses after the American Civil War, when he prescribed with abounding success removal from stress, rest and feeding up. During the Second World War it was developed for the treatment of psychiatric casualties in the Services. Sargant and Craske (1941) selected cases of good personality, who after subjection to prolonged stress had lost a good deal of weight and had developed neurotic or reactive depressive symptoms; and they found the method valuable. In civilian practice also it is sometimes useful as part of the treatment of both neurotic and depressive illnesses, where there has been exhaustion and considerable loss of weight: in the case of depressions it may be given either during or after treatment with E.C.T. Satisfactory results are also reported in the management of some cases of anorexia nervosa, and in alleviating the unpleasant symptoms of drug withdrawal in cases of addiction. There is much individual variation in response to the treatment.

The treatment promotes a gain in weight. In some cases it has also a noticeable calming effect. There is, too, an element of suggestion; and some patients accept a psychotherapeutic approach to their problems more easily if it is combined with more active, 'medical' treatment.

Technique of the Treatment. The treatment is given daily. The patient fasts overnight. At about 7 a.m. he is given subcutaneously an injection of soluble insulin: on the first day 10 Units, rising by daily increases of 5 to 10 Units, to a maximum of 40 to 50 Units each morning. He is then screened, the environment is kept quiet, and he is encouraged to relax and drowse. During this time he must be kept under constant nursing observation and details of his condition must be recorded half-hourly. The danger is that he may, while hypoglycaemic, drift into coma.

The symptoms of hypoglycaemia are feelings of weakness, emptiness, shakiness, faintness and hunger: the signs are alterations in the pulse rate, sweating and tremor. Instead of becoming drowsy the patient may become restless and disinhibited, laughing or crying. If there is muscular twitching or the patient becomes not easily rousable the treatment must be interrupted at once by giving glucose by mouth or intravenously, or 0·5 ml. of 1:1000 solution of adrenaline subcutaneously. If the treatment has to be interrupted in this way, the morning dose of insulin should subsequently be reduced by at least 10 Units.

At 10 a.m. (if a premature interruption has not been necessary) the patient is roused and given a breakfast of about 1000 calories, containing 20 to 25 G. protein.

---

[1] This, the usual descriptive label of the treatment, is somewhat misleading: the insulin is not modified.

This breakfast must be appetizing, and the patient should be encouraged to eat all of it: it should be varied as far as possible from day to day. If on account of drowsiness the patient cannot get ahead with solid food, he should be given 2 oz. glucose in a tumblerful of fruit juice and water before he starts the meal. After breakfast the patient may be allowed up and about, and it should be seen that he takes his other meals properly. In the afternoon he may again become slightly hypoglycaemic, and he should be warned of this: the symptoms can be neutralized then by eating sweets or taking a drink of sweetened tea or fruit juice.

The patient's weight should be recorded at the beginning and end of the course of treatment, and weekly during it. The treatment should be continued usually for a few weeks, until normal weight has been attained.

CONTINUOUS NARCOSIS

Woolf originated this form of treatment in 1901 and it was extensively used by Kläsi (1922), with whose name it is usually connected. It was entirely empirical and it is now rarely employed. It is mentioned here because it has not yet been clearly shown to be of no value, and because drugs which have been introduced in recent years could make this a safer form of treatment than hitherto.

The essence of treatment by prolonged sleep is the spaced administration of hypnotics at such intervals as will keep the patient asleep for 18 to 20 hours out of the 24. If thoroughly carried out, the treatment is fraught with some danger—death rates as high as 5 per cent. have been recorded: and as is the case with all treatments which demand a very high degree of skill in the personnel administering them, the risk to the patient is proportionate to the experience of the therapists.

It has been said that continuous narcosis is of value mainly in curtailing the duration of psychotic conditions which would sooner or later recover spontaneously or by other methods of treatment. One can see now no indication for its use in the affective psychoses: and in the management of acute schizophrenic excitements of the agitated fearful type, for which it was advocated, it has been replaced by the tranquillizers. Claims have also been made, more substantial perhaps, for its effectiveness in the treatment of the reactive anxiety states seen in war casualties.

The rationale of the method is that deep and prolonged sleep allows natural processes of mental healing and reintegration to take place more quickly.

Technique of the Treatment. The patient is put to bed in a quiet and darkened room. The hypnotics used most often have been *Somnifaine* (each ml. containing 0·1 G. of diethylbarbituric acid and 0·1 G. of allylisopropylbarbituric acid), amylobarbitone sodium, other longer-acting barbiturates, and paraldehyde. The average amount of *Somnifaine* required was 6 ml. in 24 hours, given intramuscularly in 2 ml. doses: amylobarbitone sodium was given in 3 to 6 gr. doses, up to a total of 30 gr. in the 24 hours. Chlorpromazine was not available when the treatment was most used, and a combination of chlorpromazine with short-acting barbiturates would be a good deal safer than *Somnifaine* (abscesses and damage to the sciatic nerve from the injections were well-recognized risks) and the longer-acting barbiturates.

Continuous, highly skilled nursing care is essential, with frequent recording of the pulse, temperature and blood pressure; charting of fluid intake and output; and repeated examination of the urine for acetone. The patient must get three full meals each day and a large fluid intake is vitally important. The bladder and bowels, too, require close attention. The treatment is continued for a week to fourteen days. Then barbiturates must be withdrawn slowly, if confusion and fits are not to be precipitated.

While under this treatment the patient is on the verge of a drug-induced toxic delirium: he may also pass into coma, become seriously dehydrated, suffer cardio-vascular collapse or develop pneumonia.

The risks are evidently very considerable, the rewards slight and inconstant, and it is perhaps time that the treatment was relegated to the histories of psychiatry.

VARIOUS DRUG TREATMENTS

Tranquillizers

This term has been introduced to describe a group of drugs which, unlike the usual sedatives and hypnotics, produce a calming effect without at the same time causing mental fogging or drowsiness. Some of these drugs appear to do more than tranquillize, and to have a distinct effect in reducing the force of psychotic delusions and hallucinations. The scope and details of their efficacy have as yet not been more than provisionally worked out. Much further research is required, in properly controlled trials, to elucidate their actions in various reaction-types and in the treatment of specific symptoms. Meantime they should be prescribed with as much discrimination as possible, and usually not in combination: though combinations of a phenothiazine derivative with reserpine for schizophrenia, and of a phenothiazine with imipramine for depressives, have been advocated. Chlor-promazine potentiates the action of barbiturates. Tranquillizers have usually to be given for a period of one to three months, before their effectiveness can be properly assessed.

The tranquillizing drugs can at this stage be separated into three main groups: 1. the phenothiazine derivatives; 2. reserpine; and 3. a group which includes benactyzine (*Cevanol*), meprobamate (*Equanil*), and chlordiazepoxide (*Librium*).

1. The phenothiazine derivatives include, in the dimethyl subgroup, chlorpro-mazine, promazine hydrochloride and prochlorperazine (*Stemetil*): and in the piperazine subgroup, perphenazine (*Fentazin*) and trifluoperazine (*Stelazine*).

Of the phenothiazines, chlorpromazine is both the most generally useful and the most toxic. It was introduced by Delay and Deniker in 1952 for the treatment of schizophrenia: and it has proved of great value in controlling turbulent schizo-phrenic behaviour, with the result that mental hospitals have in recent years become much less disturbed by the outbursts of noisy and aggressive patients, and many chronic schizophrenics have been enabled to leave hospital and live in the community. It is also useful in controlling the agitation of depression, the excitement of mania and delirium and the restlessness of senile patients.

The drug is given orally usually, in doses of 25 to 150 mg. three times a day. Larger doses have been given to schizophrenics: and the drug may also be given intramuscularly (chlorpromazine injection, B.P., in 25 to 50 mg. doses). The side-effects are many and may be serious: they include obstructive jaundice, agranulocytosis, skin reactions (including photosensitivity), dryness of the mouth, constipation, hypotension, convulsions and extrapyramidal symptoms. Of the most serious toxic effects, jaundice (1 to 2 per cent. cases) is the commonest, and occurs most often in the first two months of treatment: this, and agranulocytosis, call for immediate stoppage of the drug. Extrapyramidal symptoms often disappear if the dosage is reduced, and they may be suppressed with appropriate drugs (for example, benztropine methanesulphonate, 2 to 6 mg. daily), without impairing the efficacy of chlorpromazine. General guidance cannot be given about the duration of treatment advisable in schizophrenia: it has usually to be extended over months, and one must find out by trial and error if the drug can be withdrawn without precipitating relapse.

The piperazine subgroup of the phenothiazines are thought to have a more marked effect on the delusions of schizophrenics: they also produce extrapyramidal symptoms earlier and more severely, and in some cases severe anxiety and restlessness. Trifluoperazine is perhaps the most potent of this group of drugs. It has appeared to be of particular value in the treatment of chronic, withdrawn schizophrenics. Favourable effects, it is reported, become evident usually within ten days. Patients who respond to the drug become less impulsive and more co-operative in their behaviour, are less troubled by delusions and hallucinations (these may even be abolished), and show a renewal of interest in the world around them.

The average maintenance dose required is 15 to 25 mg. daily, and the drug is administered twice daily by mouth. Treatment should commence usually with a small dose, e.g. 10 mg. daily, and this can be increased to 15 mg. after a week. For rapid, initial administration a preparation is available for deep intramuscular injection: the dose by this route should be small, 1 to 3 mg. daily. Treatment may have to be extended over months.

The main side-effects are neurological. They appear usually in the first few weeks of treatment and become more frequent as the dosage rises above 20 to 25 mg. daily. The symptoms are extrapyramidal and may be florid: motor restlessness, jitteriness and agitation ('akathisia') are common; classical Parkinsonian signs may be developed—mask-like facies, salivation, tremor, rigidity and shuffling gait; and rarely dystonic features, spasms of limb and pharyngeal muscles and oculogyric crises. These extrapyramidal side-effects, and the less common nasal congestion and drowsiness, subside usually within a few days if the drug is reduced or withdrawn. Jaundice and blood dyscrasias have not been reported with trifluoperazine.

2. Reserpine is the main alkaloid of *Rauwolfia serpentina*. Kline first drew attention to its value in psychiatric practice in 1954. Both the phenothiazines and

reserpine have a blocking action on cerebral serotonin and noradrenaline, and reserpine is thought to inhibit the sympathetic vasoconstrictor centre in the hypothalamus. Reserpine was used much initially to sedate schizophrenics, but has recently been replaced by other tranquillizers for this purpose. Its main use now is probably for the control of mania: it may also in some cases diminish the abnormal movements of Huntington's chorea.

The usual dose of reserpine is 0·75 to 1·5 mg. daily: but in cases of mania considerably larger doses may be given, up to at least four times the usual dose. As side-effects, reserpine, like the phenothiazines, may produce extrapyramidal symptoms: it may also cause troublesome nasal stuffiness (due to oedema of the nasal mucous membrane), gastro-intestinal upset, lethargy, bradycardia, dyspnoea at rest, and depression. The latter effect is particularly important, the depression may be severe and suicides have been precipitated.

3. The third group of tranquillizing drugs is heterogeneous, and includes benactyzine, meprobamate and chlordiazepoxide. These drugs are not effective in the psychoses, but they have been advocated in treatment of neurotic reactions. There is, however, as yet no definite evidence that in the control of neurotic symptoms they are more potent than amylobarbitone sodium, and that they should be preferred to the barbiturates. Neither reserpine nor the phenothiazines are useful in the neuroses.

For further details the reader is referred to reviews by Jacobsen (1959) and Kline (1959).

Antidepressant Drugs

Of the recently introduced antidepressant drugs, imipramine and a group of hydrazine derivatives, which are amine-oxidase inhibitors, are the most important, and the former in particular has constituted an important advance in treatment. These drugs are, however, in general less potent than E.C.T., and in cases of acute, severe depression E.C.T. is usually to be preferred. They appear to lessen the severity of the illness, often markedly so, but usually not to cut short its duration: and these drugs have therefore to be prescribed normally for a period which approximates probably to the natural course of the depressive illness.

Kuhn in Switzerland introduced imipramine hydrochloride (*Tofranil*) in 1957 as a drug for the treatment of depression. It is an aminodibenzyl derivative, chemically closely related to chlorpromazine but with different properties. Its mode of action is unknown. It is undoubtedly effective in the treatment of depressive psychoses: some milder cases can be treated throughout satisfactorily in this way, so also cases which are unsuitable for E.C.T. on account of physical disease or injury, and some chronic depressions which have not responded to E.C.T.

Imipramine is prescribed in a dose usually of 25 to 75 mg. three times a day. The following is a typical full dosage schedule: 25 mg. three times a day on the first day, 25 mg. four times a day on the second and third days, and 50 mg. three times a day on the fourth and subsequent days for a month. If the drug is going to produce improvement, this is seen usually in the first 10 days of treatment: but in some cases the drug appears to be very slow in producing its effects, and continuance of it for a month at least is often advised. As the patient improves, the dose can be gradually reduced. Imipramine's side-effects include hypomanic reactions, increased agitation, sweating, dryness of the mouth, skin eruptions, and falls in old people: hallucinatory episodes have also been described, and suicide may be precipitated by reducing a depressed patient's retardation.

The amine-oxidase inhibitor drugs now on the market include iproniazid (*Marsilid*), phenelzine (*Nardil*), nialamide (*Niamid*) and isocarboxazid (*Marplan*). Their sphere of effectiveness is said to overlap that of imipramine, but most of the published papers on their use have reported that they are of particular value in the treatment of atypical, neurotic and reactive depressions.

Iproniazid is the most effective but also the most toxic, causing in some cases a fatal hepatitis: its dosage is 50 mg. three or four times a day. Phenelzine is given usually in 15 mg. doses, nialamide in 50 mg. doses and isocarboxazid in 10 mg. doses thrice or four times a day. Apart from jaundice, the most troublesome side-action with these drugs has been found to be postural hypotension. Good effects, if they are to appear, do so usually within two weeks.

Much work is currently being done on these antidepressant drugs and the sphere of their usefulness can only be indicated in rather general terms at the present time.

NARCO-ANALYSIS

This inelegant term, coined by Horsley (1943), has been used to describe the method in which the intravenous injection of a sedative drug is employed to produce a disinhibited state of mind, so that the patient becomes more communicative and has less emotional control—in fact a temporary state of veritable intoxication, similar to that produced by alcohol. The drugs most used have been *Evipan*, thiopentone and amylobarbitone sodium.

The chief usefulness of the method is in the treatment of hysterical conversion symptoms, and the rapid recovery of memory in cases of psychogenic amnesia. It is more certain to work than hypnosis and gives, therefore, more confidence to the doctor; but with sufficient patience and time, the same and probably better results can nearly always be obtained with persuasion, without either hypnosis or drugs. The method gives the patient something tangible that he understands more easily than the purely psychological method of approach, and it has, in consequence, considerable value as a vehicle of suggestion. It also provides some individuals with a welcome and apparently honourable excuse for divulging what they profess to have forgotten. It is doubtful whether it ever leads the patient to disclose what he still means to conceal. On the other hand, the productions are not necessarily factual—some patients produce phantasies in this state: it is not a 'truth drug'.

The method is also of value in promoting 'abreaction' in neurotic cases, the patient giving his story and recalling memories with more emotion than he is able to do in the ordinary therapeutic setting. It may help to clarify the diagnosis or content of a psychosis, by eliciting symptoms from a stuporous or negativistic patient. It may also be useful occasionally to get over difficult situations where the patient's tension or shame make it impossible for him to co-operate in discussion of his problems.

Technique of the Treatment. It is essential that treatment should be entered on in an atmosphere of optimism and faith in the method. It is extremely likely that usually what is really effective in the situation is the doctor's confidence in the treatment.

If amylobarbitone sodium is used, $7\frac{1}{2}$ gr. of the drug dissolved in 5 ml. of distilled water are injected intravenously, slowly, usually at the rate of about 1 ml. of the solution per minute; the patient counting backwards meanwhile until drowsiness and disinhibition are produced, without however seriously disturbing articulation. It has been said that if the narcosis is pushed beyond this, rapport is lost and is not fully restored in the state of emergence from narcosis; but this has not been our experience.

If the method is used for abreaction, a number of treatments may be required.

Excitatory abreaction, by the use of intravenous methedrine or ether on a mask, has been introduced by Sargant and Shorvon. Emotions of anger and fear particularly are aroused. A crescendo of excitement is induced, reaches a climax and is followed by collapse. Persistent neurotic reactions following traumatic incidents, in men of stable personality, may be helped in this way (see Sargant and Slater, 1954).

REFERENCES

Ackner, B., Harris, A., and Oldham, A. J. (1957) *Lancet*, i, 607.
Corsellis, J. A. N., and Meyer, A. (1954) *J. ment. Sci.*, **100**, 375.
Freeman, W. (1949) *Proc. roy. Soc. Med.*, Supp. **42**, 8.
Freeman, W., and Watts, J. W. (1950) *Psychosurgery*, Illinois.
Fulton, J. F. (1951) *Frontal Lobotomy and Affective Behaviour*, London.
Gottlieb, J. S., and Houston, P. E. (1943) *Arch. Neurol. Psychiat. (Chicago)*, **49**, 266.
Greenblatt, M., and Solomon, H. C. (1953) *Frontal Lobes and Schizophrenia*, New York.
Horsley, J. S. (1943) *Narco-analysis*, London.
Jacobsen, E. (1959) *Bull. Wld Hlth Org.*, **21**, 411.
Kläsi, J. (1922) *Z. ges. Neurol. Psychiat.*, **74**, 557.
Kline, N. S. (1959) *Bull. Wld Hlth Org.*, **21**, 397.
Knight, G. C., and Tredgold, R. F. (1955) *Lancet*, i, 981.
Lingley, J. R., and Robbins, L. L. (1947) *Radiology*, **48**, 124.
Meyer, A., and Beck, E. (1954) *Prefrontal Leucotomy and Related Operations*, Edinburgh.
Meyer, A., and McLardy, T. (1948) *J. ment. Sci.*, **94**, 555.
McKissock, W. (1943) *J. ment. Sci.*, **89**, 194.
McLardy, T., and Davies, D. L. (1949) *J. Neurol. Neurosurg. Psychiat.*, **12**, 231.
Polatin, P. (1939) *J. Amer. med. Ass.*, **112**, 1684.
Roth, M. (1952) *J. ment. Sci.*, **98**, 44.
Russell, W. R. (1948) *Lancet*, i, 356.
Sakel, M. (1936) *Wien. klin. Wschr.*, **49**, 1278.
Sargant, W. (1953) *Brit. med. J.*, **2**, 800.
Sargant, W., and Craske, N. (1941) *Lancet*, ii, 212.
Sargant, W., and Slater, E. (1954) *Physical Methods of Treatment in Psychiatry*, Edinburgh.
Scoville, W. B. (1949) *J. Neurosurg.*, **6**, 65.
Ström-Olsen, R., and Northfield, D. W. C. (1955) *Lancet*, i, 986.
Ziegler, L. H. (1943) *Amer. J. Psychiat.*, **100**, 178.

15

THE ORGANIC REACTION-TYPES

Two organic reaction-types can be differentiated, the acute and the chronic. There are also transitions between them.

The pathological difference lies in the fact that the acute organic reaction is usually the result of a temporary toxic process affecting the brain substance, *e.g.* the delirium of acute fevers, or acute alcoholism, while the chronic organic reaction is the expression of a more severe tissue change, usually a progressive degeneration, as in general paralysis and the senile psychoses.

The organic reaction-type as a whole comprises the following changes:

1. In the intellectual sphere there is impairment of comprehension, interference with elaboration of impressions, defects in orientation and retention, difficulty in activation of memories and marked fluctuation of the level of attention.
2. Affective disorder in the form of emotional instability, the patient laughing or weeping without sufficient cause, and often in an explosive way.
3. Character-change in the form of conduct foreign to the patient's natural disposition, *e.g.* indecent behaviour in a hitherto self-respecting individual.

All these disorders must be taken together as constituting the organic syndrome, although in a given case one set of symptoms is preponderant. The acute reaction consists usually of a delirium, *i.e.* disorientation with false perceptions (illusions) and hallucinations, and with a memory defect involving chiefly recent memory, but without the profound change in the personality seen in the chronic types. The chronic reaction, on the other hand, shows a defect chiefly in comprehension and memory, both recent and remote, and with marked changes in personality and in emotional responsiveness. Further, the chronic reaction is usually progressive, and the changes occur in a state of relatively clear consciousness.

ALCOHOLIC PSYCHOSES

The aetiological significance of alcohol has been discussed at length in Chapter 4, and we are now concerned only with the clinical manifestations associated with alcohol.

Symptoms of alcoholism may complicate many psychoses, *e.g.* general paralysis, manic-depressive psychoses, schizophrenia. Alcoholism may even be a symptom of an anxiety state. There are, however, various types of disturbance which are peculiar to it.

Alcoholism as a complication of subnormality (mental defect) is of particular importance, owing to the antisocial reactions which it is specially apt to release in such circumstances; and partly in relation to this, alcohol is a factor which in a medico-legal case should always be as accurately determined as possible.

Alcoholism *per se* is not, of course, a sufficient defence in law in questions of criminal responsibility.

The three main clinical types of alcoholic psychosis are delirium tremens, Korsakow's psychosis and chronic alcoholism. An alcoholic hallucinosis, an alcoholic pseudoparesis, a pseudoparanoia and an alcoholic epilepsy have also been described. Alcoholic pseudoparesis was used to designate some obscure cases of organic disease, the causation of which was not sufficiently differentiated, and where probably alcohol was only one factor among many. Alcoholic hallucinosis and alcoholic paranoia are probably misnomers, alcoholism being a symptom of an underlying instability which gives rise to the syndrome, rather than a cause of the latter. Kirby says in this connection that alcoholic hallucinosis is not a specific toxic disorder, but belongs rather in the category of reaction-types dependent on constitution and on emotional situations. We have certainly known precisely similar hallucinoses to occur in the absence of alcoholism. According to Schneider, the constitutional basis is essentially the manic-depressive one; but in a small proportion of cases (15 per cent.—Kirby) the alcoholism and the hallucinosis alike are episodes in the course of a schizophrenic illness. It is generally recognized that epileptiform episodes occur in alcoholism, but they do not constitute monosymptomatic disorders, and there is no reason why they should be placed in a separate group as 'alcoholic epilepsy'.

It has been suggested that the polyneuritis and, by inference, the cerebral alteration in alcoholism, are due not to the direct effect of alcohol on the nervous tissue but to a 'conditioned deficiency' resulting from faulty absorption of vitamins from the chronically inflamed stomach, and also from the limited diet which the habitual alcoholic allows himself. On this theory large doses of vitamin B (as much as 3000 I.U.) by injection have been administered in delirium tremens, with, it is claimed, almost immediate subsidence of the delirium; but these claims await confirmation. Even in alcoholic polyneuritis, the response to administration of vitamin B is apt to be disappointing.

Mania à Potu

Mania à potu is a state of pathological intoxication, consisting in extreme excitement, sometimes with homicidal attacks, and resulting from the ingestion of comparatively small amounts of alcohol in a susceptible individual. This condition has occasionally been advanced as a defence in murder trials. Such a case concerned a man, 38 years old, who in a fit of jealousy and after having taken a small quantity of liquor, murdered a man and a woman by shooting. When arrested he was found in bed, but whether asleep or not is unknown. Following his arrest, while in his cell he fell into a deep sleep from which he was roused only with difficulty; the profound nature of the sleep was considered to be a most significant feature. His history showed that there was a hereditary predisposition to mental illness, while he himself had suffered from a head injury when 14 years old, had had sunstroke in India, and during the war had been blown up and buried. The defence in this case was not sustained (*Transactions of the Medico-Legal Society*, vol. 22, 1928).

Dipsomania

This, a state of acute intoxication occurring at intervals, the intervening periods being free from any alcoholic indulgence, is sometimes symptomatic of recurrent attacks of a manic-depressive psychosis, and sometimes of epilepsy. In other cases the pathological basis has not been discovered.

Delirium Tremens

The condition is rare before 30 years of age. It usually arises after a debauch, but may occur in a chronic alcoholic as the result of intercurrent disease or injury. The immediate withdrawal of alcohol from a chronic addict may lead to a delirium. This is the so-called 'abstinence' delirium. Inquiry into some cases of 'abstinence' delirium will show, however, that the patient had left off drinking some days previously because of feelings of nausea; this suggests that an alcoholic illness was already developing, and that the distaste that led to abstinence was a premonitory symptom. The question of the existence of an 'abstinence' delirium is not yet settled.

The chief prodromal symptoms are great restlessness, sleeplessness and fear—the patient starting at the least sound—and profuse perspiration. If he does sleep he has vivid nightmares, and wakes up repeatedly in terror. Unless one can induce sleep at this stage, it rapidly passes into a typical delirium, during which hallucinations, visual, haptic and auditory, make their appearance. The visual hallucinations are the most common. Illusions are prominent and can be easily suggested, e.g. spots on the counterpane which the patient mistakes for animals and attempts to catch. Given a blank piece of paper and asked to 'read' it, he may proceed to do so. The usual visual hallucinations are of snakes and rats. Haptic hallucinations (probably based on paraesthesiae, and therefore more correctly called illusions) are usually of animals crawling over the skin. Sometimes the delirium is occupational in character—the busman drives his vehicle, and a stationmaster's wife constantly sees trains approaching, and crawls all over the bed to get away from them. In response to the hallucinations there may be impulsive conduct, the patient seeking to flee from his supposed persecutors, or attacking them, with the result that he may make suicidal or homicidal attempts. At the height of the delirium the patient is more or less completely disoriented, and the affect is nearly always one of great fear—of being taken away to be punished, for example, or of meeting some dreadful fate. Rarely the affective state is one of amusement or mild indifference to the hallucinations, or even euphoria. The talk is incoherent and shows distractibility, usually in response to the hallucinatory experiences. The delirious patient is very suggestible, and can be readily made to confabulate. Kraepelin and Aschaffenburg pointed out that external stimuli play an important rôle in the character of the delirious content, and that the tendency to rhyme and to form sound associations is well marked. Misidentification of persons is striking, total strangers being recognized as intimate friends. Retention of immediate impressions is almost non-existent; the patient's attention can be obtained momentarily, but it is impossible to hold it.

Physically, there is a generalized tremor, coarse in type, and affecting chiefly

2 A

the fingers, facial muscles and tongue. The temperature is usually slightly raised, the pulse is quick and the patient perspires freely. The tongue is coated, the breath foul, there may be sordes on the lips and the patient has no appetite whatever. Mild transitory albuminuria occurs in about 50 per cent. of cases. Epileptiform convulsions may occur. The pupils are often widely dilated, and may be sluggish in their reaction. The tendon reflexes are in some cases diminished or absent.

Course and Prognosis. The usual duration is from three to six days. Improvement and recovery occur when sleep has been obtained. It has also been frequently noted that when auditory hallucinations are present the duration of the illness is likely to be more prolonged. In uncomplicated cases death is rare (3 or 4 per cent.) but may occur from heart failure. In cases complicated with pneumonia and other infections the outlook is more serious.

Morbid Anatomy. Besides the changes belonging to chronic alcoholism, punctiform haemorrhages in the brain substance and degeneration of nerve cells have been described.

Korsakow's Psychosis

This psychosis, first described by Korsakow, consists in deficient power of retention for recent events, with a tendency to confabulate, and disorientation for time, place and person. It is usually of toxic or vitamin deficiency origin, and is often associated with a polyneuritis, but there are cases where no neuritis exists, as Korsakow himself recognized. Alcohol, other chemical poisons such as lead and arsenic, and bacterial toxins have all been held responsible. Probably the commonest cause is a deficiency of B-group vitamins. Clinically the psychosis is seen most often to develop in the course of chronic alcoholism, usually following an attack of delirium tremens.

The retention defect, and confabulation compensatory for it, is shown, for example, by a patient who assures the physician morning after morning that he has just returned from London that day; or by another who peruses the same book again and again. The retention defect can be clearly brought out by giving them short stories to read. Memory for remote events is usually good. Disorientation for time is more completely affected than disorientation for place or person. Korsakow patients commonly are aware that they are in hospital, and they usually recognize doctors and nurses, although not by names. They suffer from both visual and auditory hallucinations. There is a mixture of euphoria and irritability—they are affable at one time, and at another querulously demand their release. Usually their conversation is clear and intelligent, and they are extraordinarily plausible in their confabulations. Insight is completely lacking, and after recovery, although they recognize they have been ill, it is extremely difficult to persuade them that their condition has been due to alcohol.

Physically, the signs are those of alcoholic polyneuritis, with diminution or abolition of the tendon reflexes, tenderness over the nerve trunks and, in pronounced cases, wrist- and foot-drop. Any of the peripheral nerves may be affected. Ocular palsies may occur, and nystagmus is very common. There is marked tremor of the outstretched fingers.

Course. These cases run a prolonged course. Some begin to show an improvement during the first six weeks. The neuritis may disappear entirely, and usually the physical health improves to a greater degree than the mental. The memory sometimes does not entirely recover. There is also some residual emotional deterioration evidenced by an easy suggestibility, emotional facility and lack of efficiency.

Morbid Anatomy. There are the usual polyneuritic changes in the peripheral nerves. In the cerebrum there are degenerative changes with a central chromatolysis in the ganglion cells, especially of the large pyramids. There is a loss of tangential fibres. In the more chronic cases there is neuroglial proliferation. As in Wernicke's encephalopathy, foci of haemorrhage and softening may be found in the corpora mammillaria.

Chronic Alcoholism

Chronic alcoholism develops in a wide variety of persons—in some because of opportunity (barmen), in others because of the social environment, and in others it begins as a reaction to difficulties, or as the expression of an unstable disposition (manic-depressive, for example).

By the chronic alcoholic we mean to designate the habitual drinker in whom there develops insidiously a change in intellect and character. He is often able to carry on his ordinary work sufficiently well to make a fair appearance to the casual observer; but he never reaches a high pitch of energy or efficiency, and his history is one of gradual deterioration, moral and intellectual. To his companions he is usually pleasant, sociable and sympathetic, entering boisterously into his alcoholic enjoyments, and shedding a ready tear in commiseration of others' misfortunes. At home, on the other hand, he is irritable and careless of his family's welfare. 'They are not mad enough to be regarded as dangerous, so they merely ruin the home in an undramatic way' (MacCurdy). Sometimes the chronic alcoholic goes so far as to sell his home and furniture, thrash his children and strike his wife. It is at this more advanced stage that sexual crimes and indecent assaults are especially frequent.

The affect is a very shallow and labile one, and is closely related to the disorders of conduct just described. Some chronic alcoholics become depressed, and attempt or commit suicide. The alcoholic is very frequently jealous of his wife. There is usually also a generalized persecuted attitude—the patient is never to blame, he is always the worst-used man in the world, constantly bewailing his fate and saying that every man's hand is against him. He is very untruthful, and is always making promises to reform which he never fulfils. He is cunning, evading arrangements made for his guardianship and twisting facts to suit his own ends. 'His heart is soft, and his head is full of deceit.' The memory tends to be faulty, but orientation is for a long time unimpaired. The chronic alcoholic is apt to be litigious. There is no insight of any kind.

In the terminal state of alcoholic dementia the moral and intellectual deterioration reaches an extreme degree. Arteriosclerosis may then complicate the clinical picture.

The following is a typical example:

CASE NO. 48

R. P., a married man 50 years of age. He had always been of unusual temperament, having a difficulty in mixing with other people, so that even his own relatives did not visit him. He was always restless, never being able to enjoy a holiday because he wanted to get back to work. He owned a wine and spirit business, and had at one time a dozen retail shops of his own. Five years before his admission into hospital his disposition began to change. He commenced to grumble about everything at home, became irritable at trifles, swore volubly at his wife and children—a thing he had never done before. For some indefinite time he had been drinking secretly. Three years after this he fell into the hands of the police while drunk, and lost some of his licences in consequence. His ordinary daily programme at that time consisted in going out after breakfast, and returning drunk at midday, sleeping in the afternoon, going out again and returning drunk once more. He showed no care whatever for his family. His son, who was delicate, had sometimes to carry him home. While drunk he exposed himself to his family, including his daughter. During their convalescence from influenza he turned his children out of the house. He would send his wife on errands and refuse to readmit her till she had obtained what he happened to want— usually more alcohol. He took no interest in anything, neglected his business and threatened suicide but made no real attempt at it. In hospital he was antagonistic and resentful, saying that he was unjustly detained, refusing food at times, doing his best to find fault with the ward arrangements. Occasionally, however, he was affable, making caustic jokes. He boasted of his athletic prowess (he was a puny unpleasant-looking little man). He showed no shame at his conduct, denied most of it and lied readily, often contradicting himself. A slight memory defect was revealed by the more difficult tests. He was persistently unco-operative and lacking in insight.

The physical signs result from the effect of alcohol on all the bodily systems. Gastritis, cirrhosis of the liver and polyneuritis are characteristic. Tremors may be prominent, and paraesthesiae and impotence are commonly reported.

Course and Prognosis. The course is slowly but progressively downhill. Permanent arrest of a well-established chronic alcoholic deterioration must be extremely rare (outside of institutions).

Morbid Anatomy. In the cerebrum there is chronic nerve-cell degeneration: both the cortex and the basal ganglia, periaqueductal grey matter and corpora mammillaria are usually damaged.

Psychopathology. It is doubtful whether general statements can be made about the psychopathology of chronic alcoholism. It is commonly stated that chronic alcoholics as a class are essentially homosexual, either consciously or unconsciously. Alcoholic habits lead to a close association with others of the same sex, and at the same time offer a refuge from other situations which, on account of the homosexuality, are unsatisfactory. Marital jealousy is explained on this basis, as a projection of the married alcoholic's unfaithful tendencies. It may equally be the psychological result of the impotence induced by the physical effects of alcohol. Support for the homosexual theory can be obtained from a study of the content of the delirium usually only with the aid of extravagant symbolic interpretation. The content of the auditory and haptic hallucinations in cases in which these are prominent, lends some support, since it is sometimes clearly homosexual; genital paraesthesiae, for example, being interpreted by the patient as evidence of actual homosexual assault. But these cases are in a very small minority, and it has already been remarked that in them usually the alcoholism and the hallucinosis alike are symptoms, and do not stand in the relationship of cause and effect. In general, homosexuality is only one of many possible factors.

The psychological understanding of a chronic alcoholic is an individual affair, and each case must be tackled as a special problem on its merits. The factors which have helped to precipitate a chronic alcoholic habit and to sustain it do not differ in any kind from those which may produce other morbid mental reactions; and sufficient weight should be given to the influence of habit, to the influence of nagging friends and relatives in accentuating it and to the manner in which the alcoholism becomes a part of the ego-ideal, so that to keep on drinking becomes a point of honour.

Treatment of Alcoholism

There is no specific cure for alcoholism, but in the earlier stages of the illness, before dementia has developed, much can be effected and the patient given a new start.

Delirium Tremens. The chief aims of treatment are to alleviate the excitement, to maintain the patient's strength, to promote the natural functions and to procure sleep.

A patient of this sort does much better with strangers and, particularly if he is to be treated satisfactorily in his own house, nurses experienced in the management of delirious patients should be provided. Alternatively and preferably, treatment may be carried out in a nursing home or in the psychiatric ward of a general hospital. Recovery is so likely to occur quickly that there is no justification for compulsory admission to a mental hospital. No patient should be certified while he is under the influence of liquor. The delirious patient should be nursed in bed, constantly supervised, and reassured by changes and disturbances in his environment being reduced to the minimum.

There is general agreement that the amount of alcohol given must be carefully controlled, but disagreement about the advisability of an abrupt cessation of alcohol intake. In our view, it is illogical to continue to give a drug which, if it has not produced, has at least materially contributed to, a dangerous state of intoxication; and we have not seen ill-effects from stopping the intake of alcohol as soon as the patient comes under treatment. Where the provision for nursing care is less adequate and the patient less confused, some compromise may have to be made until the patient comes under the control of sedatives: and some physicians make an exception of the elderly patient, giving small quantities of alcohol in the belief that a sudden cessation of the drug might precipitate collapse.

Sedatives to produce sleep are essential, and a large dose of whatever drug is chosen should be given initially. Cyclobarbitone, B.P., 6 gr. with a further 3 gr. in four hours if necessary, or pentobarbitone sodium, B.P. (*Nembutal*), 3 gr. with a later 3 gr., we have found satisfactory hypnotics in many cases. Paraldehyde, 3 to 4 drachms by mouth (or fluid 5 to 10 ml. by intramuscular injection), has many advocates, but in some cases it seems to increase the excitement, and there is also some risk of the alcoholic becoming addicted to it. Chlorpromazine (*Largactil*) either intramuscularly or by mouth is most helpful in controlling excitement. Several drugs or combinations of drugs may have to be tried before successful control of the restlessness is obtained. Sedation during the day is also required; chloral hydrate, 20 gr. twice or thrice a day, may be sufficient. In an emergency of great restlessness, a hypodermic injection of hyoscine hydrobromide, B.P., $\frac{1}{100}$ gr., may be given. If the patient is sufficiently co-operative, warm baths are helpful in procuring relaxation and sleep. As a further aid to relaxation, soluble insulin in doses of 5 to 30 Units may be prescribed twice or thrice daily; sopor must be immediately interrupted with glucose.

When there is much gastritis, it is well to begin by washing out the stomach. Food should be liquid or semi-solid, and in small quantities to obviate vomiting: it must have as high a caloric value as possible, with plenty of carbohydrates. Tube-feeding may be necessary. Since the patient suffering from delirium tremens sweats profusely, he becomes dehydrated. This lost fluid must be replaced and an intake of around 3 litres per day should be ensured. If the sweating is very profuse and particularly if it is accompanied by vomiting, an important deficiency of sodium chloride as well as of fluid results. This can be corrected by preparing beverages with 0·2 per cent. saline instead of plain water, or by giving sodium chloride, 2 G. in capsules four-hourly. Constipation is usual, and should be treated by giving initially 2 to 3 gr. of calomel at night, followed by magnesium sulphate, 1 ounce, in the morning.

It is probable that vitamin deficiency plays a significant rôle in the genesis of delirium tremens, and it is customary therefore to prescribe B group vitamins. At least 20 mg. thiamine should be given intramuscularly, and 500 mg. nicotinic acid parenterally or by mouth daily. In cases where the intake by mouth is unsatisfactory the vitamins should always be given parenterally, and it has been claimed that B group vitamins given intravenously have an almost specific effect in cutting short the delirium. The value of ACTH in aborting the illness is still *sub judice*.

Cardiac failure and pneumonia are two of the chief causes of death. Where there is evidence of commencing congestive failure, fluid intake must be carefully controlled and the patient should be rapidly digitalized. Any chest infection should be promptly treated with an antibiotic.

Korsakow's Psychosis. Many patients suffering from this disorder have to be treated in mental hospitals, as the condition is prolonged, and difficult to manage at home. While acute symptoms of neuritis are present, the patient should be nursed in bed and care taken to minimize the effect of peripheral neuritis: massage, passive and active movements are advisable after the acute symptoms have subsided. The general physical state is usually considerably enfeebled and should be restored by giving a full diet, with Marmite. The prescription of additional specific B group vitamins is of doubtful value.

Chronic Alcoholism. The kind of treatment to be adopted, and the hope entertained for it, depends partly on the type of chronic alcoholic with whom one is dealing and partly on the stage at which he comes (or is brought) for treatment.

Careful investigation from a physical and a psychiatric view-point is an essential preliminary. Where alcoholism is found to be a symptom of some disease, mental or physical, such as general paralysis or a recurrent manic-depressive psychosis, the treatment is that of the underlying disease. When the alcoholic habit itself is in the forefront, the chief line of attack is a thorough investigation of the factors of the patient's life and personality. Usually the first step that should be insisted on is that the patient should place himself in a nursing home or in a hospital where he can be adequately supervised. This, of course, is usually what the patient refuses to do, but with the exercise of tact and patience it is often possible in the early stages to get the patient's co-operation. In our experience, the psychological view-point is usually a revelation to the patient, and the physician who places it before him is at once at an advantage; for always the patient has been taught by his friends that his condition is simply one of moral turpitude, and nearly always he has personally come to regard his alcoholism as mysterious and inevitable. The patient's goodwill having been gradually obtained in this way, it is usually possible to show him the factors, psychological and circumstantial, which have contributed to his illness; and to show him how they can be more satisfactorily dealt with. Abstinence should be insisted on, and the patient has usually to be taught that it is not unmanly to be abstinent. An avoidance of unnecessary opportunity for drinking is extremely important; for example, it is unwise to send him back to work as a bar-tender or an exciseman. The cultivation of hobbies and social recreation of a healthy kind, to replace the discarded alcoholism, is also important. When the immediate treatment is finished, and the patient returns to work, he should be encouraged to keep in touch with his medical adviser for a year or two. With the more advanced chronic alcoholic, in whom definite and irreversible moral and intellectual deterioration has set in, the case is different; compulsory admission to a mental hospital is always necessary to prevent further deterioration. This in ordinary cases is very difficult, on account of the patient's plausibility and good superficial appearance.

The emetic effects of apomorphine and emetine have been used for some years in the *conditioned aversion therapy* of chronic alcoholics: the latter drug is now usually preferred. Emetine hydrochloride is given by intramuscular injection to produce nausea and vomiting, and is usually combined with pilocarpine hydrochloride which produces intense sweating and with ephedrine sulphate which is supposed to provide cardiac support. As nausea develops, the patient is plied with alcoholic drinks, and encouraged to smell, taste and consume them despite vomiting. The procedure lasts about twenty minutes and is repeated on about five successive days. Careful preliminary physical examination is necessary to judge the patient's fitness to undergo the rigours of the treatment. It is uncertain how strong a true conditioned aversion is created: probably suggestion is important in the results obtained. Details of the treatment are given by Lemere, Voegtlin *et al.* (1942). It has been claimed that 55 per cent. of those treated have remained abstainers for three years or more (Voegtlin and Broz, 1949). Conditioned aversion therapy should not be considered more than an adjunct to the psychotherapeutic and social methods of treatment.

Tetraethylthiuram disulphide (*Antabuse*, disulfiram, I.N.N.) was introduced by Hald and Jacobsen (1948). This drug interferes with the normal oxidation of alcohol, and in doing so causes an increased liberation of acetaldehyde in the body. It is acetaldehyde poisoning that produces the symptoms upon whose discouraging effects the treatment depends. If an individual who is taking *Antabuse* takes alcohol within 24 hours of the last dose of *Antabuse*, he develops usually within 20 minutes a highly unpleasant reaction, which is characterized by intense flushing of the face, neck and upper chest, tachycardia and palpitations, headache, dyspnoea, nausea and vomiting, and in some cases cardiovascular collapse. In rare cases, acute right-sided heart failure has led to death. Other toxic symptoms have been reported, notably dizziness, diplopia, skin rashes, peripheral neuritis and delirium. At first it was thought that the *Antabuse*-alcohol reaction was the cause of these, but more recently it has been recognized that the drug itself, although relatively non-toxic, may produce side-effects. These are usually mild and include drowsiness, fatigue, headache and reduced libido. *Antabuse* has, however, been very widely used now with relatively few serious ill-effects and very few fatal ones, and though one must know the possible toxic effects of the drug their importance should not be overstressed. The individual who is given the drug must of course be in reasonably satisfactory physical condition: cardiac decompensation is an absolute bar to this treatment, as is any serious damage to the liver or kidneys. *Antabuse* should never be given while the individual has alcohol in his body, and must never be given surreptitiously. A suitable commencing dose is 0·5 G. on the first day, then 1 G. daily for three days, followed by 0·25 to 0·5 G. daily as a maintenance dose which may have to be continued for many months. On the fourth or fifth day after the commencement of the treatment, a test dose of half to one ounce of alcohol may be given, to indicate to both doctor and patient whether or not the treatment is effective: some workers now omit this as unnecessary and to some degree dangerous, and if it is carried out the patient should be in bed and equipment for his resuscitation must be at hand in case his reaction should be severe. *Antabuse* is particularly helpful in the treatment of intelligent and co-operative alcoholics, who come for treatment early in their illness and who feel that they require some extra safeguard in the early months of their abstinence, particularly on social occasions. The success of the method depends obviously on the degree of the patient's co-operation.

Unless and until a correctable metabolic disorder is found to be the cause of certain cases of alcoholism, the use of drugs in this field is likely to be a superficial method of treatment and of limited value. An approach through correction of the alcoholic's defective personal attitudes and relationships holds out more promise, and it is this which the group movement known as *Alcoholics Anonymous* (A.A.) has some success in effecting. Launched in 1934 in the U.S.A., A.A. now has groups in more than thirty countries (the location of groups in Britain may be learnt by communicating with BM/AAL, W.C.2). In voluntary association the members meet regularly, discuss experiences and problems and the tenets of their movement, and work actively in the reclamation of other alcoholics. Against the 'defiant individuality and grandiosity' of many alcoholics, they set a belief that the alcoholic can overcome his trouble only by surrender and by accepting some power greater than himself. The essential element is therefore a form of religious conversion (Tiebout, 1944). Certain criticisms may be made of the movement; that it depends rather too much on emotion, and that its conversions are not always followed by a real maturing of the personality. But, in a field where the psychiatrist so often fails, its successes may be outstanding.

OPIUM AND MORPHINE ADDICTION

The effects of opium and its alkaloid morphine are so much alike that they may be described together.

It has already been stated that the percentage of psychoses attributable to opium and its derivatives is very small indeed. The continual use of opium, however, leads to a chronic change in personality, although this seldom goes to the extent of gross mental disorder.

It has been observed that morphine in sufficient dosage can produce necrosis and softening in the brain. This is considered to be anoxaemic in origin from interference of the morphine with oxidation processes. Similar results occur with carbon monoxide and narcotics (Alfred Meyer). But in all these instances it can only be with very large and not with therapeutic doses that such irrevocable changes occur.

The habit begins in some cases accidentally, the drug having been prescribed for the alleviation of physical suffering, but the large number of opium addicts are people originally of a psychopathic make-up. In all cases a character-change, directly attributable to the use of the drug, sets in as soon as the habit is established for its own sake. The change consists in a gradual deterioration of the personality. There is a general falling off in efficiency, partly because the higher intellectual faculties become impaired, and partly because there is a lowering of aims, ambitions and energy. The whole life of the addict revolves round the procuring of an adequate supply. Ethical deterioration is a prominent feature; the sense of responsibility diminishes, and is lost; the addict becomes untrustworthy in all directions, and untruthful, especially regarding the drug habit itself. He is suspicious and furtive in his manner, perhaps on account of the social disapproval entailed by his addiction. His suspiciousness may develop into actual ideas of persecution. The mood is very variable, the degree of well-being varying inversely with the time that has elapsed since the last dose, and irritability and restlessness appearing as the time for the next dose draws near. Memory, attention and grasp of current events all deteriorate, partly as the result of progressive restriction of interest to the problem of obtaining and using the drug. When delirium (an excited hallucinatory episode with fear) occurs, it is very often because the patient has been taking some other drug as well, such as alcohol or cocaine.

Sudden withdrawal or deprivation of the drug may lead to the occurrence of a delirium, with horrible hallucinations, and with more or less restlessness, amounting sometimes to mild psychomotor excitement. In other cases the delirium may be of a quiet, dreamy type, with disorientation.

Physical Symptoms. The typical drug addict is a feeble, debilitated and emaciated creature, with sallow, greyish complexion, whose skin may show numerous marks of hypodermic injections which have been allowed to go mildly septic. Tremors and, in severe cases, slight disturbances of co-ordination affecting speech or even the eye muscles, diminished general sensibility, small pupils, impotence and paraesthesiae are the principal nervous symptoms. The tongue is dirty, the breath foul and the appetite lacking, and there is constipation, alternating with diarrhoea. There is some secondary anaemia. The skin and hair are dry.

The addict deprived of his drug, or obtaining it in insufficient doses, is miserable, restless, sleepless and full of malaise and aches and pains.

Prognosis. The outlook is always very serious. Spontaneous abandonment of the habit is very rarely successfully maintained. Treatment, even when temporarily successful, is usually followed by relapse.

Treatment. The patient must be removed to a hospital or to a nursing home, where all access to drugs can—theoretically at least—be definitely prevented. Gradual withdrawal, with the gradual substitution of other drugs, followed by their withdrawal in turn, is probably the best treatment. Sudden withdrawal is unnecessarily distressing, and may produce a collapse. The substituted drugs should be used for procuring sleep and for comfort, and may consist of codeine in doses of $\frac{1}{4}$ or $\frac{1}{2}$ gr. not oftener than at four-hour intervals, methadone, B.P., 10 to 50 mg. twice daily, or barbiturates. They should be given only in sufficient quantity to procure relief from the symptoms of gradual withdrawal, and should themselves be gradually diminished in quantity after all morphine has been discontinued. The nature of the individual dose should be concealed from the patient. After all morphine has been stopped he can be informed of the fact.

Warm baths are useful in allaying discomfort and also help to produce sleep. The nutrition must be sustained by diet appropriate to the state of the digestive system. Ample fluids should be given.

When withdrawal has been accomplished, it is important to keep the patient under supervision and to endeavour to build up his morale as well as his physique. Psychotherapy in the sense of investigation into his history and make-up, and discussion of the factors which have led to his addiction, with encouragement and general guidance, should be employed for as long a period as possible.

COCAINISM

Cocaine is not so much indulged in as opium and its derivatives, but is chiefly used as an accompaniment or alternative to other drugs of addiction. It is, perhaps, the most rapidly pernicious of all forms of drug addiction.

The results of a dose of cocaine are slight dizziness and headache, quickly followed by a feeling of well-being, during which period the patient feels more active mentally. This increased mental activity is real, but does not endure. In this stage the addict is garrulous, witty, writes a great deal and has no sensations either of hunger or fatigue. Vivid illusions and hallucinations of a pleasant kind occur, and are often of diminutive objects ('Lilliputian' hallucinations). In this stage of intoxication the illusions and hallucinations and the phantasies generally are in the nature of wish-fulfilments. After the acute effects wear off, there is a general diminution in activity, with some inco-ordination, and the mood fluctuates from well-being to irritability, moroseness and suspicion.

The addict, usually constitutionally psychopathic or of abnormal personality, becomes increasingly depraved morally, neglecting his family, his work and his social obligations. He tends to associate with other addicts and with prostitutes, and may indulge in sexual crimes and crimes of violence.

Impotence appears quickly in men, but in women libido is said to be increased, and to lead to perversions. Dilated pupils, dryness of the mucous membranes (leading to excessive drinking), anorexia, palpitation and emaciation are the common physical signs.

The end may come from cardiac failure, or paralysis of respiration, or inter-current disease, to which his feeble physical condition makes the addict peculiarly susceptible.

Abstinence produces unpleasant paraesthesiae, especially creeping sensations under the skin ('cocaine bug'), gastric disturbances, depression and fearful hallucinations.

Other types of mental disturbance have been noted by Bleuler in cocaine addicts. He described a disorder resembling a Korsakow psychosis, but with irritability, flight of ideas and ineffective preoccupation with small tasks. Co-ordination disturbance (tremor, ataxia), sleeplessness, impotence and emaciation, may appear, and the picture may resemble general paralysis.

Delusions of persecution, especially of jealousy, and with hallucinations of similar content, occur in a few patients. In this type, and in the Korsakow-like variety, orientation is not impaired, and the persecuted cocaine addict may be dangerous.

The treatment is the same as for opium addiction. There is said to be less danger of collapse from withdrawal.

Organized methods of treatment for larger groups have so far failed to justify themselves, partly on account of the failure to provide means of social rehabilitation after discharge, and partly on account of the character and personality of the addicts themselves, especially their reactions to and with each other when treated in a group—their 'code', not to give each other away and to regard addiction as a sign of manliness; and their suggestibility, so that older addicts influence the others detrimentally, and the weaker take their code from the disgruntled.

MARIHUANA INTOXICATION

Parts of the Indian hemp (*Cannabis indica*) plant have been used for centuries in many parts of the world to produce a pleasurable intoxication. Hashish is a form of the resin of the plant; marihuana consists of the dried leaves of the female plant, which in Europe and America are smoked as cigarettes ('reefers'). The number of marihuana users in the U.S.A. is not known, but according to Maurer and Vogel (1954) most experts agree that marihuana addicts there far outnumber the combined total of the users of all other addicting drugs with the exception of alcohol. Marihuana seems to have a special attraction for young people in the large cities. In Britain the problem is a small one, nearly confined to foreign immigrants and to the ports.

Intoxication produces a state of often hilarious elation, with disinhibition and increased suggestibility, and distortions in time and space perception. Depersonalization and disturbances of body image may also occur. Appetite is typically increased, the breath has a characteristic odour, and the conjunctivae are reddened. Motor co-ordination is not seriously impaired. It is not specifically an aphrodisiac. Excitement is usually followed by 'delicious' lassitude and sleep. No marked degree of tolerance of the drug is built up, the addict does not develop a physical dependence such as is found with the opiates, and there is no abstinence syndrome. A temporary toxic psychosis may, however, be precipitated in a susceptible individual.

Like alcohol, the disinhibiting effects of marihuana may lead to crime. Maurer and Vogel state that most marihuana users suffer from basic personality defects similar to those which characterize the alcoholic. They consider that the drug has received a disproportionate share of publicity as an inciter of violent crime, and that its use presents a very minor problem compared with alcoholism. Perhaps its most dangerous aspect is the fact that it may lead to the use of heroin.

BROMIDE INTOXICATION

Bromide salts used to be prescribed so indiscriminately in nervous and mental disorders, and in epilepsy, that prior to the Second World War cases of bromide intoxication were common. They are now rare, because doctors have been so thoroughly warned of the toxic effects of bromides: one feels sometimes that the drug is now so held in awe that it is not prescribed when it helpfully might be. Very occasionally now one encounters an individual who has become addicted to a bromide and chloral mixture, and rarely also an old person with failing heart who has become confused by a bromide hypnotic. Some individuals can tolerate a serum bromide level of 200 mg. or over. Mental symptoms are unlikely unless the serum bromide is at least 150 mg. per cent., but this toxic level may be lower if renal function is impaired (as it commonly is in old people).

The delirium produced by bromide does not differ from that caused by other toxic agents. The individual becomes in the earlier stages of the intoxication forgetful, irritable and generally sluggish. Later, as confusion increases, he shows a fear reaction in association with hallucinations and disorientation. He does not recover as quickly as a case of delirium tremens does, but more gradually over many days or even weeks, depending on the degree of intoxication and the rate of elimination of the drug.

Physically, the patient looks unwell and has commonly lost weight. Often he has a notably sallow complexion and he may (but does not always) have an acneiform rash on face and back. The breath may be fetid, the tongue is usually coated with a thick brown fur, and the bowels are constipated. Speech may be slurred, tremors and inco-ordination may be marked, and the pupils react sluggishly to light, so that in severe cases the clinical picture may resemble general paralysis.

The blood bromide should be estimated in all patients in whom the diagnosis is suspected. Treatment is by immediate stoppage of the drug and by giving plenty of fluid and sodium chloride.

AMPHETAMINE INTOXICATION

The amphetamine group of drugs give a stimulus and feeling of euphoria which the temperamentally unstable person may find irresistible. Multiple addictions, to alcohol, barbiturates and amphetamines are not uncommon: and the drug addict may go from one drug to another. He may have been attracted to the drug by hearing of its pep-producing qualities, or originally been prescribed it by his doctor to counteract obesity, or to relieve depression or fatigue.

Any of the amphetamine group of drugs may cause addiction—amphetamine, dexamphetamine (*Dexedrine*), methylamphetamine (*Methedrine*) and phenmetrazine (*Preludin*). Doses which give mental stimulation may produce little or no evidence of sympathetic overaction. Psychotic symptoms may result from a single large dose, but are unusual unless the daily intake of the drug is more than 50 mg. The most prominent mental symptoms of intoxication are commonly delusions of persecution, with auditory and visual hallucinations. There is often little or no clouding of consciousness, and the toxic reaction is commonly misdiagnosed as a paranoid psychosis or paranoid schizophrenia: it is, however, transient usually, responding in a few days to withdrawal of the drug. With higher doses of the drug a frank delirium may be produced. While acutely intoxicated, the patient may be violent towards others: and in the withdrawal phase there is a suicidal risk particularly in cases where the amphetamine has been prescribed for an existing depression.

The drug-addicted individual commonly dissembles about his use of drugs, and it is therefore fortunate that amphetamine intoxication may be diagnosed in the laboratory by the methyl-orange test. A 10 ml. specimen of urine should be forwarded to which 2 ml. of glacial acetic acid has been added. This test should be employed in the differential diagnosis of all acute paranoid reactions.

The features of amphetamine intoxication are not peculiar to this intoxication, and an 'amphetamine psychosis' should not be described as a clinical entity. A full description of the condition has been given by Connell (1958).

CARBON MONOXIDE POISONING

Carbon monoxide poisoning is of psychiatric importance, not only because inhalation of coal-gas and of car exhaust gases are common forms of attempted suicide, but more particularly because the mental after-effects of this poisoning may be so severe that the patient comes under psychiatric care.

In the blood, carbon monoxide combines readily with haemoglobin to form carboxyhaemoglobin, the blood's capacity to take up oxygen is thus reduced and anoxaemia results. Symptoms do not usually develop until the blood is more than 10 per cent. saturated. Headache, weakness, nausea and vomiting precede the collapse which may be fatal. In the cases of more severe poisoning which are not fatal, the patient is usually first seen in a state of delirium or coma, with a cherry-red complexion and often pulmonary oedema. This acute confusional state may clear in a few days and the patient go on to make a satisfactory recovery, or a chronic organic mental reaction may ensue if there has been severe brain damage.

There is a third possible development, as Kraepelin first pointed out, which is typical of carbon monoxide poisoning. The patient may make an apparently good initial recovery; though this recovery, if a careful mental examination has been made, will usually be seen not to have been complete, some persisting defect at least in mental grasp and concentration being usually found. The patient may be discharged home from hospital. One to three weeks later relapse occurs, and this may be acute, severe and even fatal. The patient may then pass into a state of akinetic mutism, of dementia with parietal lobe symptoms, or (and this is usually a somewhat later development) may develop Parkinsonism. The prognosis of these later-developing mental and physical sequelae is very variable and on the whole bad: dementia and Parkinsonism may persist, the akinetic mute state may be transient.

Pathologically, the main damage is seen in the cerebral cortex and in the basal ganglia. The two main factors producing the cerebral lesions are believed to be anoxaemia and vascular damage. Most typical is a bilateral and symmetrical necrosis of the globus pallidus (Meyer, 1958). More rarely lesions elsewhere in the extrapyramidal system have been reported—in the putamen and substantia nigra. The cortical softening may be widespread.

The emergency treatment of coal-gas poisoning is to take the patient into the open air and apply artificial respiration. Then oxygen and carbon dioxide should be administered by mask, and shock actively combated.

LEAD POISONING

The effect of the long-continued absorption of lead in producing peripheral paralysis, alimentary disturbances and anaemia is well known. Mental effects in the form of the so-called lead encephalopathy have also been described but are rare. The lead may be swallowed (*e.g.* by children or by those working with lead paint), or inhaled in dust and fumes in industry. Delirium and fits precede coma: death or permanent cerebral damage may result. Volatile tetra-ethyl lead, used in the blending of petrol, may produce from inhalation an acute poisoning: the sequence of symptoms described by Yandell Henderson (1926) was insomnia, visual hallucinations and violent excitement, soon leading to death. Inhalation of lead dust leads to the slower and more usual forms of poisoning.

INFECTION-EXHAUSTION PSYCHOSES

By the infection-exhaustion psychoses are designated conditions accompanying or following on infective illness, poisoning by some exogenous toxin, severe physical strain, such as haemorrhage and prolonged parturition, and any other severe stress of a physical kind. The infection-exhaustion psychoses belong principally to the organic reaction-type, but in any infective-exhaustive state a latent reaction-type of another kind (for example, manic-depressive psychosis, schizophrenia) may be unmasked. There is no unitary correspondence between variety of toxin or infection and type of clinical syndrome. All sorts of different toxic agents may produce closely similar or identical clinical pictures, and the same toxin can lead to the outbreak of very different psychoses, depending on the make-up of the individual affected.

Of the infections, those which seem most commonly to produce psychoses, both in the acute stages of the infection and in the convalescence afterwards, are malaria, influenza, pneumonia, smallpox, acute rheumatism, scarlet fever, typhoid and typhus.

Mental symptoms may appear in the prefebrile, the febrile or the post-febrile stage. The symptomatology in all three stages is closely similar, and attempts to differentiate between the mental symptoms of the various stages have not been satisfactory. The main clinical forms at any stage are delirium, epileptiform, dazed and stuporous conditions, hallucinoses, hallucinatory katatonic and incoherent confusional states (Bonhoeffer).

In the later (post-febrile) states one may see amnesia, sometimes of the Korsakow type, apathy, or other emotional change such as depression, and defects of attention. Children may suffer an arrest of mental development which may or may not be made up later.

The commonest syndrome is a delirium, usually ushered in by complaints of physical exhaustion, restlessness, sleeplessness, irritability, headaches and giddiness, terrifying dreams and a feeling of being mixed up in the head. The prodromal period of the delirium may last for several days. Disorientation for time and place follows, with illusions and hallucinations of sight and hearing, and considerable fear. The illusory manifestations are of a fearful kind, and involve sights and sounds in the environment. Suicidal attempts are not uncommon, often as a reaction to hallucinatory experiences. Wild excitement, closely resembling an acute manic excitement, is sometimes the first symptom. These are the characteristics of delirium at the height of the fever. In very severe infections the symptoms begin to indicate a still greater impairment of mental and psychomotor activity. Speech becomes still more incoherent, low and mumbling. The drowsiness may now amount to coma, often with open eyes (coma vigil), which nevertheless reveal no comprehension of the surroundings. Jactitation, *subsultus tendinum* and involuntary passage of urine and faeces occur. Cases of this type usually end in death. Less severe cases continue in the delirious state till the fever begins to subside. 'Lucid intervals' of brief duration—*i.e.* variations in the level of consciousness in the direction of clearness—may occur in the course of the delirium.

The post-febrile stage is essentially one of invalidism, with depression or apathy, disinclination for exertion and easy fatigability, mental or physical, and memory defects. This condition may appear immediately; but sometimes it does not appear for some considerable time afterwards. Convalescence is remarkably slow. After influenza, depression is especially common and there is the risk of suicide.

It is in the post-febrile period that reaction-types of a constitutional kind—manic-depressive and schizophrenic—are especially apt to appear.

Morbid Anatomy. The morbid changes in the brain are not well known. Oedema of the pia arachnoid has been seen in some cases. Some vascular congestion of the brain substance has been described. The nerve changes are such as would naturally accompany a pyrexia and toxaemia. There is a peripheral chromatolysis, especially of the large nerve cells of the cortex.

Prognosis. The great majority of infective-exhaustive psychoses get well. Death occurs, of course, in conditions of very acute or prolonged physical illness. A small number suffer a lasting impairment of intellect, especially of memory.

It may be said that the prognosis of a schizophrenic reaction occurring in a delirious setting is, on the whole, more favourable than a similar reaction occurring in a setting of clear consciousness.

Diagnosis. In the great majority of cases the diagnosis is clear, because the temporal relation between the mental symptoms and the onset of the fever is usually obvious. The differentiation of manic, schizophrenic and other reactions can only be made by following the progress of the case. Wherever delirium, often in its main manifestation more loosely called 'confusion', is present, it is a working rule to search for a physical, especially a toxic or septic, basis. Here, if anywhere, when no clear cause of a psychosis of the acute organic reaction-type presents itself, is the legitimate application of the focal infection theory. In such instances it sometimes happens that a hitherto unsuspected sinus infection, for example, usually of the 'closed' type, is the principal or at least a contributory agent. Psychogenic deliria (hysterical) having their origin in a wish-fulfilment can usually be differentiated by their much greater internal consistency, and sometimes by the grotesque absurdity of their content and their relation to recent emotional stress. The post-febrile stage of invalidism, described above, includes the 'hyperaesthetic emotional state' of German authors, and has to be differentiated from 'neurasthenia' of psychological origin by the history, the previous personality and a proper evaluation of the individual symptoms.

Treatment. This is for the concomitant physical condition. Otherwise it is symptomatic, and on the same lines as the treatment of delirium tremens [see page 361].

PUERPERAL PSYCHOSES

Jacobs (1943) has shown that a septic puerperium in itself is relatively unimportant unless it is complicated by the presence of other predisposing and precipitating factors. She makes it clear that in manic-depressives the likelihood of a psychosis following childbirth is considerably greater than in other groups. The particular precipitating factors stressed by her are: 1. aversion towards childbirth; 2. a neurotic attitude towards motherhood based on experiences in the parental home; 3. an unsatisfactory married life. The importance of the husband's attitude towards the pregnancy and birth is not enough appreciated as regards its effect on the woman. It may be very pathological indeed; for example, in one of Jacobs' cases the husband identified himself with his wife in the puerperium, suffered from hyperemesis and thus illustrated a reversion to the rite of the *couvade* in the manner to which E. Jones has called attention.

In cases of pregnancy the psychological condition of the woman should receive considerable care. The physician should not only inculcate a healthy attitude towards childbirth, but should also attempt to deal with any psychological conflicts arising out of the marital situation.

Recurrent psychoses arising in relation to childbirth are apt to lead to considerable mental deterioration, and when such a tendency exists, the possibility of termination and sterilization should be considered.

WERNICKE'S ENCEPHALOPATHY

In 1881 Wernicke described a series of cases of acute superior haemorrhagic polio-encephalitis which were regarded as dependent on chronic alcoholism. Since then Neuburger and Campbell and Biggart have pointed out that the same condition may occur as a complication of other conditions in non-alcoholics. The pathological lesions consist of foci of vascular stasis and parenchymatous degeneration occurring symmetrically in the corpora mammillaria, and in other parts of the hypothalamus, the fornix, the juxtaventricular zone of the thalamus, the peri-aqueductal grey matter of the midbrain, the posterior colliculi and the floor of the fourth ventricle. Lesions may also be found in the corpus striatum, the substantia nigra, the anterior colliculi, the optic nerves and, rarely, in the cerebral cortex.

Campbell and Ritchie Russell (1941), in an analysis of 21 cases, pointed out that Wernicke's encephalopathy was not an uncommon condition, that it occured as a complication of a wide range of other diseases, and that it could be diagnosed clinically. Eight of the cases were associated with alcoholism, but following Neuburger's suggestion regarding its occurrence in cases of gastric carcinoma and chronic gastritis, Campbell and Russell carefully investigated a series of cases of fatal gastro-intestinal disease associated particularly with a history of disturbance of memory or consciousness before death. In addition to alcoholism their case material comprised cases of gastric carcinoma, pyloric stenosis, chronic dyspepsia, macrocytic anaemia, chronic septic peritonitis, hyperemesis gravidarum, pernicious anaemia, pregnancy with vomiting, bronchiectasis, chronic pyosalpinx, meningo-vascular syphilis and a child of $3\frac{1}{2}$ years dying from (?) whooping cough. Their investigations indicate that the association of Wernicke's disease with alimentary disturbance and polyneuritis suggests a vitamin deficiency.

The clinical symptoms were described as falling into two groups: 1. disturbances of consciousness and of higher cerebral functions; 2. focal neurological signs and symptoms.

The first group of symptoms was a constant feature. The picture was of

2 B

drowsiness, delirium and Korsakow features, *e.g.* disorientation, amnesia, hallucinations and confabulation. Their experience confirmed that of Krant, who stated that he had never seen a case of fatal Korsakow's psychosis without Wernicke lesions; this referred to both alcoholic and non-alcoholic cases. Epileptiform convulsions are an occasional accompaniment. Optic nerve lesions are said to be a significant part of the Wernicke syndrome.

Oculomotor disturbances were present in 10 cases and constituted the most frequent and most important group of focal neurological signs and symptoms. Unequal and irregular pupils, the Argyll Robertson phenomenon, paralysis of conjugate eye movements, diplopia, strabismus and nystagmus were all noted.

There may be respiratory paralysis of central origin and pyramidal tract involvement, while polyneuritis was present in 9 cases.

Campbell and Russell, and others, stress the important aetiological factor as a deficient intake of some part or parts of the vitamin B complex; most probably of thiamine.

Previously usually fatal, recovery may take place in these cases if large doses of vitamin B complex are given parenterally. At least 50 mg. of thiamine hydrochloride, B.P., must be given parenterally, daily.

PSYCHOSES DUE TO SYPHILIS

Syphilitic diseases of the nervous system consist of two main types, mesoblastic or interstitial, and the parenchymatous. Clinically, pathologically and serologically, it is often impossible to draw a hard and fast line between them.

General paralysis of the insane or dementia paralytica and cerebral syphilis are examples of the organic reaction-types, the former corresponds to the chronic type of organic reaction and the latter to the acute type. In addition we will describe, briefly, a sub-type—locomotor ataxia or tabes with psychosis.

Dementia Paralytica

The successful treatment of organic affections of the central nervous system due to syphilitic infection has constituted one of the triumphs of twentieth century medicine. It has been a hard won struggle, a long process which has necessitated the correlation of observations derived from a variety of sources. Psychiatrists, neuropathologists, neurologists, ophthalmologists, serologists, and other research workers have all played a significant rôle; each has contributed from his specialized knowledge. It was not until 1913 that we could talk with confidence regarding the aetiology of this condition. It was then that the brilliant Japanese research worker Noguchi, working in association with Moore in the Rockefeller Institute, New York, announced that he had been able, in fourteen out of seventy cases of dementia paralytica, to demonstrate the presence of *Treponema pallidum* in the brain cortex. Their results were soon confirmed by other investigators, and now, with improved staining methods, organisms can be demonstrated in almost all cases. The categorical statement 'no syphilitic infection no paralysis', has become true. Syphilitic infection, however, does not necessarily lead to an affection of the central nervous system; only 1–2 per cent. are so involved, and even that percentage may be diminished as the facilities for early treatment become more available, *e.g.* by the rapid development of venereal clinics for the disease, and by the use of more potent remedies. Why some people's nervous systems are more susceptible than those of others is still unknown. Is a special neurotropic strain of organism to blame, or are some nervous systems much more vulnerable than others? Evidence *pro et contra* is available. For instance we know of numerous patients who have been infected from the same source, whereas in other cases the explanation may be consistent with von Pirquet's conception of an 'allergic' hypothesis. Fildes and McIntosh came to the conclusion that all tertiary or parasyphilitic manifestations were the expression of the reaction of hypersensitive tissues. They suggested that during the early stages of infection the tissues became altered so that they reacted more violently to a smaller spirochaetal infection or its toxins. For instance, meningitis with gummatous inflammation is simply the reaction of the hypersensitive connective tissues and blood vessels, while in dementia paralytica the involvement affects the nerve elements and neuroglia. The nerve cells and fibres are destroyed and there is proliferation of the neuroglia.

Whatever the real explanation may be, it is necessary to discuss in some detail how a disease formerly so prevalent has become so much less of a scourge. Let us start with a definition: dementia paralytica is a diffuse organic parenchymatous disease of the brain cortex, resulting in mental, physical and serological changes which can be arrested, and in many cases successfully treated. That is a very different state of affairs from that which existed earlier. Up until 1917 the wards of every mental hospital were crowded with cases of syphilitic disease of the nervous system in various stages of mental and physical deterioration. The remedies we had were unable to stem the progress of a killing disease which achieved its purpose in five years or less. Death came as a happy release from a life of intense misery.

The situation was rendered even more poignant by the fact that such cases accounted for 5 to 15 per cent. of the admission rate to mental hospitals. Th majority of those involved were in the prime of life, and there was the added danger that if the syphilitic infection was transmitted to their offspring, juvenile general paralysis might result; as a precautionary measure the blood serum, and cerebrospinal fluid of all children of parents suffering from dementia paralytica should be examined.

It was in 1798 that John Haslam, the apothecary at Bethlem Hospital, published the clinical report of a case characterized by a state of mental euphoria or well-being which was completely out of keeping with the paralytic symptoms and bodily enfeeblement from which the patient suffered. In the early years of the nineteenth century a number of French investigators—Esquirol, Georget, Bayle, Calmeil—made relevant observations which helped us to come to a clearer idea of the definition and progress of this disorder. In 1805 Esquirol noted 'that paralysis was a common complication in cases of mental disorder and added considerably to the gravity of the prognosis'. Georget agreed with Esquirol's observations and suggested that it might more suitably be described as 'chronic muscular paralysis'. In 1822 Antoine Bayle, in his thesis for the Doctorate of Medicine of the Faculty of Paris, established a correlation between the clinical and neuropathological findings from which he concluded that general and incomplete paralysis accompanied by mental disorder was due to a chronic meningitis. It was that correlation which led to a series of further discoveries. In 1826 Calmeil confirmed Bayle's findings but demonstrated that it was not merely the meninges but the brain substance itself which was seriously affected by a chronic encephalitis.

These discoveries acted as a spur. While the clinical symptoms were becoming more clearly delineated, Charcot, Babinski, and many other neurologists were accumulating information of changes affecting the reflex arc. The Edinburgh ophthalmologist, Argyll Robertson, found that in a high percentage of cases of organic brain disease the pupils did not react to light but reacted on accommodation—a phenomenon known as the Argyll Robertson pupil. The neuropathological investigations of Nissl and Alzheimer, and the serological examinations culminating in the Wassermann reaction constituted a series of brilliant advances which led to the final elucidation of this disorder—the demonstration of *Treponema pallidum* in the brain cortex.

Time of Onset. This is often difficult to determine owing to the fact that the patient may never have known of his syphilitic infection, and there may have been no residual signs of primary or secondary syphilitic lesions. From the available evidence it was reckoned that a period of five to twenty years elapsed after infection before the symptoms of dementia paralytica showed themselves. Some cases were of shorter duration than others but the usual period was from ten to fifteen years. It was thought that those who had suffered from a mild type of primary infection were more likely to develop dementia paralytica, due perhaps to less thorough treatment, but the exact correlation was not easy to determine; the organisms may have been of an especially virulent neurotropic variety.

Symptomatology. The disease is usually insidious in its development and is characterized by episodes of strange behaviour which are at variance with the previous good character of the individual. A man who had attained a position of great trust and had been of irreproachable character disgraced himself by trying to steal golf balls from a club-house in which he was a guest. Another who had been an indulgent husband and father became irritable and cantankerous, drank to excess, was unfaithful to his wife, and ill-used his children.

Changes in character and mood may be the first signs of the disease. Even at the earliest period of the illness there may be a pronounced dulling of comprehension so that questions may require to be repeated, and even then the patient may quickly forget what he has been told or asked to do. Aesthetic feelings become dulled or lost, and the alterations in the patient's personality may be such that his relations and friends are puzzled and regard him as a changed man. This rapid deterioration of personality in dementia paralytica is in striking contrast to its preservation in most other forms of organic brain disease. Its fundamental characteristics were well summarized by Campbell (1912) when he said: 'The change in the personality, which at a later stage becomes obliterated by the grosser disorders, is first shown in a loss of that special responsiveness which distinguishes the individual as a social unit. The responsiveness to ethical, aesthetic, intellectual and certain conventional standards is involved; the patient no longer shows the same judgement, the same sense of value, a function different from that of mere intellectual activity, and one upon which depends the attitude of the whole individual in the face of actual situations.'

A few patients, however, are aware of a change in themselves. They may appreciate that they are not so competent as formerly, that they cannot apply themselves to their work, are lacking in attention and concentration, are easily fatigued mentally and bodily, and are prone to make mistakes in dealing with the simplest tasks.

In another group the condition may be ushered in by physical symptoms, *e.g.* a transitory loss of speech, a hemiparesis, or a convulsive attack with unconsciousness.

During the progress of the disease one of the most significant features is the progressive loss of memory both for recent and more remote events. The main facts of the patient's life may be given correctly and relevantly but it is more usual for the patient to be unable to correlate important sequences in his life so that gaps can be demonstrated covering a number of years. The memory defect may be so great that knowledge acquired in school, including the ability to do simple calculations, becomes faulty, particularly when these calculations involve sustained concentration, as for instance in subtracting serial sevens from one hundred. There is disorientation particularly for time. An outstanding feature is the patient's complete lack of insight into his own deficiencies. He may resent attempts to correct him, or suggest a trivial explanation, or excuse. It is not long before he lapses into a state of facile, contented dementia.

Grandiose delusions of a bizarre type may be conspicuous, but are not now so common as used to be described. Indeed in some cases instead of a feeling of well-being and euphoria a state of intense depression is present even amounting to stupor with mutism. Otherwise the depressive state may be characterized by the expression of nihilistic delusions. They claim that they are dead, that their blood has ceased to circulate, that they have no pulse, or that their bodies are utterly destroyed. The delusional ideas in the depressive phase may be as fantastic and grotesque as those of the grandiose variety. During such periods of depression attempts at self-mutilation and destruction are not uncommon. As the disease progresses the memory becomes more and more disordered, but in certain atypical cases (Lissauer-type), where focal rather than diffuse involvement occurs the memory may be wonderfully well preserved. A more profound mental degeneration gradually occurs so that in the course of time the patient leads a vegetative existence requiring to be cared for and nursed in every way.

The above description gives a reasonably accurate picture of the tragic mental and physical state which may develop if, for one reason or another, treatment should prove ineffective. It requires to be understood that anomalous or extraneous symptoms may be grafted on, so that hallucinations, delusions or even alternating mood changes may appear. We only regard the mental symptoms as pathognomonic of dementia paralytica when they occur in conjunction with the neurological signs and serological findings which will be mentioned later.

Physical Signs. It has been stated above that the first evidence of this disease may be the occurrence of a convulsive seizure. It is more usual, however, for the seizures to occur during the course of the illness. In some cases convulsive states may never develop at all, but when they do they are either epileptiform or apoplectiform in type. The epileptiform conditions do not differ materially from those associated with idiopathic epilepsy; perhaps they persist for a longer time and the tonic and clonic stages are not so clearly differentiated. Even after consciousness is regained muscular twitchings may continue for many hours or even days. In contrast the apoplectiform attacks are followed by focal symptoms such as hemiplegia, monoplegia, hemianopia and dysarthria which may persist for a few days or even longer. It is not necessary that a vascular lesion should be responsible for the above conditions as they may result from a more severe involvement of certain specialized areas of the brain tissue. On the other hand there are cases in which a cerebral haemorrhage leads to permanent residuals, and not infrequently to the death of the patient.

The facies is distinctive; the features become smoothed out so that the patient looks considerably younger than his years, and has a vacant or even mask-like expression. The cranial nerves are seldom involved, but pupillary changes should always be carefully noted. These consist of inequality of the pupils, irregularity of outline, and most striking of all, sluggishness or total absence of the light reflexes. It has been stated, although the evidence is not convincing, that the consensual light reflex is lost before the direct response disappears. The Argyll Robertson phenomenon, characterized by the absence of the light response and the preservation of the accommodation response, is present in from 50 to 60 per cent. of cases. In some cases the light response can be described merely as sluggish, and the amount of excursion as smaller than normal. When the accommodation response is absent as well as the light response (internal total ophthalmoplegia) then the disease process is usually associated with locomotor ataxia.

Primary optic atrophy occasionally occurs but more especially in cases associated with locomotor ataxia.

The speech is characteristic. In the early stages the patient slurs his words, but as the disease progresses the difficulties of pronunciation become so intense that words are distorted beyond recognition. An easy and rapid way of demonstrating speech difficulties is to ask the patient to repeat, consecutively, three times, certain test words such as 'hippopotamus', 'particular popularity', 'Methodist Episcopal', 'British Constitution'. Great effort is often required to articulate at all so that, finally, it may become impossible to understand what the patient is trying to say; the effort to enunciate is accompanied by gross facial tremors.

The writing is tremulous, syllables are missed out or transposed and the words become distorted. Generalized tremors affect the hands, tongue and facial muscles; the tremor of the tongue has been described as of the trombone type.

We recognize two main types of physical involvement—the cerebral and the tabetic. In the cerebral type the tendon reflexes are equally exaggerated on the two sides, but if focal symptoms are present the exaggeration is greater on the affected side. In the tabetic type the tendon reflexes are absent or diminished. It is only in cases with focal lesions that ankle clonus and an extensor plantar response can be elicited.

Loss of control of the organic reflexes may occur during the course of the disease so that particular attention should be paid to the possibility of retention of urine, or overflow from a full bladder, and incontinence of bladder or bowel. It is only by careful nursing and cleanliness that bed-sores and contractures can be prevented, especially after the patient has become bedridden.

Serology. Ever since Heinrich Quincke, in 1891, first performed spinal puncture to relieve intracerebral pressure in the case of a hydrocephalic child, it has become a routine procedure in all forms of organic disease of the nervous system. The special cytological, chemical and serological examinations which can now be made are an enormous aid in the diagnosis, treatment and research of many diseases.

The operation of lumbar puncture is so much a part of medical practice that it requires no detailed description. In all cases other than those for the relief of intracranial pressure no more cerebrospinal fluid should be withdrawn than is necessary for examination purposes. If the clinical examination indicates that a syphilitic involvement of the nervous system is probable 10 ml. of cerebrospinal fluid may be withdrawn, but in those cases in which the diagnosis is doubtful it is wise to limit the amount to 5 ml. The reason for precaution is to avoid the unpleasant after-effects such as nausea, headache, dizziness which often occur in cases with negative findings. After the lumbar puncture has been performed the patient should be advised to be recumbent for a period of 24 hours.

It was Widal, Sicard and Ravaut, in 1900, who emphasized that an increase in the number of lymphocytic cells in the cerebrospinal fluid might prove an invaluable diagnostic aid. Less than 5 cells per c.mm. is regarded as within normal limits, from 5 to 10 cells is doubtful, and more than 10 cells per c.mm. is regarded as abnormal. In dementia paralytica there is nearly always a moderate pleocytosis, but in acute syphilitic reactions, particularly with meningeal involvement, there may be as many as 200–300 cells per c.mm. or more.

We recommend counting the cells by the Fuchs and Rosenthal counting-chamber method; this avoids the necessity of centrifuging, and the form of the cells is thus preserved. The Fuchs-Rosenthal slide has a depth of 0·2 mm. and the rulings are 4 mm. a side. The pipette is similar to that used for counting leucocytes. The cell types can be differentiated by using the following stain:

Methyl violet	0·10
Distilled water	50·0
Glacial acetic acid	2·0

The stain is drawn up to the mark 1 on the pipette, and the cerebrospinal fluid to the mark 11. The fluid is thoroughly mixed with the stain by shaking the pipette for 3–4 minutes; the first two or three drops are discarded, the next drop is put on the slide, and the number of leucocytes per c.mm. can be estimated. The whole sixteen sets of sixteen squares are counted and to obtain the number per c.mm. the total number is multiplied by 11 and divided by 32, *e.g.* (X = 11 a/32—approximately a/3). Two or three slides should be counted so as to get an average.

In 1907 Alzheimer introduced a more refined method of cell differentiation which has certain advantages. It consists of centrifuging 3 or 4 ml. of cerebrospinal fluid with double the quantity of 96 per cent. alcohol; depending on the speed of the centrifuge this may take from half an hour to an hour. A hardened plug is formed which is further dehydrated by adding absolute alcohol, then absolute alcohol and ether, and finally ether, each for a variable number of hours depending on the thickness of the plug. The plug is finally loosened from the tube by a fine platinum needle, is embedded in celloidin and cut in sections of from 1 to 5 μm. in thickness. The cut sections can be stained with Pappenheim's pyronin-methyl green or with Unna's polychrome methylene blue.

Henderson and Muirhead modified the above technique by using dextrin as the freezing medium so that the sections could be cut with an ordinary freezing microtome. A greater variety of cell types were demonstrated in general paralysis than in any other condition except tuberculous meningitis. Plasma cells and gitter cells were characteristic features of both diseases.

Protein is present in the healthy cerebrospinal fluid in small amounts ranging from 15 to 50 mg. per 100 ml. In inflammatory affections of the meninges and in dementia paralytica the quantitative protein content is increased and may reach three times its normal level. In syphilitic conditions of the nervous system a protein increase is usually accompanied by a pleocytosis.

Qualitative protein reactions are a simple and rapid way of estimating whether or not the protein content is increased. The fact that they are related to the globulin present does not constitute any objection 'because the increase in the protein in the cerebrospinal fluid is often due solely and exclusively to an increase in globulin' (Lups and Haan, 1954). The following may be used:

Nonne-Apelt: Two millilitres of saturated ammonium sulphate solution are mixed with 1 ml. of cerebrospinal fluid. The two solutions are shaken together, and the result is read off after three minutes. An opalescence or turbidity constitutes a positive reaction.

Ross and Jones modified the above reaction by performing it as Heller's nitric acid test is performed with urine. 1 ml. of cerebrospinal fluid is allowed to flow gently on top of 2 ml. of saturated ammonium sulphate. The formation of a ring at the junction of the two fluids indicates a positive reaction. The ring is described as 'clear cut, thin, greyish white, and has the thickness of a thin piece of paper. It should form within three minutes.'

In Pandy's test 1 drop of cerebrospinal fluid is mixed with 0·5 ml. of Pandy's reagent (7 g. of phenol in 100 ml. of distilled water). If turbidity appears then globulin is present.

It may be of considerable diagnostic importance to make an accurate estimation of the degree of cerebrospinal fluid pressure. Only a very rough estimate can be made by observing the rapidity of flow through the lumbar puncture needle. It is advisable therefore to use a manometer, and a puncture needle with a three-way tap and attachment for the manometer. The best type of manometer is a vertical glass tube which has a diameter of 1mm. and is graduated in millimetres. The patient should lie in a horizontal position with his head raised, by a small pillow, to the level of his spinal column. His body should be completely relaxed.

Before the needle penetrates into the spinal canal the tap should be opened, and when the cerebrospinal fluid begins to flow it should be turned so that the fluid is able to rise in the tube, and the result can be read off. In adults the normal lumbar fluid pressure may vary between 60 and 180 mm. of water. A reading of between 180 and 200 mm. is regarded as suspicious, and if over 200 mm. it is abnormal.

Clinically an increase of cerebrospinal pressure is likely to be found in cases of meningitis, dementia paralytica, cerebral haemorrhage, or brain tumour. A decrease of pressure is noted when the flow of fluid into the lumbar space is obstructed by spinal cord tumours, or in cases where the subarachnoid space has been obliterated by a meningitis.

In 1906 Wassermann, Neisser and Bruck applied the Bordet-Gengou phenomenon of complement fixation as a test for the diagnosis of syphilis. In dementia paralytica the blood serum gives a positive reaction almost invariably, and the cerebrospinal fluid is positive in 95 per cent.

Lange introduced a physico-chemical test, the colloidal gold test, in 1906. It consists of a colour change due to the dispersion of a gold colloid, and can be viewed in a series of test tubes. The shades selected as standard for reading the results are red, reddish blue, or purple, blue, grey blue and colourless. These shades are given the numbers from 0 to 5 respectively and the results are given in a series of figures, always beginning with the figure for the 1 in 10 dilution.

Three types of curves are differentiated:

1. *The Paretic Curve.* The reaction is of the '5' type, *i.e.* there is a clear colourless fluid with a deposit of blue granules in each of the first three to six tubes, and a typical curve would read:

$$5\ 5\ 5\ 5\ 5\ 4\ 2\ 1\ 0\ 0$$
$$\text{or}\quad 3\ 4\ 5\ 5\ 4\ 3\ 2\ 1\ 0\ 0$$

In addition to being characteristic of dementia paralytica a similar curve has been observed in tabes, disseminated sclerosis, and brain tumour.

2. *The Luetic Curve.* The reaction occurs in the first six tubes but is not so complete as in the paretic curve. It can be represented as follows:

$$1\ 1\ 2\ 3\ 2\ 1\ 0\ 0\ 0\ 0$$
$$\text{or}\quad 2\ 2\ 3\ 3\ 2\ 1\ 0\ 0\ 0\ 0$$

This curve is seen in cases of cerebrospinal syphilis, secondary syphilis and tabes.

3. *The Meningitic Curve.* Here the reacting zone is in the higher dilutions, and shows no reduction in the first three or four tubes.

$$0\ 0\ 0\ 1\ 2\ 3\ 4\ 4\ 3\ 2$$

This curve occurs most frequently in cases of purulent meningitis.

The fact that neurosyphilitic diseases have become much less frequent is supported by Hare (1959) who states that deaths due to dementia paralytica in England and Wales were first recorded by the Registrar General in 1901 when they amounted to 2,272, whereas in 1957 there were only 68. We must, however, resist being lulled into a state of false security because a recrudescence may occur and that is why we have described the symptoms, signs and serological reactions in so much detail; they should be familiar to all practising physicians. For instance Steel (1960) examined 18 cases of general paralysis during the eighteen months from April 1957 to September 1958. While his clinical records are not completely convincing yet in all the cases the serological examinations were positive. Bockner and Coltart (1961) have reported a similar series. One of us (I.R.C.B.) has, since 1958, had a series of 13 cases under observation and treatment of which the following are examples.

CASE No. 49

A married woman, 40 years old, four months previous to admission to hospital showed a character change as evidenced by her conduct and conversation. In hospital she was confused, forgetful, facile and expressed grandiose delusions. Treatment with penicillin resulted in good recovery.

She was an average pupil at school. At the age of 15 years she had an illegitimate child before marrying another man when she was aged 17. Later she married again. Her work record as a waitress had been satisfactory. She denied any history of venereal infection.

Her relatives had noticed a marked change in her disposition and behaviour during the four months previous to her admission to hospital in 1958. She 'made silly remarks and did silly things', and told lies. Her gait was unsteady, her appetite voracious. At her brother's shop she had made a nuisance of herself, and on several occasions she had gone, unexpectedly, for long, solitary, motiveless walks; on one occasion the police brought her back from a railway line. In the month before admission she had twice been arrested for soliciting. Two days before admission to a mental hospital she had complained of acute abdominal pain, but examination in a general hospital proved negative. The pain subsided and she explained this by saying that she had had an appendectomy on the previous evening. She was mentally confused, gave a wrong home address, and stated that she had been working until the day before admission, when in fact she had not done outside work for several years.

In hospital she was in a foolish, happy, facile state. She was indifferent to her surroundings and answered questions at random. She announced that she was pregnant and expected a baby in two months; shortly afterwards she said she had had a menstrual period one month ago. Asked to name the capital cities of Europe she said that when in Rome she had gone, dressed in ermine and diamanté, to dinner with Mussolini's son, and added, 'The Mussolinis did very well during the war'. Her memory was faulty, she lacked concentration and was disorientated.

Physically the pupils were unequal, the right was small, irregular and did not react to light. Her tongue was coarsely tremulous. The Wassermann reaction was positive both in blood and cerebrospinal fluid. The Lange curve was of the paretic type 5 5 5 5 5 3 2 2 1 0; there was no pleocytosis.

The patient was treated with procaine penicillin, 24 million Units.

At the time of her discharge she was mentally well, and no organic mental defect could be demonstrated. Her serological abnormalities persisted and arrangements were made so that her condition could be constantly reviewed.

CASE NO. 50

An unmarried, middle-aged woman began to show a character change, becoming irritable, forgetful and at times confused. Later she claimed that she was married and had an adopted child. On admission to hospital was found to be euphoric and demented. There was neurological and serological evidence of general paralysis. Dementia was advanced before treatment could be commenced.

This patient had suffered from acute rheumatism in childhood, with both carditis and chorea. She was a below-average scholar. After leaving school she had various jobs as a clerk and shop assistant. She was described as being of an aggressive and dogmatic nature, and as having few friends and interests outside her home. There was no family history of mental illness, or personal history of venereal infection.

A progressive change in her character had been noted for a year before her admission to the psychiatric observation ward. She had become very irritable, complaining, abusive and difficult to get on with. She seemed unable to concentrate on the newspapers and made numerous mistakes, frequently giving wrong answers to questions, forgetting messages, handing shopkeepers the wrong coins and returning from shopping with the incorrect change. In the six months before admission her confusion and memory impairment had become gross. She had also become unable to knit because of 'nerves in her hands'. Two days before admission she got out of bed at night declaring that she was going to live with her husband, that she had been married for a number of years and had an adopted child one year old. She packed a suitcase. On the following day she screamed and shouted at her mother, or sat disinterested by the fire. On the way to hospital she said, 'Will you bring my baby here now? Where are they taking me? There's nothing wrong with me. I'll have to be home in time for John's dinner. Put the baby in the basket, will you, and keep it till I get home this evening.'

In hospital the patient was at times agitated and wanted to leave, but mostly she displayed a fatuous euphoria and was pleased to recount details of her wedding ring and wedding dress and of the child she alleged she had adopted. She told the examining doctor that he had nice glasses, and asked 'Don't you think I have a nice face?' Mental examination showed that she was suffering from an advanced organic dementia. She was disorientated in time and place, said she was born in 1958, and failed to carry out correctly the simplest tests of retention and calculation. At times she perseverated. She had no insight.

Physically she showed slurred speech, Argyll Robertson pupils, a coarse tremor of her hands and was sometimes incontinent of urine. Blood W.R. was positive. C.S.F. W.R. was also positive, protein 140 mg. per cent. and the Lange curve 5 5 5 5 5 4 4 4 3 3; there was no pleocytosis. She had an enlarged heart and multiple valve lesions.

The patient was transferred to a mental hospital, where she was treated with bismuth and three full courses of penicillin. She has improved only slightly, is still after two years grossly demented and the blood W.R. is still positive.

Juvenile Dementia Paralytica

This condition, the result of congenital syphilis, was described in 1877 by Clouston. It usually becomes manifest at the end of the first decade but flagrant symptoms may not appear until adult life. The number who can be reasonably successful at school, and even set up a good work record are more numerous than might be suspected. According to Mott who reported an impressive series of 22 cases of a juvenile type, 16 of which were confirmed at autopsy, the disease does not differ, essentially, from the adult form. A case which was under our observation was that of a young man, 21 years old, who had been accused of stealing money from a friend. A mental examination disclosed that he was seriously incapacitated. He was talkative, excitable, expressed delusions of grandeur saying that he had been awarded the V.C., the D.S.O., M.C. and D.C.M., that the Boys' Brigade had made a collection for him and had presented him, on account of his distinguished gallantry, with a cheque for £2,000,000. His intellectual faculties were also seriously impaired. Physically, his features were smoothed out, his teeth were notched, his pupils were of the Argyll Robertson type, tendon reflexes exaggerated, marked tremor of tongue, facial muscles and hands, and his speech showed distortion of test words. His serological reactions were positive.

Neuropathology. The brain membranes are thickened, and areas of pachymeningitis may be present. The pia-arachnoid is affected as well as the dura; the frontal tips are adherent, and the temporal tips may be tacked down to the under surface of the brain. When the pia-arachnoid is stripped it causes decortication of the brain substance. The Pacchionian granulations are increased. The brain looks smaller than usual, and the brain weight is diminished. The convolutions, particularly in the frontal and parietal areas, are atrophied, and in consequence there is a widening of the sulci. A frosted-glass appearance due to granulations is visible on the ependyma of the lateral ventricles and fourth ventricle.

The histopathological changes which have been described so fully by Alzheimer affect the blood vessels of the cerebral cortex, as well as the nerve elements. In the former there is a proliferation of the endothelial cells with a tendency to the formation of new vessels through sprouting and vascularization of the proliferated intima. There is also a thickening both of the elastica and adventitia; the lymph spaces are widened and are infiltrated by plasma cells, lymphocytes and mast cells. In cases which have been of long duration regressive changes are present in the vessel walls.

In the brain cortex long or short rod-shaped cells are present; these are histiocytes with enlarged and elongated oval nuclei. The cell layering is disorganized, and the nerve cells show a great variety of degenerative forms; in some cases many of the nerve cells disappear altogether, while in others the Nissl granules are absent. The axis-cylinder processes are also degenerated. As a compensation phenomenon for the destruction and disappearance of nerve cells there is a marked proliferation of neuroglia. This may be so great that dense masses of glial fibres may be formed; the most marked increase is usually along the vessel sheaths.

Another characteristic change is the large amount of free iron, which stains readily with Prussian blue, deposited in the cortex.

In addition areas of focal softening can be demonstrated, and *Treponema pallidum* is invariably present in the brain substance. Dunlap found it most commonly in the anterior part, and in the middle and deeper layers of the frontal cortex. Sometimes they may occur in swarms or colonies especially in those cases in which convulsive seizures have been prominent.

Prognosis. Up until the introduction of successful treatment by malarial inoculation and penicillin the course of the disease was rapid, the prognosis was poor, and death normally resulted in a period of from two to five years. Now we can hope to arrest the progress of the disease, to cure the symptoms, to prolong life, and to effect a recovery whereby the patient can return home, and resume his work and responsibilities. The earlier the case is recognized, and the more quickly treatment is instituted the better the result. We still hesitate to speak in terms of a complete recovery. In a disease often so insidious in onset and causing such extensive destruction of nerve tissue we require to realize that complete regeneration is not possible. It is advisable, therefore, to follow up treated cases, and re-examine them from time to time so as to ensure that no recurrence of symptoms is taking place. In juvenile cases the prognosis is by no means as satisfactory as in the adult types.

Diagnosis. The suggestion that a patient may be suffering from dementia paralytica has so many serious implications that it is unwise to come to a final conclusion until the mental, physical and serological examinations have been completed, and found consistent with one another. When they are all positive then the diagnosis can be made with certainty, and treatment started without delay.

Sometimes it may prove difficult to differentiate dementia paralytica from other types of cerebrospinal syphilis but in the latter group we emphasize the acute inflammatory nature of the disorder, its onset within 5 years of primary infection, and the presence of headache, delirium, involvement of the cranial nerves, and the prominence of focal symptoms due usually to a syphilitic endarteritis.

In arteriorsclerotic brain disease—non-syphilitic in origin—the onset is usually ushered in by an apoplectiform seizure with ensuing emotional instability, but gross deterioration of the personality is not likely to occur until a late stage ; the serological findings give negative results.

Before discussing the treatment of dementia paralytica we have considered it advisable to describe the other syphilitic affections of the nervous system as the same treatment is more or less applicable to all.

Cerebral Syphilis

This type of syphilis affects the interstitial and mesoblastic tissues and gives rise to acute organic mental symptoms. It occurs, usually, from 6 months to 5 years after primary infection. For instance Naunyn in a series of 325 cases reported that the most common time was during the first year after infection. Other observers, *e.g.* Erb, Mott, Kahler, obtained similar results, and in a series of personally examined cases (D.K.H.) the average interval elapsing between infection and onset of symptoms was 6 years—the shortest period being 5 months, the longest 22 years (confirmed by autopsy).

Symptomatology. The mental symptoms are of an acute delirious nature characterized by hallucinations, sleeplessness, fear, disorientation and inability to concentrate. There may have been premonitory symptoms such as difficulty in thinking, a sense of uneasiness and emotional instability amounting to euphoria or depression. Once the condition becomes more fully established the memory may be found to be faulty especially for more recent events, but more diffusely as well. A confabulatory state of the Korsakow type is not unusual.

In those more unusual cases, described by Nissl and Alzheimer, as an endarteritis affecting the small vessels supplying the basal nuclei the clinical features may vary considerably, and may be difficult to recognize. In some instances they resemble a Parkinsonian state, and the patients suffer especially from a lack of sustained attention and concentration; there are none of the gross symptoms consistent with a meningitis, gumma, or large vascular lesion.

Subjective symptoms are often most distressing. There are complaints of severe headache, dizziness, a tendency to faint, a feeling of nausea, and sometimes vomiting unaccompanied by nausea. Such symptoms are indicative of increased intracranial pressure especially when accompanied by stupor and a slow pulse giving rise to the habitual sub-vertiginous state described by Fournier.

The physical signs are manifold, and particularly involve any of the cranial nerves. Eye symptoms of all kinds and degrees are among the earliest and most characteristic. A blurring and dimness of vision, diplopia, squint, ptosis may all be complained of. It is the coming and going of such symptoms, their transitoriness, which is so characteristic. It used to be estimated (and it may still be true) that in the absence of head injury, upwards of 90 per cent. of all cases of ocular palsy in adults are caused by syphilis or brain tumour. The pupils are frequently irregular in outline, and unequal, but in contrast to cases of dementia paralytica the Argyll Robertson pupil is rarely present; in a series of 26 cases it was only present in two. Optic neuritis is common, and not infrequently precedes an optic atrophy; primary optic atrophy points to a more chronic process. The third cranial nerve is the one most frequently affected, but the fourth and sixth also suffer. Oppenheim's investigation of 100 cases showed that the third nerve was affected forty-four times. Of the other cranial nerves the seventh and eighth are more commonly affected than the others.

Convulsive seizures occur especially in cases of endarteritis, but they are by no means infrequent in meningitic and gummatous cases as well. In the endarteritic group the residual focal symptoms may be of a permanent nature. When the small vessels of the basal nuclei are involved bilateral softenings may result in the production of cases of pseudobulbar paralysis with their characteristic spastic gait, slurring speech, and emotional instability.

Serology. With the exception that the colloidal gold reaction is less complete in the first six tubes as compared with the paretic curve, the findings in the blood serum and cerebrospinal fluid are, more or less, identical to those in dementia paralytica.

Pathology. Three main types of cerebral syphilis can be differentiated—meningitis, endarteritis and gumma—but in any one case all these forms may co-exist. The endarteritic type is further subdivided into:

1. Syphilitic endarteritis of the large cerebral blood vessels described by Heubner in 1874 in a classical monograph.
2. The small, or terminal vessel form of endarteritis described by Nissl and Alzheimer.

It may be very difficult to make an absolute histopathological differentiation of cerebral syphilis either from dementia paralytica or from arteriosclerotic brain disease. Dunlap stated that cerebral syphilis and dementia paralytica can come so closely together as to be almost indistinguishable. If the cortex becomes involved in cerebral syphilitic cases, he suggested that the lesion had probably extended from the pia inwards whereas in dementia paralytica the primary change is in the cortex.

In differentiating an endarteritis syphilitic in origin from an atheroma the former shows a more limited, less opaque involvement than the latter.

As an example of how one condition may merge into another we can instance the case of a man 38 years old who developed a right-sided hemiplegia ten months after syphilitic infection. He recovered, worked for five years and then on account of depressive symptoms again came under observation. A few months later he had a convulsive seizure and afterwards began to express grandiose delusions. His serological reactions were all positive, and eventually he died following a number of general convulsions. Autopsy showed that in addition to a syphilitic meningitis and endarteritis he had a focal general paralytic process affecting the left temporal, supra-marginal and angular gyri regions.

Diagnosis. The difficulty of differential diagnosis between this condition and dementia paralytica has already been referred to. We need only mention again that an acute onset accompanied by severe headache and cranial nerve palsies almost invariably means a syphilitic involvement of the meninges, rather than a parenchymatous change.

In relation to vascular involvement, arteriosclerotic brain disease is a disease of later life, usually after the age of fifty years, and the negative serological reactions would rule out the possibility of syphilitic endarteritis.

Prognosis. Four main factors merit consideration:
1. The early recognition of the disease.
2. The age of the patient.
3. The pathological type.
4. The amount of treatment.

The most hopeful prognosis can be given in cases which occur a few months after primary infection, but good results can be expected even in cases which have developed over a period of several years. If the patient is over 40 years old the prognosis may require to be more guarded as he may have accompanying arteriosclerotic changes which will reduce his recuperative power.

The meningitic and gummatous types respond to treatment more quickly than cases of endarteritis. In the latter, areas of softening may have been caused giving rise to permanent damage so that we may only be able to arrest the progress of the disease.

Tabes with Psychosis

There are certain patients who already may be suffering from tabes dorsalis but who at a later date may develop dementia paralytica. Other cases occur, however, in which tabetic cases show mental symptoms which are not of a dementia paralytica nature. Kraepelin and Otto Meyer described such cases, and one of us (D.K.H., 1911) reported a series of 5 cases in which there was no evidence of a paralytic process; in two cases the diagnosis was confirmed by autopsy. Two of the cases presented an hallucinatory state closely akin to the clinical picture described by others; two were accompanied by depression; one was characterized by hypochondria.

The clinical features which distinguish such cases from dementia paralytica are the absence of memory defect, and on the physical side the absence of tremors and of speech and writing defect.

Treatment

Ever since inflammatory and degenerative affections of the nervous system were recognized, strenuous attempts were made to treat them by a variety of methods. It was not, however, until syphilitic infection was proved to be the most frequent and potent cause that more specific methods were used so as to arrest the course of the disease even although a cure might prove impossible. Mercurial preparations and the iodides, arsenicals in the form of salvarsan as originally suggested by Ehrlich, tryparsamide and salvarsanized serum were all utilized. They were administered by mouth, by inunction, by intravenous or intramuscular injection, or directly into the spinal canal. Our efforts proved unavailing, and we were forced to admit that all the above-mentioned methods of treatment were unable to modify the course of a progressive disease which almost certainly resulted in the death of the patient in five years or less.

The credit for the introduction of the successful treatment of syphilitic diseases of the nervous system rests with Wagner Jauregg of Vienna who in 1917 recommended the use of malaria therapy. Initially he inoculated 9 cases of dementia paralytica with malaria of whom 6 were greatly benefited, and 3, five years later, were maintaining themselves at work, and showed no signs of the disease. These were better results than ever previously had been recorded. Similar good results obtained by other workers from many different parts of the world confirmed Wagner Jauregg's findings.

The induction of one disease to cure another was a novel form of treatment. Its rationale depended on the observation that mentally ill patients who suffered from an intercurrent febrile illness seemed, for the time being, to become more normal and co-operative. They relapsed again, however, as soon as the fever had subsided. The temporary improvement, however, raised the hope that an artificially produced pyrexia might be prolonged for a longer time and give correspondingly better results. Injections of tuberculin, sodium nucleinate and phlogetan were employed but the results were disappointing. Wagner Jauregg's courageous idea of using malaria infection was based on the belief—later disproved—that dementia paralytica did not exist or at least was extremely rare in those countries in which malaria was endemic; the pyrexia was regarded as the potent agent.

Plasmodium vivax (benign tertian) was the parasite used. Infection was induced either by allowing mosquitoes to bite the patient, or by the inoculation of blood from a malaria infected person. The method now employed is to use 5 ml. of heparinized blood which is injected intramuscularly just below the scapula; the incubation period is usually 10–16 days. If the blood is injected intravenously the incubation period may be only 2 or 3 days, and the fever uncomfortably severe.

The fever in about 86 per cent. of cases is quotidian in type, the peaks of pyrexia may reach 104° F. or even higher. The usual practice, depending on the strength and resistance of the patient, is to allow 8–12 uninterrupted febrile attacks. If the patient can only tolerate a few bouts of pyrexia the infection can be stopped, and another inoculation can be given at a later date. For termination of the fever, F. G. Shute, Malarial Reference Laboratory, Horton Hospital, advises either proguanil, 0·2 G. daily for 10 days, or mepacrine, 0·3 G. daily for 7 days, or quinine, 5 gr. daily for 15 days. If the fever is quotidian in type it is usually advisable to change it to tertian or to abort it temporarily. A single intramuscular injection of 0·2 G. of *Thio-Bismol* is usually sufficient for that purpose.

As soon as the course of treatment has been completed a marked improvement is likely to have occurred both in the mental and physical symptoms; the serological changes may prove more difficult to modify but the progress towards recovery can be gauged by repeated examinations of the blood serum and cerebrospinal fluid.

The general nursing care is similar to that necessary in any acute febrile state. When the pyrexia is at its peak the temperature should be recorded at frequent intervals so that hyperpyrexia, signs of collapse, or other serious complications can be avoided. Copious glucose drinks will combat dehydration. The patient's position in bed should be changed constantly so as to avoid bed-sores, and the possibility of contractures. Bladder and bowel functions require to be most carefully attended to.

The results obtained through malaria treatment have been remarkable; a killing disease has been transformed into one which can be completely arrested even although it is not cured.

Hyperpyrexia has also been produced by means of the Inductotherm Fever Cabinet and the Kettering Hypertherm but neither method has been so successful as malarial therapy.

The use of penicillin has, however, constituted a further advance in the treatment of syphilitic affections of the nervous system. Penicillin is extremely potent, is non-toxic, and is the method of choice in cases of the acute organic reaction type, *e.g.* cerebral syphilis. It is also most valuable in cases of dementia paralytica in doses of half a million Units twice a day for 28 days. If necessary it may be repeated at a later date. There is not sufficient evidence as yet to suggest that penicillin will entirely supersede malaria or other pyrexial methods of treatment. It can, of course, be supplementary to them.

DISSEMINATED SCLEROSIS WITH PSYCHOSIS

The most frequent mental symptom in disseminated sclerosis is a mild elation (euphoria). It is present in the great majority of cases, and, according to Cottrill and Wilson, is more frequent than any other single symptom, not excluding the

2 c

physical ones. Coupled with the euphoria, and probably, in fact, dependent upon it, there is a lack of insight for the seriousness of the illness. There has also been described a feeling of physical well-being ('eutonia'—Cottrill and Wilson) which is said to be only less frequent than the euphoria, but it is hard to differentiate the two. Disseminated sclerosis is often mistaken in the early stages for hysteria. The characteristic mental attitude in the latter is the *belle indifférence*, which contrasts to some extent with the positive euphoria of disseminated sclerosis.

In a smaller proportion of patients there is mild depression. In most cases the mood varies readily, but a few are dull and apathetic, and some are irritable and cantankerous. Outbursts of laughing and crying, of an uncontrollable character, and not necessarily accompanied by an appropriate change in mood, are not infrequent. As would be expected in an organic condition, the memory is affected in a proportion of cases. That it is not more often affected depends presumably on the limitation of the sclerotic process to lower levels of the nervous system. The intellectual defect is sometimes very great. In one patient there was complete amnesia for important dates in his life. His knowledge of current events was very poor. His school knowledge was largely lost, and his power of immediate retention was very slight. Orientation also suffers in such a case. A Korsakow syndrome appears rarely. Judgement may be very poor, partly as the result of such defects as these, and partly in consequence of the mood disturbance.

Persecutory and grandiose delusions, sometimes of a bizarre type, occur in some cases. Hallucinations, auditory and visual, have been reported.

Epileptiform convulsions sometimes occur. Wilson and MacBride reported 15 cases, 7 of which were personally observed. One of our patients used to call out for her mother and brother in general tonic-clonic attacks from which it was impossible to rouse her. She died recently, and the diagnosis of disseminated sclerosis was confirmed by autopsy.

EPIDEMIC ENCEPHALITIS

During and following the First World War, epidemic encephalitis, first described by von Economo in 1917 and also called lethargic encephalitis and Type A encephalitis, occupied an important place in psychological medicine. For example, 3350 fresh cases were notified in England and Wales from January 1, 1919, to December 31, 1922, and in February 1925 there were 140 patients in the mental hospitals of England and Wales suffering from the after-effects of encephalitis, with a further 60 in mental deficiency institutions. Though the majority of cases of the disease showed mental symptoms of some degree, most of them did not require admission to mental hospitals. However, those that did require psychiatric care often presented difficult problems: in the case of adults the disability was prolonged, and in children the after-effects were of a type peculiarly difficult to manage. It was in order to facilitate the care of adolescents suffering from chronic epidemic encephalitis that the Mental Deficiency (England) Act of 1927 made it possible to certify a mentally defective person in whom the defect had arisen as late as 18 years of age.

The greatest incidence of this disease, which was probably a virus infection, was between the ages of 15 and 50.

Very few, if any, certain cases of epidemic encephalitis have been reported since 1925. However, the disease is still of considerable interest, because of its protean clinical manifestations; and most mental hospitals still care for a few of the chronic cases. The description of this infectious disease will also serve to draw attention to the very various general and focal symptoms in the central nervous system which may be caused by neurotropic viruses. Sporadic cases of virus encephalitis, which are not cases of epidemic encephalitis, are at present not uncommon.

Symptoms

Only the mental symptoms will be described here.

They are best considered in two stages, the acute and the chronic; but the two varieties of symptoms merge into one another both in type and in time. The symptoms in both stages belong chiefly to the organic reaction-type, as might be expected, but there are some symptoms not ordinarily associated with the organic reaction-type which occur in some cases of epidemic encephalitis, and give it its striking and exceptional mental colouring.

Acute Stage

Delirium, stupor and psychomotor excitement have all been reported. It was from the frequency of stupor in the cases recognized in the early epidemics that the name 'lethargic encephalitis' was derived. The stupor is of an unusual type, in that the patient can be roused for brief intervals, and can respond clearly to questions. An exceptional symptom which we have seen in the acute febrile stage in a youth is 'pressure of talk'—the patient talking rapidly and incessantly, but with complete coherence and *rapport* with his environment, and without mood alteration. Neurotic symptoms have also been noted at this stage, *e.g.* anxiety (Bonhoeffer), which may not have been a specific effect but a reaction to physical malaise (as it certainly can be in the chronic stage).

Sleep disturbances of all kinds are present, and insomnia is much commoner than the usual descriptions of 'lethargic' encephalitis would lead one to believe. It is not unusual for several nights of complete insomnia to precede the onset of lethargy. Complaints of headache are common. The mental symptoms of the acute stage may overshadow the neurological signs, and in a few cases have been the only symptoms detected during life. Delater and Rouquier reported a case in which autopsy confirmed the diagnosis of epidemic encephalitis from mental symptoms only, neurological signs being absent. The lesions were confined to the cortex and meninges. In rare instances, behaviour disorders (which are common in children in a setting of clear consciousness in the chronic stage) have occurred in the early part of the illness.

The absence of mental symptoms in the early stages, or at least of a history of mental symptoms, does not make it impossible for them to appear in the chronic stage. The disease is so protean, even in its forms of onset, and the history given is often so vague, that the diagnosis of encephalitis has not infrequently to be made from the signs and symptoms of the later stages, both neurological and psychological.

A subacute form was described by Truelle and Petit. In this form they reported mood and character disturbances, with polymorphous delusional ideas and psychomotor excitement, especially at night. These were succeeded by somnolence and stupor. Death in from two to six months, or a chronic condition, ensued.

Chronic Stage

There are very considerable clinical differences between the symptoms seen in most adults and in most children affected by the disease. The symptoms common in adults will be described first. It is impossible to make positive statements as to the relative incidence of certain symptoms, as in small groups there is always an error of sampling. Thus in a series of 8 long-standing cases, we observed apathy (emotional indifference) as a leading symptom in 7, but in another series of 23 chronic patients apathy was present only in 3.

The behaviour of adult post-encephalitic patients is usually in consonance with their affective condition. Thus the apathetic patient is usually inactive—a patient in whom consciousness is perfectly clear often lies motionless in bed, or sits staring out of the window for hours on end, with only a casual type of mental content, *i.e.* the inactivity does not depend on preoccupation. In the Parkinsonian syndrome, however (and it is mostly, but not at all exclusively, in association with this syndrome that mental symptoms occur), there is a definite physical handicap to the patient's activity. His ordinary voluntary movements are slow ('bradykinesis') although he can sometimes perform movements of rapid phase with apparent ease, *e.g.* he can play tennis with facility when it is laborious for him to walk ('paradoxical movements' of Souques). He has to devote a good deal of conscious attention to his movements, and this has a mental effect—it means a sense of unusual effort and a restriction of interest when movements normally automatic require much voluntary reinforcement. The restriction in interest can in itself be depressing, in addition to the discouraging effect of the knowledge of the presence of a chronic disabling disease. The patient may become irritable and bitter, in part because of his clear realization of his infirmities (Naville). In our experience the infirmities more commonly produce depression. Corresponding to the physical slowing and lack of spontaneity ('bradykinesis'), there is a psychic viscosity ('bradyphrenia'). Naville described this post-encephalitic bradyphrenia, which is confined to Parkinsonian types, as consisting in a diminution of voluntary attention, of spontaneous interest, of initiative and of capacity for effort and work, together with objective and subjective fatigability and slight memory impairment. Extreme cases of this sort lead a purely vegetative existence, like the patients mentioned above who remain motionless for hours. Wimmer observed atypical psychoses with a history of 'Spanish influenza' and consisting in fatigue, anxiety, sleep disturbance, depression, hypnagogic hallucinations, slight fever and myoclonic jerkings.

Psychomotor excitement occurs sometimes. We have known 'pressure of talk' to persist for three years after the onset, accompanied by mild euphoria and lack of insight.

Emotional Reactions

There is no affect which can be regarded as having a specific relation to encephalitis, unless it be the remarkable apathy found in some cases. The apathy cannot be related directly to the Parkinsonian type of after-effects of encephalitis, since it occurs also in non-Parkinsonian cases, and Parkinsonian cases may not show it; nor is it a feature of true Parkinsonism (paralysis agitans). Many other types of emotional reaction can occur. In a series of 23 cases we observed depression in 14 (with a suicidal attempt in 1 case), euphoria in 5, anxiety in 4 and emotional instability in 1. Depression is not to be regarded as specific. It is certainly in many cases a reaction to the physical disabilities, and can sometimes be removed by psychotherapy. A post-encephalitic patient of Parkinsonian type of three years' standing, who was extremely depressed and anxious, and had had to leave work, became confident, happy and efficient again after three months' simple psychotherapy. He had hyoscine also, but his physical improvement was slight. Euphoria is more difficult to explain, in the face of physical disability. It may be a specific effect of the toxin, akin to what occurs in phthisis. Wimmer remarks that this type of emotional disorder is 'essentially different' from that in manic-depressive psychoses, and, with the reservation that we do not see why epidemic encephalitis should not sometimes unmask a latent manic-depressive predisposition, we are inclined to agree.

Volitional Disorders

'The subjective (and objective) phenomena of the chronic stage seem sufficient, even after allowing for physical impediments, to indicate a profound mental change in the volitional sphere, with which emotional deterioration is closely connected.' This applies especially to adult patients with apathy, and to children in whom aggressive behaviour disorder is the prominent feature.

Trend Reactions (delusions, hallucinations, ideas of reference)

These are not very common in the chronic stage (6 out of 31 patients in our series). They are consistent with the prevailing mood. Thus a woman with marked euphoria had an obvious wish-fulfilling delirium for several months—she was exalted and believed herself pregnant, and had hallucinations and illusions confirming her delusional belief. True hypochondriasis (excessive preoccupation with bodily functions in the absence of physical disease) is not common. Very frequently, however, the motor difficulties give a persistent direction of attention to the bodily functions, which readily becomes in excess of what is necessary and justified.

Organic reactions, such as disorientation, with or without hallucinations, memory defect and weakness of attention, are absent in the majority of chronic cases. They were present in 6 patients out of our series of 23. A Korsakow syndrome may rarely occur (Wimmer).

Intellectual Functions (comprehension, apperception, calculation, reasoning)

Impairment of these, as such, is probably rare in adults, but lack of interest may give an impression of intellectual impoverishment. There is evidence that in children the intellectual level is lowered in the chronic stages and in some instances a progressive deterioration occurs (Dawson and Conn, 1931). Naville and Claparède found that simple intellectual operations were not impaired in quality or rapidity; but wherever a certain amount of reflection and concentration was necessary the intellectual operations experimentally demanded were slower. This slowing seems to be independent of the physical motor 'viscosity'.

Sleep

All disturbances are possible—insomnia, hypersomnia, inverted rhythm, etc. Hypnotics are of very little use. We have noticed that these patients do not seem to feel the lack of sleep to the extent that a normal person does.

Chronic Stage in Children

In children the chronic stage is noteworthy for the preponderance of behaviour disorders of a restless and aggressive kind. This is in obvious contrast to what is the rule (with some exceptions) in adults.

The characteristic change—it can be called characteristic since there is no other physical disease affecting children which leaves after-effects of this kind and degree and in such a large proportion of cases—is the appearance in a child, hitherto of normal decorum, of impulsive, unruly, shameless activity. Very rarely a reverse change has been noted. Grossman recorded the case of a very unruly child who became docile after epidemic encephalitis. The psychic disturbances in children are said by Wimmer to set in late and slowly, and are given by him as follows: restlessness, garrulity, meddlesomeness, excessive curiosity, erratic but active attention, foolish mirthfulness, irritability, temper-tantrums, scolding, mischievousness, destructiveness, abusive language, smearing with faeces and urine, micturition on surrounding persons, violence, attempts at murder and arson, cruelty to children and to animals, truancy, vagrancy, begging, dishonesty, pilfering and precocious erotism (sometimes with precocious puberty) with obscene language and conduct, including attempts on adults and small girls. The children seem to be very literally transformed into 'little devils'. Punishment has no effect whatever. Asked why he does these things, the child will answer that he does not know, or that 'something in me makes me want to do it', as one expressed it. There is, in some cases, no evidence of shame or of a sense of responsibility for their actions; others express apparently genuine regret.

Inverted sleep rhythm is very frequent, and the nocturnal wakefulness is accompanied by great psychomotor excitement. In some cases there is psychomotor excitement in the daytime as well as at night.

Intellectually, there arises a secondary intellectual deficiency from lack of concentration and interest, and fatigability with consequent unreliable perception and imperfect retention, so that at school these children appear backward. There are, in addition, evidences of a temporary arrest of intellectual development, such as may result from any prolonged severe debilitating illness in children. This may sometimes prove permanent.

Tics, in the sense of habitual more or less complex co-ordinated movements occurring without reference to any apparent external need, are more common in children than in adults. Many of these encephalitic and post-encephalitic tics are more complex than those that have usually been considered 'functional'—*i.e.* not dependent on organic change. Hohman gives a list which includes spitting, nose-picking, forced respiratory movements (sniffing, snorting, coughing), touching the shoe and putting the hand in the mouth, wetting the finger and rubbing the cheek and ear with it, shaking the hand, making the sign of the cross and stretching the arms laterally in rhythms of some multiple of three.

There is no evidence that behaviour disturbances are commoner in children of psychopathic inheritance or make-up than in children without this handicap. The prognosis of behaviour disorders in children is variable. Some go on to develop Parkinsonism, often with recession of the behaviour disturbance, others improve considerably but often with some form of instability remaining (Gibbs). Much depends on the early institution of training in a skilled environment, and on the age of the patient, those under 12 having a better chance (Bond).

Cerebrospinal Fluid

The changes in the cerebrospinal fluid are never great. In the acute stages there have been reported lymphocytosis, increased globulin and precipitation in the 'luetic zone' in the colloidal gold test. In the chronic stages the changes are slight or absent.

Histopathology

The macroscopic post-mortem findings are frequently insignificant, but there may be congestion of the pial blood vessels, oedema of the brain and superficial haemorrhages. The most constant histopathological lesion is a perivascular infiltration, so that in sections the blood vessels in the affected region appear congested, with their walls packed with lymphocytes, plasma cells, adventitial cells, and in very acute stages polymorphs ('cuffing'). These infiltrations persist even in chronic cases. The parts chiefly affected are the basal ganglia and the region of the Sylvian aqueduct (especially the subthalamic region). Less frequently the grey and white matter of the cortex, and the medulla and spinal cord, are involved. Whether true parenchymatous infiltration occurs is not definitely decided; but extensive nerve cell degeneration does occur, and is very important. McAlpine has drawn attention to the narrowing of the zone occupied by the substantia nigra and its paleness of colour; microscopically he found a marked decrease of cells.

Psychopathology

We have already pointed out that in apathetic or depressed cases the volitional disturbance and the apparent intellectual impairment can be considered to depend

on the emotional alteration, and that while the latter may often be partly explained as a reaction to the physical disabilities, it appears in some instances at
least to be a primary effect of the disease process.

The greater instability in affect and behaviour found in children as compared
with adults has to be related to the stage of development of their psychophysical
organization.

Prognosis

The prognosis of the mental symptoms is intimately connected with that of the
physical signs, but is not inseparably bound up with the latter. Death in the acute
stages has been estimated variously as occurring in 10 to 50 per cent. of the cases.
The course of the mental symptoms is very changeable, so that in a single case
there may be a sequence of *e.g.* delirium, stupor, exaltation and psychomotor
excitement, with (later) hallucinations and delusions, a lethargic phase and
finally recovery or (in another case) initial psychomotor excitement followed by
apathy and depression with retardation, inactivity and flexibilitas cerea. The
delirium of the acute stage usually subsides after a few weeks, or may be followed
by complete recovery, or by other mental symptoms.

The initial sleep disturbance may continue or disappear, or may show as
heterogeneous a succession as the other mental symptoms, *e.g.* hypersomnia,
followed by hyposomnia, or by inverted sleep rhythm with sometimes a return
later to hypersomnia.

It is impossible to make a prognosis in an individual case, even in the acute
stage, and very difficult in the chronic stage. We have known a patient recover
symptomatically and return to his work, only to have Parkinsonian signs and
affective changes appear nearly five years after the onset.

The adult patients coming under the notice of the psychiatrist in the chronic
stage have usually a more or less extensive Parkinsonian syndrome. Parkinsonian
cases are prognostically very unfavourable from the physical point of view, but
when the affective symptoms are depressive or anxious, the mental prognosis is
not necessarily bad. We have known anxiety and depression to disappear, and a
return to work be possible. When euphoria accompanies the Parkinsonism, useful
occupation is possible. The euphoria, like the other affective changes, may persist
indefinitely. Apathy accompanying Parkinsonism, we have not known to disappear. In children, Wimmer recorded that of 25 acute cases, 11 died, 2 were
untraced and 12 displayed psychic sequelae (chiefly behaviour disorders). We
have not seen complete recovery occur from the behaviour disorder. The onset
of Parkinsonism, however, is sometimes, but not invariably, associated with a
cessation of impulsive conduct. Hohman recorded marked improvement or recovery in 6 out of 11 juvenile cases. Gradual deterioration and death can also
happen.

Differential Diagnosis

The apathy and lack of spontaneous movement in certain patients have led to
an erroneous diagnosis of schizophrenia, and as such some of them were classified

in mental hospitals. But closer investigation of such cases shows a normal grasp of the immediate environment without distortions, and no disorder of talk or of thought or other evidence of 'splitting' of the personality. There is rarely any doubt of the true condition. Of course, epidemic encephalitis, like any other stress, may precipitate a schizophrenic reaction.

Treatment

Specific treatment in the acute stages is lacking. Hydrotherapy (baths or packs) for excited patients was sometimes the only helpful measure. The usual hypnotic drugs are not very successful as a rule in producing sleep, either in the acute or chronic stages. In the chronic stage of Parkinsonian cases, hyoscine hydrobromide, B.P., is the most useful drug, in doses by mouth up to $\frac{1}{50}$ gr. four times a day. Hypodermic injection is no more effective. A small dose is often as effective as a large one. The indication for the administration of hyoscine is Parkinsonian rigidity; the mental attitude is affected indirectly by the diminution of the rigidity so produced. Tincture of stramonium in doses of from 20 to 90 minims three times daily or oftener is effective in lessening rigidity and in increasing the ability to perform fine movements. It may be necessary to begin with a small dose and increase gradually to avoid discomfort. The more recently introduced drugs ethopropazine hydrochloride (*Lysivane*) in daily oral doses of 50 to 500 mg. and benzhexol hydrochloride (*Artane*) in daily oral doses of 2 to 10 mg. may be similarly helpful. Simple occupation is useful both in adults and children. The juvenile cases, if at all severe, got on much better if segregated in a hospital ward specially designed for their reception; a sympathetic but firm régime and occupation were beneficial. Psychotherapy in adults undoubtedly has its uses in certain cases, and in the anxious, depressed group especially, sympathy and understanding produce an improvement both in mental and physical performance.

PSYCHOSES OF SENESCENCE AND SENILITY

The care and treatment of the ageing members of the population who are no longer able to manage for themselves constitutes a national medico-social issue which can only properly be met by the co-operation of Local Authorities, Government Departments (health and national insurance) and charitable voluntary organizations, *e.g.* Nuffield Foundation, British Red Cross Society, Salvation Army, etc. As we advance in years we become more vulnerable to physical and mental incapacity, the machine slows down, it loses something of its resistance and elasticity, and there is no longer the spontaneous vigour and buoyancy of earlier times. There are, however, a favoured few whose physical and intellectual powers remain intact almost to the end of their days, but a far greater number, of a different habit, become old in mind and body long before their appointed time. Why such a difference exists we do not know. Heredity, constitution or diathesis, prolonged stress and strain, toxaemia, the ductless glands, may all come in for their share of blame. But in addition there are many socio-economic reasons, *e.g.* poverty, loneliness, faulty nutrition, poor living conditions, and family disharmony, any or all of which may be of equal if not greater importance. The pride and responsibility of maintaining a family group spirit appears to be dwindling in favour of a somewhat selfish individualism.

The problem, therefore, of ageing with its accompanying incapacity is in urgent need of much greater sympathetic understanding and more intensive research than ever has been accorded to it. It is one of the most important aspects of preventive medicine which should be familiar to and within the scope of every well-trained doctor, nurse, almoner or social worker. It is a mistake to regard it as a specialist geriatric issue which requires expert personnel. Such over-emphasis narrows the concept instead of encouraging everyone to play his or her part in helping to remedy it. For instance, it is imperative, whenever possible, to decrease the admission rates to all hospitals, and to expend every effort in caring for and treating elderly patients in their own homes, or in residential units which have been made suitable for that purpose. To ensure the success of such schemes an accurate medical diagnosis should be made as rapidly as possible so that an appropriate assessment can be made of the probable course of the illness, and the extent of the help required.

Thomson, Lowe and McKeown (1951) in their valuable and notable survey in Birmingham estimated that approximately 12 persons in every thousand aged 65 years and over were in hospitals for the chronic sick. They suggested that in order to reduce the demand for expensive hospital beds for the aged three things are necessary: 1. the provision of better social services in the home (nursing, domestic help, laundry, beds and bedding, and meals); 2. housing designed for the elderly; 3. residential institutions (other than hospitals) which afford domestic services and simple nursing (washing, feeding and dressing). All such amelioristic measures have met with universal approval, and should confer a great benefit. Their necessity becomes even more apparent as we become aware that the number of persons over pensionable age continues to show a continuous increase. In Great Britain the ratio has advanced from 1 in 17 of the population in 1900, to 1 in 6 in 1961; a total of approximately 8,000,000 pensioners. As a further commentary it may be noted that the admission rate to mental hospitals of persons over the age of 60 years has doubled since the beginning of the century. These grave facts call for immediate consideration and action.

We may now direct attention to the various clinical senescent states which demand a more detailed description. They will be considered under three headings: 1. the pre-senile; 2. the cerebral arteriosclerotic; 3. the senile.

Pre-Senile Psychoses

Three types are differentiated:
1. Alzheimer's disease.
2. Pick's disease.
3. Jakob-Creutzfeldt's disease.

Alzheimer's Disease

This condition is an organic brain disease with focal manifestations, due to a primary parenchymatous change, occurring in persons between the ages of 40 and 60 years; certain persons may be affected in youth or early manhood. For instance Malamud and Lowenberg reported the case of a child who when 7 years old had contracted scarlet fever and subsequently showed a lack of physical and mental development. After his death at the age of 15 years the histopathological investigation of his brain revealed the miliary plaques and nerve cell changes which are regarded as characteristic of Alzheimer's disease. And Biggart quotes Hallevorden as reporting that in 10 cases of post-encephalitic Parkinsonism, whose ages ranged from 10 to 50 years, he had been able to observe the presence of typical Alzheimer 'tangles' in the substantia nigra and tegmentum of the pons. It is evident, then, that Alzheimer's disease has a wider spread than was thought and that a variety of aetiological factors may be implicated. We have not seen any cases under the age of 40 years, and believe, with Grünthal, that any such should be investigated with the most careful scrutiny. Women are thought to be more frequently affected than men.

Alzheimer's original observation, in 1906, concerned a woman, 51 years old, whose clinical state was marked by a severe failure of memory so that she was unable to find her way in her own house. She was perplexed and puzzled, disorientated for time and place, and experienced states of transitory confusion and delirium accompanied by hallucinosis. She exhibited a paraphasic state with perseveration, and had difficulty in understanding spoken speech. Her illness progressed over a period of four and a half years; at the time of her death she was greatly enfeebled, and her limbs were contracted. Alzheimer described the histopathological changes in the brain as follows: 'In an otherwise normal cell there appear at first one or more fibrils which on account of increased thickness and stainability stand out prominently. In the further course of the alteration many neighbouring fibrils are similarly affected. These then form thick bundles which gradually come to the surface of the cell. Finally the nucleus and cell disintegrate and only a tangled bundle of fibrils remain to indicate the site of a former ganglion cell'. In addition to the so-called 'tangles' or 'baskets of fibrils' which were so characteristic, many miliary plaques were demonstrated throughout the brain cortex. It had been known that such plaques were usually present in the brain of elderly persons, but in cases of senile psychoses their number was always considerably increased.

Clinical Symptoms and Morbid Anatomy. The clinical symptoms are so insidious in onset that it is only at a later date that their significance is fully realized. A previously capable and intelligent person may appear to lack concentration, to be absent-minded, to make mistakes in doing the simplest tasks. There is emotional instability which varies from facility to irritability. Such symptoms are apt to be made light of, a rest, a change of air, a tonic may seem to be all that is required. Gradually, however, it becomes recognized that the above symptoms are much more persistent and serious than was originally thought. The difficulties in attention, concentration and comprehension seriously interfere with the person's ability to perform the ordinary daily tasks, and the tendency is to blame others for the growing incapacity; ideas of reference, suspicion and even transitory, unsystematized delusions of persecution may be expressed. As the illness pursues its slow and ominous course forgetfulness, both for recent and remote events, becomes a more notable feature. The power of sustained attention becomes less and less, the person's whole life may be wiped out so that there is complete disorientation for time and place and person; they become unable to name or recognize their most intimate relatives. They regress to that stage of infancy when all one's bodily and emotional needs have to be provided for by others.

Grünthal in his clinical analysis of 14 cases divided the course of the illness into three stages:

1. A stage of gradual loss of memory, and disturbance in perception, carelessness in work and appearance, place disorientation, weakness or epileptiform attacks, some loss of words and slurring speech.
2. Complete disorientation for time, place and person, dulling of comprehension, restlessness at night, inability to read, write or do simple arithmetic.
3. A stage of irritability, with paraphasia, uncleanliness and stereotyped movements.

We would stress that in addition to what has been said, more specialized disturbances may occur depending on the site or sites of the pathological lesions. When the association tracts are diffusely affected all manner of sensory-motor aphasic disorders are easily demonstrated. Furthermore, the E.E.G. changes are characteristic, and though not pathognomonic are unusual in other conditions. Letemendia and Pampiglione (1958) reporting on 17 histologically verified cases of Alzheimer's disease, record the common E.E.G. findings as follows: 'Absent or scanty alpha rhythms; generalized 2 to 7c./sec. activity poorly affected by sensory stimuli, slightly increased by overbreathing but clearly diminished during drowsiness; well-preserved responses to photic stimulation; and poor fast activity response to barbiturates. Sleep spindles were recognizable though often of low amplitude; K-complexes were only infrequently evoked by sensory stimuli. The E.E.G. abnormalities were fairly uniform in all cases without constant relationship to the duration and severity of the clinical picture, the presence or absence of fits, or the patient's age.'

There is a coincidental bodily impairment with inco-ordination of movement, emaciation and bodily enfeeblement so that the patient becomes bedridden.

The brain is atrophic and similar to that seen in senile dementia. Atheroma is not usually present in the cerebral blood vessels.

Histopathologically the nerve cells are replaced by neurofibrillary tangles arranged in the form of whorls or baskets. Senile plaques are also present as well. There is proliferation of neuroglia.

The following cases are illustrative:

CASE NO. 51

An unmarried woman in her fortieth year began to suffer from a marked failure of memory, and was restless and excitable. She gorged herself with bananas and sweets and gained considerably in weight in a few months. In hospital she helped herself to the food provided for other patients. She was happy, facile, lost interest in her former pursuits and was completely lacking in appreciation of her seriously disordered mental state. She did not resent adverse criticism but merely giggled in a mirthless way. Her memory for recent events was much more seriously impaired than for remote ones. She repeated the same story over and over again, and confabulated. She had difficulty in understanding spoken speech, and in finding the words she wanted to say (word amnesia).

A post-mortem examination showed a generalized brain atrophy more pronounced in the frontal lobes, particularly the left. The histological examination showed a band of vacuolation in the layer immediately above the large pyramidal cells; this band was peculiar to the frontal area. In the occipital and other regions the vacuolation was less localized and encroached in some places on the white matter. Senile plaques were scattered throughout all the cortical areas examined. They were most abundant in the hippocampal region, and seemed to prefer the second and third layers of the cortex. The nerve cells throughout the cortex had undergone the profound degenerative changes described by Alzheimer.

CASE No. 52

A woman, 48 years old, exhibited a profound memory defect. She had forgotten the personal details of her life, where she was born, her age on leaving school, the date of her marriage. She was irritable, emotionally labile and wept without provocation. She expressed ideas of a persecutory nature. An examination for aphasia revealed defects both in the receptive and emissive spheres. There was word amnesia with paraphasia and perseveration. On the receptive side she was unable to understand and comply with simple commands, e.g. 'touch your nose with your right hand'. She was unable to compose words spelled to her, or copy print in capital letters. The above condition had developed insidiously for two years.

In addition to the main symptoms she constantly kept informing the police that her personal belongings were being stolen when she had merely mislaid them. Her conduct became so unpredictable that arrangements had to be made for her admission to hospital.

A post-mortem examination showed a general atrophy of the cerebral convolutions, especially affecting the frontal lobes. Microscopically a band of vacuolation was present in the frontal gyrus, and similar bands occurred in other areas as well; in Ammon's horn the band of vacuolation ran along the plexiform layer of the gyrus. Senile plaques and Alzheimer cells were seen throughout the cortex and interspersed with the latter were the granulo-vacuolar degenerative cells which Simchowicz had described. The cells in the basal ganglia had also undergone extensive degenerative changes of the granulo-vacuolar type.

Pick's Disease

In 1892 Arnold Pick of Prague described a *circumscribed* atrophy of the frontal and temporal lobes which contrasted with the diffuse involvement of the Alzheimer group. The persons affected are between 40 to 60 years old, and the illness may persist from fifteen to twenty years. The aetiology is obscure but in some cases there is a familial history of heredo-degenerative traits. Grünthal, for instance, reported its occurrence in two brothers, and in two generations of another family.

Clinical Symptoms. The clinical picture bears a close resemblance, especially in its early stages, to Alzheimer's disease. The onset is usually most insidious, and in general the symptoms correspond to those which are characteristic of organic brain disease, e.g. intellectual disorganization with a change in character and affect. The earliest indication of the disorder may be a failure of attention and concentration leading to forgetfulness, and apparent lack of interest. The previously capable, efficient person seems to be unduly casual, is perplexed and confused, and a constant source of worry and anxiety to relatives and friends. The true significance of the illness does not usually become appreciated until even more gross symptoms develop. These usually consist of a complete loss of spontaneousness and initiative so that the ordinary everyday tasks such as dressing, eating, attention to bodily habits, and the simplest tasks cannot be accomplished without much assistance. There is a regression to a childhood level with lability of mood and stereotypy of speech and conduct. Disorientation becomes complete, memory for recent and remote events disappears, and life is continued at a purely automatic level. Aphasic, alexic, agraphic and dyspraxic phenomena occur depending upon the localized area of brain tissue involved. Epileptiform attacks occur occasionally but are not a special feature.

The terminal stage is one of mental and bodily enfeeblement so that the patient becomes bedridden.

Morbid Anatomy. The brain shows a circumscribed atrophy particularly affecting the frontal and temporal lobes; there may also be a shrinkage of the corpus callosum. The left hemisphere of the brain is the one more usually affected. The motor cortex and cerebellum usually remain intact.

Microscopically, the nerve cells in the third layer of the cortex disappear first, and are replaced by neuroglial proliferation. The cells in the three first cortical layers are more intensely involved than the others. Many of them become swollen, 'ballooned', and show deep argentophilic staining. The chromatin substance of the cells disappears, the nucleus is displaced to the periphery of the cell, is pale in colour and vacuolated. Occasionally senile plaques and Alzheimer's cells may be present but they are not a conspicuous feature of the disease. The white matter may also atrophy.

Differential Diagnosis. Clinically it is extremely difficult—and sometimes impossible—to differentiate Pick's disease from Alzheimer's. They occur at the same age period, run a more or less identical course, and exhibit similar phenomena. Sjögren and Lindgren (1952) compared and analysed the symptoms in a group of 18 cases of each disease. The average age of onset in each group was 54 years. Amnesia and progressive dementia were especially prominent in Pick's disease, while the Alzheimer group showed an increase in muscle tone, unsteady gait and space disorientation.

In each group 3 of the 36 parents had suffered from senile or pre-senile dementia, and one sibling in each group was likewise involved. The risk of parental involvement was estimated as 10 ± 4 per cent. for Alzheimer's disease as compared with 19 ± 5 for Pick's; the risks for brothers and sisters was $3 \cdot 8 \pm 2 \cdot 1$ per cent. and $6 \cdot 8 \pm 2 \cdot 9$ per cent. Sjögren suggested that a dominant gene of incomplete penetrance was the important factor in Pick's disease, and that a multifactorial inheritance was responsible for Alzheimer's disease. A familial tendency appears to be a feature of both diseases. It is only *post mortem* that an accurate distinction can be made. In Pick's disease the lesions are circumscribed, and the basal ganglia are rarely affected; in Alzheimer's disease there is a diffuse atrophy of the cerebral cortex, and changes are usual in the basal ganglia.

Jakob-Creutzfeldt's Disease

This syndrome differs from the other pre-senile states by the predominance of pyramidal and extrapyramidal involvement. At various times the syndrome has been described as a 'spastic pseudo-sclerosis'; 'encephalo-myelopathy with disseminated lesions'; 'cortical pallidospinal degeneration'.

It is a disease of middle life, but in some instances cases have been reported with autopsy findings in which the patients were not 30 years old. The aetiology is not known. It has been suggested that it may be a variant of epidemic encephalitis, a deficiency disorder or a familial hereditary degenerative state. Anxiety and depression are prominent clinical features, but the emotional picture varies considerably and sometimes a state of euphoria and incurable optimism is in marked contrast to the obvious physical and mental disabilities. A progressive deterioration of the intellectual faculties involving memory, judgement and insight occurs, and is sometimes accompanied by confabulation of the Korsakow type. The terminal stage is one of complete dementia.

Physical Symptoms. A sense of tiredness and of weakness in the legs is an early sign. There is difficulty in raising the legs, so that the patient will walk round rather than step over any obstacles. Later considerable ataxia develops so that walking is a matter of great difficulty. The tendon reflexes are markedly exaggerated, ankle clonus can be elicited, and the plantar responses are extensor. The muscles of the arms and legs may show the atrophy and fibrillations which are so commonly associated with amyotrophic lateral sclerosis. Extrapyramidal signs take the form of spontaneous movements, tremor, athetosis, disturbance of muscle tone. Parkinsonian symptoms may be present, and dysarthria is almost invariably present. Death may occur in a period of two to five years.

The pathological change consists of a symmetrical frontal lobe atrophy which sometimes extends back to the parietal and temporal lobes. The histopathology shows a diffuse diminution of the cortical ganglion cells with moderate neuroglial proliferation. Similar destructive changes occur in the basal ganglia, ventral-medial nucleus of the thalamus, bulbar motor nuclei, and anterior horn cells. The myelin sheaths and axis cylinders of the pyramidal and extrapyramidal tracts are seriously affected.

Psychoses in Cerebral Arteriosclerosis

Arteriosclerotic brain disease occurs, for the most part, in persons over the age of 50 years. In those families, however, in which there is a distinct tendency to early arterial degeneration the members of the 30 to 40 age group may not escape.

There are many persons who may have a generalized peripheral arteriosclerosis for many years but their cerebral vessels may never become affected. Under such circumstances the patient's subjective complaints are usually of a bodily rather than of a psychological nature. The general personality and character of the individual is fully maintained. But mental symptoms may be ushered in with the dramatic suddenness of an apoplectic seizure. It may be of a minor nature—an arterial spasm—causing a state of mental confusion, a clouding of consciousness with word amnesia and paraphasia which may only persist for an hour or two. It should be taken as a warning, as an indication that, for a time at least, the strain and stress of life should be curtailed. No further untoward symptoms may develop and the patient may be able to lead a happy and efficient life. If, however, the apoplectic seizure should be of a major type accompanied by unconsciousness and followed by paralytic symptoms the situation is much more ominous. It is true that the patient may make a good recovery, that all residual symptoms may disappear, and that the patient's personality will continue to be well preserved; he is still the man he used to be. Sometimes, however, and this is more usual than not, his confidence in himself has been disturbed, he fears another 'stroke', is inclined to be introspective and obsessive so that there is a noticeable loss of efficiency. Such patients are very loath to give in, they struggle against their disabilities, and if frustrated in their efforts, bouts of anger and irritability occur which may precipitate another cerebral incident. Emotional instability in a middle-aged man who has never previously suffered from temperamental diffi-culties is most likely to be organically determined. In such states laughter and tears are never far apart—the one succeeds the other in an almost explosive way. Suspicion, jealousy, delusions of persecution, leading to violent outbursts which may have dangerous consequences occur especially during periods of clouding of consciousness and disorientation. After these episodes have passed the patient may have a complete amnesia for their occurence. In his more lucid moments he expresses great regret and sorrow to those who have been caring for him for causing so much trouble. His condition, however, may vary from day to day, or from week to week, and there is a gradual weakening of his personality structure, and an inability to contend with the tasks of everyday life. Accompanying his emotional lability and personality change, forgetfulness, lack of concentration, and memory failure particularly for recent events, become conspicuous features. This may be so much the case that it may become imperative to appoint an attorney or curator to look after his business affairs so that the interests of the family are properly protected. In contrast to his forgetfulness for recent events, his memory for the events of his childhood and early days may be retained to the end of his days. In those cases suffering from a repetition of 'strokes' the mental and physical disorganization may be much more rapidly completed. A pseudobulbar paralysis may occur due to a bilateral involvement of the pyramidal tracts above the medulla.

Physical Symptoms. Headache, dizziness, tinnitus and nose bleeding are among the earliest symptoms. The pupils are small and sluggish in their reaction in about 25 per cent. of cases. The hands are tremulous, the gait is unsteady and tottering, and paraesthesias of the lower extremities are a fairly constant occur-rence. The tendon reflexes are usually exaggerated, and in those cases with a residual paralysis there is an extensor plantar response, and ankle clonus. In addition to the production of monoplegias, hemiplegias and a bilateral spastic state, all varieties of sensory-motor aphasia and apraxia may be in evidence.

An ophthalmoscopic examination will often reveal a sclerosis of the vessels of the fundi, even when there is no indication of a peripheral arteriosclerosis. An increase of blood pressure is a usual, but not invariable, concomitant. The heart is often enlarged, with accentuation of the second sound, and there may be slight albuminuria, and glycosuria. The cells in the cerebrospinal fluid and its globulin content may show a slight increase.

Morbid Anatomy. In addition to the involvement of the cerebral blood vessels arteriosclerosis may be evident in the aorta, and coronary vessels. The heart is hypertrophied and dilated, and infarctions may be present in the kidneys and other bodily organs.

The brain membranes are thickened and often adherent to the cortex. The brain itself may show localized or more general atrophy. Evidence of subdural haemorrhage is not uncommon. Cyst formation and dilatation of the brain-ventricles occur.

Three main types of arterial degenerative change have been described: 1. atheroma; 2. colloid-calcareous degeneration; 3. arterio-capillary fibrosis.

1. Atheroma is distinguished by its 'signet ring' appearance—the whole circumference of the vessel is not uniformly affected. The degenerative change occurs first in the elastica and media, and then proliferation of the intima occurs, in the form of a plaque, to strengthen the weakened vessel wall. There is no formation of new blood vessels to the proliferated intima which in its turn may readily undergo degeneration. This type of sclerosis is particularly common in the large cerebral blood vessels and gives rise to gross lesions, *e.g.* hemiplegia, hemianopia.

2. In this type colloid-calcareous material infiltrates into the media, and ultimately replaces the muscular coat. The vessel ultimately becomes obliterated, and 'softenings' in the surrounding tissues result. The vessel may rupture before the obliteration is complete. This is the type of involvement which is apt to produce degeneration in the white matter (*vide infra*).

3. Arterio-capillary fibrosis is a uniform thickening of the vessel walls, and affects, chiefly, the small vessels supplying the nerve cells.

In 1902 Alzheimer gave a more comprehensive account of the degenerative brain changes which may result from the above arterial lesions and which we have summarized as follows:

1. Arteriosclerotic brain atrophy. This is a diffuse degeneration of the brain tissue with pigment-atrophy of the ganglion cells and proliferation of glial tissue. Clinically the symptoms may be comparatively mild, and consist principally of mental fatigue, headache and dizziness. There is, however, a more severe type with marked intellectual impairment, progressing to dementia; the physical impairment is determined by apoplectiform seizures, and focal symptoms.

2. Subcortical encephalitis was described originally by Binswanger and consists of an atrophy of the white matter resulting from sclerosis of the long medullary arteries. The anatomical defects characterized by foci of softening may involve the basal nuclei and brain stem as well as the white matter.

In some cases the cortical vessels may be affected as well as the medullary ones. In such circumstances irritative symptoms, *e.g.* twitching, choreiform movements, mild seizures, are likely to preponderate.

3. Perivascular gliosis caused by the progressive obliteration of small vessels

2 D

and creating nerve cell atrophy with compensating neuroglial proliferation occurs much more frequently than is generally recognized. It is a basal nuclear phenomenon, and demonstrates its presence clinically by a history of headache, dizziness, fatigue, lack of concentration and a terrible sense of frustration. The memory impairment may never become unduly troublesome, but there is a slow progressive impairment of intellectual and bodily symptoms, *e.g.* a Parkinsonian state. Throughout the course of the illness no gross involvement of the large cerebral vessels need occur.

4. Senile cortical devastation is usually associated with senile brain atrophy and is characterized by wedge-shaped foci or areas of softening which are spread throughout the brain cortex. The particular clinical symptoms are determined by the localization of the lesions.

Senile Psychoses

The medico-social problem of making adequate arrangements for the ageing members of the population is an ever increasing one and is receiving the most sympathetic consideration. There are very few families who are unaware of the unhappy, distressing, and even tragic circumstances which, sometimes, can constitute a great trial and grief not only to the patient but also to relatives and friends. Many of our most famous essayists, poets and novelists have portrayed the characteristics, the vagaries of conduct, and the foibles of the elderly. For the most part they have done so in a sophisticated, kindly, understanding manner so that ample allowance can be made for the ultra-conservatism, arbitrariness and obstinacy which constitute so much of the clinical picture. Senescence is a slow progressive process. At first the changes may be very slight, and may not consist of more than a mere modification or caricature of the normal personality which can be maintained for a considerable time. A complete transformation or distortion of the personality only occurs coincidentally with a severe involvement of the brain tissue. It is only then that the disorganization of the intellectual faculties and the physical changes give cause for alarm.

One of the most prominent—and even irritating—features of the senescent state is inflexibility, a resistance to change, an inability to adapt to what are regarded as 'new-fangled' ideas, or other ways of living. It is this lack of insight, this inability to recognize one's short-comings and limitations that may have led government departments, local authorities, universities, big business organizations, and the services to ordain compulsory retirement at the 60–65 age level. Sometimes such arbitrariness may seem a little unfair, and may even be a means of accelerating the senescent process rather than of retarding it. Judges, ministers of religion, members of parliament, and some business executives remain exempt from the above strictures—and it is difficult to understand why—it must be assumed that they have inherited the wisdom of the ages!

But when all aspects are taken into consideration it is probably an excellent plan to fix a compulsory retiral age. It provides the younger person with the opportunity and incentive for promotion, for the infusion of new blood, or the elimination of dead wood, whichever process seems to be the more appropriate.

Elderly persons whose mental powers are showing a noticeable failure, and yet who persist in maintaining a senior position often provide a sad spectacle. It is, of course, natural enough to want to maintain prestige, and to be proud of past achievements, but it is wearisome in the extreme to listen repeatedly to the same old story no matter how richly it is embellished in the re-telling. The refrain is always the same—how much better the old days and ways were, children respected their elders then, the world is going to the dogs, the wisdom and experience of age is being neglected.

In other words senescence creates a one-track mind so that any departure from the daily routine (the 'misoneism' which is so characteristic) becomes anathema. To live in the past, to indulge in reminiscences, anecdotes, clichés and platitudes may be taken as indicative of inability to cope with present-day affairs. Lack of attention and concentration results in the repetition of questions the answers to which are forgotten almost in the same breath. Such states of absentmindedness and forgetfulness may cause books, business papers, dentures, spectacles, etc., to be mislaid, and those in attendance are blamed for stealing them. Such accusations and suspicions are usually transitory, but sometimes they lead to an alienation of affection which may influence testamentary capacity. That is a matter which should always be kept carefully in mind not only so as to safeguard personal property, but to prevent the exploitation of those whose minds may be easily influenced.

Also at this stage there may be a difficulty in remembering intimate relatives and friends, and of naming objects which are in constant use, *e.g.* watch, knife, scissors, fork, hair-brush. Despite such obvious failures and disabilities the person retains his personality as known to his friends. At one time he may be kind, gracious and charming, but at the other extreme cantankerous, ill-tempered, pompous, a tyrant to everybody associated with him; there are many intervening shades. Finally, as an indication of the progressive senile disorganization which is taking place, sexual anomalies may occur as a futile compensation for impotence and failing manhood. In many instances such offensive conduct, especially when directed to children, has led to apprehension by the police and court proceedings. We would suggest that in all persons over the age of 50 years accused for the first time of sexual offences, the possibility of beginning organic brain disease should always be suspected.

There is loss of weight, the body is stooped and bent, the features are fine-drawn, the hair is white and sparse, and the skin is wrinkled, dry and often discoloured by purpuric patches and petechial haemorrhages on the backs of the hands or other parts of the body. There may be tremor of the head and hands, shaky hand-writing, and difficulty of articulation; the gait is of a shuffling character (marche à petits pas). Subjective complaints of headache, dizziness, fatigue are common.

Senile Dementia. A diffuse involvement of memory both for recent and remote events marks the further progress of mental disorganization. It is coincidental with a general shrinkage of the brain, and with extensive atrophy of the cortical nerve cells. A charming, elderly gentleman who was well over 80 years old used always to say that he was only one day old. Obviously he lived in a 'day-tight' compartment so that neither the past nor the future disturbed his blissful equanimity. Disorientation for time, place and person becomes complete. Night and day cannot be greatly distinguished, the days, weeks, months and years pass unnoticed; he cannot recognize his own home; he fails to recognize intimate relatives with whom he has been on the most affectionate terms. The above symptoms can prove most troublesome and even dangerous especially at nighttime. On awakening from a restless, disturbed sleep he may be in a confused bewildered state. In attempting to determine his whereabouts he may fall from his bed and sustain a fracture of his femur or pelvis, or he may wander aimlessly about the house or set it on fire, or leave it altogether. Such episodes are most alarming. Personal habits become faulty, he is unable to dress himself properly, stuffs his pockets with rubbish, and becomes uncleanly in his bodily habits. The emotional disorganization is punctuated by bouts of explosive anger which have resulted in suicidal or homicidal attacks for which there is clouding of consciousness amounting to complete amnesia. Inevitably the intellectual and emotional life is reduced to a state of childish fatuity, a prattling mindlessness, and a purely vegetative existence.

Some writers have been inclined to emphasize the melancholic, maniacal and paranoid states which may show themselves during the progress of the senile illness. We see no reason or purpose in doing so because the above states differ in no way from similar states occurring at any other period of life. They merely reflect the underlying constitutional make-up which has been exposed or laid bare by the profound organic disturbance.

Senile Delirium. Symptomatically senile delirium is closely akin to that which occurs in toxic-exhaustive states. It is characterized by hallucinosis, fear, disorientation and exhaustion. In senile states we see it most commonly as a postoperative phenomenon, *e.g.* following prostatectomy, excision of cataract, or as an after-effect of head injury. Insomnia may be extreme, and great care should always be exercised in choosing an appropriate hypnotic; injudicious medication may aggravate the condition we hope to cure. Delirious states may also occur more or less spontaneously as a result of the ageing process. For instance, a gentleman, 86 years old, who had experienced a birth phantasy, requested that his congratulations should be conveyed to one of his male nurses. He stated that during the night he had given birth to twins, and that the male nurse in attendance had assisted their delivery in the most skilful way imaginable. Another, when found lying under his bed, explained that he was fishing for pearls in a private loch the property of a person in whom he had been intensely interested. Physically all the changes which have been described become greatly intensified, and in the final stage the patient becomes bed-ridden, requires to be fed, and to be assisted in his natural functions.

Morbid Anatomy. The brain is small, and its weight may be diminished by as much as 200 g. The skull is thickened, and the membranes may be adherent to the tips of the frontal and temporal lobes. Internal haemorrhagic pachymeningitis is frequently seen. The Pacchionian bodies are increased. The convolutions of the brain are shrunken, the sulci are widened, and the ventricles dilated. The cerebrospinal fluid is increased. The blood vessels may exhibit a degree of sclerosis but not sufficient to cause areas of softening.

Microscopically there is atrophy of the nerve cells with an increase of lipoid substance, and a disturbance of cortical layering. The neuroglia is proliferated but it may also undergo atrophy. The tangential fibres diminish in number and become atrophied. Fischer's 'plaques' occur normally in every senile brain but in dementia their number is considerably increased. They consist of a mixture of neural and glial elements and form a conglomerate mass. In addition to being present in the superficial cortical layers they also invade the optic thalamus. Both Achucarro and Bonfiglio described basket-like formations of fibrils of the Alzheimer type particularly in the frontal lobes and pes hippocampi.

Prognosis

We must accept the fact that, once degenerative changes have occurred in the brain tissue and in the cerebral blood vessels giving rise to objective clinical symptoms, the prognosis must be viewed with grave concern. The probability is that the degenerative process will be progressive in nature and will lead to a state of mental and physical enfeeblement. While this, eventually, is the final outcome yet we are impressed by the frequency with which temporary betterment can be effected. This is particularly the case in cerebral arteriosclerotic states. For example, a man of 62 years had an apoplectiform seizure followed by inability to speak, and a right-sided hemiplegia. He became so difficult to manage that treatment in a mental hospital was imperative. Under skilled medical and nursing care a great improvement was effected, and in three months he was able to be discharged. He had regained his ability to converse, his paralytic symptoms disappeared, and he acquired good insight into his illness. His memory and general efficiency were only slightly impaired.

Apart from post-apoplectic states we have been gratified to see how frequently, as a result of improvement in nutrition and general management, irritable, suspicious, aggressive delusional states become so greatly modified that the patients may be able to live comfortably in their own homes.

These transitory improvements occur much more frequently than is generally recognized.

Treatment

The medico-social preventive aspects of the treatment of the elderly have been stressed by all who have studied the problem. It is of paramount importance and constitutes a challenge to our skill and humanitarianism. Elderly, lonely people with slender material and economic resources are often in a sorry plight and are in urgent need of all the assistance friends, relatives, voluntary organizations, and the Welfare State can provide. Such assistance must have been visualized when the National Assistance Act (1948) made it incumbent on the local authority to provide 'residential accommodation for persons who by reason of age, infirmity or other circumstances are in need of care and attention not otherwise available to them'. That Act has not, so far, been implemented to any appreciable extent but certain local authorities are recognizing that it is applicable to the case of many elderly persons. There is, however, so much to do that governmental and local authority departments would make little impression on it unless they had the enthusiastic support of all the magnificent personnel engaged in voluntary and charitable work. Those bodies recognize that if their efforts are to meet with the reward they deserve they must not be squandered in an haphazard way. The actual individual situation requires to be carefully defined, and an accurate diagnosis established so as to determine the best procedure. The family doctor may be able to do this, or if necessary he may refer his patient to a specialist for a domiciliary consultation, or to a hospital. We believe that in the first place if it is practicable every effort should be made to provide home care; to remove an elderly person from his accustomed surroundings may constitute an additional hazard. The help of relatives, friends, neighbours, may require to be enlisted, and for special services, home helps, almoners, district nurses and 'meals on wheels' can prove invaluable. Some elderly persons are very independent, they prefer to have their freedom and not be beholden to anyone. So long as they do not constitute too much of a danger to themselves or to their neighbours it is a good plan to reduce interference to a minimum. The family doctor, a social worker, a relative or friend, should be encouraged to maintain contact, not so much for a specific purpose as for security reasons.

If home-care is considered inadvisable it may be possible to arrange for the patient's admission to hospital pending the next step. Special units for elderly persons who do not require specialized nursing care have won the support of many private individuals, religious organizations and charitable agencies, *e.g.* British Red Cross Society, National Old People's Welfare Council and the King Edward's Hospital Fund for London. Such special units have much to be said for them. The patients lead a community life, have their own room, or may be in a small dormitory with others, are well nourished and maintained, and in many instances are able to go in and out with freedom and safety. In other cases, depending on the condition of the patient, it may be considered advisable to recommend admission to a mental hospital. This is not the formidable procedure it used to be. It can be arranged informally and the patient can be assured of receiving skilled attention, kindness and understanding to an extent which the public do not sufficiently realize. Here the patient will find all that modern science can do to make life easier and more pleasant. Attention is paid to nutrition, sleep, hygienic habits, there is plenty of indoor and outdoor space to move about in, there is companionship, occupational therapy, radio and television, church services and social parties, so that life can be at a much fuller but yet more protected level than under home conditions.

Organizations such as have been detailed implement the recommendations which Thomson and his co-workers in Birmingham have stressed. Contractures of the limbs, deformity of the feet, the immobility of the paralysed, and the investigation and control of the natural functions, are all matters for urgent attention. Their correction can create immense relief. The great advantage of hospital treatment of the elderly is the constant supervision both night and day. Private nursing home organizations and small specialized residential units are apt to be much more expensive, and good nursing and night supervision hardly exist. In hospital there is much less chance of serious accidents, and if they should occur an efficient medical and nursing service is at hand to deal with them. From the mental view-point the interests of the patient are much more safeguarded than under other conditions, and the wider preventive research aspects are always kept in close relation to psychiatric and general medical problems.

General nursing measures which materially add to the comfort and contentment of the patient are warm clothing, a comfortable bed, a well-heated room, easily masticated food, a warm drink at night-time. Wet beds, bed-sores, faecal impaction, incontinence of urine, and the possibility of becoming bed-ridden should be avoided. Bed exercises, simple occupations, getting the patient up each day, and not tucking in too tightly at night-time may all help enormously.

Restlessness and sleeplessness may be greatly modified by improving nutrition with ascorbic acid tablets (vitamin C), four daily. Parenteral vitamin B_{12} has been strongly recommended in those states where fatigue and lassitude are complained of; its effect can be maintained by fortnightly injections. Nicotinic acid by mouth (100 mg. daily) or by injection can also prove most helpful. In irritable, cantankerous states chlorpromazine hydrochloride (*Largactil*) in 25 mg. doses two or three times daily may be most effective.

For those who have been accustomed to alcohol a glass of whisky or sherry or beer may be a source of pleasure. Chloral hydrate, 30 gr., combined with tincture of opium, B.P., 5 minims, or nepenthe, 10 to 15 minims may ensure a good night's sleep. Paraldehyde by mouth or injection, butobarbitone (*Soneryl*), *Amytal Sodium*, pentobarbitone sodium (*Nembutal*), 1½ gr., are all efficacious. It is wiser to induce sleep than to allow sleeplessness to become a habit.

HUNTINGTON'S CHOREA

Huntington's chorea is a familial disease, occurring usually between the ages of 30 and 50, characterized by general choreiform movements and by gradually increasing mental deterioration dependent upon organic disease of the brain. It is inherited directly from parent to child [see page 37]. The one psychiatric condition in which a simple Mendelian transmission is held to be demonstrated is Huntington's chorea. It is a simple Mendelian dominant and every patient heterozygous for the disease has to expect an average of 50 per cent. of affected offspring. Cases have rarely been recorded without demonstrable inheritance. In a few instances it has occurred before the age of 30. The average length of life after the onset is about sixteen years (Hughes, 1925).

The physical and the mental symptoms are alike progressive: but arrest rarely occurs. The mental changes may precede the physical signs by years. The early mental symptoms consist in deterioration of behaviour—slovenliness in dress, hoarding of useless articles, carelessness of social conventions, *e.g.* the use of obscene language, expectoration on the floor, great irritability issuing in altercation or in actual assault. Usually the patient is depressed; a few are euphoric. There is poverty of thought, a failure of memory, defective attention and defect of judgement. Delusions, persecutory or religious or jealous, and often absurd in their content, are frequent.

Physically, there are continuous movements of the head, trunk and limbs—stretching, jerking and grasping, reminiscent often of athetosis rather than of chorea. The movements begin usually in the lower limbs, and are often unilateral for a time. They cease during sleep, which is usually broken. The voluntary movements are irregular and inco-ordinate. Speech is hesitating and stumbling, and interrupted by clicking sounds, or so thick that it cannot be understood. Writing shows much irregularity. Swallowing may be impaired, and spasmodic jerking of the respiratory muscles may occur. The tendon reflexes are increased, but the sphincters are intact.

The usual termination is dementia and physical helplessness, so that the patient is bedridden. The constant jerking movements continue to the last, and produce irritation of the skin, resulting in bed-sores.

Morbid Anatomy. In 1911 Alzheimer emphasized the occurrence of degenerative changes in the cortex, but also demonstrated extensive changes in the corpus striatum which, he believed, were responsible for the motor phenomena. Dunlap (1927) reported a diminution in size of the cerebral hemispheres, while the cerebellum was of normal size; the average Huntington-chorea brain weighed 980 g. as compared with 1153 g. for the average control case.

As a result of widespread neuronal degeneration, there is a gross generalized cerebral atrophy involving both the cortex and the basal ganglia, and both the white and the grey matter. The caudate nucleus and the putamen are usually particularly severely damaged, with a great reduction of their nerve cells. There is some compensatory ventricular dilatation.

Treatment. With the exception that reserpine may in some cases diminish the abnormal movements, symptomatic treatment is unavailing, but provided suitable legislative measures were enacted so as to ensure the sterilization of all those potentially liable to develop this disorder, it could be diminished. The problem is by no means a small one. Stone and Falstein have given particulars regarding the spread of the condition, and state that as a social and eugenic problem it appears to be out of control.

An account by Pleydell (1954) of the occurrence of Huntington's chorea in Northamptonshire supported the above findings. The incidence was approximately five cases per 100,000 of the population. It is suggested, if that figure holds good, that there are at present more than 20,000 people suffering from Huntington's chorea in England and Wales.

PELLAGRA

Pellagra was described in the eighteenth century as occurring in Spain and in Italy, and in the nineteenth century cases were recognized in France, Rumania,

Egypt, the United States and in the British Isles. In 1866 Howden of Montrose described the first case in the British Isles, but no further mention was made in British literature until in 1909 Brown and Cranston Low described a second case. Since that time numerous cases have been described by other observers in many countries. Since from 4 to 10 per cent. of all pellagrins show mental symptoms, its psychiatric importance is considerable in countries where poverty and malnutrition are common. It may also result from malabsorption secondary to some lesion of the alimentary tract; and it occurs, though uncommonly, in cases of mental illness, where the diet has been defective. We have seen it complicating cases of senile dementia, alcoholism, involutional melancholia and schizophrenia.

Aetiology. At one time it was thought that this disease was caused by the excessive use of corn, or by corn that was diseased. But it affects persons who have never eaten corn or corn products, and, moreover, pellagra is occasionally absent from districts where corn preponderates in the diet. In 1915 the experimental work carried out by Goldberger, Waring and others of the U.S. Public Health Service proved that pellagra is due neither to diseased maize nor to an infective agent, but to a defective diet. Goldberger's conclusion that the disease was dependent on some fault in the diet has been amply confirmed by later work, which has demonstrated that pellagra can be promptly cured by administration of the appropriate vitamin, nicotinic acid, the pellagra-preventing (P.-P.) factor of the vitamin B complex. A suitable dose is 500 mg. per day orally or 40 mg. intramuscularly thrice daily, but it should be accompanied by a well-balanced, nourishing diet, since other vitamin deficiencies are commonly associated with deficiency of nicotinic acid. Most protein foods are sources of nicotinic acid, especially yeast, fresh or canned salmon, and some liver extracts. In more severe cases larger doses of nicotinic acid (niacin) are required. Sydenstricker advised 100 mg. of niacin every hour for 10 hours during the first 2 days and believed that most patients improve within 48 hours after beginning the treatment.

Symptomatology. Pellagra is characterized by a combination of cutaneous, digestive, nervous and mental symptoms, which may show remissions and recurrences over a long period of years. Occasionally the disease may run an acute course and proceed quickly to a fatal termination.

The skin lesions consist of an erythema, followed by a dermatitis, and discoloration of the skin, resembling a severe sunburn. This condition involves the backs of the hands, extending as a band round the wrists, and in some cases involving the palms of the hands. The face, the neck, the elbows, the knees, the scrotum or vulva may show a similar condition.

The mucous membranes of the mouth and tongue become inflamed, so that the mouth is painful, and the tongue has a glossy, red, raw appearance. Associated with this condition there may be gastric symptoms, and a history of alternating diarrhoea and constipation.

The nervous symptoms are of a general nature, and consist mainly of paraesthesiae occurring throughout the body, tremor, increased or diminished reflexes, and occasionally convulsions.

The mental symptoms associated with pellagra are usually either in the nature of a depressive state, a chronic organic reaction (memory-loss, etc.), or a delirium. The last is the most frequent. The depression is probably based on the fact that the patient realizes he is suffering from a severe physical illness, while the delirium shows no peculiar features.

Morbid Anatomy. The principal histopathological finding in cases of pellagra is an axonal reaction affecting especially the Betz cells of the motor cortex. This type of axonal reaction was described by Adolf Meyer and termed by him 'central neuritis'. The probability is that his cases of central neuritis were really cases of pellagra. The axonal reaction consists of a swelling of the cell body as a whole, while the centre of the cell exhibits a pale, more or less homogeneous appearance of the protoplasm, with a loss of stainable substance, which might or might not be well preserved at the periphery of the cell, and displacement of the nucleus towards the border of the cell body (Dunlap).

Treatment. We have already stated that pellagra is due to faulty nutrition, and the best way to prevent its occurrence is to give the patient an abundance of fresh milk, eggs, fresh lean meat, peas and beans. In mental hospitals special care should be taken to see that patients who are being tube-fed have a varied diet, and that patients who are less able to look after themselves are protected from those who are inclined to steal their food from them. It is largely as the result of insufficient diet from such causes that pellagra develops in mental hospitals. The necessary dosage of nicotinic acid for treatment has been indicated above.

MENTAL SEQUELAE OF HEAD INJURY

Mental symptoms may be precipitated by injury to any other part of the body as well as to the head, and in that event we are concerned with the psychological effects of the traumatic experience in precipitating either a neurosis or a psychosis, according to the nature of the pre-existing personality or to the special circumstances. The symptoms are not different from those of neurotic and psychotic forms of reaction in general.

Head injury may precipitate or cause mental symptoms in one or both of two ways: either it acts as a non-specific psychological stress like injury elsewhere in the body (though associated perhaps with greater fear of the consequences) and precipitates a 'functional' reaction, a neurosis or a psychosis; or it causes organic mental symptoms as a result of damage to the brain. To put it in other words: an abnormal mental state following a head injury may be due to the physical effects of the injury on the brain, or to the psychological effects of the experience on the personality, or to a combination of the two.

It is only the organic sequelae of head injury that are in any way specific, and with which we are mainly concerned here. A convenient clinical subdivision of the mental after-effects is as follows:

1. Post-concussional and post-contusional syndromes; including deliria and transient dysmnesic states.
2. Post-traumatic dementia; including personality changes and Korsakow's psychosis.

3. Other neurological sequelae; including epilepsy, aphasia and subdural haematoma.

After a minor head injury with concussion, the mental symptoms are transient, disappearing usually in a few days. In addition to complaining of headache, the patient may be dazed, irritable, restless and for some time confused. The effects of cerebral contusion, which implies a more significant degree of organic damage to the brain, are more severe and tend to be much more persistent. The patient may proceed through the phases of stupor, delirium and confusion as he slowly emerges from coma following a major trauma. He may then recover completely, or show residual disabilities of lesser or greater severity.

Post-contusional Syndrome. After cerebral contusion, the patient is apt on recovering full consciousness to complain for some time of a group of symptoms which has been called the post-contusional syndrome. These symptoms include headache, which is usually throbbing and aggravated by stooping and physical or mental stress; dizziness or giddiness; increased fatigability; impaired concentration; slowing of thinking processes, and forgetfulness; irritability and over-sensitivity to noise; and a decreased tolerance of alcohol. Headache is not always present: Guttmann (1943) found that only 46 per cent. of his series of cases complained of headache at any time. The patient realizes that he is ill and is often anxious and depressed. Typically he prefers to keep away from all forms of amusement as well as from work, since the one is nearly as great an effort as the other: this distinguishes him from the malingerer.

The following case illustrates the typical physical complaints as well as the typical mental symptoms following minor head injury.

CASE No. 53

The patient's previous career suggests an instability which may be related to the subsequent symptoms.

He fell 30–40 feet from a girder and remembers the first part of the fall. He states he was unconscious for about half an hour, but his amnesia covers about an hour, except for two incidents which he remembers—asking for a cigarette and going into an ambulance. When he came to, he ached all over and had a headache, having received two scalp wounds. He discharged himself from hospital after 5 to 6 hours, stayed in bed at home for 4 days and then got up and walked about. Headaches, which had been slight when he was in bed, became worse when he commenced getting about. They have persisted more or less up to the present time, but have been more severe for the last 2 to 3 months and occur every day more or less continuously. The pain is situated across the frontal region, is worse when he stoops and is also accompanied by dizzy feelings. It is aggravated by drill and running, but unaffected by coughing or straining. It is relieved by aspirin.

He has also become more irritable, particularly with regard to noise. The least noise, such as that of a typewriter, irritates him. He has become moody, depressed and apathetic. On a few occasions he has felt that he could sit down and cry, for no reason at all. He has no inclination for any kind of games. He cannot concentrate well, and has tried to make himself study, but 'just cannot be bothered'. His memory, he thinks, is as good as ever. He has noticed an increased susceptibility to alcohol, and 'cannot hold his beer so well'. He used to be able to 'hold quite a lot' but now gets 'tight' on half the quantity.

He feels unable to cope with his work and does not feel like doing anything; but he has periods when he feels quite pleased with himself. He was euphoric at times during the interview and tended to treat the accident as a joke.

Personal History. No neurotic traits are recorded. He never suffered from headaches before. School 5–14 Secondary. He was average at his work. He played the usual games and did much cycle racing. When he left school he seems to have lived a carefree existence, having had three to four jobs until he was 18, and up until about 4 years ago, when he married and settled down, he had had about twenty changes in all. He changed either because he got 'fed up' or because he wanted more money. His work for the last four years has been engineering. He describes his temperament as happy-go-lucky.

He has suffered from duodenal ulcer for the last 3 to 4 years. He was told to go on a diet but did not bother to stick to it. He has had recurrences of pain after food, occurring at about 3-monthly intervals.

The post-contusional syndrome is often accompanied by anxiety, and this complication is responsible for difficulty in diagnosis and prognosis, as well as for some of the confusion in terminology which has existed. When the majority of the above symptoms are complained of, there is no difficulty in concluding that true cerebral damage has been sustained and persists; but when the patient complains only of lack of concentration and difficulty in memory, and of headache not influenced by posture or by some movement, as well as of dizziness of an ill-defined type, and when he is obviously anxious, the diagnosis is much more difficult. The apparent mildness of the original injury is not conclusive: there may be little or no evidence of loss of consciousness after cerebral injury.

The previous personality is of importance. Symptoms are more likely to be due to persistent brain damage if they occur in a person of previously stable personality. It is essential to find out if the patient has domestic or other such worries, which may be complicating the situation. Questions of compensation favour neurotic developments. It is interesting that neurotic syndromes appear to be rare after head injuries sustained in the hunting field.

Many have emphasized that head injury is particularly apt to be followed by anxiety, since the individual attaches special importance to his head and brain; moreover, in those who have to earn their living by intellectual work, damage to the head is mentally disturbing. Schilder (1943) pointed out another source of anxiety in the feeling of insecurity produced by repeated experiences of dizziness.

The *pathological* physical effects of brain injury are both focal and diffuse, immediate and delayed. The focal lesions consist at first of capillary haemorrhages and oedema; and later in the occurrence of secondary degeneration, demyelination and the formation of scar tissue. Diffuse effects of the same kind are also produced. The circulation of the cerebrospinal fluid is usually disturbed, the pressure being either raised or lowered.

The *prognosis* is determined by a number of factors. The time taken for convalescence to be completed varies more or less directly with the length of the post-traumatic amnesia (measured from time of injury to time when continuous awareness is re-established). Where the P.T.A. has been less than 2 hours the patients are usually back at work within 3 months. Where it has been less than

48 hours they are usually back inside 4 months, but if it has been over 48 hours the time taken to return to work varies from 3 to 6 months, and in some cases longer, depending largely on personality and circumstances.

The prognosis depends also importantly on the adequacy of the previous personality. It has been said that what is often spoken of as the prognosis of head injuries in the post-contusional group is more accurately the prognosis of willingness to return to work in spite of the persistence of such symptoms as headache. Ritchie Russell (1934) recorded that of 120 patients whose symptoms persisted longer than 2 months, 66 per cent. still had symptoms after 18 months, but in many cases work, even heavy manual labour, was not interfered with. Some patients are driven back to work too soon by economic and other pressures.

Anxiety about compensation hinders recovery. Ritchie Russell reported that after 18 months 35 per cent. of his compensation cases had not reported fit for work, while in the non-compensation group only 9 per cent. had failed to do so.

The prognosis is also influenced by age, those over 40 being less successful in getting back to work quickly.

Details of the *treatment* of head injuries will not be discussed here: they can be read in textbooks of neurosurgery. Rest in bed is imperative at the beginning, but how far it should be prolonged is a matter for judgement. If his headache has gone the patient may usually be allowed up, by gradual stages, soon afterwards. Explanation of the symptoms and encouragement in what is often a long convalescence, are needed. Occupational therapy and graduated physical exercise prepare the way for a return to other normal activities and to work.

Post-traumatic Dementia. Gross and permanent dementia following head injury is rare: and one should not conclude that damage is permanent until at least 18 months after injury. The slighter degrees of residual disability are more frequently seen but are still uncommon. The brain-damaged individual may develop a post-traumatic personality change, in that he becomes more labile emotionally and mentally slower and forgetful, shows a diminished sense of moral responsibility, neglects his personal hygiene and may have outbursts of episodic violence. Frontal lobe damage is particularly apt to be associated with this sort of deterioration in the personality which is revealed in loss of the finer feelings, in childishness and in emotional decay. A less common sequel is a persistent dysmnesic syndrome or Korsakow's psychosis, with euphoria, gross memory retention defect, disorientation and confabulation, which may last for weeks or months following the injury or become permanent. This, and other severe types of damage, may so incapacitate the patient that long-term mental hospital care becomes necessary.

Other Neurological Sequelae. Epilepsy may be a late complication of closed head injuries, but follows more often cases in which the dura has been penetrated. There may be an interval of years before fits commence, due to scar formation.

Lesions involving cortical areas associated with speech functions interfere more or less with the mental functions also, since the individual is so dependent on speech and allied functions, both receptive and expressive, for his contact with the environment, and on verbal symbols for his thinking. Aphasic syndromes resulting from such lesions may on superficial examination be mistaken for a diffuse dementia.

The signs and symptoms of subdural haematoma may not develop until some weeks or months have passed, and the head injury itself may have appeared so slight as to have caused little concern at the time: the latter perhaps most often happens in the cases of old people and alcoholics. Intense headache, with the development of a state of fluctuating consciousness, is typical. Neurological signs are often slight, inconstant and misleading in localizing the site of the haematoma. If the haematoma is bilateral, a fairly rapidly progressive dementia results. It is of great importance to make the correct diagnosis and to make it as soon as possible. The response to surgical drainage through burr-holes is usually excellent.

Tests of Mental Deterioration

Various psychological tests have been devised which can be of much assistance in confirming and refining clinical observations in brain-damaged patients.

Wechsler (1952) points out that the measurement of mental deterioration involves three separate problems: 1. the reliable measurement of the individual's actual or present functioning ability; 2. the evaluation of his previous functioning level; 3. the expression of the difference between the two in meaningful, quantitative terms'. He developed a differential-test-score method of measuring mental deterioration, which uses the fact that some abilities decline relatively little during adult life and others to a considerable degree: abilities tapped by performance tests, for example, decline more rapidly with age than those involved in verbal tests; general information and comprehension are maintained better than the memory span for digits. Tests are allocated to two groups, those which 'hold up' with age and those which do not. Tests which hold up with age are: 'information, comprehension, object assembly, picture completion and vocabulary'. Tests which do not hold up with age are: 'Digit span, arithmetic, digit symbol, block design, similarities'. To obtain a measure of deterioration, one compares the sum weighted scores of the two groups of tests. Pathological deterioration is defined by Wechsler as follows: 'An individual may be said to show signs of possible deterioration if he shows a greater than a 10 per cent. loss, and of definite deterioration if a loss greater than 20 per cent. than that allowed for by the normal decline with age'.

The observation that the formation of new associations is hindered has also been utilized in a small group of tests adapted by Zangwill (1943). In the first test the total memory span with a series of digits, such as 3.1.7.2.9.4., is contrasted with the time taken to learn to repeat gradually a series which is one digit longer than it is possible for the patient to reproduce immediately without error after one reading by the examiner. Thus a patient with a basal digit span of six digits may be unable to learn a sequence of seven digits even after ten consecutive trials.

The second test is adapted from Babcock's scale and consists in counting the trials necessary for the patient to learn a sentence of rather unusual syntax:

'One thing a nation must have to become rich and great is a large secure supply of wood'.

The sentence is repeated alternately by the examiner and the patient until the latter gives two consecutive word-perfect versions.

While an intelligence test may show no appearance of intellectual defect yet the deteriorated patient may not be able to learn to repeat the sentence perfectly even after ten trials. Even this test, however, may show nothing when the patient has been originally of superior intelligence.

The assessment of minor degrees of organic impairment should depend on a combination of total clinical impressions and the results of specific tests. Taken together these give a more accurate picture than either in isolation.

BRAIN TUMOUR

Tumours of the brain are amongst the commonest of tumours and in the majority of cases are primary, originating in the brain itself or in its coverings. In less than a quarter of the cases the tumour is a secondary deposit, and then often multiple: of these the primary focus is most often in the lung. It is important to note that the primary lung cancer may be more or less clinically silent, while the secondary deposits are giving rise to symptoms of confusion or dementia. Brain (1958) reports that bronchial carcinoma itself may give rise to fluctuating clouding of consciousness and dementia, apparently without metastasizing to the brain. The chest should therefore be X-rayed in all cases of suspected brain tumour.

Mental symptoms are usually stated to be present in upwards of 60 to 85 per cent. of all cases of brain tumour, and in 100 per cent. of patients with tumours of the corpus callosum. Mental symptoms may be the earliest and presenting symptoms, and it is unfortunate that usually they are of a general and indeterminate character, not specific to tumour and without localizing value, being those associated with any condition producing an increase of intracranial pressure. The very earliest symptoms are often very slight—undue fatigability, difficulty in concentration, indefinite malaise and anxiety: they may easily be thought neurotic or depressive. If an epileptic fit occurs in such a setting, or indeed for the first time in adult life, whether or not there are accompanying symptoms, brain tumour should always be considered in the differential diagnosis.

The less equivocal symptoms and signs which are developed as the tumour grows fall into two groups: those due to the widespread effects of increasing intracranial pressure, and those due to the local effects of the tumour itself. Raised intracranial pressure causes typically headache, throbbing or bursting, at its worst often on wakening and increased by stooping or coughing; vomiting, with or without nausea; and papilloedema. In old age, when the shrunken brain leaves more space within the skull, this triad of symptoms of increased cerebrospinal fluid pressure may be unusually late in developing. The mental symptoms are those of confusion or dementia. The patient becomes dulled, irritable and forgetful, later apathetic and somnolent: disorientation and incontinence usually precede the terminal lapse into coma.

The nature of the local symptoms depends of course on the location and mode of spread of the tumour. Metastatic tumours, which are commonly multiple and rapidly growing, tend to cause mental confusion.

If the tumour is in a frontal lobe, or involving by pressure one of the frontal lobes, the presenting clinical feature may be a personality change, a frontal lobe deficit syndrome. The patient may become mildly euphoric, with a tendency to pun or joke (the so-called 'witzelsucht'), facile, tactless, degenerate and unconcerned. His behaviour deteriorates as his dementia progresses and he remains without insight. A grasp reflex may be pathognomonic. The mental symptoms do not help to locate the side of the lesion.

Mental symptoms may also be the earliest symptoms of a temporal or temperoparietal lobe tumour. The clinical picture depends on whether or not the lesion is in the dominant hemisphere. If the lesion is anterior, in the non-dominant hemisphere, the symptoms may be similar to those described above as typical of frontal lobe lesions and may precede the development of neurological signs. A left-sided lesion in a right-handed individual is likely to cause aphasia. The most frequent other neurological signs are a homonymous visual field defect and slight hemiplegia (initially most often a lower facial weakness): hemianaesthesia is less common. The patient with a temporal lobe tumour is often notably moody, intermittently depressed and irritable. Psychomotor seizures are also characteristic signs of tumours in this area. They may last for minutes or much longer, even for days: the patient is clouded mentally, and experiences hallucinations of taste or smell and feelings of unreality or *déjà vu*. In this clouded state he may act bemusedly or violently, or go off in a fugue.

Tumours of the occipal lobe are much rarer. Visual field defects are characteristic, and if the patient has fits the seizures may be prefaced by a visual hallucinatory aura.

Corpus callosum tumours are also very uncommon. Mental disorganization is a prominent feature and memory disturbance may be particularly severe. There is usually also early damage to the pyramidal tracts.

For a full description of the symptoms and signs of tumours in the various cerebral areas, the reader is referred to a textbook of neurology, such as Russell Brain's (1955).

PERNICIOUS ANAEMIA

Cabot, Woltman, McAlpine (1929) and others have described the mental symptoms which may be found in cases of pernicious anaemia. Depressive reactions are not uncommon. Confusion and dementia may also occur, in association with E.E.G. changes (Walton *et al.*, 1954) and due apparently to similar lesions of degeneration and demyelination in the white matter of the brain as are found in the cord in cases of subacute combined degeneration. The essential aetiological factor in the production of these organic mental symptoms is vitamin

B_{12} deficiency: and it is noteworthy that mental symptoms, like the signs of subacute combined degeneration of the cord, may be apparent before anaemia is observed. The mental symptoms also respond to treatment with adequate doses of vitamin B_{12}.

PORPHYRIA

The intermittency of the symptoms of porphyria is one of its clinical characteristics which may make diagnosis difficult. So also is the fact that the urine may not be port-wine in colour. The peak incidence of the disease, which may be inherited as a Mendelian dominant, is in the third decade. The affected individual comes under medical observation for abdominal, neurological or psychiatric symptoms. Attacks of colic may mimic acute obstruction and the patient not uncommonly bears the scars of several laparotomies. Various neuropathies may occur, with paraesthesiae and muscle weakness. The mental symptoms, if wrongly diagnosed (and they are not at all specific), are probably most often described as hysterical: there may be much emotional instability, irritability and apparent hypochondriasis. A crisis may be precipitated in a susceptible individual by the giving of barbiturates.

A history of recurrent attacks of emotional instability and colic should suggest the diagnosis, and the urine should be screened for porphobilinogen, uroporphyrin and coproporphyrin. A comprehensive account is given by Kark (1955).

REFERENCES

Alzheimer, A. (1907) *Zbl. Nervenheilk. Psychiat.*, **30**, 449.
American Journal of Psychiatry (1931) **10**, 433.
Anderson, W. F. (1957) *Care of the Elderly Sick in General Practice*, Royal College of Physicians of Edinburgh.
Bockner, S., and Coltart, N. (1961) *Brit. med. J.*, **1**, 18.
Brain, W. R. (1955) *Diseases of the Nervous System*, 5th ed., London.
Brain, W. R. (1958) *Lancet*, ii, 971.
Campbell, C. M. (1912) *Nervous and Mental Disease Monograph Series*, No. 9, New York.
Campbell, C. M. (1914) *Focal Symptoms in General Paralysis*, New York.
Campbell, C. M. (1916) *Psychiat. Bull. (Utica)*, **9**, 316.
Campbell, A. C. P., and Russell, W. R. (1941) *Quart. J. Med.*, **10**, 41.
Ciba Foundation (1955) *Colloquia on Ageing*, Vol. 1, London.
Connell, P. H. (1958) *Amphetamine Psychosis*, London.
Dawson, S., and Conn, J. C. M. (1931) *Spec. Rep. Ser. med. Res. Coun. (Lond.)*, No. 162.
Dunlap, C. B. (1911) *J. nerv. ment. Dis.*, **38**, 486.
Dunlap, C. B. (1912) *State Hosp. Bull. (N.Y.)*, **5**, 452.
Dunlap, C. B. (1914) *Amer. J. Insan.*, **71**, 249.
Dunlap, C. B. (1927) *Arch. Neurol. Psychiat. (Chicago)*, **18**, 867.
Fuchs, A., and Rosenthal, R. (1904) *Physical, Chemical, and Cytological Examination of Cerebrospinal Fluid*, Vienna.
Guttmann, E. (1943) *Lancet*, i, 10.
Hald, J., and Jacobsen, E. (1948) *Lancet*, ii, 1001.
Hare, E. H. (1959) *J. ment. Sci.*, **105**, 594.
Henderson, D. K. (1911) *Rev. Neurol. Psychiat.*, **9**, 529.
Henderson, D. K., and Muirhead, W. (1913) *Rev. neurol. Psychiat.*, **11**, 195.
Henderson, Y. (1926) *Brit. med. J.*, **1**, 41.
Hughes, E. M. (1925) *Amer. J. Psychiat.*, **4**, 537.

Jacobs, B. (1943) *J. ment. Sci.*, **89**, 242.
Jones, E. (1909) *Rev. Neurol. Psychiat.*, **7**, 379.
Kark, R. M. (1955) *Med. Clin. N. Amer.*, **39**, 11.
Lemere, F., and Voegtlin, W. L. (1942) *Quart. J. Stud. Alcohol*, **3**, 322.
Letemendia, F., and Pampiglione, G. (1958) *J. Neurol. Neurosurg. Psychiat.*, **21**, 167.
Lups, S., and Haan, A. M. F. H. (1954) *The Cerebrospinal Fluid*, Amsterdam.
McAlpine, D. (1929) *Lancet*, ii, 643.
Maurer, D. W., and Vogel, V. H. (1954) *Narcotics and Narcotic Addiction*, Illinois.
Meyer, A. (1960) in *Neuropathology*, ed. Greenfield, J. G., London.
Mott, F. W. (1909) *Brit. med. J.*, **1**, 454.
Mott, F. W. (1910) in *A System of Syphilis*, ed. Power, D'A., and Murphy, J. K., Vol. 4, London.
Noguchi, H., and Moore, J. W. (1913) *J. exp. Med.*, **17**, 232.
Plaut, F. (1911) *Nervous and Mental Disease Monograph Series*, No. 5, New York.
Pleydell, M. J. (1954) *Brit. med. J.*, **2**, 1121.
Robertson, G. M. (1922) *Brit. med. J.*, **2**, 1120.
Rudd, T. N. (1953) *The Nursing of the Elderly Sick*, London.
Russell, W. R. (1934) *Edinb. med. J.*, **12**, 129.
Schilder, P. (1943) in *Injuries of the Skull, Brain and Spinal Cord*, ed. Brock, S., 2nd ed., Baltimore.
Sjögren, T., Sjögren, H., and Lindgren, A. G. H. (1952) Morbus Alzheimer and Morbus Pick, *Acta. psychiat. (Kbh.)*, Supp. 82.
Steel, R. (1960) *Lancet*, i, 121.
Stewart, C. P., and Dunlop, D. M. (1958) *Clinical Chemistry in Practical Medicine*, Edinburgh.
Stone, T. T., and Falstein, E. I. (1939) *J. nerv. ment. Dis.*, **89**, 795.
Thompson, A. P., Lowe, C. R., and McKeown, T. (1951) *The Care of the Ageing and Chronic Sick*, Edinburgh.
Tiebout, H. M. (1944) *Amer. J. Psychiat.*, **100**, 468.
Voegtlin, W. L., and Broz, W. R. (1949) *Ann. intern. Med.*, **30**, 580.
Walton, J. N., *et al.* (1954) *Electroenceph. clin. Neurophysiol.*, **6**, 45.
Wechsler, D. (1952) *The Measurement of Adult Intelligence*, 3rd ed., Baltimore.
Zangwill, O. L. (1943) *Proc. roy. Soc. Med.*, **36**, 576.

16

EPILEPSY

The term epilepsy has for long been used to designate a heterogeneous group of symptoms, of which the most prominent feature is the repeated occurrence of convulsive attacks. But it is now generally recognized that it is more accurate to speak of 'the epilepsies', or to consider epilepsy a symptom rather than a disease. The essential feature is not the convulsive seizure or the disturbance of consciousness, but the episodic sudden disturbance of function in the central nervous system. Hughlings Jackson from his clinical observations pointed to the nature of the neuronal process as an active discharge at some level of the central nervous system anywhere from the cortex to the diencephalon, with accompanying phenomena, such as automatisms following a major fit, conceived as release phenomena. That a neuronal discharge is the primary condition is supported by Penfield and Erickson's observation that an attack which seems to the patient and observer to be identical with the customary seizure can be provoked by electrical stimulation of the appropriate part of the brain. Both the physical and the mental phenomena can be conceived in the same way. For example, one of Penfield and Erickson's novel discoveries was that a visual memory of some old experience, which may have appeared also in a nightmare, as well as forming part of a seizure, could be elicited by electrical stimulation of a temporal lobe.

Epilepsy is a most important condition in the psychiatric field for a number of reasons. Abnormal mental symptoms and disturbed behaviour may either accompany, or follow, epileptic seizures; and may be so severe or prolonged in some cases that the label epileptic psychosis is merited. Major and minor seizures must often also be distinguished from other disturbances of consciousness or motility due more purely to psychogenic causes. While in interparoxysmal periods the sufferer from epilepsy may show certain anomalies of personality or temperament which, apart from his overt fits, impair his social adaptation.

Recent research has increased the number of cases of epilepsy in which a causal lesion can be found by detailed physical examinations which include X-rays, air-encephalography, angiography and electroencephalographic recordings. However, the hope expressed by some that soon there will be no need for such a category as 'idiopathic' epilepsy, in which no physical basis for the attacks can be discovered, is probably illusory; and we are coming to appreciate better the importance of hereditary factors, which though they may be called physical are unlikely soon to be dissected.

AETIOLOGY

The aetiology of epileptic seizures is certainly a multiple aetiology, and much remains unknown, particularly about the so-called idiopathic group. We shall set out the causal factors under three main heads—constitutional, predisposing and precipitating. These are not to be understood as distinct or mutually exclusive categories, but as a means only of ordering the data. In cases where the constitutional factors appear to be of greatest importance, or the aetiology is unknown, the epilepsy is usually described as idiopathic, or genetic (Lennox): when predisposing factors predominate, it is called symptomatic or acquired. The precipitating or eliciting factors are common to both groups.

Constitutional Factors

Among constitutional factors we may include the rôle of heredity, the influence of the endocrine system, and age.

There is convincing evidence that *genetic* factors are important in the production of epilepsy. The incidence of epilepsy is higher amongst the near relatives of epileptics than it is in the general population. Lennox (1951), reviewing near relatives of 4231 epileptics, found that 3·2 per cent. had a history of one or more seizures; whereas the incidence of epilepsy amongst the young adult population of the U.S.A. (those of draft age) is about 0·5 per cent. Lennox found a positive family history of epilepsy in 1·8 per cent. of cases of symptomatic epilepsy, and in 3·6 per cent. of cases of idiopathic (metabolic) epilepsy. He also reported that the incidence of epilepsy amongst relatives declined progressively with increasing age of the patient at the time of the first seizure: thus in cases of idiopathic epilepsy which began in infancy, 6·4 per cent. of relatives were found to be affected, while amongst those cases with onset at age 30 years or over, the family incidence of epilepsy fell to 1·3 per cent.

Twin studies have been employed to elucidate the relative importance of hereditary and environmental causal factors. Lennox and Jolly (1954) studied 173 twin pairs subject to seizures. Concordance of epilepsy among 77 monozygotic pairs was 70·1 per cent., among 96 dizygotic pairs 12·5 per cent. If cases with acquired brain damage were excluded, the concordance among 51 monozygotic pairs rose to 88·2 per cent. Concordance for epilepsy among monozygotic pairs of around 60–70 per cent. has also been reported by Rosanoff (1934) from the U.S.A., and by Conrad (1935) from Germany. Figures for concordance among dizygotic pairs have a much wider scatter, from 3 to 24 per cent. Lennox and Jolly not only found a high concordance of epilepsy in monozygotic twins, both absolutely and in comparison with dizygotic twins, but reported that this high concordance extended to the type of seizure and particularly to the three per second wave-and-spike pattern of the E.E.G. The rôle of heredity appears to decrease progressively in the three groups, *petit mal*, *grand mal* and psychomotor seizures.

Though only a small percentage of the near relatives of epileptics have epileptic seizures, a considerable percentage have abnormal E.E.Gs. Lennox, Gibbs and Gibbs (1940) reported abnormal E.E.Gs. in 54 per cent. of the parents, sibs and children of epileptics, whereas only 6 per cent. of a control group unrelated to epileptics exhibited similar abnormalities. It has therefore been suggested that what is inherited is a cerebral dysrhythmia, a tendency or predisposition to abnormal cerebral discharge, which may show itself as fits or as anomalies of temperament, or may not manifest itself clinically at all.

The mode of inheritance of epilepsy has been much debated, and the action of single genes, recessive and dominant, as well as that of polygenes, has been postulated by various workers. Such discrepancies in the opinions expressed are not unexpected, since epilepsy is not a nosological entity and research has been much hampered by the great difficulty experienced in obtaining case samples for investigation which have not been in some way biased in their selection.

One may say in summary that hereditary factors appear to play a part in the genesis of both idiopathic and symptomatic epilepsy, but more particularly in the former, and especially in idiopathic cases with *petit mal* seizures; and that the mode of inheritance is not yet known.

The incidence of epilepsy is approximately equal in the two sexes. In women, there is an important relationship of fits with menstruation, seizures tending to occur in some cases shortly before or at the menstrual periods. Pregnancy may have no influence on the frequency of seizures: on the other hand, they may temporarily disappear during a pregnancy, or become more frequent.

Idiopathic epilepsy usually becomes manifest before adult life is reached. It is said that three-quarters of the cases have their onset in the first two decades, often about puberty. A history of infantile convulsions is obtained in about 20 per cent. of epileptics, compared with 4 per cent. in a control group (Patrick and Levy).

Predisposing Factors

Factors which predispose to epilepsy are those which cause directly tissue damage in the brain, or indirectly interfere with its normal functions. They are very numerous.

Amongst local cerebral causes may be mentioned tumour, arteriosclerosis, meningitis, cerebrovascular syphilis and general paralysis, cysticercosis and head injury. The latter may be inflicted at birth, by trauma or asphyxia; or in adult life, when epilepsy is most often a complication of penetrating injuries. The incidence of epilepsy after closed-head injury is 6 per cent. (Phillips, 1954), but may rise even to 45 per cent. if the dura has been penetrated (Ascroft, 1941). Epilepsy may also occur in cases of subnormality (*e.g.* in cerebral palsy, tuberous sclerosis); and in some cases of pre-senile dementia (*e.g.* Alzheimer's disease).

General causes include infections, intoxications and other illnesses leading to profound metabolic or circulatory changes. In infancy, epilepsy may be a symptom of an acute infection with high fever, or of tetany, for example; in adult life, of uraemia, eclampsia, delirium tremens, hypertensive encephalopathy, heart block.

Precipitating Factors

These may be primarily emotional or physical. Frustration may produce a fit in a susceptible individual; so may other strong emotions. Specific sensory stimuli are effective in certain rare cases—*e.g.* music, or visual flicker. Metabolic changes are especially important: hydration, hyperventilation leading to alkalosis, and hypoglycaemia are common precipitants. So also is sleep; and, less commonly, general anaesthesia. Ketosis, on the contrary, tends to inhibit seizures.

Relationships with other Syndromes

Some writers have claimed an association between epilepsy and migraine, which others have denied. Migraine has been said to occur in the heredity of 60 per cent. of epileptics, compared with 17 per cent. in normals. A clearer relationship may be seen between epilepsy and aggressive psychopathic states, particularly the so-called 'epileptoid' group of the latter, whose intermittent outbursts of violent conduct often closely resemble clinically psychomotor seizures of temporal lobe origin: and in both conditions E.E.G. abnormalities may be found in recordings from the temporal lobes.

PHYSIOLOGY OF THE SEIZURES

The brain has a continuous spontaneous electrical activity and it is these changes in electrical potential which are recorded by the E.E.G. When sensory stimulation is reduced to a minimum the cortex shows a resting rhythm while the individual is conscious. The origin of the resting activity is not known: it has been suggested its pace-maker may be situated in the central grey matter, perhaps in the reticular system of the brain stem. This resting rhythm is markedly altered by incoming stimuli, and if the individual increases his mental alertness by concentration and attention or emotional excitement, or if he diminishes it by falling asleep.

In epileptic seizures the neurones discharge paroxysmally, and there is excessive electrical activity, which tends to be hypersynchronous. This epileptic discharge may be initiated either in the grey matter of the cerebral cortex or in the subcortical ganglia. The reasons for this abnormal activity are not clearly known. It is recognized that the metabolism of the neurones is very easily disturbed. They are particularly sensitive to changes in cerebral blood flow causing ischaemia or hypoxia, and this may be a common factor in causing epileptic discharges. The rôle of diminished H-ion concentration is uncertain.

Penfield and Jasper (1954) state that experiments indicate the following functional characteristics of epileptogenic nerve tissue:

1. Increased tendency to spontaneous activity and to self-sustained paroxysmal discharge.
2. Decreased synaptic resistance.
3. Increased and more prolonged discharge in response to afferent nerve impulses.
4. Hypersynchrony—greater number of cells firing together, though excessive discharge may also be relatively asynchronous.
5. More intense, higher frequency, discharge of impulses from each cell.
6. Spread of paroxysmal activity from a focus to adjacent tissue with progressive recruitment of larger masses of cells in synchronous discharge.
7. Projection and distant spread of paroxysmal activity over two-way neuronal conducting pathways between the cortex and subcortical structures, and over association pathways between distant cortical areas, and between the two hemispheres.

8. Non-synaptic spread of excitation by electrical field effects between adjacent areas of grey matter due to heightened facilitation and high-voltage discharge.

PATHOLOGY

In assessing the relevance of post-mortem findings in cases of epilepsy, it is necessary to remember that the changes found may be either the cause or the result of the epileptic process, whatever it is. There are no constant pathological findings.

Alzheimer discovered pathological changes in 'idiopathic' cases, notably sclerotic changes in the cornu ammonis (hippocampus) and superficial gliosis of the hemispheres. Many other workers have reported Ammon's horn sclerosis, laminar atrophy, particularly of the third cortical layer, and disseminated cerebellar sclerosis. These changes, which may be slight or severe, have usually been ascribed to anoxia.

In 'symptomatic' cases various lesions are found, according to the nature of the causal disease.

Recent research has been focussed on lesions of the temporal lobes. Penfield and Baldwin (1952) found that in case after case of temporal lobe epilepsy the cortex was tough in the anterior and deep portion of the first temporal convolution, extending into and growing more marked in the uncus and hippocampal gyrus. This condition was named 'incisural sclerosis', and Penfield and Jasper (1954) have given the following explanation of it: 'It seems likely that, at the time of the passage of the infant head through the birth canal, the mesial portion of one or both temporal lobes may be squeezed downward through the incisura of the tentorium. Thus, the margin of the lobe, including uncus and hippocampal gyrus, would be subjected to greater ischaemia than other portions of the brain. It also seems likely that the artery of supply, the choroidal artery, and even, at times, the posterior cerebral artery, might be compressed against the incisural margin.' Penfield and his colleagues believe that incisural sclerosis is the commonest cause of temporal lobe epilepsy.

Other causes of temporal lobe epilepsy are tumours, porencephalic cysts, angiomas, and the scars of penetrating head injuries and infections. Meyer, Falconer and Beck (1954), reporting the pathological examination of 14 operative cases without gross structural lesions which could be demonstrated before operation, found that birth injury as the cause of the temporal lobe epilepsy was proved or likely in at most 3 cases: on the other hand, 3 cases followed a cerebral complication (probably vascular accident or encephalitis) during measles, 'status epilepticus' following 'teething', and chickenpox respectively; which draws attention to events in infancy, childhood and early adolescence whose significance has perhaps been previously overlooked. Meyer and his colleagues (1955) have also described the interesting case of a boy, aged 9 years, suffering from Still's syndrome, who became demented after a status epilepticus and died one year later. His brain showed lesions in the first temporal convolution and hippocampus of a type which Penfield and his colleagues have attributed to incisural sclerosis. It is therefore still an open question whether, and how often, sclerosis of Ammon's horn and associated lesions precede or are secondary to severe major epileptic seizures.

SYMPTOMS

These can, for convenience, be divided into paroxysmal and interparoxysmal.

Paroxysmal

The clinical features depend on the site of origin and the spread of the cerebral disturbance.

Some epileptics become aware some hours or even days before a seizure occurs, that one is impending; they may feel that they are 'working up' to it; they are usually depressed, restless and irritable, have sensations of tension or fullness in the head, or experience muscular twitchings. This is a true warning of a seizure. Gowers, from the examination of more than 2000 cases of epilepsy, concluded that 57 per cent. of the cases had some kind of warning. The 'aura', sensory, motor, visceral or psychic, the common immediate precursor of major seizures, is not a true warning but is in fact the first few seconds of the seizure itself. In some cases the epileptic discharge consists of a sensory aura alone (sensory fit). There are numerous varieties of aura, depending on the locus of discharge. Probably the most common is a sinking feeling in the epigastrium. Vertigo is also common. There may be headache, diffuse or one-sided, or feelings of heat or cold, or numbness or tingling of a limb. The special senses may be involved, the aura being a hallucination, *e.g.* of taste or smell (in temporal lobe seizures). Visual phenomena (occipital lobe discharge) may be specks or lights in front of the eyes; or they may be elaborate hallucinations, which may be grotesque and reach always a certain stage of development at which the loss of consciousness occurs. Hallucinations of sound (temporal lobe discharge) are usually simple, such as humming, but may be elaborate, as music; they are most often associated with dizziness. Motor aurae may be sudden muscular twitches or complicated movements, such as running. A psychic aura may take the form of sudden disturbance in the use of words, or of obsessive thoughts, with irritability. It is of much importance in every case where there is an aura, to obtain from the patient a clear description of it, since this may assist the discovery of a focal lesion.

Grand Mal. The classic major epileptic attack, *grand mal*, consists of four stages. 1. The patient, falling to the ground with sudden and complete loss of consciousness, may injure himself. As he falls, there may be a cry. This is followed immediately by 2. the stage of tonic spasm, involving the entire body-musculature. In this stage, which lasts usually from ten to thirty seconds, respiration is arrested by spasm of the muscles of expiration and the muscles closing the glottis, so that cyanosis occurs and is sometimes extreme. The individual lies rigid, arms flexed, legs extended. This is followed by 3. the clonic stage, which may last for as long as three to four minutes and in which there is clonic jerking of the muscles which have hitherto been in tonic spasm. The jerking of the face muscles may cause the tongue or lips to be bitten. Froth often appears at the lips. Urine and faeces may be passed involuntarily. 4. There follows the stage of coma, during which the subject remains in a condition resembling sleep for a varying period of time, usually not more than an hour or two. In some patients the stage of coma is replaced or followed by a stage of (post-ictal) automatism.

During the seizure the plantar responses are extensor, the corneal reflexes absent. At first the pupils are usually small; then they dilate widely, and remain rigid until the attack ceases. Babinski's sign may be present for some hours. Usually there is no recurrence of the fit for some time, but occasionally fits succeed one another without intermission: this status epilepticus, if not treated, may go on to exhaustion and death. Major fits may be nocturnal or diurnal only, or occur at any time in the twenty-four hours. When the fits are nocturnal, suspicion of their presence may be aroused by the fact that the patient awakes in the morning feeling unduly tired, or because he finds that he has wet the bed, or that the bed-sheets have been torn.

After a fit, and recovery from the coma, the patient is usually transiently confused, and complains of headache and fatigue. In this phase of only partial consciousness and some bewilderment, he may perform acts which are semi-automatic: he may, for example, undress, or wander off, and if opposed may respond with violence. The automatic acts performed under these circumstances lack motive and no attempt is made at concealment.

After a major fit the patient's mental condition is usually temporarily improved —he is less irritable, and may even be unusually affable and pleasant for a time, in comparison often with his behaviour before the paroxysm.

Petit Mal. The typical seizure ('true *petit mal*') consists in a momentary loss of consciousness with which are associated few or no convulsive phenomena. There is no aura. The subject turns pale, suddenly becomes silent and halts in what he is doing, seems to stare blankly and may exhibit some slight twitching of his facial muscles. The attack is over in a few seconds, and he resumes his previous activity as if no interruption had occurred. He commonly also has other types of epileptic seizure.

The associated bilaterally synchronous wave-and-spike rhythm in the E.E.G. is very characteristic. On the analogy of an epileptic discharge occurring in a speech area which produces silence and not words, Penfield argues that an epileptic discharge at the 'highest level' of integration, *i.e.* consciousness, should also produce loss of function, in the form of a loss of consciousness such as occurs with a lesion of the diencephalon and in the electrical stimulation of this region, without evidence of loss of function in the cerebral hemispheres such as would be shown by an extensor plantar reflex. The conclusion suggested is that the focus of origin of the discharge in *petit mal* is probably in the diencephalon.

Related conditions include pyknolepsy and akinetic and myoclonic seizures. *Pyknolepsy* was first described by Friedmann in 1906 in a paper entitled 'Non-epileptic Absences or Short Epileptic Attacks'. Papers have been contributed also by Heilbronner and Adie. The attacks are of a uniform mildness, and consist in an inhibition of the higher mental processes, lasting from five to ten seconds: speech and voluntary movements cease, but automatic movements remain and consciousness may not be completely lost. The attacks begin suddenly in healthy children between the ages of 4 and 10 years, and may number 100 daily. After persisting for a number of years they may disappear entirely, and neither the physical nor mental development of the patient is in any way affected. The contrast between the prognosis in these cases and cases of ordinary epilepsy is remarkable. Akinetic seizures, sudden losses of muscle tone causing falling, and myoclonic seizures are also most commonly seen in children.

Psychomotor Seizures. Various other names have been given to this rather common group of seizures, in which psychological symptoms predominate— 'psychic epilepsy', 'psychic equivalents' or 'epileptic equivalents': but the term equivalent is particularly inappropriate, since the disturbance is indubitably an epileptic seizure. These psychomotor fits are episodic disturbances (not losses) of consciousness, usually without detectable convulsive phenomena, but commonly associated with automatic motor acts. The clouding of consciousness may last for seconds, minutes, hours or, exceptionally, days.

A typical form of psychomotor seizure is the so-called 'uncinate' fit, in which the focus of the epileptic discharge is in a temporal lobe. This variety of epilepsy was first described by Hughlings Jackson in 1888. In 1898 he and Colman published further details of the case of a medical man who, after death, was found to have a small patch of softening in the left uncinate gyrus. This patient's seizures were in the nature of 'dreamy states', during which he had vivid *déjà vu* experiences and a slight feeling of dread; he would act for a minute or two in a semi-purposive, confused way, and on occasion he smacked his tongue and moved his lower jaw; and afterwards he would behave apparently normally for a period for which he subsequently had amnesia. Further symptoms which may occur in this type of seizure are hallucinations of taste and smell, feelings of unfamiliarity or unreality, panoramic memory (in which the patient feels that he remembers forgotten stretches of his life) and forced thinking or 'crowding thoughts'.

In other psychomotor seizures the dream-like (twilight) state is more prolonged, and the disturbance of behaviour much more severe. In his clouded state the individual may be vividly hallucinated, auditorily or visually usually, and the affective change may be extreme, the patient experiencing intense fear, depression, rage or ecstasy. He may be immobile, dazed and retarded, or impelled to violent action. It is this state of epileptic ictal (seizure) automatism, and the clinically similar state of post-ictal automatism which may follow a *grand mal* fit, which are associated with the most gross acts of violence against others. These acts lack any conscious motive, the individual makes no attempt to cover his tracks and subsequently he has an amnesia for what he has done. Under these circumstances the epileptic is of course not legally responsible, and may be found insane. In other cases, during his seizure the individual wanders away in a fugue.

A differential diagnosis from hysteria must be made in many of these cases. There are symptomatic as well as aetiological differences. The epileptic fit exhibits a stereotyped uniformity on repetition, a relative simplicity as a rule, and a lack of adaptation to the immediate environment (*e.g.* a complete disregard for social conventions—as in indecent exposure) which are foreign to the hysterical attack.

The mechanism behind the hysterical fugue is not so much a release, in Hughlings Jackson's sense, as a dissociation of cortical activity—*i.e.* the activity of the attack can be of just as high an order as that of ordinary life. But the fundamental psychological distinction between co-ordinated epilepsy and a hysterical fugue is that in the latter a search for personal emotional factors will reveal adequate cause for the condition, which is then seen as purposive from the point of view of the patient's personality, whereas in epilepsy no such cause can usually be discovered. Some epileptic automatisms are however very complicated, and the diagnosis is particularly difficult if the epileptic fugue has occurred in the setting of some emotional crisis, when it may look like an hysterical (avoidance) phenomenon rather than an epileptic one. The diagnosis is also complicated by the fact that in a mainly psychogenic fugue one usually finds evidence of a temperamental instability, dependent often on a manic-depressive or epileptic inheritance (Stengel).

The individual who has psychomotor seizures commonly also has *grand mal* seizures.

Recent research has shown that in many cases psychomotor seizures are associated with an abnormality of one or both temporal lobes. This abnormality is manifest in the E.E.G., which shows a commencing disturbance in a focus in the anterior part of one or both temporal areas. The underlying lesion may be, *e.g.*, atrophic, a scar, angioma, cyst or tumour. It has been stated that about half the cases of temporal lobe epilepsy are associated with a personality disorder or a psychosis. Lundervold (quoted by Penfield and Jasper, 1954) investigated 112 patients suffering from temporal lobe epilepsy. In 75 per cent. the E.E.G. abnormality was unilateral, in the remainder bilateral. Forty-three patients showed mental or behavioural abnormality, which was more than twice as common in those with bitemporal E.E.G. abnormalities. '23 patients complained of poor memory; 19 showed some mental retardation; 12 presented behaviour problems; 11 were apathetic; 10 irritable; 10 over-impulsive; 7 emotionally unstable; 6 depressed; 4 stuttered; 3 were alcoholic; 2 paranoid and 1 manic. Three had been under psychiatric treatment.' Mulder and his colleagues (1954) have investigated the locus of the lesion in 100 cases of epilepsy with visceral symptoms in the fit (including aura): in 75 of 83 cases where the lesion could be found, it was in the temporal lobe.

There is thus a close relationship, but not an identity, between psychomotor seizures and temporal lobe discharges. They are notoriously difficult to treat satisfactorily with drugs: and control of the fits may be associated with a deterioration in the individual's behaviour.

CASE No. 54

A case which is of considerable medico-legal interest is that of a young man, 26 years old, who was convicted on a charge of murdering his mother, and also his nephew and niece, aged respectively 12 years and 2 years and 11 months, by cutting their throats with a razor. This crime was committed on the day on which he had been discharged from a general hospital where he had been a patient for seven months, during which time he had had a foot amputated. His history showed that ever since infancy he had a deformed leg, for which he had had considerable treatment. When quite a child he had been in a Home for crippled children, and while there he had caused trouble by turning younger children out of their cots, by reversing the pictures on the walls and so on. When about 16 years old he was a patient in a colony for mental defectives, but ran away. On one occasion, in his adolescence, he had attempted to commit suicide by throwing himself into the canal, from which he was rescued with great difficulty. During his adult life he had frequently been in trouble, and had served terms of imprisonment for assault and for theft. On one occasion he set the house on fire.

He stated that ever since the age of 14 years he had suffered from 'turns' of a peculiar nature, during which he felt strange. These 'turns' were accompanied by headache, and occasionally vomiting. After he lay down, the attack would gradually wear away, and he would feel better. In these attacks he was not completely conscious. During the seven months he had been in hospital previous to the commitment of his crime, he had two such attacks. In one of these the sister in charge of the ward stated that he had behaved in a strange way, tearing his bedclothes, and strewing cigarettes all round in great disorder. On another occasion, when on leave from the hospital, he was overcome by a feeling of dread, hurried home, asked his mother if he looked peculiar and, after having vomited, came to himself and realized that he had had a 'peculiar turn'. After the crime with which he was charged had been committed, he gave himself up to the police. He knew that something dreadful had happened, but he denied knowledge of the actual details. During the time he was in prison he behaved in a perfectly normal, rational way. His general intelligence was well up to the level of one of his social class.

His history indicated clearly that he was an unstable, irritable, impulsive man, who had been subject to peculiar episodes which he himself described as 'turns'. His physical deformity had no doubt helped to accentuate his character traits. It seemed reasonable to suggest, since the crime was committed without motive, and there was no attempt at concealment, that his condition was one of psychic epilepsy. The plea of epilepsy was not sustained in bar of trial, but his sentence was modified to one of penal servitude. In the course of a few months he made an unprovoked assault on a warder, was certified as insane and removed to a criminal asylum.

CASE No. 55

H. B. A patient, 39 years old, was admitted to the Glasgow Royal Mental Hospital in July 1922, with a history of having been ill since October 1921. His mother had died in a mental hospital. Two sisters had suffered from attacks of mental illness, from which they had made good recoveries. The patient himself was a nervous child, and a sleepwalker. He was clever at school, and after leaving, learned the trade of an engineer, at which he worked steadily. For three years during the war he acted as chief engine-room artificer.

His disposition was that of a sensitive, reserved man, inclined to be rather self-depreciatory.

He married in 1911 a woman who was twenty-one years older than himself.

In October 1921 he had a cycle accident, but escaped with a severe bruising. A fortnight later he told his wife that he had seen a bicycle accident: he seemed peculiar, and his wife went to get a doctor. He followed her to the doctor's surgery, and pulled her out of it. During that night he was in a very confused mental state. He attempted to throw his wife out of the bedroom window, burned a Bible and ill-treated a cat of which usually he had been very fond. He rushed from room to room shouting that the house was on fire, that he saw flames leaping up the bathroom walls. This period of confusion continued during the following day, and he stripped himself and sat naked on the kitchen floor for two hours.

He was admitted to a mental hospital, and there his condition was described as one of acute confusion. He was discharged in the course of four months as recovered. On one occasion while in that hospital he had been allowed to leave on probation. He visited his mother's grave, and for two days afterwards he was acutely depressed, and expressed delusions of sin. He was sure that he would go mad and die in a mental hospital as his mother had done.

He remained fairly well for a period of time, but then again became confused and excited, so much so that one night he ran about the house putting out the gas and lighting candles. He put his wife out of one room after another. He talked in an incoherent way, and he finally locked himself in a room and turned on the gas.

When admitted to this hospital his physical condition was carefully investigated. The results were entirely negative. His blood gave a negative Wassermann reaction, his cerebrospinal fluid was negative in all respects. His mental condition was characterized by recurrent periods of confusion. During such periods he seemed to have little idea of where he was or what he was doing. It was impossible to engage him in conversation. He wandered aimlessly about, picking up match-ends and pieces of paper, and anything that he could get his hands on. He would put such articles in his mouth and chew them, or would attempt to stuff them into his ears and nose. While in this condition he made several attempts to injure himself by suffocation and by strangulation. When interfered with, he became excited and violent, and was dangerous to other people. This peculiar state would pass off just as abruptly as it had started, and he would become perfectly clear and rational. He apparently had no recollection of having been in such a confused state, as he always asserted that he felt quite well, that he was normal and that there was no reason for his detention. Sometimes he had periods when he remained clear for several weeks on end, but at other times periods of confusion would recur regularly every day. His memory, his power of retention and his grasp on general knowledge were all well retained. His family undoubtedly had shown psychotic tendencies; the patient had been greatly attached to his mother; he had been a sleep-walker; his mother's death created a severe psychic trauma; his illness seemed to have an exacerbation following a visit to her grave; the only reason for his marrying a woman twenty-one years older than himself seemed to be that she was going to take the place of his mother rather than be a wife to him. We were inclined to look on this condition, even in the absence of any history of epileptic convulsions at any time, as in the nature of a psychic epilepsy.

CASE No. 56

G. H. A second case, very similar in many respects, was that of a man, aged 60 years, who was admitted to the Glasgow Royal Mental Hospital in March 1924, and was discharged in April 1924.

The patient had come from a healthy stock, and had developed normally. He was a master mariner. He tended to be of a rather jealous, suspicious temperament, and was touchy, sensitive and ambitious.

In June 1923, while abroad, he had a fall, due to a sudden loss of consciousness. He was unconscious for a minute or two, and then seemed quite himself. He was in hospital for a month, and then came home as a passenger. On the voyage home he communicated with his owners, asking permission to take charge of his own ship, but it was considered advisable for him to return home. Following his return in August 1923, his wife noticed that he had 'turns' of some kind. In the 'turns' which he had previous to October 1923 he would turn his eyes up, his limbs shook, but he did not fall. He did not himself seem to be completely conscious of these. During the six weeks previous to his admission to this hospital, it was noticed that he had 'turns' during which he became pale, complained of headache and was perturbed and in a state of great anxiety. On one occasion when the doctor was present he had such a turn, and during it he wished to kiss the doctor, and seemed to be quite unaware to whom he was speaking. He became much more irritable and jealous; he constantly recapitulated an incident when one of his owners had said to him that he had had many accidents, and he was inclined to feel that he had a grievance. On one occasion, while in one of these peculiar confused spells, he lifted a knife with the intention of striking his wife. His wife gradually became more and more frightened of him, because in his violent outbursts he was very threatening and dangerous to her.

Physically he was a big, deep-chested, well-nourished man. His blood pressure was 150–110. No abnormalities were detected in his nervous system. His blood Wassermann reaction was negative.

Following his admission, it was noted that there were short periods of time during which he became greatly confused. On one such occasion, observed by the medical officer, his face became flushed, his eyes were staring, he addressed the medical officer as 'dear' and apparently was quite unaware of his identity. In a few seconds this attack had passed off, and he talked to the point. These attacks occurred practically every day. Apart from them he was able to give an excellent account of himself, and his memory was good; he was inclined to be diffuse in his conversation, but there was no evidence of any intellectual disturbance.

Other Types of Seizure. Most seizures can be categorized as belonging to one or other of the three main types whose characteristics have been outlined above. This classification cannot, however, be claimed as entirely satisfactory, and it is certainly not comprehensive though it is useful enough in practice. There are various forms of motor and sensory seizures which we have not described, and brief comments only will be made here on a few symptom-complexes of some psychiatric importance.

Narcoleptic attacks, paroxysms of sleep, are commonly associated with cataplexy, paroxysmal attacks of loss of muscle tone often without loss of consciousness. Both types of attack tend to follow emotional excitement. The propriety of including narcolepsy in the category of the epilepsies is debated on the grounds that in epilepsy there is a spread of abnormal excitation in the central nervous system, while in narcolepsy there is apparently a spread of inhibition the aetiology and nature of which is in most cases unknown.

Rare and complicated fits, in which all the manifestations are autonomic, have been described by Penfield as *diencephalic autonomic seizures*. They are characterized by vasodilatation, lacrimation, sweating, salivation, pupillary alteration, slowing of pulse rate and respiration, and hiccoughing, and have been attributed to a disturbance originating in the diencephalon, on two grounds: namely, the discovery in such a syndrome of a tumour in this region, and the possibility of eliciting the same appearances by electrical stimulation of the diencephalon.

Such cases and other epileptic seizures accompanied by feelings of great dread may have been included by Gowers in the category of what he called 'vaso-vagal attacks'. It is, however, probable that the majority of the attacks which have been called vaso-vagal have not been epileptic, but acute anxiety attacks, determined by psychological causes, characterized by emotional and physical tension and vasomotor symptoms such as palpitation, pallor and sweating and accompanied by a feeling of impending death (*angor animi*). The term 'vaso-vagal attacks' is neither precise nor descriptively accurate, and might well be dropped.

The 'affect epilepsies' described by Bratz and Leubscher also appear to have been not epileptic seizures, but panic reactions of a primitive type produced by psychic situations; *e.g.* the so-called 'prison rage' which Kretschmer classified among his explosive, hypobulic reactions. A young man who suddenly realizes that the key is turned upon him in prison for a life-sentence may beat against the bars and rush aimlessly about, tearing his clothes. Hallucinations may occur in these attacks, and amnesia may follow, although consciousness is not entirely lost in them.

Interparoxysmal

Everything that has been described in association with the fits may appear in an individual who shows no detectable abnormality between the attacks. In those cases where a more persistent abnormality is present at the outset or develops later, the clinical features are usually described under the headings of the 'epileptic personality' and 'epileptic dementia'.

The Epileptic Personality. It has been held by some that there is a characteristic epileptic make-up in which the disorder called epilepsy develops. Thus certain traits have been described as constituting the 'epileptic character' or 'epileptic personality': rigidity and egocentricity; moodiness and irritability, with a proneness to explosive reactions of rage and resentment; pedantry, circumstantiality, argumentativeness and religiosity. The egocentricity is said to lead to shallow professions of interest in others, and to a selfish kind of religious devotion, so that 'they are considerate without being kind, and are religious without zeal, and . . . they will work for praise but not for love' (MacCurdy). Clearly these particular traits are not peculiar to epileptics: and while it is true that in a proportion of persons developing idiopathic epilepsy an unusual degree of egocentricity and sensitiveness can be demonstrated, it is certainly not usually possible to demonstrate this type of make-up.

Since these traits were most commonly observed in individuals who had been epileptic for some years, the epileptic character was for long looked upon as secondary to 'the disease', *i.e.* to the fits: and indeed it could in many ways be considered the result of comprehensible responses to the frustration, insecurity and social ostracism which so often has been the lot of the epileptic. It is now recognized that the epileptic character can sometimes be shown to have existed before the fits began; and evidence is accumulating that in many of these instances the personality traits have been the first evidence, the earliest symptoms of temporal lobe epilepsy. It is particularly in temporal lobe epilepsy (though not confined to it) that transitory disturbances, especially of mood, are frequent in the interparoxysmal period. The patient becomes excessively irritable, and picks quarrels with great facility. Assaults on bystanders occur in such a mood, with slight or no provocation, and sometimes on the basis of hallucinatory experiences, often with a religious colouring. Depression occasionally reaches such a pitch that suicide is attempted. Paranoid trends are common. In the episodic attacks on others the patient gives full rein to his primitive tendencies and may have an impulsive desire for sexual satisfaction, while he lacks any objective sexual interest.

Epileptic Deterioration and Dementia. This is a state of very gradual mental decline and enfeeblement found most often in those cases where the epilepsy has begun in childhood or at an early age and has been very severe, leading to institutional care becoming necessary. It is therefore encountered only in a small minority of epileptics, and particularly amongst those with frequent fits whose condition has not responded to treatment..

The affected individual becomes more self-centred as he loses interest in his environment. In the earlier stages this slump in interest may be interrupted by special efforts at arousing the epileptic's attention, but spontaneously he pays less and less regard to what is going on around him. Hence his mental content becomes very limited, and his memory poor both for recent and for remote events —for recent ones because passing events are not registered, and for remote events ultimately for the same reason, and also because, in the absence of interest, associative thinking is reduced to a minimum. The defect of remote memory is not so great as at first appears, since special effort at recollection often improves it remarkably. Some patients have insight for their memory defect, but others fabricate to fill the gaps. Related to the effort of recall in memory, there develops sooner or later in many cases a functional aphasia—words are brought up and used with increasing difficulty, while in extreme instances there is mutism. In contradistinction to organic aphasias, reading, writing and spelling may be surprisingly well done. Composition is rambling and pedantic. Speech and thinking become slower, and perseveration is sometimes present in excessive degree. Speech may lose its normal inflections—the so-called 'plateau speech' resulting.

Pari passu with this intellectual deterioration, which is secondary to the affective defect—the loss of interest—there occur other changes also directly referable to the increased egocentricity. The patient becomes more susceptible to flattery; he indulges more and more in boasting, the childishness of which is in direct proportion to the degree to which insight and judgement in general have deteriorated; his vanity increases, and yet his care of his personal appearance decreases; he becomes less amenable to discipline; and he is increasingly inactive and lazy. His interest becomes exclusively centred on his body (hypochondriasis).

In the final stage of epileptic dementia the patient leads a purely vegetative existence, reminiscent of the helpless infant, but displaying much less spontaneity. He has to be fed, clothed and cleaned, is unable to control his sphincters, does not utter a word and has a vacuous expression.

The cause of the cerebral damage which underlies this terminal state is not certainly known, but recurrent anoxia due to frequent fits or status epilepticus is probably an important factor. Deterioration of interests and habits may also be produced by prolonged, excessive medication with drugs. The milder early symptoms of deterioration may be organically determined, but they are not necessarily so. The epileptic may lose contact with his environment because it fails to stimulate or has rejected him: without a job or confined to an institution he may become oppressed by a settled hopelessness about his future, and his pessimistic inertia may then be misinterpreted as an organic deterioration in his behaviour due to his disease.

ELECTROENCEPHALOGRAPHY

The interpretation of E.E.G. tracings requires specialized training and knowledge, and no attempt will be made here to explore the complexities of the subject. Reference may be made to the texts by Hill and Parr (1950) and by Penfield and Jasper (1954). There are two main aspects of the examination: 1. assessment of the types of wave form, and their frequency, occurring during seizures and in the interparoxysmal period; and 2. their localization in the brain.

Gibbs, Gibbs and Lennox (1938) described the electrical discharges in the three main clinical types of epilepsy as follows: ' *Grand mal* is characterized by extreme acceleration of the electrical activity of the cortex, psychomotor attacks by extreme slowing of this activity, and *petit mal* by the alternation of fast and slow activity. With these disorders of frequency, there are associated abnormally high amplitudes.' Though these distinctions remain apparently generally valid, further work has shown that the identification of specific features in the E.E.G. with specific types of clinical seizure is not so simple. Of the three types of discharge described above, the 3 per second wave-and-spike form is the most distinctive; but though characteristic of *petit mal*, it is not confined to it and may be found during some psychomotor seizures. Psychomotor seizures may have other accompaniments, *e.g.* spike discharges or high-voltage slow waves from the temporal lobe. *Grand mal* seizures usually commence with paroxysmal 20 to 30 per second waves of abnormally high voltage.

The E.E.G. is usually only of confirmatory value in the diagnosis of epilepsy, and rarely does the E.E.G. record alone provide a reliable diagnosis. About 10 per cent. of the normal population show anomalies in their E.E.G. tracings, mild irregularities of unknown origin and debatable significance: while about 20 per cent. of epileptics are said to have normal tracings. This latter figure can be reduced somewhat if methods of eliciting seizures are employed (*e.g.* hyperventilation, barbiturate sleep, photic stimulation): but a remainder still show normal tracings, and a normal E.E.G. does not, therefore, rule out the diagnosis of epilepsy.

An unequivocally epileptic type of record will clinch a clinical diagnosis of epilepsy, and assist the differential diagnosis in cases of supposedly hysterical attacks and other episodic disturbances of consciousness. Some so-called faints and some fugues are revealed as epileptic by the E.E.G.

E.E.G. records are of particular value in assisting the localization of acquired cerebral lesions in cases of symptomatic epilepsy.

COURSE AND PROGNOSIS

The prognosis depends considerably on the stage at which the patient seeks treatment, and of course on the efficacy of the treatment he receives. If treatment is begun early there is considerable hope that the fits may at least be made very infrequent, if they are not stopped altogether. Fits may disappear for a long period of time, and sometimes cease entirely.

2 F

The great majority of epileptics never display mental symptoms; and amongst those who do, many never require institutional care and remain at their occupations throughout their lives. Mental deterioration is more common and more severe in symptomatic epilepsy following brain injuries than in idiopathic epilepsy, and is more commonly associated with psychomotor than with other types of seizure (Lennox, 1942). It is only a very small minority of epileptics who have to be admitted to mental hospitals, and the average course in these cases is steadily downhill.

DIAGNOSIS

One must determine first if the patient's symptoms are due to epilepsy: and, if they are, the cause of the epilepsy must then be sought.

Epilepsy is characterized by a set of phenomena which in most cases differentiate it clearly from hysteria—the onset in many cases in early childhood, the tonic and clonic succession in the convulsion, the unconsciousness and the other symptoms of the *grand mal* attacks (often nocturnal, the sphincter incontinence, Babinski's sign) are characteristic. Other typical features are the occurrence of the attack when the patient is alone, or in a position of danger (*e.g.* on a bicycle or driving a car), actual self-injury in the fall, the performance of some stereotyped action, drowsiness, headache and prolonged sleep afterwards. Hysterical fits are diurnal, there is always an audience, and if attempts are made to restrain the patient he responds with wild struggling: self-injury is unusual. Other hysterical symptoms may resemble epilepsy—hysterical amnesias and disturbances of consciousness, including fugues, stupors and so-called twilight states. The attack is not often seen by the physician and he has to rely much on the history obtained from the patient and from his relatives, on witnesses' descriptions of the attacks, on an assessment of the individual's make-up and recent circumstances, and on the results of both mental and physical examinations (including the E.E.G.). The typical hysterical personality differs considerably from that of the epileptic, but the latter is often not demonstrable. A history of mental stress immediately preceding the first attack is not necessarily in favour of hysteria, since epileptic seizures can also be precipitated by obvious psychological causes. In any instances where there is doubt, prolonged observation is desirable. When the description of the attack is not typical of major epilepsy or of *petit mal*, it is a good working rule to accept nothing as idiopathic epilepsy until a very thorough search has been made for psychological and for physical causes.

Where automatic acts follow an obvious seizure (are post-ictal, in Penfield's terminology) as a release phenomenon, the diagnosis is much easier than in the instances where the automatic acts are the seizure (ictal automatisms). When an epileptic clouded state is prolonged, the condition may be described as an epileptic psychosis, and may be mistaken for schizophrenia. The diagnosis may be for some time in doubt, and then revealed by the re-establishment of clear consciousness, without evidence of residual schizophrenic disorder. The occurrence of major seizures may also clarify the situation.

There is a close clinical resemblance between certain cases with psychomotor epilepsy and certain aggressive psychopathic states. In both conditions there occur explosions of disturbed behaviour, which may come suddenly or be prefaced by a period of increasing tension and irritability; which may be precipitated by emotional frustration, alcoholism or fatigue; and which may be accompanied by some clouding of consciousness and followed by a rapid recovery of equilibrium. The differential diagnosis often depends on the E.E.G. findings.

Some cases of migraine resemble epilepsy in having a well-marked sensory aura with a slow and distinctive 'march', *e.g.* from the finger up the arm; but the aura is much more prolonged than in epilepsy, and there is usually no consequent loss of consciousness.

When the diagnosis is in doubt, it is sometimes possible to induce a seizure for the purpose of immediate inspection, by voluntary over-breathing. In two or three minutes afterwards in some cases, the epileptic attack occurs, instead of the tetany which would occur in the non-epileptic person in the same circumstances. Other ways of inducing epileptic activity have been mentioned in the discussion of electroencephalography.

When a diagnosis of epilepsy has been established, the cause of the epilepsy must be sought: at least, it must be determined whether or not it is symptomatic. A careful general physical examination is as necessary in every case as a meticulous clinical examination of the nervous system. Where there is any doubt the blood Wassermann reaction, lumbar puncture, skull X-rays and E.E.G. must be carried out. Epilepsy occurring for the first time after the age of 30 years should be assumed to be symptomatic, until this has been disproved. Epilepsy in adult life is commonly associated with brain tumour, general paralysis, and cerebral arteriosclerosis, and there are many other causes, both general and local (cerebral). Advances in brain surgery make the early diagnosis of focal brain lesions a major responsibility for the clinician.

TREATMENT

The epileptic should not have his life made dull and miserable by unnecessary restrictions. The great majority of epileptics are capable of living normal lives with the exception of driving motor-cars and the like, swimming in deep water, or indulging in any other occupation or recreation in which a fit would definitely endanger the lives of others or of themselves. The mortality of epileptics from accidents arising during fits is, in fact, exceedingly small. Wherever possible the epileptic should be gainfully employed: but excessive fatigue should be avoided since it tends to precipitate fits. The more stable, the less frustrating, the individual's emotional environment, the better.

Attention to the individual's general physical health and hygiene are important. Physical disease, major and minor, should, of course, be promptly treated: and Lennox and Cobb have drawn attention to the need for eliminating any nasal obstruction. Meals should be regular. Bowels should be kept open. Alcohol should not be taken in any circumstances.

Since we know little as yet about the hereditary transmission of epilepsy, it is difficult to give satisfactory advice about marriage. The hereditary factor is of considerably more significance in idiopathic than in symptomatic cases. From the eugenic point of view it is evident that one epileptic should not marry another; and it is probable that an epileptic should not marry an individual who has an abnormal E.E.G. The presence or absence of a positive family history is also important on both sides. Each case must be considered on its merits, and present evidence indicates that one is not justified in most cases in being too rigorous in prohibition of marriage and child-bearing.

The chief indications for the treatment of an epileptic in an institution (colony or mental hospital) are pronounced irritability, or frequent and prolonged psychomotor seizures, tending to violent assaults; and general mental deterioration. The settled régime of an institution is in itself helpful—the sources of irritation are lessened, meals, etc., are regular, and the patient is among people who are accustomed to dealing with epileptics. It is of particular importance that the epileptic in a clouded state should not be treated in an arbitrary, excited or aggressive way: he will only respond with greater violence to such clumsy handling. Further, in an institution suitable outlets can easily be provided for the development of the epileptic's interests, and this retards the progress of deterioration as well as lessening the frequency of the fits. Occupation should be a main part of the treatment from the beginning.

The drugs which have been tried are legion, and year by year more, and more effective, anticonvulsants are becoming available. Whatever drug is used the doses should be arranged so that a maximum saturation with the drug will be produced during the hours at which the fits most regularly occur; for example, if the fits occur during the night, the patient should have the largest dose in the evening. Often anticonvulsant treatment has to be continued for life: it should certainly be maintained until the individual has been without fits for at least three years. Sudden cessation of anticonvulsant treatment must always be avoided, since status epilepticus may be precipitated and the individual's life thus be put in danger.

Phenobarbitone (*Luminal*) has now replaced bromide as the sheet anchor of treatment in the average case, and especially when the seizures are *grand mal* in type. The commencing dose should be ½ gr. twice a day. If control of the fits is not obtained with 2 to 3 gr. phenobarbitone daily, a combination of a smaller dose of phenobarbitone with one of the hydantoins should be tried.

The most commonly used of the hydantoins is sodium diphenylhydantoin (phenytoin sodium, B.P., *Epanutin*): 3 gr. daily may be given initially and the dose raised gradually as required to 7½ gr. daily or until intolerance develops. Toxic symptoms are fairly frequent in the skin, gastro-intestinal tract and nervous system: namely, skin rashes, anorexia, indigestion, nystagmus, ataxia, and (if dosage is prolonged, in some cases) hypertrophic gingivitis and hirsutism.

Primidone (*Mysoline*) is also a valuable anticonvulsant: 0·5 to 1·5 G. may be given daily in tablet form. Toxic effects, commonly drowsiness and ataxia, are usually mild and transient. This drug is of particular value in cases with *grand mal* attacks, but it appears that psychomotor seizures may also be diminished.

Petit mal seizures usually respond to trimethyloxazolidine dione (*Tridione*). An initial dose of 0·3 G. thrice daily may be raised to 2 G. daily. Toxic effects include rashes, nausea, visual glare and agranulocytosis. The latter, most serious complication is better guarded against by warning the patient to cease taking the drug immediately if he develops fever, malaise and a sore throat, than by carrying out routine blood counts at monthly intervals.

When satisfactory control has not been gained by the use of the above drugs, alone or in various combinations, and in cases where there have been toxic or allergic reactions to these drugs, bromides should be tried. Potassium bromide may be given in a commencing dose of 15 gr. twice daily and the dose increased up to 100 gr. in twenty-four hours. Acneiform rashes and mental dulling, which may develop into a delirious reaction if the blood bromide passes a figure around 150 mg. per cent., limit the usefulness of this drug, which is probably most effective in cases with *grand mal*.

Psychomotor seizures are the most difficult fits to control with drugs. The patient should if possible be coaxed to go to bed: and if he is violent thiopentone, B.P., or amylobarbitone sodium, B.P.C., may be given intravenously. A prolonged clouded or twilight state may be interrupted by inducing a major fit electrically (E.C.T.).

Status epilepticus always endangers life and must be treated urgently. The series of convulsions can usually be interrupted successfully by giving 3 gr. sodium phenobarbitone, B.P., intramuscularly, or 5 to 10 ml. sterile paraldehyde intramuscularly, or $7\frac{1}{2}$ gr. amylobarbitone sodium intravenously. Further injections of sodium phenobarbitone, B.P.C., or paraldehyde may be required if there is relapse.

To all these drugs the individual response varies, and to a large extent the physician must proceed by trial and error until he finds the most suitable drug or combination of drugs. Furthermore, it must always be remembered that drug treatment is symptomatic treatment only. In every case, if it is possible, one should of course seek to attack the cause rather than the symptom.

The appropriate treatment of cases of symptomatic epilepsy depends, of course, on the nature of the causal disease. The discovery and surgical treatment of focal brain lesions has of recent years assumed an increasing importance in this field, and Penfield and his colleagues have pioneered the operation of temporal lobectomy for the treatment of temporal lobe epilepsy. In most of his cases Penfield removed the anterior part of a temporal lobe only when there was a demonstrable macroscopic lesion: others have operated on the basis of symptoms and E.E.G. findings alone. The short-term results have been promising, but it is too early yet to state the indications for and pros and cons of this radical treatment. Detailed information may be obtained from Penfield and Jasper's textbook and from an article by Murray Falconer and his London colleagues (1955).

REFERENCES

Ascroft, P. B. (1941) *Brit. med. J.*, **1**, 739.
Conrad, K. (1935) *Z. ges. Neurol. Psychiat.*, **153**, 271.
Falconer, M., Meyer, A., Hill, D., and Mitchell, W. (1955) *Lancet*, i, 827.
Gibbs, F. A., Gibbs, E. L., and Lennox, W. G. (1938) *Arch. Neurol. Psychiat.* *(Chicago)*, **39**, 298.
Hill, D., and Parr, G. (1950) *Electro-encephalography*, London.
Lennox, W. G., Gibbs, E. L., and Gibbs, F. A. (1940) *Arch. Neurol. Psychiat. (Chicago)*, **44**, 1155.
Lennox, W. G. (1942) *Amer. J. Psychiat.*, **99**, 174.
Lennox, W. G. (1951) *J. Amer. med. Ass.*, **146**, 529.
Lennox, W. G., and Jolly, D. H. (1954) *Res. Publ. Ass. nerv. ment. Dis.*, **33**, 325.
Meyer, A., Falconer, M. A., and Beck, E. (1954) *J. Neurol. Neurosurg. Psychiat.*, **17**, 276.
Meyer, A., Beck, E., and Shepherd, M. (1955) *J. Neurol. Neurosurg. Psychiat.*, **18**, 24.
Mulder, D. W., Daly, B., and Bailey, A. A. (1954) *Arch. intern. Med.*, **93**, 481.
Penfield, W., and Baldwin, M. (1952) *Ann. Surg.*, **136**, 625.
Penfield, W., and Jasper, H. (1954) *Epilepsy and the Functional Anatomy of the Human Brain*, Boston.
Phillips, G. (1954) *J. Neurol. Neurosurg. Psychiat.*, **17**, 1.
Rosanoff, J. A., Handy, L. M., and Rosanoff, I. A. (1934) *Arch. Neurol. Psychiat. (Chicago)*, **31**, 1165.

17

SUBNORMALITY AND SEVERE SUBNORMALITY (MENTAL DEFECT)[1]

In the Mental Health Act, 1959, 'mental defect' has been renamed 'subnormality' and conditions of arrested or incomplete development of mind have been divided into two newly designated groups, the 'subnormal' and the 'severely subnormal'. The subnormal group corresponds to what was previously termed 'feeble-mindedness' or high-grade mental defect. The severely subnormal group includes those who were previously named 'idiots' and 'imbeciles', and replaces the category of low-grade mental defect. The main distinction still lies between the slighter degrees of mental subnormality manifest by the dullest members of the general population, and the more gross syndromes often associated with the stigmata of frank physical abnormalities, which render the affected individuals childishly or helplessly dependent on others.

The Mental Health Act's definitions are as follows: '"Severe subnormality" means a state of arrested or incomplete development of mind which includes subnormality of intelligence and is of such a nature or degree that the patient is incapable of living an independent life or of guarding himself against serious exploitation, or will be so incapable when of an age to do so.'

'"Subnormality" means a state of arrested or incomplete development of mind (not amounting to severe subnormality) which includes subnormality of intelligence and is of a nature or degree which requires or is susceptible to medical treatment or other special care or training of the patient.'

With regard to the phrasing of these new legal definitions, it may be pointed out that the term subnormal is clearly more applicable to those cases which border the normal, and it is difficult to see why care, training and medical treatment should be mentioned in relation to only one of the two main categories of subnormality. It may also be objected that these new definitions are for clinical purposes rather lacking in specification.

The use of the terms subnormality and severe subnormality should be confined to those cases in which there is clear evidence of intellectual defect. Emotional instability, with or without social maladjustment or antisocial trends, may complicate the clinical picture, being either products of the same physical causes as have determined the intellectual defect or secondary developments, traits acquired by a limited individual in failing to come to acceptable terms with his environment. The diagnosis of intellectual subnormality can of course be made without the use of intelligence tests, but it must be able to stand up to and be confirmed by detailed testing. For medical purposes intelligence may be taken to mean the

[1] In the Mental Health (Scotland) Act, 1960, the term mental deficiency is retained, but the terms idiot, imbecile and feeble-minded are abandoned. The category of Mental Deficiency in Scotland comprises Subnormality and Severe Subnormality.

ability to understand one's environment and to make use of one's understanding to earn a living or manage a home. The individual's social failure may be so gross, childish and persistent that the diagnosis is never in doubt. In other cases, where the subnormality is of slight degree and particularly where emotional instability is in the foreground or neurological defects disturb the individual's performance, detailed psychological testing is necessary to determine accurately the patient's intellectual resources. In general, mental testing in cases of subnormality is of more importance in helping to gauge what the individual may be capable of and in pin-pointing special disabilities in the mental sphere, than in coming to the diagnosis itself. What the individual can achieve as a social being is of greater importance than his test scores.

Subnormality is most conspicuous during the school age period, when the individual's intellectual performance first comes under really close scrutiny. Technical difficulties in the accurate measurement of mental abilities, differing views of what should be considered a state of subnormality, and the considerable problems involved in making a full tally of the cases in any community, have made the prevalence of subnormality a matter of some dispute. In Great Britain probably a little less than one per cent. of the population are mentally subnormal. Lewis in a most painstaking and accurate investigation of a population of 600,000 individuals in England and Wales in 1929, reached the figure of 0·86 per cent. He found, as have others, that the incidence was considerably higher in rural than in urban areas. Similar results were obtained in Baltimore in 1942 by Lemkau and his colleagues, and have been reported from Scandinavia. In all these countries subnormality preponderates over severe subnormality. In England and Wales in 1957 there were approximately 126,000 ascertained subnormal individuals.

'Moral defectiveness' and 'moral imbecility' are terms which have been applied to individuals who have shown antisocial conduct from an early age. They should not be perpetuated since classifications arrived at by moral judgements, which tend to be subjective, relative and changeable, cannot be securely translated into medical categories. If the delinquent individual is intellectually defective, we class him as a case of subnormality: if he is not intellectually defective, he may be suffering from a psychopathic state [see Chapter 13].

In Britain 'amentia' has been a synonym for subnormality. In drawing a distinction between amentia and dementia, Esquirol said, 'The demented man is deprived of the good that he formerly enjoyed: he is a rich man become poor. The ament has always lived in misfortune and poverty.' In other words, the ament lacks something, while the dement suffers from a disorder of that which he possesses. In Europe the term amentia has been applied to confusional states on a toxic-infective basis. Where there is risk of muddle, the term is best avoided: it is anyway *de trop*.

THE AETIOLOGY OF SUBNORMALITY

This is complex, varies very much from case to case and is probably often multiple, an admixture of genetic and environmental factors. In our present state of knowledge the aetiology in the majority of individual cases cannot be ascertained. This ignorance challenges us and points to the necessity for far more research than has so far been done in this field of medicine, where there has been often too fatalistic an acceptance of the facts of disability and too little curiosity about their antecedents.

There are broad and important differences between subnormality and severe subnormality. In the former there is usually a familial concentration of cases; in the latter much less markedly and infrequently so, and usually only in the proportions which might be expected from single-gene inheritance. The subnormal group, which cannot be sharply distinguished from the general population, have also been called the 'sub-cultural' and 'aclinical'. Most of the severely subnormal group suffer from clearly pathological syndromes, and have considerably damaged brains.

Probably at least three-quarters of the subnormal belong essentially to the normal population, though they are the dullest members of that population. Intelligence in the general population shows a normal or Gaussian distribution, a smooth bell-shaped curve: the subnormal constitute the lower end of this curve, down to about I.Q. 50. This quantitative variation of intelligence is largely genetically determined, it is thought, by numerous genes (polygenes) of small individual effect. Many of the parents and relatives of these subnormal individuals are themselves mentally dull or subnormal: about one-quarter of their siblings are said to be so. In the aetiology of these familial cases of subnormality it should be noted that adverse environments, which are very common, also play a part. The mentally poorly endowed tend to provide for their children not only a defective genetic inheritance, but also an environment which is neither intellectually stimulating nor educative: the term 'sub-cultural' could be applied as well to their homes as to their intelligence.

A significant number of cases of subnormality, perhaps as many as one-quarter of the total, are due to pathological causes, either genetic or environmental. This is also the situation with nearly all the cases of severe subnormality; the possible exceptions here occurring at the borderland between severe subnormality and subnormality.

For purposes of description it is convenient to distinguish between genetic (intrinsic) and environmental (extrinsic) aetiological factors, but we should not be misled into thinking that they are separated in nature. Though the genetic factors are present at conception, it is also important to recognize that their presence may not be obvious at birth: in every child, subnormal as well as normal, genetic and environmental factors continue to interact to produce the characteristics and complexity of the developing personality.

Both polygene (as explained above) and single-gene inheritance occur in the aetiology of subnormality, the former in the subnormal cases, the latter mainly in the severely subnormal. Syndromes due to dominant and recessive (single gene) types of inheritance will be described: and the recently discovered associations between subnormality and chromosome abnormalities.

The environmental factors producing mental subnormality are numerous, distributed in time from conception through the intra-uterine period of gestation, and continuing past birth and infancy to childhood itself. The clinical outcome depends not only on the nature and location of the injury to the brain, but also significantly on the time and period of development at which the injury is done.

Amongst the environmental factors acting during the intra-uterine period, which may cause mental subnormality, maternal infections are important: particularly rubella, syphilis and (much less commonly) toxoplasmosis. Radiation of the mother may also do profound damage to the developing embryo, causing microcephaly. Eclampsia and dietary deficiencies in the mother may possibly cause subnormality. Other traumata to the mother, physical and possibly psychological, may be considered speculatively.

At the time of birth, traumata due to obstetrical complications which may do most damage by causing intracranial haemorrhage and asphyxia, are important causes of subnormality as they are of cerebral palsy. The premature infant is especially at risk. The dangers also in these cases of giving oxygen in excess, and of thus producing retrolental fibroplasia (fibroplastic overgrowth of vascular tissue in the eyes) and possibly also serious brain damage, are now well recognized.

After birth, hazards of course continue to crop up but they are different. Severe neonatal jaundice with kernicterus may cause subnormality as well as other serious permanent neurological damage. Some endocrine disorders, which may have had their origins at an earlier time, become important aetiologically, notably hypothyroidism. An attack of encephalitis lethargica, or one of the other encephalitides (complicating, for example, measles or mumps), may so permanently damage the brain that the child becomes subnormal: so may a meningitis, tuberculous or septic. Lead poisoning is the classical instance of a metallic poisoning of aetiological importance in this field. Head injury is much more often claimed by parents to be the cause of a child's subnormality than the facts warrant, and in infancy and childhood is probably an uncommon cause.

THE DEGREES AND SYMPTOMS OF SUBNORMALITY

Severe Subnormality

This category spans a wide range of mental incapacity, extending from those who cannot guard themselves even against common physical dangers to those who, though capable of a certain amount of constructive work, are yet unable to earn a living independently. These intellectually very limited individuals do not at best have an I.Q. of more than about 49, or a mental age of more than 7 years. They number about one-quarter of the whole subnormal population.

At its most severe, severe subnormality represents the lowest form of mental development and is readily recognizable from a very early age. Physical deformities, paralyses and fits are very common. The affected individuals can do almost nothing for themselves. Their incapacity ranges from bedridden helplessness, to walking imperfectly and speaking a few monosyllables. If the child can feed himself, it is only clumsily: he cannot care for himself in the way of washing, dressing or keeping himself clean. His incontinence is a major problem in his nursing care. Most of these cripples die before reaching adult life.

The least disabled in this category can do a simple routine job, and simple tasks and cleanliness can be expected of the majority of those whose I.Q. ranges from 20 to 49. Some learn to write and read a few monosyllabic words, but further scholastic attainments are beyond them. Neurological defects and other physical stigmata are common, and they are characteristically ungainly. Often suggestible and easily exploited, they cannot manage their own affairs or be taught to do so. Their life span is below average.

Subnormality

Those who fall into this group do not usually exhibit the physical stigmata or the evidence of brain damage which are so common amongst the severely subnormal. In scholastic attainments they may not be any worse than the more poorly educated type of constitutionally normal child: and a considerable proportion of those who are educationally subnormal prove capable of supporting themselves socially on leaving school. Indeed, in routine and menial jobs they often prove industrious workers and as stable citizens as their fellows. But more often than is the case with the population of average intelligence, the subnormal are unstable in their aims and occupations, impulsive and lacking in common sense. This instability may be revealed in a poor work record, criminality or sexual promiscuity. Those amongst them that become criminal are responsible for many petty offences and indiscriminate violence: some, too readily suggestible, become the dupes of more practised criminals. The unstable subnormal woman may become illegitimately pregnant or drift into prostitution: as a mother she is usually incompetent and as a housewife slatternly. But it must be emphasized that gross social failure is the fate of only the minority of the subnormal.

The subnormal child cannot derive benefit from instruction in ordinary schools and requires special educational care and training.

The subnormal constitute about three-quarters of the whole defective population. Their I.Q.s range from about 50 to 69, their mental ages from 8 to 11 years.

SOME PHYSICAL ABNORMALITIES COMMONLY ACCOMPANYING SUBNORMALITY

Many different varieties of nervous system lesion, of cerebral developmental malformations, and of congenital abnormalities in other systems of the body are found in the subnormal, and naturally most frequently in those who are severely subnormal. The severely subnormal have usually, in fact, a constitution defective in many respects. Impairment of vision and hearing, aphasia of various types and specific reading disabilities may all complicate subnormality: and these disabilities, in the normal child, may occasionally lead to a misdiagnosis of subnormality. No attempt will be made here to give a comprehensive account of all the pathological conditions which may occur, but a brief review will be made of the commoner and more important varieties.

Cerebral Palsy

This is a relatively common condition, occurring in 1 to 2 per thousand of the school population. It is frequently associated with some degree of subnormality, and particularly with severe subnormality. Kirman (1956) reported that in the Fountain Hospital, which cares mostly for severely subnormal cases, 23 per cent. of the patients were affected.

The physical symptoms range from clumsiness and speech difficulties to such severe motor involvement that the child is helpless. Various clinical types and admixtures of types occur: they include spastic diplegia, hemiplegia, choreo-athetosis and ataxia, the first of these being the commonest. Epilepsy is a common accompaniment of cerebral palsy and is said to be found in as many as half the hemiplegic cases.

Many varieties of pathological damage and aberrant brain development produce cerebral palsy. Some forms of spastic diplegia are inherited as recessive defects: damage early in intra-uterine life may lead to atrophy of both cerebral hemispheres: porencephaly, hemiatrophy or microgyria may result in hemiplegia: haemorrhage and asphyxia at birth are well-recognized causes: and in a much smaller number of cases the damage is sustained in early childhood. Cerebellar atrophy may be found in the ataxic varieties, and the commonest antecedent of choreo-athetosis is kernicterus with its lesions in the basal ganglia.

Epilepsy

Epilepsy is not a cause of subnormality but a symptom which commonly accompanies it, and which may be an expression of the same pathology as has determined the mental retardation. Both idiopathic and symptomatic types occur. In the former group genetic factors are important: in the latter some structural or metabolic abnormality disturbs brain function, and understandably epilepsy is most common in cases of severe subnormality with neurological deficits. Epilepsy is, for example, frequently associated with cerebral palsy. 10 to 15 per cent. of the subnormal in institutions are epileptic. All types of seizure are manifest—*grand mal*, *petit mal*, psychomotor and myoclonic.

Epileptic fits may aggravate a child's mental backwardness by interfering with his schooling: so may the dulling effect of anticonvulsant drugs, particularly if these are prescribed in excess.

Microcephaly

Microcephalic is a descriptive term for those subnormal individuals who have abnormally small heads. Microcephaly is not a clinical nor a pathological nor an aetiological entity: primary (genetic) cannot be separated from secondary (environmental) types. In a recent comprehensive and valuable review of the topic Brandon and his colleagues (1959) have proposed that microcephaly should be defined as 'cases with a cranial circumference smaller than three standard deviations below the mean for the age and sex'. Fairly satisfactory norms are available.

Microcephaly is found in about one-fifth of the severely subnormal. The individual's skull is characteristically dolichocephalic, *i.e.* the breadth of the skull is less than four-fifths of the length: and the vertical measurements are also much reduced. In the most severe cases the microcephalic's appearance is most odd and bird-like. The forehead and chin are sharply receding, the nose appears like a beak, and the ears are out of proportion. The scalp may lie loosely, in longitudinal furrows.

The brain in these cases is also abnormally small, and light, and many other abnormalities of brain structure are common, *e.g.* microgyria, porencephaly. Other gross physical defects are frequent: dwarfism, cerebral palsy, epilepsy, cardiac and ophthalmic lesions: and the prognosis for life depends not only on the development of the brain but also largely on these other defects. Microcephalics tend to die earlier than those with larger heads. About one-third of mongols are microcephalic: so also are many phenylketonurics.

The degree of subnormality is as variable as the size of the head, and is not directly correlated with head size. The majority of microcephalics are severely subnormal. There is no characteristic temperamental type.

The aetiology is very various. Familial cases occur, and the risk of a sib being affected was estimated by Brandon from his series to be 6 per cent. Cases due to single gene (recessive) inheritance are probably very much in the minority, and not clearly separable from those of different aetiology. Traumatic environmental factors probably operate most commonly early in intra-uterine life: only two of these extrinsic factors so far are known—irradiation of the mother during pregnancy, and maternal rubella.

Hydrocephalus

This is a common finding in cases of subnormality, especially among the severely subnormal: like microcephaly, it is not a disease entity but a symptom of various pathologies. Its immediate cause is a disturbance of the formation, circulation or absorption of cerebrospinal fluid. In the congenital cases obstruction is the commonest cause, in the Sylvian aqueduct or at the foramina of Magendie and Luschka or elsewhere in the circulation pathway; and the abnormality of structure probably originates in the first three months of intra-uterine life. Obstetrical difficulties are likely then to be produced by the over-large head and such children may die during birth. In most congenital cases the subnormality is severe and other physical abnormalities are common: the hydrocephalus, for example, may be associated with spina bifida and lumbosacral meningocele. In infancy a meningitis, especially of the meningococcal variety, may produce hydrocephalus. Later causes such as tuberculous meningitis may lead to hydrocephalus without gross enlargement of the head.

In severe early cases the head becomes enormous, globular, the forehead bulging, the veins of the scalp visibly congested, the eyes pushed forward and downwards: cranial circumferences of 25 to 30 inches have been recorded. The cerebrospinal fluid pressure is increased, the ventricles are greatly dilated, the cortex stretched, thinned and deformed, and the skull itself may become very thin, with gaping sutures and greatly enlarged fontanelles. The inadequately protected brain is of course also vulnerable to external trauma: and the large head itself incapacitates the child, unbalancing it. Not only subnormality usually results: blindness, epilepsy and paralyses are common, and deafness only less so.

Hydrocephalus may be rapidly progressive, producing early death: or it may be self-arrested at any stage. The various surgical operations which have been devised to alleviate it have been of limited value.

Much more rarely, an abnormally large head in a subnormal individual may be due to megalencephaly or Paget's disease of the skull.

INHERITED SYNDROMES

Cases of single gene inheritance, dominant and recessive, are rare. There is greater variability of the clinical picture in the case of the dominant defects. Both dominant and recessive syndromes are associated usually with severe subnormality.

Dominant Syndromes

Tuberous Sclerosis (Epiloia). Tuberous sclerosis is inherited as a dominant, and sporadic cases seem to be evidence of a rather high mutation rate. Its incidence is probably about the same as that of phenylketonuria; that is, about 1 in 30,000 of the population (England and Wales). Incomplete forms of the syndrome occur, and it is found associated with all degrees of subnormality; occasionally even with mental normality. The pathological lesions are numerous. Most characteristic is the adenoma sebaceum—a brownish red, acneiform rash in a butterfly distribution on the cheeks and adjoining parts of the face, which develops usually about the time the child reaches school age.

In the brain there are multiple gliotic nodules with giant cells (tuberous sclerosis), which may become calcified and demonstrable radiologically. Similarly benign tumours occur in many other organs, including the retina (phakomata), heart (rhabdomyomata) and kidneys (hamartomata). All these tumours are prone to become malignant.

The affected individual is usually epileptic, his mental condition commonly deteriorates, and he has a reduced expectancy of life.

Neurofibromatosis (von Recklinghausen's disease). This is another syndrome probably due to an irregularly dominant gene, which has similarities to tuberous sclerosis, and may be related. It is less common and it is not necessarily associated with subnormality. At least 10 per cent. of the cases are, however, subnormal. Skin lesions of two types are seen—*café au lait* patches of pigmentation, and subcutaneous neurofibromata. As in tuberous sclerosis, tumours of the retina (phakomata) also occur.

Naevoid Amentia (Sturge-Weber syndrome). Naevoid amentia occurs in families and is thought to be a dominant defect. It is characterized by the concurrence of subnormality and angiomatous developments. Typically there is a large port-wine coloured naevus on one side of the face in the distribution of the trigeminal nerve, and an intracranial haemangioma on the same side which may become calcified. The affected individual is usually both severely subnormal and epileptic: he may also have a hemiplegia on the side opposite to the intracranial angioma.

Von Hippel-Lindau's Disease. This shows a similar association of subnormality and naevi.

Recessive Syndromes

Clear-cut syndromes are to be found in this group of the subnormal. A single gene appears typically in these syndromes to produce its effect by dislocating an enzyme system (an enzyme normally present may be absent): an 'inborn error of metabolism' results.

Examples of the following types of metabolic disorder will be briefly described: disorders of amino acid metabolism—phenylketonuria and hepatolenticular degeneration: disorders of carbohydrate metabolism—galactosaemia and von Gierke's disease: and disorders of lipoid metabolism—amaurotic idiocy, Niemann-Pick's disease, and gargoylism. Already more than two dozen familial metabolic disorders associated with mental retardation have been described, and doubtless many others await discovery.

It is with the study of the biochemical abnormalities manifest in some of these cases that a new era in psychiatric genetics opened. Though the group is still a small one numerically, we are reaching with them such a fundamental understanding of the pathological mechanisms underlying the mental retardation that rational control and treatment are becoming possible. The paradigm is phenylketonuria.

Phenylketonuria. This condition was discovered in 1934 by Fölling, a Norwegian biochemist; in the U.S.A. it occurs once in every 25,000 to 30,000 births (Jervis), in this country in about one per 30,000 of the population. The essential feature is the excretion daily in the urine of about one gramme of phenylpyruvic acid. Due to the absence of an enzyme phenylalanine hydroxylase, phenylalanine is not converted to tyrosine, phenylalanine accumulates in the blood, and phenylpyruvic acid, phenyllactic acid and phenylacetic acid are voided in the urine. It is uncertain precisely how the subnormality is caused and what the neuropathological changes are.

The affected individual is usually severely subnormal: rarely he is mentally normal or near normal. The diagnosis may be suspected on clinical grounds alone, but the clinical features described by Penrose, Jervis and Cowie are not pathognomonic and the urine must be tested to confirm the diagnosis. Nearly all the subjects have fair hair, fair skin and blue eyes. The head measurements are slightly reduced and the incisor teeth are widely spaced. The posture is usually stooping and flexed, the gait stiff, the limbs hypertonic with very brisk tendon reflexes. The children tend to be hyperkinetic, to show digital mannerisms (such as flicking, twiddling, pill-rolling), and to suffer from epilepsy particularly in their earlier years. They also seem to be unusually prone to eczema and dermatitis.

The diagnosis can usually be made in the first 4 to 7 weeks of life. To a sample of urine which has been acidified a few drops are added of 5 per cent. ferric chloride solution: a characteristic light green reaction quickly develops and darkens to deep bluish green. Lately a quick stick test for phenylketonuria (*Phenistix*) has been introduced, facilitating the diagnosis in babies: the stick is simply pressed against a wet nappy, and if the test is positive a grey or grey-green colour appears on the stick within 30 seconds. The diagnosis may be confirmed by estimating the blood phenylalanine.

Attempts to treat the condition by feeding the infant with a diet low in phenylalanine have been made by Bickle, Wolf, Moncrieff, Coates and others. Treatment must begin as soon as the abnormality is detected. Phenylalanine free casein-hydrolysates are used, supplemented by milk. Dietary control must be checked by serial estimations of blood phenylalanine levels. The diet is expensive and unappetizing, and it is not yet known if it has to be continued indefinitely. Moncrieff and Wilkinson (1961) reviewing the present position state that the treatment offers 'a reasonable chance of preventing mental retardation'. While the chemical balance can be restored, the effects on the developing brain are much harder to gauge. Coates (1961) reports that of 28 cases treated at The Hospital for Sick Children, 22 (79 per cent.) showed improvement; in 12 (43 per cent.) this improvement was marked—a rise in I.Q. points of 9 or more.

Hsia and his colleagues (1956) have claimed that the heterozygous carriers of phenylketonuria can be detected by phenylalanine tolerance tests. If confirmed, this is an important finding, which would have eugenic implications. Known carriers could be advised not to inter-marry and have children.

Hepatolenticular Degeneration (Wilson's Disease). Kinnier Wilson in 1911 first described this very rare condition, in which retardation is associated with lesions of the liver and corpus striatum.

There is in these cases a complex disturbance of copper metabolism. Copper is excreted in large amounts in the urine, and it is deposited in many organs, especially in the basal ganglia and in the liver: the blood copper is low. These changes appear to be due to a genetically determined deficiency of a plasma copper protein, ceruloplasmin, which normally binds 90 per cent. of the copper in the blood.

The onset of the disease may be in childhood, but more usually it is in adolescence: it may also be delayed until adult life. There is then a progressive development of extrapyramidal symptoms and dementia over the usually few years of remaining life. Tremor is often the earliest symptom, preceding the generalized development of a rigidity of Parkinsonian type, with progressive limitation of voluntary movement and interference with speech and swallowing. Choreo-athetoid movements are also typical, and there may be torsion spasms. The dementia is of a non-specific type, with emotional lability. In some cases the cornea shows a characteristic change, due to the deposition there of copper: this is the Kayser-Fleischer ring, a golden-brownish staining of the periphery of the cornea which can best be seen with the aid of a slit-lamp. There are the usual systemic symptoms of cirrhosis.

The lesions in the brain, which consist of degeneration of ganglion cells, neuroglial overgrowth and deposition of copper, are found in the basal ganglia, the cortex and elsewhere: they are concentrated in the corpus striatum and particularly in the lenticular nucleus. The liver shows a multilobular cirrhosis.

Treatment with dimercaprol (B.A.L.), which aims to eliminate the excess copper in the body, has had uncertain results: but here again we have a disease the aetiology of which we are beginning to understand, and we may reasonably hope for more definitive treatment.

Galactosaemia. In these rare cases there is an inability to metabolize galactose, due to the absence of an enzyme, phospho-galactose-uridyl transferase: hence galactose accumulates in the body in toxic amounts, and appears in the urine in excess. Symptoms usually begin in early infancy, with vomiting and jaundice. Progressive wasting, enlargement of the liver, cataract and brain damage follow: and there is a high mortality.

All cases of severe subnormality associated with cataract should be investigated for galactosuria. Treatment will arrest the damage and the clinical signs may recede. Lactose and galactose must be eliminated from the diet: that is, the child must not be given milk, and other sugars must be substituted.

Glycogen Disease (Glycogenosis, von Gierke's Disease). This is another rare abnormality of carbohydrate metabolism, which may cause mental retardation. There is a disorder both of the storage and of the liberation of glycogen, due apparently to the deficiency of a specific glycolytic enzyme, glucose-6-phosphatase. Glycogen accumulates in various bodily organs, usually particularly in the liver and in some cases particularly in the heart.

The child fails to grow and develop normally, the liver is grossly enlarged (its cells being distended with glycogen), and there is a low fasting blood sugar, with ketonuria. There is no splenomegaly.

Amaurotic Idiocy (Cerebromacular Degeneration). Infantile (Tay-Sach's disease), late infantile (Bielschowsky-Jansky disease), and juvenile (Vogt-Spielmeyer's disease) forms of this very rare condition have been described. It is not known what biochemical anomaly leads to the infiltration and distension of the brain cells with lipoid, which is mostly ganglioside. There is no effective treatment.

In the infantile form the onset is usually in the latter half of the first year of life, severe subnormality results, and death occurs in a year or two. The progress of the disease is marked by nystagmus, optic atrophy, epileptic fits and paralyses. In the retina, a cherry-red spot develops in the region of the macula where the choroid vessels become visible. The late infantile form, as its name indicates, begins later and develops more slowly; the macular spot may be absent. The juvenile form starts at the age of about 6 years and may run a course of 10 years or so, before it too is fatal.

Niemann-Pick's Disease. This is another of the very rare cerebral lipoidoses, which has not yet been clearly differentiated from amaurotic idiocy. Distinguishing features are said to be the gross enlargement of the liver and spleen, where there are lipoid deposits: and the lipoid is said in these cases to be sphingomyelin. The condition may also arise in adult life, and then cause dementia.

Lipochondrodystrophy (Gargoylism, Hurler's Disease). The term gargoylism,

2 G

though neatly descriptive, should perhaps be abandoned as likely to cause distress to relatives. The precise nature of the metabolic fault has not yet been defined. There appears to be a disturbance in the metabolism of lipo-polysaccharides, and the brain and many other organs become the site of abnormal intracellular deposits of polysaccharides. Subnormality does not always result but severe retardation is usual. There is no known treatment.

The appearance of these children is striking. The face is coarse, craggy and un-childlike. The head and face look heavy, bony prominences are large, the bridge of the nose is sunk, the eyebrows and lips are thick. The cornea may be misty or opaque. Deafness is common. The skeletal abnormalities include dwarfing, thoracic or lumbar kyphosis, and limitation of joint movements. The abdomen is swollen due to severe enlargement of the liver and spleen. There may be hypertension and cardiac enlargement: and early death from respiratory infection is common as it is in mongolism.

Sex-linked recessive cases have been described in males.

Nephrogenic Diabetes Insipidus. This condition in males is transmitted as a sex-linked recessive. The patient has polyuria from infancy, and if his fluid intake is not increased sufficiently death or severe subnormality commonly result. The polyuria is resistant to vasopressin. The carrier state can be identified in female relatives by a simple urine-concentration test (Carter and Simpkiss, 1956).

SUBNORMALITY ASSOCIATED WITH CHROMOSOME ABNORMALITIES

Only in the past five years has it become possible to count accurately human chromosomes, to identify individual pairs of chromosomes, and to ascertain the nuclear sex. In normal men and women the diploid number of chromosomes is 46:22 pairs of autosomes and one sex chromosome pair. Males and females have different numbers of X chromosomes, and the male has a Y chromosome which is absent in the female. In man this Y chromosome appears to be the male determinant: males are XY, females, XX. The nuclei of chromosomal females possess sex chromatin (are chromatin-positive), those of chromosomal males lack it.

As a result of researches which have used new techniques of somatic cell culture (from bone marrow and skin biopsies), and of separating, spreading and staining the chromosomes, it is now known that certain cases of subnormality have an abnormal chromosome constitution.

In *mongolism* there is usually a single extra chromosome, a third member of one of the autosome pairs: the mongol is hence said to be trisomic for this autosome. The condition is described in greater detail on page 455.

Chromosome counts have revealed also abnormalities in the sex chromosomes in some human intersexes associated with subnormality.

Some patients with *Klinefelter's syndrome* (seminiferous tubule dysgenesis) are mentally subnormal. This type of male hypogonadism is characterized clinically by leg lengthening without corresponding lengthening of the arms, testes much smaller than normal, reduced facial and abdominal hair, and enlarged breasts

(Stewart *et al.*, 1959). Both chromatin-positive and chromatin-negative cases occur. Chromatin-positive cases have been found to have usually an extra sex chromosome, *i.e.* 47 chromosomes and an XXY sex chromosome complex (Jacobs and Strong, 1959).

Turner's syndrome is commonly associated with mental subnormality. In this condition girls with gonadal dysgenesis fail to develop secondary sex character-istics at puberty and commonly show other developmental anomalies—small stature, webbed neck, congenital heart lesions. Most of these patients are chro-matin-negative, and in this group one sex chromosome is usually missing, *i.e.* there are 45 chromosomes, and an XO sex chromosome complex (Ford *et al.*, 1959*b*).

In both the above syndromes the nuclear sex is at variance with the phenotypic sex.

A human 'super female' has also been described, with a chromosome number of 47 and a chromosomal sex of XXX (Jacobs *et al.*, 1959). This individual, who presented with secondary amenorrhoea, showed hypoplasia of the uterus and ovaries, and was mentally below average.

Ford and his colleagues (1959*a*) have reported a severely subnormal individual with both mongolism and the Klinefelter syndrome. He has two supernumerary chromosomes (total 48), including an extra small acrocentric in addition to two X chromosomes and a Y.

Mongolism

The mongolian variety of subnormality was so designated by Langdon Down in 1886 because of the resemblance of the physical characteristics of the patients to those of members of the Mongolian race. The resemblance is, however, super-ficial, and the physiognomy of the mongol can still be recognized when the individual is Mongolian by race.

Mongolism is a common type of subnormality, occurring in about one of every 700 births and comprising about 5 per cent. of the subnormal cared for in hospitals and colonies. There is a low familial incidence, though familial cases do occur, two or more affected sibs or other near relatives then being found in a family. According to Penrose, pairs of affected sibs occur about once for every 100 single cases randomly collected. The frequency of mongolism in twins is similar to that in other children, and there is a frequent concurrence of normal and mongoloid babies in the same twin pregnancy (Allen and Baroff, 1956).

Aetiology. Mongolism has recently been demonstrated to be associated usually with, and presumably to be due to, trisomy of one of the smallest chromosomes—No. 21 in the Denver classification (Lejeune *et al.*, 1959). There is a small extra chromosome, giving a total of 47 chromosomes. This extra chromosome is an acrocentric chromosome in the smallest size range: it belongs to one of the two short autosome pairs that resemble the Y, and it is probably the result of tripling of one of these normal pairs.

The risk of giving birth to a mongol child is closely related to increasing maternal age, the incidence of the syndrome rising rapidly in women over 30.

Penrose (1949) and others have reported that the mean age of the mother at the birth of a mongol averages about 37 years, compared with a mean age of 29 years for all births. Between the maternal ages of 45 and 49, the incidence rises to 2–3 per cent. Probably usually the primary disorder lies in oogenesis, the trisomy being the result of 'non-disjunction' at one of the meiotic divisions of parental gametogenesis producing a gamete with 24 chromosomes instead of 23 —a defect which apparently becomes more frequent as the gonad ages.

More recent research suggests that mongolism may occasionally arise from chromosomal mechanisms other than the trisomy of chromosome No. 21. There may in these rare cases of mongolism be only 46 chromosomes.

Clinical Features. Mongolism is characterized by a number of physical anomalies which when found together give an unmistakable clinical picture: these are found especially in the skull, eyes, tongue and hands. The skull is small, rounded and so diminished in its antero-posterior diameter (brachycephalic) that the antero-posterior and lateral measurements are nearly equal: both the face and the occiput are flattened. The tongue is large, with hypertrophied papillae and transverse fissures (the 'scrotal tongue' of French writers), the mouth is often slightly open and the lower lip commonly protrudes. The palpebral fissures of the eyes are oblique, narrowed and slit-like, often there is a marked epicanthic fold, and other abnormalities are frequently found, *e.g.* ectropion, strabismus, cataract and blepharitis. There are abnormalities of the creases and dermal ridges of the palms and soles: typically a single transverse palmar crease and a single crease on the little finger, while the dermal ridges also tend to be more transversely arranged than normal. The little finger commonly curves inwards, the terminal phalanx being atrophied and the middle phalanx shortened: and the joint ligaments are very lax, giving a greatly increased range of movement to the fingers and toes. The individual is dwarfed in stature, with generally scanty, dry and straight hair, congenital cardiac abnormalities are common, and he is prone to catarrhal infections. Unlike many other subnormal individuals, mongols are not unduly prone to epilepsy: but they have a raised mortality from leukaemia.

Mentally, the mongol is usually severely subnormal. The majority have a mental age of between four and seven years. Many observers have described the mongol as usually good natured and easily amused, and as giving the appearance of being more alert and bright than he or she really is, because of a quick imitativeness and mischievousness: other authorities have denied that there is a characteristic personality. The brain is usually smaller and the convolutions simpler than usual.

Many mongols die during the first few months of life, and at birth the expectation of life is less than ten years. Acute respiratory infection is the commonest cause of death. Some live into adult life.

ENDOCRINE DISEASE AND SUBNORMALITY

Of the endocrine disorders which may cause mental subnormality, cretinism is the commonest (though not itself common) and most important. Much less common causes are idiopathic hypoglycaemia and idiopathic hypoparathyroidism.

Cretinism. There are several distinct types, of different aetiologies. McGirr and Hutchison (1956 and subsequently) in Glasgow have contributed much to their understanding.

Endemic cretinism is almost always associated with endemic goitre which is due to iodine deficiency in the diet. It is found in certain goitrous regions of the world, but very rarely now in Britain or the U.S.A., and it has in recent years also become rare in Switzerland which used to be an affected area: mass prophylaxis with iodized salt has proved very effective.

Sporadic cretinism may occur with or without goitre. Where there is no goitre, there is a deficiency of thyroid tissue: some thyroid tissue is however usually present, though ectopic or undescended owing to some defect in the development of the thyroid gland. In sporadic goitrous cretinism, a rare condition, there is apparently usually some intrathyroid enzyme deficiency causing a block somewhere along the pathway of the synthesis of thyroid hormone. The condition may be inherited as a recessive disease and it is probably another of the inborn errors of metabolism.

Cretinism may be associated with any degree of subnormality: it also produces characteristically traits of placidity and unaggressiveness. It is upon the physical signs that the diagnosis is based. The body is dwarfed, the neck short and thick, the abdomen protuberant, the limbs short, podgy and often clumsy. The skin is dry, the hair coarse. The head is large, with swollen eyelids, pug nose, thick lips and protruding tongue. Ossification and dentition are delayed. The basal metabolic rate is low.

It is of the greatest importance to make the diagnosis as soon as possible and attention must therefore be directed to the earliest symptoms. Lowrey and his colleagues (1958) have given a helpful description of 49 cases, from this point of view. They state that in 50 per cent. of their cases, three or more of the following cardinal symptoms were present during the first month of life: lethargy with absence of crying; constipation; feeding problems due to somnolence and the large tongue; and respiratory difficulties (30 per cent. showed respiratory distress with cyanosis). The infant is shorter than it should be, and often has an umbilical hernia.

The diagnosis can be confirmed by laboratory tests. The serum protein-bound iodine is below normal, and hypercholesterolaemia is usual though the serum cholesterol may be normal. It may be helpful also to make a radiographic estimation of the bone age.

Early and fully adequate treatment may be curative. The child will need thyroid regularly for years, and must be given the optimum dose to ensure mental and physical growth. In the first year of life the dose of thyroid may begin at $\frac{1}{8}-\frac{1}{2}$ grain daily, but it must be raised soon to a level which is just below that which produces symptoms of toxicity. If treatment is delayed or intermittent, some degree of subnormality is inevitable.

Idiopathic Spontaneous Hypoglycaemia. This, in children, is probably not a clinical entity and it is not the only syndrome in this age group of which hypoglycaemia is a symptom: hypoglycaemia in an infant may also, for example, be due to adrenocortical insufficiency, glycogen disease or islet cell adenoma. The syndrome has been reviewed recently by Haworth and Coodin (1960). Symptoms begin in the first two years of life, and in 60 per cent. of cases under the age of 6 months. Generalized convulsions are associated with pallor, sweating, limpness or stupor: the fasting blood sugar is usually below 45 mg. per cent. Half of those children who develop the syndrome in the first six months of life become mentally retarded as a result of hypoglycaemic brain damage; paralyses and athetosis may be other neurological sequelae. Some cases respond to treatment with ACTH or adrenocorticosteroids; others which have resisted medical treatment have been cured by partial pancreatectomy; more than 10 per cent. die. The aetiology of these cases, as the name given to them implies, is still unknown. This is another syndrome the early recognition and treatment of which may forestall the development of subnormality.

Idiopathic Hypoparathyroidism. This, a rare disease in children, is due to the congenital absence or destruction of the parathyroid glands. Tetany is the characteristic symptom, presenting at first as paraesthesiae or cramps of the limbs: other features are weakness, epileptic seizures, defective skin, hair, nails and teeth, cataract and occasionally cerebral calcification; in addition to mental retardation. The plasma calcium is lowered, the plasma phosphorus raised. Treatment is based on calciferol (vitamin D_2) or dihydrotachysterol (*A.T.10*).

SOME OTHER CLINICAL SYNDROMES

Subnormality due to Rubella. Rubella infection of the pregnant mother during the first twelve weeks of her pregnancy may cause profound damage to the developing foetus; a situation which was first reported by Gregg from Australia in 1941. The risk of death for the baby *in utero* and up to 2 years of age is about doubled. In those that survive, subnormality, blindness due to cataract, nerve deafness, pyloric stenosis and congenital heart lesions may all result. Of these congenital defects, deafness is the commonest, affecting about 19 per cent.: subnormality occurs in 1·8 per cent. against 0·4 per cent. in controls (Manson *et al.*, 1960).

Congenital Syphilis. This is now an uncommon condition in this country, because of scrupulous antenatal care. In cases where the infection is transmitted by the mother before birth, the child shows usually subnormality and specific serological abnormalities, with or without other neurological signs of meningovascular lesions such as paralyses. The classical stigmata of congenital syphilis, the frontal bosses, keratitis, saddle nose, perioral scars and malformed teeth, may not be present. Later in childhood a congenital syphilitic infection may produce juvenile general paralysis (juvenile G.P.I.).

Subnormality due to Blood Incompatibility. Rhesus factor incompatibility is the commonest variety, though the minority of Rhesus-positive children of Rhesus-negative mothers develop these complications. Severe neonatal jaundice in this syndrome is associated with kernicterus and lesions of the basal ganglia, especially the caudate and lenticular nuclei. Convulsions and coma occur early, and many of the affected infants die: later spasticity and choreo-athetosis are associated with subnormality and often epilepsy to form a rather distinctive clinical picture.

Diffuse Sclerosis (Schilder's Disease and Allied Syndromes). Both familial and sporadic cases of these demyelinating diseases occur: their aetiology is unknown. The disease process begins usually in the white matter of both the occipital lobes symmetrically and spreads forwards: in the affected areas both myelin sheaths and axis cylinders degenerate and are replaced by gliosis. In nearly half the cases, symptoms begin in the first ten years. Visual impairment, inco-ordination, bilateral spastic paralysis, and dementia are progressive. The child becomes helpless and blind, with spastic diplegia and fits, and dies within a few months or years. The cerebrospinal fluid shows usually no abnormality.

NEUROSES AND PSYCHOSES IN ASSOCIATION WITH SUBNORMALITY

This is a subject which would repay further investigation. We should know more than we do about symptomatology and response to treatment. The general situation seems to be that subnormal individuals are subject to the same abnormal reaction-types as intellectually normal individuals: but their abnormal reactions tend to be more easily precipitated by the environment and to be more transient. There is also some difficulty, particularly in the case of subnormal children, in classifying these reactions in terms of the classical psychiatric syndromes of adult life.

THE DIAGNOSIS OF SUBNORMALITY

In coming to a diagnosis, the doctor should seek more than a short answer to the simple question, is this child or adult subnormal. He should try to determine also the degree of the subnormality, the mental fields in which the patient is subnormal, and the cause or causes of his subnormality. Both the patient and his environment will have to be carefully reviewed.

In the case of the severely subnormal the diagnosis of subnormality may be easy, one may have only to look at the individual's odd appearance or silly expression to come to the right conclusion. In cases of borderline subnormality, on the contrary, and in infancy and early childhood, the correct diagnosis may be much harder to reach. The subnormal child may be blamed and criticized for failures in performance for which he is in no way to blame, and the recidivist be given repeated prison sentences for crimes which are symptoms of his unrecognized subnormality.

The earlier in life the diagnosis can be made the better: and in the case of certain syndromes of severe subnormality, such as cretinism or hyploglycaemia, which are susceptible to treatment, early diagnosis is of critical importance.

A detailed history must be obtained from the patient's near relatives: this will include a family history of subnormality or other relevant illnesses; a detailed account of the mother's health during her pregnancy with this child, and of any obstetrical difficulties; and a comprehensive description of the child's develop-ment and total behaviour from infancy. Inquiry must be made about the times at which this child developed various skills, in comparison with the progress of the average child: as a baby at what age could he sit up unsupported, when did he begin to stand, walk and talk, when could he use a spoon, dress himself, gain control over his bladder and bowels, and when did his teeth erupt. Various 'developmental scales' have been devised for assessing the normality of mental and physical growth in the pre-school child, of which Gesell's and Griffith's are perhaps the best known, and these may be of some service: but a knowledge of what may be expected of the average pre-school child, critically applied in appraisal of the possibly subnormal child's performance, is usually a reasonably reliable guide to the doctor. The doctor must always keep in mind that the small child's mental growth is often uneven and that normal children show very wide individual differences in their modes and rates of maturation. Repeated examina-tions of the child, at intervals of some months, may be necessary when the diagnosis is doubtful.

When the child goes to school he is inevitably critically assessed: his intelli-gence is usually formally tested, his capacities are further revealed in his class-room work, and his normality or backwardness become more apparent as he mixes and competes in various ways with other children. In gauging the mental status of a child of school age, it is of great assistance to have a report from his head- or class-master. An educational psychologist's report, if available, should of course also be obtained: the results of mental tests given by an expert are much more reliable than the amateur's.

Intelligence tests are of great value in the diagnosis and assessment of mental defect. In most cases their results serve to refine the diagnosis rather than to establish it. They must be used critically always, with knowledge of their limita-tions. Below the age of three years intelligence tests are grossly unreliable. From school age their reliability is established.

The most commonly employed quantitative measure of intelligence is the Intelligence Quotient (I.Q.). The individual's Mental Age (M.A.) is the age at which the average child would have passed the tests the examinee has passed. The individual's I.Q. is the ratio of his Mental Age to his Chronological Age (C.A.), expressed as a percentage: that is, $I.Q. = \dfrac{M.A.}{C.A.} \times 100$. For adults, the C.A. is taken to be 15 or 16 years. The I.Q. is only one of the possible measures of intelligence, and though the best known it is perhaps not the most satisfactory. Many authorities would prefer to use percentile scores, as the indices of intellec-tual brightness or dullness.

The intelligence tests most commonly used are the Terman-Merrill revision of the Binet-Simon tests, and the Wechsler Intelligence Scales for Adults and for Children. The Terman-Merrill is probably the most useful test for the severely subnormal child and *faute de mieux* for the severely subnormal adult also. The Progressive Matrices is a valuable non-verbal test which is easily given and scored: it assesses the subject's capacity to reason by analogy. Various performance tests are also available, which do not depend on verbal or symbolic material: these are psychomotor tests of such special abilities as speed of manipulation, spatial ability and manual dexterity. While intelligence and manual dexterity are usually fairly closely allied and are alike necessary for any manual work which requires skill, their measurement alone cannot be used to predict success at such work. The temperamental qualities of the individual, his behaviour and emotional stability, are always of paramount importance. Further details of tests should be sought in such a textbook as Cronbach's (1949).

It is important to recognize that the I.Q. is by no means a constant like the individual's finger-prints. It is only relatively constant, and the reliability of its assessment depends on the skill of the tester. It may change even by 20 points or more, revealing fluctuations in the individual's performance not due to any change in his native capacity. It may show a marked and permanent improvement in cases where the mental retardation has been due considerably to an adverse upbringing and deprivation of education.

If intelligence tests are to produce the fullest and most reliable information, they should be administered by an expert; a psychologist's advice should certainly be sought in any difficult or marginal case. Mental testing should be used to reveal not only the patient's general intellectual level, but also his more specific aptitudes and disabilities, since knowing these we can then plan much more effectively an educational programme or give vocational guidance. It is deplorable that so many hospitals for the subnormal in this country are without psychologists on their staff.

In addition to the assessment and measurement of his intelligence, the subnormal child's or adult's personality must be appraised. His temperamental traits, his emotional stability, his persistence and reliability, his capacity to come to terms socially with normal children or adults, all these qualities must be elicited. These aspects of his make-up are often of major importance in gauging how best he can be helped, stimulated or cared for. And the subnormal individual must be seen in his family or social setting, his environment's normality, inadequacy or detrimental aspects must be known: in this part of the investigation of the case, the social worker who can visit and report on the family situation has a key rôle.

The doctor must in every case carry out a detailed physical examination, paying attention to abnormalities of physical constitution and development, to congenital lesions and stigmata, and particularly, of course, to the state of the nervous system. The child is often handicapped in more ways than intellectually, and these additional handicaps must be defined. Examination of the urine should be carried out routinely; blood samples may be required for laboratory examination if, for example, syphilitic infection or hypoglycaemia are suspected; X-rays and other specialized investigations may be indicated. The correct diagnosis of a subnormal child's clinical syndrome will often test the doctor's knowledge of general medicine at many points.

The biochemist has now an important and rapidly growing part to play in the diagnosis of syndromes of subnormality. Moncrieff (1960), in a valuable survey of the biochemistry of subnormality, has calculated that between 2500 and 4500 of the 126,000 ascertained subnormal individuals in England and Wales may have a biochemical factor in their aetiology; and he suggests that this may be an underestimate. Furthermore, if the subnormal individual is found to have a biochemical abnormality, study of this abnormality may necessitate laboratory examination of his relatives.

In conclusion, it must be emphasized that the diagnosis and evaluation of subnormality frequently requires the collaboration of all those concerned with the child's health and education, if it is to be made in a way which will facilitate constructive planning for the individual's future. And when the diagnosis has been made, the facts and their implications must be placed before the parents or guardians with great tact and sympathy, to elicit their co-operation and to minimize any feelings of family stigma or of personal failure which the diagnosis may have caused.

DIFFERENTIAL DIAGNOSIS

It is of course a most serious error, fraught with grave complications for the child's future, to diagnose a child as subnormal when he is not. Such a mistake is fortunately rare. Much more often the diagnosis of subnormality is missed, or for social or other reasons is rejected or glossed over.

Two groups of conditions may be wrongly diagnosed as subnormality: sensory, perceptual or aphasic defects, and psychoses. The deaf or deaf-mute child, the child with impaired vision or with some motor defect involving speech, the child seriously limited by a specific reading or calculating disability, may be misdiagnosed as intellectually backward and the true reason for his poor performance may not be recognized. The only way to avoid such errors is to make examination in every case meticulous, with attention both to the medical and the psychological status of the child.

A schizophreniform psychosis or early infantile autism may be misdiagnosed as subnormality. There are of course symptomatic differences [see p. 518]: and the history of a more or less normal beginning to life with subsequent deterioration would strongly suggest psychosis, if a state of subnormality due to an extrinsic cause such as encephalitis could be ruled out. Frequently cases of subnormality have been wrongly labelled 'childhood schizophrenia' by psychiatrists ignorant of the syndromes of subnormality.

PREVENTION AND TREATMENT

Preventive measures which are rational and effective can be based on a knowledge of aetiology and as our understanding of the aetiology of subnormality grows more opportunities for mental hygiene therefore present themselves. Much can be done, and is being done, to diminish some of the causes of subnormality. This is effected most directly through control of environmental factors which may injure the child before, during and after birth. The maintenance of high standards of antenatal care, skilled attention during childbirth, satisfactory nutrition and vastly improved control of infection in the infant, all these have been and will continue to be of great importance; and the medical services have been supported in these advances by a public better educated in health matters than its forebears.

Negative eugenic measures are harder to apply and are at present of slight practical importance; though our increasing knowledge of the genetics of subnormality provides data which can be used in genetic counselling, at least in connection with some of the clear-cut syndromes of subnormality. In cases of single gene inheritance, where the mode of inheritance of the clinical entity is known, intelligent and inquiring adults may be given the facts about the expectation of abnormality in their offspring which will enable them to decide for themselves about marriage and birth control. Our ability to reduce the incidence of recessively inherited syndromes depends on the identification of carriers of the abnormal genes, and here progress has been slow. The important work already referred to on the carrier-states in phenylketonuria and idiopathic diabetes insipidus should be followed up.

Early medical treatment is of prime importance in those syndromes where treatment is possible; for instance in cretinism, galactosaemia, phenylketonuria, diabetes insipidus, syphilitic infection. It is interesting that the specific treatment consists in several syndromes simply in giving a special diet, but unfortunately the control here is often still a matter of considerable technical difficulty. Once significant cerebral damage has been done it is usually irreversible; though one must note that hemispherectomy has sometimes proved a successful operation in carefully selected cases of subnormality which have been associated with hemiplegia and epilepsy. For the early diagnosis upon which effective treatment so often depends, the maternal and child health services carry a particular responsibility.

Many educational, social and medical agencies are available to help the subnormal: special schools and special classes, occupation centres, out-patient psychiatric clinics for children and adults, and colonies and hospitals for those who need in-patient care and treatment. Specialist psychological testing and vocational guidance are available to orientate the treatment and management. We have developed the services, but all too often we lack the staff to make full use of them: the most serious shortage is perhaps in teachers for the educationally subnormal: it is impossible in over-large and insufficiently differentiated classes to give to backward children the individual attention they need and to which they will often respond rewardingly. Doctors, teachers, psychologists, social workers, health visitors and voluntary associations of lay people have all their parts to play. But it must be said that the activities of those who seek to help the subnormal have not always been well co-ordinated: and the medical contribution to the problems of subnormality has been impaired by the inability of the specialist services to attract many of the best medical talents. In the last year or two, however, there has been a most welcome resurgence of interest and enthusiasm: biochemical and genetic researches in this field have aroused widespread medical interest, and there has been a much more optimistic attitude towards the rehabilitation of the subnormal. Both paediatrics and neurology have major contributions to make, and specialists in these disciplines should be encouraged to work in the health services for the subnormal.

Many of the severely subnormal require admission to hospital. Those with a mental age of less than 3 years demand skilled nursing care above all in their management, and this is probably the only group of the subnormal who should be considered ineducable. Much attention has been paid recently in this country to the training of the severely subnormal. Many will respond to patient and encouraging guidance: and some can be trained in repetitive mechanical tasks in sheltered workshops to such a degree of competence that they can contribute financially to their keep. They are, of course, much slower and less dexterous than the normal.

Subnormal children and adults should if possible be retained in the community. Many never need any medical care on account of their subnormality. If they are failing to adapt themselves socially many agencies are at hand to give them support, and full use of these should be made before hospitalization is decided upon. Admission to hospital cuts into the child's schooling, breaks the loving ties that exist in nearly all but the very worst homes, and marks the child off from his fellows: it should therefore be recommended only after careful consideration and for positive reasons, never as the easy way out. Some unstable subnormal adolescents and adults, who by reason of their delinquency or sexual promiscuity have become serious social problems, have, of course, to be segregated in hospital for prolonged periods: but hospital should for most of the subnormal be considered not as a place of segregation from the community but of preparation for it. It is with the subnormal that the greatest progress can be made; naturally so, since they are at, or not far from, the borderland of normality: and the fact that about one-half of the patients in mental deficiency hospitals in this country fall into this group, presents a great challenge to the medical profession in whose care they have been placed. Major contributions to the rehabilitation of the subnormal in hospital have recently been made by psychologists, and this work has been reviewed by O'Connor and Tizard (1956): the authors themselves have been pioneers in the research they describe. A detailed description of their work will not be attempted here. We will only say in brief that subnormal patients in hospital must get, not only a kindly discipline which will inculcate regular habits and acceptable social attitudes, but also a schooling that will attempt to teach them at least reading, writing and simple calculation and a realistic training in work which will fit them to take jobs in the community. And when they leave hospital, subnormal patients must never be allowed to drop unsupported into a social void. They may be helped to progress to community life via a hostel. Finally, the homes to which they will return will often need the supervision and assistance of the local social services if further breakdown is to be prevented. It is the obtaining of suitable employment which is often the most difficult hurdle in rehabilitation and it is entirely fortunate that there is a state of nearly full employment in this country which makes gainful occupation easier for the subnormal.

REFERENCES

Allen, G., and Baroff, G. S. (1956) *Acta genet.* (*Basel*), **5**, 294.

Brandon, M. W. G., Kirman, B. H., and Williams, C. E. (1959) *J. ment. Sci.*, **105**, 721.

Carter, C., and Simpkiss, M. (1956) *Lancet*, ii, 1069.

Coates, S. (1961) *Brit. med. J.*, **1**, 767.

Cronbach, L. J. (1949) *Essentials of Psychological Testing*, New York.

Ford, C. E., Jones, K. W., Polani, P. E., Almeida, J. C. de, and Briggs, J. H. (1959*a*) *Lancet* i, 711.

Ford, C. E., Polani, P. E., Briggs, J. H., and Bishop, P. M. F. (1959*b*) *Nature*, **183**, 1030.

Hawarth, J. C., and Coodin, F. J. (1960) *Pediatrics*, **25**, 748.

Hsia, D. Y. (1956) *Nature*, **178**, 1239.

Jacobs, P. A., Baikie, A. G., Brown, W. M., MacGregor, T. N., MacLean, N., and Harnden, D. G. (1959) *Lancet* ii, 423.

Jacobs, P. A., and Strong, J. A. (1959) *Nature*, **183**, 302.

Kirman, B. H. (1956) *Arch. Dis. Childh.*, **31**, 1.

Lejeune, J., Gautier, M., and Turpin, R. (1959) *C.R.Acad.Sci.* (*Paris*), **248**, 1721.

Lewis, E. O. (1929) Report of the Mental Deficiency Committee, London. H.M.S.O.

Lowrey, G. H., Aster, R. H., Carr, E. A., Ramon, G., Beierwaltes, W. H., and Spafford, N. R. (1958) *Amer. J. Dis. Child.*, **96**, 131.

Manson, M. M., Logan, W. P. D., and Loy, R. M. (1960) *Rubella and Other Virus Infections during Pregnancy*, London, H.M.S.O.

McGirr, E. M., and Hutchison, J. H. (1956) *Lancet*, i, 106.

Moncrieff, A. (1960) *Lancet*, ii, 273.

Moncrieff, A., and Wilkinson, R. H. (1961) *Brit. med. J.* **1**, 763.

O'Connor, N., and Tizard, J. (1956) *The Social Problem of Mental Deficiency*, London.

Penrose, L. S. (1949) *The Biology of Mental Defect*, London.

Stewart, J. S. S., Mack, W. S., Govan, A. D. T., Ferguson-Smith, M. A., and Lennox, B. (1959) *Quart. J. Med.*, **28**, 561.

18

PSYCHOSES AND NEUROSES IN WAR

GENERAL CONSIDERATIONS

The First World War taught several valuable psychiatric lessons, although it produced no novel type of mental disorder. It proved, with great prodigality of example, that purely psychological factors can produce mental illness. This should hardly need such proof; but just as there were many who could see only physical commotion as a cause of 'shell-shock', so there are many who find in endocrinopathy and sepsis the principal cause of its civil equivalents. It is therefore useful, for this as well as other reasons, to review the psychiatric experience of war: for in war the reactions are superficial and transient and more readily understood than the more complicated illnesses of ordinary life. 'We find in these cases', says MacCurdy, of the neuroses, 'a great simplicity in the psychic mechanisms operating to produce symptoms.' The war also demonstrated the validity of certain important psychological hypotheses and disproved some others. Thus the unconscious influence of a wish in determining symptoms was well shown. But it also showed that a 'sexual' aetiology for war neuroses could only be hypothecated by using 'sexual' in the widest possible sense to denote any emotional investment of an object. If any doubts remained from the First World War as to the share of pre-existing personality in the causation of war neuroses, as well as of psychoses, they were removed in the second one. A predisposition of some kind is evident in most cases, except when the external stress has been very severe, in which event it is possible that anyone may develop symptoms. It is illuminating also to find that predisposition, as far as it can be quantitatively estimated, and external stress act together in a more or less additive way. It is broadly true that the more predisposition the less stress is necessary, and vice versa.

The nature of the predisposition is various and often composite, or, more precisely, its ascertainment depends on taking account of a diversity of facts and qualities. The most frequently recurring of these are a family history of mental illness of neurotic or psychotic form, or of a neurotic or psychopathic personality; a history pointing to personal insecurity, as from the early loss of a parent, or, on the other hand, to too much security and self over-valuation, as in the case of the precious only child; psychological immaturity, arising often from the background just described; a history of nearly lifelong neurotic anxiety, such as is heralded by pronounced fear of the dark in childhood, or of excessive real anxiety in the shape of marked anticipatory apprehension of coming events; timidity, betrayed by lack of enthusiasm for the more hazardous games and sports; seeming antipathy to aggressive action, whether against other boys in the shape of boxing, or against animals, as shown in aversion to even the mildest blood sports; fainting or other excessive visceral response in face of emotionally disturbing experiences; lack of persistence, as shown by frequent change of job for insufficient or specious reasons; a history of what might be called in a question-begging way 'physiological instability' in the form of sleep-walking, occasional insomnia, nocturnal enuresis, and manifestations of tension, such as long-continued nail-biting, and the like; lability of affect, especially a tendency to get easily depressed; extreme shyness; and indeed any of the other qualities which are known to favour psychological illness. But those which have been more particularly enumerated seem to be more often responsible for breakdown in the face of physical danger, although they are important also in breakdowns arising from Service conditions generally, such as separation from home and adaptation to community life, to financial sacrifice, to drastic alteration in the routine pattern of living, and to an unfamiliar job. It should be pointed out that some such personal characteristics may be an advantage in peace and a disadvantage in war, and vice versa; so that there will also be neuroses arising from transition back to civilian life, as indeed there were last time, although they did not provide newspaper headlines.

It should always be remembered, however, when making a psychiatric estimate of liability to breakdown under war conditions that the previous personality in its liabilities and assets is not the whole story. There is a fluctuating entity, very difficult to estimate, that must always be taken into account, namely motive. While this can be permanently strong in certain types of character and temperament, and even to a pathological degree, as in the obsessional temperament, it is, in the majority of people, subject to external influences, such as battalion or squadron spirit, leadership, incidence of casualties, the general state of the war, fatigue and so forth.

Of special note has been the occurrence of schizophrenia-like conditions in a transient way and apparently without residual deterioration. This observation is of both theoretical and practical importance, for it supports the view that in some cases schizophrenia is the psychological reaction of an individual to his environmental difficulties rather than that which regards it as the mental manifestation of some obscure 'metabolic' disorder or structural degeneration. It shows also that such a reaction need not be permanently vicious. If the stress be removed in time, recovery occurs; and the stress of war is more easily and immediately removed than the distresses of civil life. Further, war experience is much more brief, and the schizophrenic reactions were not progressively woven into the personality, so as to become habits. The following was a case of this kind:

CASE No. 57

Y. Z., 26 years, single, clerk, was admitted to hospital in April 1919.

Family history was negative for nervous or mental disease. Patient was a healthy child and developed normally. He was a sober, good-living lad, and a strict Catholic. He enlisted in May 1917, but was marked C 3 on account of his size, and never served overseas. In November 1918 he contracted influenza, but recovered, and in December 1918 came home on leave. Four or five days after returning from leave he was admitted to hospital with mental symptoms. At that time he was greatly excited, incoherent and was in a padded room. He spoke much about the Kaiser, said his brother was his father, and was under the belief that he had some scheme, and that various common-place things that happened worked in with this scheme.

Four months later he showed no disorder of conduct, answered questions promptly, spoke in rather an abrupt way and constantly asked that the question should be repeated to him. He tended to make light of his case. He told how he had enlisted in May 1917, how he had suffered from influenza and had been in hospital, and then developed mental symptoms. In this connection he stated that it was something in the meat which made him sick. He then made an incoherent statement saying it all came about through an argument with some man—'It was a sign, a puzzle'. He could not give any satisfactory explanation of the above statements; admitted having had im-aginations, and having heard 'voices', but said that these had now disappeared.

Physically he was in good condition.

On the night of April 21, 1919, he seemed rather excited; was the smartest man in the world, he told an attendant. Later, when questioned about these things he flushed up, but denied all knowledge of them. When asked why he said he was the smartest man in the world, he said, 'I am treating myself; do you not see I am different every day?' Gradually during his hospital residence he made good progress, worked with a garden party and conducted himself in a quiet, rational, well-behaved way.

In September 1919 he was discharged as recovered. This patient was looked upon as a case of schizophrenia. The features which he showed were all rather striking, while the incoherence in his speech and his vague ideas of suspicion were much more in the nature of a schizophrenia-like reaction than anything else. He made a very good re-covery, however.

NUMERICAL INCIDENCE

In considering the incidence of mental disease under military conditions, it is useful to do so at three stages: 1. at mobilization; 2. during war; 3. at demobiliza-tion. In 1. the conditions approximate to the peace-time status in the civil populace; 2. alone bears directly on the problem; while 3. is in practice a com-bination of 1. and 2., the proportion of 1. depending on the thoroughness of examination at mobilization. Figures from the First World War will be quoted except where experience of the Second World War has called for revision in any significant way. In the latter the total percentage of risk was less than in the First World War, and the more exposed sections, namely the Air Force and the Sub-marine Service in the Navy, were selected groups not likely to develop psychiatric disorders to the same degree as the generality of mankind.

1. In the U.S.A. 12 per cent. of all rejections on mobilization in the first year of the First World War were for nervous and mental diseases. Inspection at camps following mobilization led to the rejection from these causes of a further 9 per cent. of the first million recruits. Nervous and mental diseases were fourth in the list of numerical importance of all causes of rejection. Of the rejections for nervous and mental disease, psychoses constituted 11 per cent., neuroses 15 per cent., epilepsy 9 per cent., mental deficiency 32 per cent., constitutional psycho-pathy 9 per cent. and organic nervous diseases and injuries 10 per cent. We quote the American figures, because the Americans, profiting from European experi-ence, made their psychiatric examination on enlistment more complete.

2. Farrar's statistics for Canadian casualties showed that nervous and mental diseases contributed 10 per cent. of the total disabled, and that of these 58 per

cent. were neuroses, 16 per cent. 'mental disease and deficit', 8 per cent. epilepsy and 'epileptoids', 14 per cent. head injuries and 4 per cent. organic nervous disease. This illustrates very well an important conclusion: that while psychoses and mental deficiency were the most frequent cause of initial rejection for nervous or mental disease, in actual warfare neuroses were numerically a far more important cause of disablement. To the same effect May quotes Hoche, who analysed Birnbaum's summary of seventy-two German articles written up to 1915, and concluded that among service troops psychopathic conditions, various psychogenic reactions, hysterical and anxiety states and exhaustion conditions were all very frequent, whereas serious psychoses were much rarer. Wollenberg, too, found that the individuals who broke down during mobilization developed manic-depressive or schizophrenic illness or psychopathic excitements, while the cases occurring at the front were chiefly hysteria, anxiety states and conditions of exhaustion. In troops who have not seen any fighting, neurotic conditions are also the commonest. The heavier the predisposition the earlier the breakdown as a rule.

Six thousand cases of 'shell-shock' were on the average admitted annually to British hospitals during the First World War. The admission rate for nervous and mental disease was 2 per 1000 in home troops, 4 per 1000 in service troops and 1 per 1000 in the civilian population. As to the type of illness, exclusive of neuroses, it was of interest to note the large percentage of mental defectives among British troops. Among 202 home troops, Henderson found 30 per cent. mentally defective—much the commonest type. Marr claimed to find as many as 42 per cent. mentally defective among 3755 cases (exclusive of neuroses). It is clear that psychiatric examination on enlistment is a necessity.

The rôle of wounding in the production of mental illness was slight. Mental illness was rare among the seriously wounded. A minor wound might determine the localization of a hysterical disorder. In the psychoses, where wounding was found in the anamnesis, other factors could usually be discovered as well. Of 17 wound cases with subsequent psychoses examined by us, only 3 showed no other predisposing factor, and in these 3 the history was imperfect.

3. One-seventh of all discharges from the British Army in 1917 were for nervous or mental disease. After the cessation of a war, the proportions of mental illness existing among the troops previous to service reassert themselves. How this occurs was shown dramatically by the figures furnished by Ireland, who stated that of 2500 shell-shock cases awaiting transportation to the U.S., 2100 recovered within a day or two of the armistice. Hence, of the neuropsychiatric cases who in 1920 formed 27 per cent. of the beneficiaries of war risk insurance in the U.S.A., 66 per cent. were psychoses, 19 per cent. neuroses, 5 per cent. epilepsy, 2 per cent. mental defect and 8 per cent. organic nervous or mental disease or injuries. Within the group of psychoses the proportions also change, since on the whole the schizophrenics remain permanently ill, while the manic-depressives recover. Hence, in the service patients remaining in mental hospitals, schizophrenia is the commonest variety of illness (43 of 113 cases—Henderson and Gillespie, 1923). Of the psychoses persisting after demobilization, it may be

2H

said that the majority would have occurred eventually without the superaddition of the strain of war.

Among prisoners of war, neuroses are rare. Mörhen found only 5 cases among 40,000 prisoners, and Lust found 'very few' among 20,000.

PSYCHOSES

Aetiological Factors. In the psychoses, just as the types occurring in war do not differ from those of peace, so the causative factors in war and peace seem to be similar. Morbid heredity, psychopathic predisposition, previous mental illness, subnormality and excessive alcoholism were found in every one of a series of 66 cases in which fairly complete data were available to us from the First World War. It happened in these cases that the war precipitated a psychosis in a personality which (in the majority of cases) would have sooner or later become ill in civil life. Sometimes the war laid bare a latent disposition to illness which would not otherwise have been suspected and which only a post-war catamnesis confirmed. A schizophrenia-like stupor has been recorded occasionally following a severe emotional experience in an individual not apparently predisposed.

As a rule, the policy of returning mental cases to the front was a failure. Of 2429 cases, mainly psychotics, recorded by Eager, only 10 per cent. were returned to the army (not necessarily to the front) and of these only half were fit and well a few months later. Napier Pearn examined 200 cases which were considered to have recovered sufficiently from psychoses to return to duty. Only 47 per cent. were found to be well some months after.

Toxic and infectious factors were not very prominent in the aetiology of war psychoses. Of 113 cases, 19 gave a history of malaria, dysentery, enteric, scarlet or rheumatic fever. The comparative freedom from serious infectious illness of the troops in the Western theatre was largely responsible for this. In the East malaria was the most important infectious agent in the production of mental illness (First World War).

In those cases in which mental illness followed actual brain injury, the resulting disturbance, if any, was of the organic type, acute or chronic. The acute organic variety was the immediate effect of injury, and could be attributed to one or more of the following factors—brain commotion from blast; concussion with or without burial (both of these resulting in increased intracranial pressure); decompression from rarefaction of air and embolism by bubbles of nitrogen and carbon monoxide; and inspiration of carbon monoxide. Loss of consciousness was the immediate result, frequently followed by a condition of 'dipping' of consciousness, in which consciousness reappears from time to time, but is marked by disorientation, and often by incontinence, and complaints of violent headache. 'A delirium is very frequent, the content of which is constant aggression on the part of the enemy' (MacCurdy). Mott found *post mortem* in two cases of true shell-shock, *i.e.* brain commotion resulting from an explosion, congestion of the meninges, scattered sub-pial haemorrhages and congested vessels in the internal capsule, pons and medulla.

Mott described symptoms occurring after concussion and resembling those of carbon monoxide poisoning: headaches, blurred vision, visual hallucinations, blindness, giddiness, palpitation, yawning, weariness, vomiting, cold sensations, sense of oppression, loss of memory and of speech, and tremors.

The chronic type of organic brain disturbance included cases of aphasia (cf. Head's series), traumatic epilepsy (in only 5 per cent. of all head injuries—Turner) and diffuse types of memory loss. Psychotic symptoms were rare among soldiers suffering from brain injury, and conversely a history of brain injury was rarely found among psychotic soldiers. Farrar remarked that among Canadian troops with head injuries psychoses and 'traumatic neuroses' were practically never observed. He quoted also Villard and Mignard, who among 350 cases of brain injury observed no characteristic mental symptoms, but only occasional confusional states suggesting epileptic equivalents. Aschaffenberg examined 74 men recently shelled but apparently well, and found evidences of local organic lesion in 67 of them. A week later some of these evidences had disappeared, but in no case did neurotic symptoms develop. Henderson observed an unusual sequel of brain injury which was probably the result of general cerebral commotion, in the form of a Korsakow-like syndrome. After exposure to blast there may appear symptoms pointing to cerebral damage such as general intellectual impairment and especially some defect of memory, occasionally some transient aphasic disturbances, and sometimes changes in the cerebrospinal fluid.

There is no doubt that a number of men in the early stages of general paralysis were passed into the army as the result of insufficient examination. These broke down completely in a few weeks or months. On the other hand, nine men known to us who developed general paralysis within three years of enlistment had served an average of 2·1 years before breaking down.

The clinical experience of the First World War gave suggestive data on the part played by *fatigue* in the causation of psychoses. Psychoses in which 'exhaustion' was the sole or even the principal factor were extremely rare. Reliable authors have entirely denied their existence (Birnbaum, Bonhoeffer, Aschaffenberg, Farrar). Bonhoeffer pointed out that psychoses were extremely rare among Serbian prisoners who had experienced six years' continuous warfare and suffered from emaciation, diffuse muscle atrophy, cardiac dilatation, arterial fibrosis and extreme weakness. But in one group—those cases which followed a long and severe febrile illness—post-febrile exhaustion was very prominent and must be assigned a rôle in the subsequent development of a psychosis. Farrar has emphasized that the symptoms of exhaustion *per se* have to be differentiated from those of an actual exhaustion psychosis. The symptoms of exhaustion in soldiers included restlessness, irritability, sleep disorders, emotional instability and attention defects. As exhaustion psychoses there have been reported such syndromes as delirium and clouding. It seems to be going too far to deny exhaustion a principal part in producing such states, and to attribute them instead always to psychogenic factors, as Birnbaum did.

This reflection has been confirmed by experience in the last war. By far the greater proportion of casualties, other than wounds, in certain stages of the

Middle East campaigns were states of exhaustion which recovered within a few days; only a small residuum turned out to be fundamentally psychogenic.

It has to be remembered that stress, whether it be fatigue or fear, may often be a main factor in releasing psychological types of reaction which would not otherwise appear, whether they be anxiety states in those exposed to repeated danger or mild depressions, which have appeared not uncommonly in individuals of obsessional temperament as the result of prolonged overwork. The appropriate treatment is rest with sedatives at bedtime to begin with.

NEUROSES

The First World War revived the old-standing controversy about the physical or psychical origin of numerous symptoms, such as paralysis, tremor, delirium, amnesia, disordered action of the heart, etc. Oppenheim, extending his peacetime theory of the basis of 'traumatic neuroses', such as follow a railway accident, and which he believed to be caused by physical commotion of the nervous system, and consequent molecular change in it, was of the opinion that the important factor in producing such symptoms was concussion. He assumed that the latter, acting on a nervous system weakened by terror and exhaustion, produced a functional disturbance of delicate 'psychic mechanisms'. In support of this hypothesis he drew attention to the rarity of a history of previous psychopathy in the patient and in his relatives. But his hypothesis broke down before a mass of contrary evidence. As in the psychoses, so in the neuroses of war, gross brain injury was the exception. Further, recovery from neurotic disturbances was frequently sudden, and was often brought about by psychic methods such as persuasion and suggestion. Exactly similar cases developed in men never exposed to battle conditions—'shell-shock' cases, so called, were not by any means unknown at the base camps. Moreover, the wounded rarely suffered. It is true that a certain proportion of wounded developed hysterical disorder, but in many of these it was after a long 'latent' period, when they were convalescing. A limb immobilized for the purposes of healing would sometimes remain so after all necessity for immobilization had gone.

Nevertheless at the beginning of the Second World War special hospitals for D.A.H.—later called 'effort syndrome'—were opened, but it was soon found that with the exception of a small proportion of cases following an infectious illness the 'effort syndrome' was an expression of some psychological disorder, and without any peculiar feature in psychopathology to justify regarding this as a separate group. The psychopathology was that of any state of neurotic anxiety or depression, psychopathic personality, hysteria, mental dullness, or subnormality.

The reason for the inadvertent choice of this form of expression of emotional conflict lies sometimes in medical suggestion; more often in the fact that in individuals who have lived a sedentary life the unwonted physical effort demanded of them in a Service gives rise to feelings of cardiovascular distress, which naturally become the focus of any uneasiness of mind that may arise from the problem of adjustment to military life. It is the old story of morbid anxiety tending to centre round the function that is most used.

It is in line with this interpretation that effort syndrome, or D.A.H., was almost unknown in flying personnel, who are more apt to become concerned about their eyes. It might even be said, aphoristically and without much exaggeration, that heterophoria is to the Air Force what D.A.H. is to the Army.

The types of neurotic disorder which occur are the same as those of civil life, but the factors involved are much more obvious and simple. Illness can be the result of failure to adapt to military conditions at any stage from enlistment to actual fighting. Enlistment itself demands a solution of a conflict between domestic ties and social obligations, and between self-interest and social prestige. Even when this primary difficulty is surmounted, an inadequate solution often paves the way for trouble later on. An example of this is furnished in an instance which came under our notice, of a man whose father was British but whose mother was German, and who was much under the latter's domination. He delayed enlisting in the British Army as long as possible and finally did so with a feeling of disloyalty to his mother. He obtained a commission, but had not been very long on service when he became depressed and irritable, and finally exhibited a fugue, after which he was sent home.

After enlistment comes the recruit's adaptation to his comrades; there also inadequacy could be a source of difficulty, either at the time or much later, as MacCurdy has shown. The greatest difficulty occurs when the front is reached, and the soldier has to manage his self-preservative tendencies, which come into conflict with his ideas of duty, loyalty and respect in the eyes of his fellows. The thought of dependents at home also produces a desire for escape. The ability to accustom oneself to scenes of carnage has been said to depend on the success attained in giving rein to the primitive desire to kill or maim the enemy. If any of these conflicts remains unsolved, the way is paved for a neurosis; desertion and malingering being impossible (except in rare exceptions), death or wounds are longed for, and the longing is often only imperfectly repressed. Consequently, when physical symptoms (such as tremor, tachycardia, diarrhoea and insomnia) do appear, either as the result of fear and horror or of some apparently physical experience, such as partial burial or the effect of a near-by explosion, they attract undue attention. They persist long after the apparently exciting cause has passed, because the conflict already present sustains and reinforces them and because also in certain instances they present a solution of the conflict. Deafness or blindness, for example, occurring momentarily at the time of an explosion, are obviously totally disabling if they persist as the result of auto-suggestion. As regards the more detailed psychopathology, there has been a tendency in psychoanalytic teaching to see in war neuroses an expression, not so much of the conflict between group demands and egotistic demands of self-preservation, as of the revival of infantile anxiety arising from insecure relationships with real or phantasied parents or their substitutes. This is more relevant to what might be called the neuroses of mobilization than of actual conduct.

In dealing with fatigue as a cause of symptoms in war neuroses, it has to be remembered that in civil life at least fatigue is much more commonly a symptom of a neurosis than a cause, and further, that the 'fatigue' symptoms described above in discussing the aetiology of war psychoses are not different in kind from neurotic symptoms. But fatigue and general bodily discomforts probably play an important rôle in lowering the morale, increasing the desire for escape, and at the same time impairing the resistance to it. MacCurdy found that fatigue was an almost universal factor in the production of anxiety states in soldiers observed by him.

The neurotic disorders of war may, for convenience, be divided into two stages. In the *acute stage*, which might follow the bursting of a shell, or some harrowing experience, the symptoms bore a superficial resemblance to those of genuine concussion (*vide supra*), the patient being in a condition which was described by MacCurdy as expressing the acme of fear, with dilated pupils, shallow breathing, violent tremor and incapacity for voluntary movement. 'Following this there is a phase when voluntary movement is possible, during which he is dazed, inactive, confused and amnesic, and may use gestures in place of speech.' Hallucinations sometimes occur, but there is no true loss of consciousness, and the entire picture is usually very transient, the condition developing into the more chronic one of an anxiety state or of hysteria. Babinski and Froment described a 'slight confusional syndrome' with suggestibility, in circumstances of great emotion; and such a condition would presumably afford an admirable opportunity for the beginning of, *e.g.* a hysterical paralysis. It is often exceedingly difficult, however, to differentiate acute stuporous states of the functional (emotional) kind from organic stupor. Disorders of undoubtedly hysterical nature may occur in actual trauma when blood appears in the cerebrospinal fluid; and the analogous occurrence of 'neurotic' manifestations in epidemic encephalitis has to be remembered.

The *more lasting neurotic disorders* follow the stuporous state described, or, more often, gradually develop independently. Not uncommonly they seem to begin after a latent period following some physical experience of a startling kind; but it is probable that in nearly all such cases the 'affective background' is present to begin with, and the explosion or what not had simply a suggestive effect which operated when some further strain was added. They fall into two main types, anxiety states and hysteria, and their symptomatology does not differ essentially from the similar illnesses of peace. In the anxiety cases battle-dreams are frequent and are always of a terrifying description, at least until convalescence is reached. Jumpiness is usually present. In the First World War it seems to have been universally agreed that anxiety states were found chiefly among officers, and hysteria almost exclusively among the rank and file. To account for this unexpected distribution, Rivers elaborated the theory that suggestion was more potent in the private, as the result of his disciplinary training, and that sublimation and repression played a larger part with the officer, who had a deeper sense of responsibility and duty and had to repress the display of his emotions to a greater extent. MacCurdy related the difference to the type of solution desired: the officer wished for death as the only solution compatible with honour, while a disabling wound was acceptable to the private. Differences in education, as Rivers suggested, probably had a share also.

States of Fear or Anxious Tension. It seems necessary to distinguish from true neurosis, states of chronic fear with resulting bodily or mental discomfort, such as lack of concentration, headache, palpitation, etc., usually with objective signs such as pallor, restlessness, lack of facial expressiveness and a rising consumption of cigarettes and alcohol. An individual in this condition may know quite well that he is afraid and that his discomforts arise from that cause; he can hardly be regarded as psychologically ill unless his discomforts become of such intensity as to disable him in action, or unless he comes to mistake his symptoms for those of bodily illness and to utilize them, consciously or unconsciously, as a means of avoiding duty. Until that happens such conditions are more correctly designated states of fear or of tension rather than neurosis. One distinguishing mark is that the neurotic condition persists even when no immediate danger threatens, while states of fear or anxious tension tend to show mainly or only when danger is to be expected within a few hours or days. It appears, however, that with repeated experience of frightening situations the condition may become habitual and the symptoms of it may persist at all times. This would explain the restless sleep and fearful dreams, and loss of weight over a long period, of some individuals of good morale persisting in their duty.

Associative or 'Conditioned' Fear-reaction. An individual who has had some very lurid experience in which he may have conducted himself perfectly well at the time, may afterwards, when faced with any threat of a repetition of the same experience, such as getting into an aeroplane again, develop symptoms of extreme apprehension to a disabling degree in spite of all his efforts to overcome them. The closest analogy appears to be that of the conditioned reflex.

It must not, however, be supposed that the phrase 'conditioned reflex' as it is usually understood accurately describes this state of affairs. It is not a simple reflex consisting in visual stimulus followed by emotional disturbance; it is the meaning of the situation that matters, whether the situation be the sound of an aeroplane or the sight of a falling bomb, or what not. As Massermann has pointed out, no conditioned reflex can be established except in the event of some instinctive interest being aroused, and in this case the instinct is that of self-preservation and the avoidance of danger. It has been noticed that any reminder of such a situation may produce the bodily reverberations of emotion but no conscious fear so long as the reminder itself does not indicate danger *now*. For example, a pilot on a country walk found his heart bounding suddenly although he felt no fear; he then noticed a smell of burning and realized that it reminded him of an aeroplane crash in which he had been involved and some of his comrades had been burned.

Desertion is sometimes accomplished by hysterical or other morbid mechanisms, but it is an unusual solution. The following is an example:

CASE NO. 58

A private in the R.A.M.C., aged 36, who had seen fourteen months' active service and who had been sent home in a nervous depressed condition, with headaches and sleeplessness, volunteered for service again in France. On being ordered to rejoin the Field

Ambulance he again began to suffer from headache, giddiness, sleeplessness. He remembered arriving at the railway station, but then 'something came over him', and he wandered away. On recovering himself he realized that he had committed a grave offence and determined to end his life. He remembered going into a billet where there were rifles and ammunition, and maintained that a rifle went off accidentally and shot him through the foot. This was probably an attempt at self-mutilation. For many weeks he remained sleepless, tremulous and depressed about his conduct.

Desertion also occurred in soldiers suffering from previously existing but unrecognized organic disease—*e.g.* cerebral contusion, general paralysis, subnormality, epilepsy and infection-exhaustion states, and as part of a manic-depressive or schizophrenic psychosis (Henderson). Amnesia following desertion is sometimes the result of panic with failure of perception at the time; but more often it is the excuse of a weak individual for leaving the post of danger, and is then akin to malingering.

My late colleague and collaborator, R. D. Gillespie, in his last-published paper (1945) discussed the aetiology and symptomatology of a group of cases which had interested him greatly. The paper embodied his experience while employed as Air Commodore with the R.A.F. He concluded that there were at least two types of neurotic response to a terrifying stimulus—one physiological and one psychological, occurring at different levels of personality integration. The response consists of a recurring dream or nightmare, and of a conditioned or associative response to stimuli resembling or in some way recalling the original experience. While the dream state usually disappears the conditioned response is apt to persist, but no doubt it too can be made to disappear by the use of suitable abreactive methods.

PREVENTION

This falls under two main heads: 1. selection; and 2. the maintenance of morale. The need for selection was recognized in the fighting Services of most of the belligerents. All recruits in this country now have a group intelligence test, which is successful in picking out nearly all the dullards. Those scoring below the agreed level are referred automatically to the psychiatrist for individual appraisement. The psychiatrist should not be guided by the result of intelligence tests alone, since tests even of the non-verbal type are influenced by factors other than innate ability. A social record indicating ability to stand on one's own feet in spite of a minimal intelligence score will allow a man or a woman to be placed within a Service in some non-combatant job of a more or less menial kind.

Subnormal persons who are either too dull for a Service at all, or who are in a job too difficult for them, betray themselves in a variety of ways—chiefly as unreliable and erratic in their work, to the extent of being a menace in a combatant unit and a nuisance in any other; as perpetrators of repeated offences against discipline, usually of a passive rather than an active kind, such as being absent without leave; as habitual attenders at sick parades for minor ailments; and as dirty and untidy in their personal appearance and more apt than the average to acquire venereal disease.

No diagnosis is more frequently missed by medical officers of units than that of mental dullness. Placed in jobs suitable to their mental limitations and supervised by selected N.C.O.'s, most dullards improve, sometimes remarkably, in their happiness and behaviour.

The British Army placed dullards in unarmed Pioneer Corps, where they were happy and useful, doing labouring work. The other Services have been able to utilize very dull individuals as kitchenmaids, dish-washers and the like. Nevertheless it is unlikely that anyone with an intelligence quotient of less than 50 will give satisfactory service. The prospect can usually be anticipated by perusing the social record, which shows an inability to obtain a job or to keep it for any length of time. A history of frequent changes of job for unsatisfactory reasons indicates usually dullness or psychopathy or a combination of dullness with temperamental instability. A psychopathic personality, if well pronounced, should usually also preclude acceptance, even if the individual is very intelligent. This should be the rule at least in instances where the psychopathy has shown itself not in any internal suffering but in failure to make a satisfactory adjustment to civil life. The hope that some psychiatrists have entertained that a disciplined Service would stabilize psychopathic personalities is certainly often, and perhaps usually, unfulfilled. Dullards on the whole, if not too dull, and if they are stable, may do better in a selected job in a Service than they do in civil life, because the régime is regular, employment is certain, and there is no unavoidable competition; but every case has to be judged on its merits, and what sways a decision towards acceptance or rejection is often the man-power situation.

A history of prolonged incapacity from mental illness at any time or from frequent disturbances of the psychosomatic sort (indigestion, fibrositis, etc.) or of chronic complaints of the same kind should raise grave doubts about acceptance —a fighting Service is not a sanatorium.

These observations apply to acceptance for Service as a whole, including the multifarious non-combatant jobs that are a necessary part of the structural organization of a modern fighting force.

A written questionnaire even of a simple kind will succeed in picking out the majority of such individuals for a psychiatric interview.

Previous civilian experience in a specific job acquired slowly over a long period of years may compensate for lack of ability, but where a skilled trade has to be learned quickly, intelligence tests are valuable in finding out those who are more likely to make the grade than those who are not. For such purposes a battery of tests consisting of verbal and form-perception tests, as well as tests of the ability to perceive relationships, *i.e.* non-verbal reasoning tests, is on the whole more useful than one type of test used alone. Arithmetic tests, although they have a scholastic appearance, are in fact among the most valuable as tests of general intelligence. All such tests are usually given in a group fashion as paper and pencil tests. It is possible by these means to assess the probability of an individual passing a given course of trade training, and of performing satisfactorily afterwards.

When individuals intellectually unequal to the job have been eliminated, the majority of the failures are due to temperamental instability of great or less degree, ranging from chronically anxious personalities to social psychopaths.

In the elimination or 'screening' of such people from skilled trades and higher responsibilities psychiatrists can be of service in collaboration with their psychologist brethren.

At the other end of the spectrum, as it were, there are the highly skilled jobs, for which selection according to both intelligence and temperamental attributes is highly desirable, although very difficult to do.

Experience has shown that while different jobs naturally require different levels of intelligence, the range of intelligence scores among those actually doing these jobs successfully is fairly wide, and that there is consequently a considerable overlap in the intelligence scores of individuals in one group of more skilled jobs in comparison with jobs above and below them in level of difficulty.

More difficult still is the selection of individuals for posts of executive responsibility, which in a Service usually means selection for commissioned rank in the first place. The Service officer is apt to be optimistic about individuals whose intelligence is, in fact, inadequate, partly because people who are not accustomed to dealing preponderantly with the intellectually or temperamentally inadequate have greater trust than is justified in the ability of individuals so handicapped to improve themselves by effort and education.

The less obvious sorts of defects of personality may, to the less skilled observer, be successfully concealed behind a façade of good manners or good looks or a fine physique. Difficult as the matter is, selection for commissioned rank can be helped by the use of intelligence tests and by psychiatric opinion.

TREATMENT

As regards methods of treatment, these may be defined as: 1. simple rest, in the sense of removal from the scene of battle or of enemy action; 2. psychotherapy; and 3. physical methods, especially sedation. Mere removal from the scene of action for a time may be sufficient, especially where fatigue, which is so prominent in war, has played a part. It can also be enough in a certain proportion of individuals who have been exposed to a very disturbing situation and received a severe fright, provided at least that they had a good previous personality and have a sound morale.

Psychotherapy is applicable mainly to those who develop transient states of anxiety, hysterical disabilities and amnesias, while physical sedation, by means of hypnotics, usually of the barbiturate group, is indicated in states of emotional disturbance of recent origin, and sometimes in chronic anxiety states and depressions following exposure to danger.

Naturally all three methods may be usefully combined in individual cases. In states of acute fright or panic with generalized tremor, staring eyes, and sometimes total immobility and mutism, and with severe insomnia and terrifying dreams which wake the patient up very soon after he drowses off, sedation of any degree up to continuous narcosis, by any of the usual methods, from twenty-four hours upwards according to the severity of the case, is the best method. In less acute states of fear immediately following a disturbing experience, emphatic reassurance and persuasion, together with an hypnotic at bedtime, may prevent the continuance of anxious tension, or the hysterical perpetuation of symptoms.

For psychogenic amnesias brief mild narcosis with thiopentone or amylobarbitone sodium will serve as a means both of rapid recovery of the repressed memory of a traumatic experience and as a method of suggestion to remove hysterical symptoms connected with the experience. The advantages over hypnosis possessed by narcosis of this type are some saving of time, and greater certainty of success, because it gives the doctor himself more confidence. In some cases it works simply by giving the patient a tangible excuse for sharing with the doctor the memory of experiences that he professes to have forgotten. But this observation applies more to the amnesia that is protective of self-esteem and not to amnesia arising from sheer terror in the automatic attempt to protect oneself from the mental pain of it. If the patient is seen early enough after the traumatic experience, it is possible to prevent the development of amnesia by persuading him to recount the history of what he has gone through.

In some chronic states of anxiety, prolonged narcosis has been found helpful in promoting improvement, especially in those who have got into a rut, but it is not to be expected that such treatment will enable those to return to active service who would not otherwise have done so in the course of a slightly longer time; in other words, in individuals whose temperament and personality are in themselves such as to make a return to full duty unlikely.

For neurotic reactions of minor intensity simple explanation and persuasion are sufficient, at least in individuals of good morale. Very often it is not desirable to remove such people, even temporarily, from the scene of action. It has to be remembered that it was noticed in the First World War that the farther a soldier with neurotic symptoms was transported from the front, and the longer the symptoms had existed before treatment was begun, the more frequently he had to be removed also from the prospect of a return to active service: the percentage of neurotics who returned to the front from base hospitals and did not relapse was extremely small. On the other hand, of those treated at casualty clearing stations or field hospitals, 70 per cent. were said to have been returned rapidly and successfully to the front. It is obvious that discipline and the atmosphere of mass suggestion which comes from standing 'shoulder to shoulder', as Farrar puts it, are important psychotherapeutically.

It is a matter of experience to know how much firmness to combine with an understanding attitude. Clearly the medical officer has to avoid the appearance of furnishing an easy escape from duty. Some individuals will confess to the medical officer their resolve not to return to the post of danger. Such individuals frequently do not profess any symptoms. The matter then becomes one for the executive branch, unless the M.O. is fully convinced that the symptoms are of sufficient severity to constitute disablement in themselves, in which case evacuation to a hospital is justified. In a base hospital it was noticed that hysterical symptoms were very favourably influenced by the withdrawal of privileges, *e.g.* of receiving visits or of being allowed recreation outside the hospital grounds.

On the whole it may be said that the greater the external stress, the better the prognosis. Where fatigue rather than fear has been the important factor the prognosis is also usually favourable. It is, however, important to estimate the personality, both in its liabilities and its assets. The prognosis depends on this much more than on the nature of the symptoms, although on the whole it can be said that the prognosis for states of anxiety is better than for hysterical reactions, which develop very readily in people with inadequate motivation and with a special capacity for self-deception.

In special hospitals for the treatment of psychiatric casualties it is essential to have a well-organized régime of recreation, physical training, organized games and social activities. Not only is rumination thereby forestalled as far as possible but the general morale of the patient is improved. Many patients like to feel that part of their day is spent constructively, and for this purpose farming and other occupations not reminding them of the war are helpful. The prescription of a suitable occupation, however, is an individual matter. There are some individuals who are inclined to regard hospital life of this kind as a pleasant alternative to duty and develop a vested interest in remaining there. It is therefore important to establish the tradition of a fairly rapid turn-over.

In depressions of the constitutional type, electric convulsion therapy is obviously applicable, but it is necessary to consider carefully before applying it in Service personnel. A considerable proportion of the depressions that are seen are precipitated by fatigue and external stress and make a quick recovery in any event. A depressive illness is apt to recur and in its early stages to be subtle and undetected, and therefore a source of possible risk that cannot be provided against except by excluding the patient from further responsible duties.

In individuals who have lost weight, fattening by insulin has been found useful in improving both the physical condition and to some extent the mental state, where this is mainly anxious or mainly depressive in nature (Sargant, 1942).

PSYCHIATRIC CASUALTIES AMONG CIVILIANS

Psychiatric disorders attributable to air raids have been remarkably few. As far as can be measured by absenteeism during 'blitz' conditions there was no appreciable increase; absenteeism in fact was rather less in some large firms than before (Gillespie, 1942). Of 2306 patients admitted to the Sutton Emergency Hospital serving one of the London areas between September 2, 1939, and August 31, 1941, only 283 were civilian casualties, and of these only 41 were attributable to the effects of air raids (L. Minski). A survey of conditions in general practice at this time revealed only a slight increase, and that mostly among people who had previously suffered from psychological disability of some kind (Lewis, 1942).

Clinically the immediate reactions induced were terror, panic and stupor, the last being an immobility reaction, comparable perhaps to the defensive immobility of animals threatened with attack.

In children the same general observations held; they took their cue largely from the adults around them. When anxiety was displayed by children in connection with air raids it has been attributed to the reactivated fear of their own aggressive impulses and of retributory punishment for their own phantasied misdeeds. It has even been suggested that they were relatively immune from fears engendered by threats of enemy attack, since, in their games, they developed methods of mastering their anxiety during the 'blitz' period; they became interested in playing war games of bombing, etc., without any sense of fear but with a feeling of excitement.

A number of people who showed no abnormal reaction during an air raid itself developed anxiety or hysterical symptoms some days afterwards. This was related to the severity of the experience and especially to their degree of pre-disposition. It is probable that disorganization of their pattern of living, from loss of relatives, home, etc., plays a larger part in many such after-effects than the experience itself. Psychotic patients are singularly unmoved by threats to their safety.

In children the effects of separation from parents and the like are much more pernicious than the effects of exposure to danger. It has been calculated that during the Second World War there was a slight increase of neurotic disorders among children of the order of about 5 per cent. Even here, however, it was more often a question of revival of pre-existing trends than the creation of new ones. Such problems were, of course, mostly seen in areas to which children had been evacuated for safety's sake. Enuresis and behaviour disorders were what came mostly to notice, since they were the difficulties that were most evident to foster-parents and others. What the ultimate damage may be as the result of the dis-ruption of emotional ties at a crucial stage of the development of the child's emotional life remains to be seen in the future years.

As regards after-effects of air-raid experience in children it was found that about 4 per cent. of 8000 school children in Bristol exhibited symptoms. Some months afterwards it was calculated that about 11 per cent. had symptoms sug-gesting a development of disturbance after a latent period. All these were children under $5\frac{1}{2}$ years (Bodman, 1941).

Other possible effects of war conditions are suggested by Mira's observation on the mental effects of starvation. 'People who would stand their ground in the food queues in an air raid, would become desperate or hopeless when they failed to get the promised amount of bread or other nourishment. Butter was quite as important as guns.'

REFERENCES

Bodman, F. (1941) *Brit. med. J.*, **2**, 486.
Gillespie, R. D. (1942) *Psychological Effects of War*, New York.
Gillespie, R. D. (1945) *Brit. med. J.*, **1**, 653.
Henderson, D. K., and Gillespie, R. D. (1923) *Amer. J. Psychiat.*, **3**, 175.
Lewis, A. J. (1942) *Lancet*, ii, 13.
Sargant, W. (1942) *Brit. med. J.*, **2**, 574.

19

THE PSYCHIATRY OF CHILDHOOD

PRINCIPAL CHARACTERISTICS OF CHILD PSYCHOPATHOLOGY

Three cardinal points exist for discussion in the psychology of children, in distinction from adults, as far as a distinction in this field can be drawn. They are: first, the enormous influence of environment on the child's mental processes; second, the plasticity of the latter; and third, the prominence of egoistic tendencies—their substitution and frustration—in the production of symptoms.

Influence of Environment

Environment means, of course, the personal environment of parents, brothers, sisters, teachers and companions; and an important reflection occurs here, that when signs of morbidity appear, they arise at the surface of contact, so to speak, of the child's environment with his aims and desires, rather than at some locus of conflict deeply within the psyche. It is far more often a question of some direct frustration than of an intrapsychic conflict.

This is a generalization which admits exceptions, but it is of sufficient importance in theory, and especially in practice, to warrant expansive discussion. For instance, it connotes that relatively simple adjustments of the environment, after careful consideration of the tendencies whose frustration or misdirection are indicated by the symptoms, will cause the latter to disappear, and that intensive intrapsychic exploration of the child's mind is usually unnecessary. Hence the psychiatrist's method of exploring the problem principally through interviews with parents and other adults more than with the child has its justification. There is, however, a small residue of cases in which intensive exploration is desirable.

Plasticity

The second point, the plasticity of the attitude and behaviour of children, is another aspect of the first, and is of immense practical and theoretical importance, although the plasticity is limited to some degree by inborn disposition and temperament. In the adult the problem of adjustment is complicated by the existence of a long accumulation of habits and attitudes, of the origin of most of which the subject is unconscious at the time the causal factors operate. In the child this accumulation is naturally much less, and even those attributes with the longest history are comparatively unfixed. The practical importance of the consequent plasticity lies not only in the management of nervous children, but in the prevention of neurotic and psychotic disorders in later life. There are two principal psychopathological views of the aetiology of adult mental illnesses. Both of them place the primary focus in the formative influences of childhood; but one view to which much attention has been paid in this book regards the adult illness as the cumulative result of mental habits acquired and ingrained throughout childhood and adolescence; while the other regards it as a regression to particular emotional fixations or attachments of an erotic kind at the same period. The apparent divergence of views lies perhaps more in emphasis and terminology; but they certainly agree in acknowledging the importance of early factors. It seems to us, however, that in its insistence on a set pattern, the Oedipus pattern in the infantile foundation of neuroses, the second view does less justice than the first to the almost infinite plasticity of the young organism's mental and emotional equipment, the wide variety of the influences that impinge upon it, and the multiplicity of its responses. This belief receives support from an unexpected quarter—so experienced a child analyst as Anna Freud has to confess that she has failed to observe directly in the children she has treated the developmental situations in the first two years of life classically considered by psychoanalysis as at the root of adult neuroses. She meets this by saying that the material presented by the child furnishes 'clear and unequivocal clues to the foundation of the infantile neurosis', but that the absence of the reaction-formations and cover-memories of the latency period deprives the child analyst of the material which alone furnishes the psychoanalytic data. The pre-speech period remains inaccessible—the analysts would say, not because the material was not there, but because in children it has not had time to be formulated. It would also be possible to suppose that the psychoanalytic situations were not commonly important at that age, and that the memories in most instances were relevant only to later neuroses.

Whatever view be taken, the plastic trend of childhood remains highly significant for the prophylaxis of adult neuroses, but the more immediate practical importance of the plasticity lies in the improvement that follows treatment in 'nervous children' generally. This therapeutic response is so marked and so invariable where it can be expected that the reflection readily arises that so called 'nervous children' would usually get better of themselves without the aid of the clinic. Indeed, while giving proper weight to the immense effect of the child's environment in producing psychological disturbances in him, it is necessary to remember that all children are subjected to innumerable traumata, and the wonder is, not how many nervous and unstable children there are, but what a large proportion grow to be reasonably normal men and women.

Rôle of Innate Factors

But just as too much optimism may lead to a policy of *laissez faire* on the ground of the self-adjustment of the majority of psychopathological phenomena in children, so, on the other hand, may a pessimism preconceived on the score of the importance and immutability of inborn temperament and disposition lead to a failure to grasp numerous possibilities of modification, for the limitations produced by inborn factors are much less than is usually believed. It is a sound working rule to attribute nothing morbid, whether of behaviour, mood or thought, to congenital and therefore, presumably, less modifiable causes until a complete investigation has revealed nothing in the history of environmental influences and personal events that will reasonably account for the symptoms, and until the latter have proved but little modifiable by any known therapy; and even then the matter may not have been congenitally engraved.

A further point is the profound interconnection between mental and physical factors in the child. Even more than in the adult, the emotions influence bodily processes and vice versa. Not only do the various bodily functions have a lower threshold of irritability than in the adult, but the autonomic nervous system in particular appears to be less stable. Thus 'psychosomatic' reactions and disorders of various kinds are common, especially in children of sensitive, excitable disposition and often of above average intelligence. In addition to the same kinds of psychosomatic syndromes as one encounters in the adult, more superficial and transient reactions are commonly found, such as the vomiting which may precede parties or examinations.

With these general reflections we may proceed to a brief discussion of psychopathology as it applies to children. The intrinsic psychological factors are conveniently discussed first.

The Egoistic Tendencies

It is customary to designate the thinking of the young child as essentially egocentric. Quoting Piaget's example, we would say that for the child the sun or the moon appears to follow him wherever he goes; at first there is no thought of reconciling this relationship with the sun's possible appearance to other persons. But this is merely the more intellectual aspect of the general tendency and orientation of the child—he is not merely egocentric but egoistic. Growing up, psychologically, consists in a progressive diminution in egoism, and a corresponding socialization of derivatives of the instinctive tendencies, egoistic and other.

This egoism implies many things—a drive towards self-assertion in all regions of living, including therefore a desire for affection and approbation, a tendency towards self-display, a craving for personal prominence, rivalry with others and jealousy of them; and, on the other hand, a persistent awareness, dimly or not at all consciously formulated, of a lack of personal security. It is a cardinal principle of treatment that this many-sided egoism must have outlets, but they must be healthy, and such as are socially acceptable and adapted to the chronological stage of development. Mental growth is one long conflict between the demands of natural egoism and the conditions of the environment; but it need not be a painful conflict except at intervals. A very large proportion of children, and the grown-up children we call adults, who are brought for treatment are, however, suffering from the pains of this strife. Very often the pains are far more acute than is needful, since the parents, for reasons later to be explained, have begun by indulging the egoism. Hence the child finds on entering school or going among his coevals in any way, that the contrast is too sharp for him to bear, and so he develops truancy, or anxiety, or outbursts of temper, or hypochondriacal aches or pains. Along with egoism, and as an example of that bipolarity which is characteristic of so many aspects of the mind, there goes a feeling of helplessness and insignificance, the famous 'feeling of inferiority' which colours so many of the child's reactions as well as of the adult's.

The egoistic trends, like so many of the other childish characteristics, have a high degree of plasticity. It is usual to speak of this plasticity in its relationships to persons as suggestibility, and where an element of conscious volition enters as 'imitation'. The suggestibility can appear in relation to anyone in the environment, but especially towards those with whom bonds of affection exist, and towards those who are older or who for some reason possess prestige. Naturally the parents and their substitutes, as the most ordinary objects in the environment, and the mother especially as the most intimate, are potentially the mightiest factors of this kind. The nervous disorders of childhood, which are not dependent considerably or entirely on errors in parental example or attitude, and which cannot be greatly improved by modifying that attitude or example, are in the minority. The point is also usefully considered, however, from the aspect of abnormalities in the parents, which will be summarily discussed later. In the meantime, let us recall that the automatically suggested example of the parents and elders and companions becomes gradually embedded in the child's mind, sometimes reaching conscious expression as the ideal ego, but more often operating quietly and unconsciously to modify the conduct (the super-ego or the unconscious conscience, see Chapter 7). Not all, however, of parental example and precept is incorporated in this way. Some of it is rejected, and may even provoke the opposite reaction to that desired (negativism or counter suggestibility), the result of egoistic aims coming into too direct collision with environmental demands. Negativism is apt to grow and flourish upon increase in the environmental resistance, on the principle, as it were, that every action produces an equal and opposite reaction; and, like many mental reactions, negativism may continue to operate automatically as a habit, in apparent independence of any connection with its original stimulus. Hence it comes about that the most rigid disciplinarian among parents may produce the most stubborn children. This general tendency towards conflict between egoism and the environment naturally has its foci of special concentration. The regulation of any special manifestation of the self-assertive tendencies along a social channel, or the relinquishing of any form of pleasure not socially permissible, can form such a focus. In accordance with his general theory, Freud attached importance principally to the conflict produced by enforced relinquishment, especially, of activities of a sensuous or, in the Freudian sense, erotic kind. Hence weaning and the education of the bladder, and especially the bowel function, become, on this theory, the critical points of development of temperament and character, and so also in the determination of the pattern of future reactions. Thus an unusual difficulty round the relinquishment of 'anal pleasure' (either from accidental accentuation of the latter, or from innate factors) is held to lead by 'reaction-formation' to traits of obstinacy (persistent negativism). This view differs from that encouraged by observation of the reactions of children, in attributing obstinacy specially to anal erotism instead of regarding it, as we do, as a reaction which may arise and persist as the result of mismanagement of any phase of development, of egoism generally or of its specific manifestations.

Negativistic conduct, being the outcome of aroused egoism, can naturally

21

minister to egoism in a high degree. Temper tantrums, for example, serve the double purpose of avoiding some duty of accommodation of one's wishes to others, and of self-display. Some investigators consider that there is a definite crisis in the adjustment of the infantile egoism to society between the ages of three and five, and that if this stage is not properly managed, obstinacy may persist as an unusually prominent personal characteristic.

It has been a favourite phantasy of mankind that the original state was one of happiness and universal love. Mythology and religion alike tell of a 'Golden Age' when the world was young. English men of letters of the eighteenth century and later were fond of referring to the 'noble savage'. There are not wanting psychopathological grounds for seeing in this an unconscious desire for a return, on the part of those who advocate these views, to the 'Golden Age' of their own childhood, when all was (as they now believe) as they wished, and only ties of affection governed their relations to other men. It is a fact that affection is the readiest response of the infant and young child to other individuals; but as the latter do not always minister to his needs, and may even frustrate them, it is not difficult for the corresponding opposite to appear, namely, hatred or some degree of it. This may lead to a cordial death wish towards the obnoxious person. Death does not mean very much to a child; it represents disappearance as far as he is concerned; the antagonist is no longer in the path. Such feelings of hate, however, appear much more readily in relation to rivals, or, in other words, as jealousy, with results which have been exemplified above. In a wider circle than the family we find hatred combined with negativism to produce an attitude of hostility to the social group in which the child finds himself—especially his or her companions at school and the neighbouring children. Not infrequently a child is sent to a clinic with the label from school, 'Dangerous to others': we have known such a label to be attached to a six-year-old. The child had been sticking pins in others, or 'going for' their eyes or hitting them with slight or no apparent provocation. Usually such a child comes of a bad home, and is often reproducing the attitude to the world of school which it found meted out to it by its parents—hatred showing itself in verbal or corporal chastisement or in other ways. Sometimes, of course, it is a direct retaliation for attitudes assumed by school-mates towards someone recognized as not belonging to their particular herd—children coming from some other country or another race; or some personal peculiarity, especially of such a type as Fröhlich's syndrome, may produce ridicule which stings the child to retaliation. As the majority of children are timid in face of much show of physical aggression by their comrades, another factor begins to act; the aggressor finds that he can dominate in this way, and so compensates doubly for his own felt inferiority. More often than is usually suspected a desire to dominate other children shows itself also in subtle ways, as in a girl of twelve who managed to impress and frighten a class-mate and competitor in such a way that the latter was miserable and consequently did her work badly, so allowing the tormentor to bear the palm.

In vindictive behaviour such as this there sometimes enters a definite element of cruelty. There is no doubt that all children possess a capacity for cruelty, but it is not commonly shown to any marked degree, and then only transiently as a rule. There is equally no doubt that behind such manifestations of cruelty lies a certain feeling of pleasure. Cruelty, however, except in cases of certain subnormal (mentally defective) and psychopathic children, nearly always yields to kindly depreciation and provision of other outlets.

The inner development of egoistic feeling determines, almost independently of outside influences, phantasies of power and importance. The upbringing of most young children favours this, for at first the baby is usually the centre of his little world and he does not readily relinquish the feeling so engendered. The couplet,

'I do not love the human race,
I do not like its ugly face',

covers the survival in many adults of the results of the clash of reality which is felt to interfere unpleasantly with the infantile omnipotence (the Jehovah-complex, or God-complex, of the Freudians; the 'almightiness' of Adlerian usage, and the root of many phantasies and mannerisms of everyday life). But in children it is not a 'complex' in the morbid sense, but a normal state of affairs. The feeling of importance usually undergoes correction in the light of experience, as long as no close rival appears on the scene. But let a younger brother or sister appear before the elder child has outgrown the phase of wanting everything in his environment for his own delectation; then the signs of jealousy readily appear. One small girl was found to have banged her baby brother's head on the gas stove and at another time to have emptied him from his pram into the roadway, while yet another was discovered pulling the baby sister's hair and spitting on her face as the baby lay in her cot. Instances of that sort, less pronounced as a rule, are numberless.

The notion of power and omnipotence is closely linked with the unreality feelings, which are far more common in children than is usually realized. The latter present in a way the reverse side of the picture, and result from the contrast of a small being, suddenly aware of his own comparative insignificance, with the overwhelming immensity of the external world of space and time. The more intense the notion of power has been, the more intensely this contrast is felt, and the greater the resulting anxiety, reinforced, sometimes at least, by feelings of remorse for having provoked the external forces, often regarded at this age implicitly, if not explicitly, in a demoniacal light.

The Sexual Instinct and its Ramifications

Of the tendency of children to develop affectionate attachments to persons of either sex, everyone is aware, but it is difficult to differentiate their attitude to persons of the same sex from that shown towards persons of the opposite sex. The same elements of interest and regard and affectionate dependence are evident in either case, but what sex the choice is focused on seems to be a matter of circumstance. Much has been said of the tendency of a boy to prefer his mother, and a girl her father, but from infancy a strong preference for the parent of the same sex is not infrequently observed. This can sometimes depend on the attitude of the parents eliciting a differential response in the child. Similar factors can determine to some extent the attachments formed outside the family; thus males are chosen by small girls as substitutes for unaffectionate fathers.

To say, however, that any considerable proportion of the relationships just discussed have a sexual aspect, conscious or unconscious, in the sense of adult sexuality is still a large assumption; and to say further that such attachments, or the repression of these attachments upon a sexual basis, is the root cause of the symptoms of many of the persistent nervous disturbances in children is not yet justifiable. No one can deny the existence of infantile and childish sex manifestations, but their place in the psychopathology of childhood is another matter.

Parent-Child Relationships

It is a commonplace that the relationship of parent to child is of maximal importance for the shaping of character; it is of no less weight in the production of psychopathological deviations in childhood. The factors of dependence, imitation and suggestion already mentioned, with their complication in action and reaction, are of primary importance. There are two parental attitudes that are specially common, the over-anxious mother and the domineering father over-keen for the progress and advancement of his son. The father who expects his son to conform closely to his own desires and aspirations, and shows it, often succeeds in producing either a weak-kneed creature lacking in initiative, readily depressed and filled with morbid fears, or an unstable truant, or a sullen, defiant and sometimes furtive individual, who steals and goes with 'rough boys'.

The 'babying parent' is a caricature of the over-anxious one and may produce either the same namby-pamby type, or, in turn, frank rebellion. It is not very uncommon to find mothers who help at their son's bath until he is 16 or 17, and we have even encountered a father who was frequently present at the same function with his daughter of 16. A father of this type dandled his daughter on his knee and wrote poetry about her and with her, from her childhood into adolescence; her subsequent schizophrenic psychosis was strongly tinged with feelings of guilt towards him. 'Babying' of this kind has obvious sexual connotations, but at an earlier age these connotations do not usually enter. A mother's insistence on having her child sleep in the same room as the parents after the period of infancy can heighten a child's feeling of insecurity, increase his fears and fill him with an uncomfortable curiosity. It can also foster a close attachment of the child to the mother which can seriously hinder adaptation to marriage in later life.

'Spoiling' in the sense of indulgence and lack of discipline is a commonplace as a cause of childish misbehaviour, as well as of difficulty in after life. Of it are born temper tantrums, food fads, ostentation, mannerisms, tearfulness, jealousy and the like.

At the opposite extreme of these instances is that of the parent of an unwanted child, which, in consequence of the lack of love or actual spitefulness of its parent, displays similar traits in itself.

Parental dissatisfactions have, however, subtler consequences than this. A parent dissatisfied with his or her own life wants to see his or her own unfulfilled longings gratified in the children. A father expects his son to excel at games, and is annoyed, and the boy correspondingly depressed, when the expectations are not fulfilled; and at a later stage choice of occupation may be unfortunately regulated from the same motive. A young woman who has had an unhappy experience in relation to her own mother, tries to make her companionship with her offspring 'perfect', and so blocks out the possibility of her child making the fullest use of friendships with coevals. Or she may be unhappy in her marriage and seek emotional compensation in excessive devotion from her child, with a resulting conflict in the latter, and its consequences in fears or compulsions. Parental rejection, no matter how carefully disguised, is felt by the child as a lack of the affection it craves, and it is a frequent factor in producing psychological disturbances.

The grandparents (and over-indulgent uncles and aunts) can also have important formative, or, rather, deformative, influences on a child's life—especially if parents and grandparents happen to live together, as occurs fairly often in the houses of the poor. It is possible for a grandparent to be on more friendly terms with a child than its own parents, and it is equally possible for a grandparent to appear as a destructive kind of ogre and spoil-sport. It is not uncommon to find parents and grandparents differing openly in their attitude to the child, from personal prejudice and from the result of old-standing conflicts between them, with the result that the child's training and standards are impaired, and he learns to play off one generation against the other.

Difficulties found Primarily at School

Of these the most common, but even yet often undetected, is scholastic backwardness, of all degrees from mere dullness to obvious subnormality (mental defect). Naturally, cases of severe subnormality announce themselves early, and if they appear in school at all are not long left there. But not infrequently with the dull and backward, or the subnormal, the first sign of anything amiss is some form of misbehaviour. Naturally, the child who is not capable of the average school work for his years becomes either uninterested, anxious and humiliated, or openly rebellious. Rarer and more localized forms of congenital handicap, like word-deafness and word-blindness, are still more readily missed, being mistaken for subnormality.

When intelligence testing first became popular, much was made of the idea of the possible discovery by this means of hidden talent, and even of genius. Expectations of this kind are only rarely borne out, but occasional instances of persistent ill-behaviour, or even apparent scholastic backwardness, are found, which depend on a child's being included in a class where the work is far below the level of his intelligence.

Emotional factors count no less than intellectual ones in the production of symptoms of unrest at school. Naturally, emotional conflicts at home may disturb the attitude at school, but much more rarely than would be expected. The school itself affords emotional difficulties *sui generis*.' Differential behaviour', *i.e.* a good report from school as compared with a bad one from home, or vice versa, is a valuable diagnostic aid. The child has to adapt to school-fellows as well as teachers—from both he begins by expecting the same kind of attitude as he experienced from members of the family. Disappointment in some degree is inevitable and may intensify a previous feeling of uncertainty and inferiority. But this will rarely reach pathological dimensions unless the soil has been prepared by unhappy relationships at home, or unless the teachers themselves adopt a mistaken attitude. The latter is not uncommon, but should never be inevitable. Large classes, while valuable in one way in reducing the chance of perpetuating 'spoiled' and similar reactions, operate against individual understanding when any preliminary difficulties have already appeared. It is not an uncommon experience to find a child given a bad name by schoolmasters, which in itself serves the worst possible purpose.

As with parents, so with teachers—dissatisfactions and morbid attitudes of their own may produce morbid reactions in the children under their care. A love of power, or sometimes actually sadistic trends, show themselves in teasing, bullying and stupid forms of punishment. Such minor manifestations of lack of the proper relationship between teacher and pupil as impatience, frequent criticism and heavy reproof in front of others and the like, can have a considerable effect in producing difficulties both of scholarship and behaviour. An attitude of a too affectionate kind on the part of the child depends for its results on the response of the teacher, who, if wise, may turn it to good account. Such attitudes frequently have, consciously or unconsciously, an erotic basis, and more is heard of them when this basis is of a homosexual kind; but heterosexual attachments, limited naturally by the arrangements of things in schools to preferences of female teachers for certain pupils, are commoner than is supposed, and account for some instances of favouritism, which is the equivalent in school of spoiling at home. Naturally such attitudes have a specious maternal look, and the ill-effect on the child is simply the ill-effect of most-favoured-nation treatment. All these possible variants of the relationship between child and school are fraught with greater importance in boarding-school than in day-school. A general observation is opportune: that just as the usual type of scholastic education suits one child far better than another, so does boarding-school vary in its value in comparison with day-school with various types of children. The choice of a suitable school is of enormous importance for the nervous child.

METHODS OF INVESTIGATION

These differ considerably in some respects from the methods used in adult mental and nervous illness, for two principal reasons, that the average child is even less conscious of his own mental processes than the average adult, and for this reason does not readily communicate material that is of value; and secondly, that since in practice it is found that so much can be done principally by manipulation of the environment, it is not necessary as a rule to attempt to probe the child's mental life too closely or in too great detail. The general principle is to make the lines of inquiry as broad as possible, by including school reports and (in clinic practice) a report from a social worker, visiting both home and school, as well as the evidence obtained from parents and from the child himself.

Since a child practically never seeks advice of its own accord, it is from the parent or guardian, or from the school, that the information about the 'complaints' or symptoms is obtained. This should be recorded in detail, and inquiries extended to all the fields of possible unrest mentioned in the subjoined classification. A history of the child from its earliest days is then taken, both with regard to physical development and physical illnesses, and with special reference to landmarks in mental and nervous development. The times of beginning to walk and talk are of great importance, and, of a very young child, of beginning to support its head, to sit up and to crawl. Of lesser importance is the date when bladder control in the day-time was obtained. Normally a child holds up its head at four months, can sit up unsupported at six months, can walk and talk by not later than two years, and can control the bladder sphincter by day and night at the latest at three years of age. In some exceptional cases talking has been delayed even as late as five years, without subsequent intellectual retardation, but usually a very considerable proportionate retardation in any of these functions beyond the times mentioned is evidence of subnormality. The dates of more educational and less intrinsic significance are those of sleeping alone, of first being allowed out to play with other children, and of going to school.

Then follows an inquiry directed to the family relationships—the number of brothers and sisters, their personalities and the place of the child in the family—whether eldest, youngest or what. Attempts have been made to demonstrate statistically that eldest and youngest children are more prone to maladjustment than children in other positions in the family series. Levy has shown that eldest children are slightly more liable to suffer generally; while only children are more likely to be victims of parental over-solicitude and ambition.

The actual sleeping arrangements (hours of sleep and whether alone or with brothers or sisters or with parents) and the history of these is to be ascertained, and behind any peculiarities the reasons for them (accommodation or parental wishes).

It is necessary to have particulars about play—whether the child is allowed to play with other children, at home or outside; whether he prefers to play alone; and the types of play he prefers (e.g. a girl, aged 6, preferred to amuse herself by shooting and killing tin soldiers, which was on a par with her behaviour to others).

Information about the parents themselves is naturally one of the most important lines of inquiry. They should be interviewed alone, as well as together (if possible), and a kindly attitude will usually prompt confidences about their own lives which may throw considerable light on the symptoms of the child. Tact is very necessary, since they are often naturally sensitive about their failures with the child. It may be possible to discover whether the child was wanted, whether the parents co-operate in training it and in their discipline, and what place the child is occupying in the mind of each parent with regard to the other. The grandparents are also of importance, not only because they had so much to do with forming the parents' character, but because they frequently intervene, deliberately or not, in the upbringing of the grandchildren. Not uncommonly a relationship which is more pleasing to the child can be found with its grand-parents than with its own immediate parents.

Stepchildren seem, from experience, more likely to come under the psychiatrist's care than when the parents still survive and live together; and the children of 'broken homes' are also more prone to do so.

The economic status of the family, the size of house and other facts of this order are often of much importance.

In all these fields of investigation the services of a social worker are invaluable, and for carrying out parts of the treatment, in hospitals and clinics at least, indispensable. She can arrange either to do this herself or by co-operation with some social agency outside the hospital or clinic, always of course under the psychiatrist's ultimate direction.

Not least in all this routine, and in spite of the reservation made at the beginning, is contact with the child himself. We say 'contact' advisedly, because we do not plunge into an investigation of the child, but rather seek to establish a friendly relationship. After that has been accomplished, and it can be done remarkably quickly with most children, since they are naturally friendly, it is possible with surprising frequency to get the patient to talk about his difficulties. This talk may not be very free, or, if it is free, it is usually superficial, but it is often illuminating. Even when deception enters, the fact of deception itself is of great interest; its evaluation can follow in the light of discoveries from other sources. In younger children it has to be remembered that denial has the rank of phantasy—the child readily believes his own statement, once made.

A child, however, cannot stand prolonged conversations. They are boring for him after a short time, unless something else is introduced. The natural thing to introduce is play. It is also the easiest way to study the child, as he is off his guard, at least to some extent, even if it is with a doctor or a member of the clinic staff that he plays. Strictly speaking, it is not necessary to institute observation during play for the investigation of the majority of problem children, but as we desire to know as much about the children as possible, we arrange play-time with a member of the clinic staff, if not with the psychiatrist himself, wherever possible. Organized play can be of three types—games with other children, where the social reactions can be studied; games of the solitary type, such as building bricks, Meccano and the like, cutting out shapes, plasticine modelling, dolls, toy soldiers; and aesthetic and intellectual pursuits—drawing, painting and story-telling (oral and written). All these give additional sidelights on a child's character and problems, as well as providing him with outlets and modes of expression, untrammelled by criticism.

For cases not yielding to these methods, and for those not likely to be satisfactorily treated by them, such as neurotic anxiety states not dependent on environmental influences, obsessive compulsive neuroses, and some behaviour disorders (e.g. cases of truancy, and stealing not resolvable in environmental terms or in terms of personality organization), play technique, either interpretative or non-interpretative, is indicated. It is in many cases, even of the apparently obscure kind, worth trying the simpler methods first, since often they are capable of subsiding in a surprising way in response to simple measures, *e.g.* physical or psychological alteration of the environment.

Play Technique

The method of studying the child when he is playing, and of making use of well-controlled interpretations based on his play, is the method of choice in any case requiring intensive study rather than environmental manipulation. For example, if a child of a family consisting of father, mother and two daughters is supplied with dolls to represent each of these, the child may proceed to a play in which the dolls clearly represent its own attitude to its parents. For example, one little girl who was very jealous of her younger brother, when given two dolls of different ages, used invariably to smack the face of the smaller one within a few minutes. In this case the interpretation told us nothing new, but the principle involved may lead to interesting discoveries in more complicated settings.

In brief, we should always remember to take account both of environmental factors and inner mental processes, and welcome any method, however indirect, of getting at the latter; for in a child this is a specially difficult task and a direct approach is of very limited value, being handicapped in many ways by the child's reserve and his lack of verbal formulation of his problems.

Materials. The materials for a more extended use of play as a means of discovering the contents of a child's mind include such primitive materials as sand and water; plasticine for modelling into objects of interest or curiosity; articles capable of functioning as power symbols such as toy motor-cars and engines; others such as toy guns or animals capable of symbolizing aggressive impulses; objects with direct or indirect reference to excretory functions such as toy lavatories, watering-cans, etc.; and pencil and paper. Such materials give a wide range of opportunity for the expression of aggressive, excretory and sexual impulses, and together are capable of expressing most of the child's interests.

Interpretative Technique. The degree to which the use made of these materials by the child can be utilized for the understanding of his or her inner interests and conflicts, is a matter of dispute. Melanie Klein considered that the play of children is comparable with the free association of adults and that interpretation to the child can and should be made accordingly. Apart from the dubiousness of some such interpretations and the impossibility in many cases of satisfactory confirmation, the objective value of the therapist's subsequent observations is diminished by the suggestive effect on the child of such interpretations.

Relationship to Therapist. Anna Freud believes that the relationship of the child to the analyst has something essentially different from the relationship of the adult in analysis and that the classical transference situation does not exist, since the parents, the original love-objects, are still important in the patient's life and are not phantasies with which the adult can be clothed. As a corollary, she considers that the super-ego of the child is still attached to the external objects (persons) from whom it is derived, and that re-education is therefore possible and important.

As Rogerson pointed out, 'again and again one finds evidence that it is not the interpretation of a difficulty that causes it to vanish. On the contrary, the important things are the expression of it, and the reception of it without hostile criticism.' He also considered that the relationship with the therapist can be a very simple one, similar to what occurs in the shorter forms of psychotherapy in adults, but that it can be sufficient to enable the child to feel enough protection to discuss the jealousies, for example, that had been producing anxiety (Rogerson, 1939).

Modification According to Age. Play therapy in some form is the only medium of approach to the younger children. With older children, story telling, story writing, drawing and painting, the invention of and participation in little plays, and the use of a toy theatre, have all been found useful in one case or another. For group purposes, puppet shows have been found useful by Bender and Woltmann, the children tending to pick out the episodes that stimulate their inner phantasies. They are asked at critical points in the play what the persons should do and are asked to retell the story in their own words. With young adolescents discussions become possible, and for deeper investigation, free association may, in a few instances, be found practicable. Melanie Klein used their interest in games, sports, motor-cars, bicycles, etc., as symbolic of conflicts dated from earlier years and gave interpretations accordingly (sexual guilt, rivalry with siblings for mother's affection, etc.).

Allen prefers to study the child itself in its immediate relationship to him while playing and talking with him. By showing him how to deal with the mistakes in his attitude and behaviour which arise during his contact with the therapist during the session, he helps the child to manage similar emotional problems occurring in the wider setting of his ordinary life.

The types of phantasies revealed by the interpretation of play technique in Melanie Klein's hands were especially those of the sadistic pregenital stage of libido organization. Urethral-sadistic phantasies (*e.g.* of destroying by flooding, etc.) help to give the penis the unconscious significance of cruelty and to cause subsequent disturbances of potency in the male. Sadistic impulses in general are shown to be directed towards the inside of the mother's body, which may be pictured as having incorporated the father's penis, or as being the source of potential rivals (younger brothers and sisters)—both of which objects the child wishes to destroy. The child pictures his parents as 'destroying each other by means of their genitals and their excrements, which are imagined as dangerous weapons. . . . The penis, incorporated in the mother turns into a dangerous weapon or into weapons loaded with explosive substances; or . . . the vagina becomes an instrument of death, for instance a poisonous mouse-trap.' In her work with children Melanie Klein also came to the conclusion that the super-ego is a product largely of the pregenital stage, and that the destructive nature of the child's impulses at that time have much to do with the super-ego's subsequent severity (Klein, 1932).

Therapeutic Effect of Play Technique. The fact that in many instances the child improves without any interpretation being given to his play, suggests that it is the feeling of security that the child gets from expressing thoughts and impulses of which he is otherwise afraid, in the presence of a non-critical and kindly adult, that is the important medium of therapy. Rogerson instanced a child with obsessive thoughts about killing people who said to him, 'You know, it's funny I don't have these thoughts when you are here', and later she played violently aggressive games of killing and stabbing. It is not always aggressive impulses of which the patient has been afraid; sometimes it is the rebuffs that he would have experienced had he expressed his thoughts to anyone else.

Nature of Impulses Recorded in Play. In the course of play aggressive impulses may be displayed towards the therapist, and the child then oscillates between affection and antagonism. This may represent a reactivation of earlier and contemporary attitudes towards the parents. Rogerson pointed out that after an outburst of jealousy the child would call the therapist 'Daddy'. The expression of such contradictory feelings in the presence of an adult not reacting critically towards them evidently enables the child not only to get rid of the tension produced by them, but to accept them as part of himself.

Even general aggressiveness, without specific object, can lose its disturbing quality when expressed in play under the eye of the therapist. The timid child with underlying aggressive impulses which he is afraid to exhibit, derives lasting benefit from this release.

Relationship of Play Trends to Symptoms. The appearance of excretory and sexual phantasies in the play of children, does not mean that they are causally related to the symptoms. Curiosity, rivalry with the opposite sex, the difference between the sexes, and anxiety about the absence of a penis or its possible loss, all may appear without apparent relevance to the symptoms: but this is not to say that a castration fear, founded on the observation of sex differences, may not play a part in the genesis of a chronic state of anxiety later on. But Rogerson noticed in practice that anxiety connected with birth phantasies as revealed in play (e.g. building a hollow house in which babies were found) tended not to disappear till an explanation was given to the child.

We have quoted Rogerson's work at some length as it was conducted with a deliberate avoidance of interpretation (except in the last instance quoted) and seemed to demonstrate that great improvement and recovery can occur without interference by actual interpretations; and that the child's acceptance of its own impulses and interests under the protection of an older person was the potent therapeutic factor.

Melanie Klein, on the other hand, declared that she has 'never seen any advantage follow from a policy of non-interpretation'. Nevertheless interpretation is certainly not necessary in a fair proportion even of those cases in which play technique is the only likely method of approach.

We have ourselves been impressed with the relative infrequency with which specifically sexual interests are causally associated with the problems of childhood. This is a judgement based on an examination of symptoms, of the circumstances apparently producing them, and of the results of treatment devised from our observations. On the other hand—and there is no seeming contradiction here—it is equally certain that children exhibit sexual interest of some sort, in some cases from their earliest days. Masturbation, presumably with pleasurable sensation, is found even in infants, and even as early as 4 years we have known it associated with conscious thoughts of the other sex, although there had been no known precocity of education in these matters. Homburger related in detail the case of a girl of 3 who showed definite signs of erotic pleasure in genital examination and of erotic interest independently of actual stimulation. Curiosity as to the genitalia and excretory functions of children of both sexes, exhibited in looking or in actual mutual sexual play, is usually felt as wrong at the time because of the general social prohibition that is felt to surround them. Later they may become coloured with a greater feeling of guilt, from their conscious association with more adult forms of sexuality. Such associations may lead to anxiety or to obsessive-compulsive preoccupations in children, but not by any means necessarily; nor need anxiety or obsession necessarily or usually be related to erotic trends. Naturally, if as the result of unwise parental attitudes and actions, such as will be illustrated later, erotic feeling has been aroused in relation to the parents, the conflict will be more intense and the likelihood of a neurosis greater; but instances of nervousness dependent on such definitely sexual interests are much in the minority in children, and only begin to appear with any frequency in adolescents.

CLASSIFICATION

We have found the following classification useful for nervous disorders in children in general. Only the first three are additional to the syndromes, described in previous chapters, in adults.

1. Disorders of personality: Timidity, obstinacy, irritability, sensitiveness, shyness, day-dreaming, lack of sociability, emotional disturbances, etc.
2. Behaviour disorders: Truancy, wandering, temper tantrums, lying, stealing, begging, cruelty, sex misdemeanours, food fads, refusal of food, etc.
3. Habit disorders: Nail-biting, thumb-sucking, incontinence (nocturnal and diurnal), constipation, vomiting, stammering, etc.
4. Psychosomatic disorders: Migraine, asthma, cyclical vomiting, etc.
5. Neuroses: Anxiety, hysteria, obsessional states (including phobias, compulsions and some tics).
6. Psychoses: Schizophrenia, manic-depressive psychoses, etc.
7. Epilepsy.
8. Subnormality (mental defect).
9. Mental disorders occurring with, and probably dependent on, some physical disease: *e.g.* chorea, epidemic encephalitis, trauma.

This grouping is for convenience of description only. The same patient may manifest disorders in several of the above categories. The following is a brief systematic description of the various categories.

Personality Deviations

Personality traits are the outcome of the interplay of inborn and environmental factors, and it is from the beginning difficult to distinguish how much each of

these types of factor shares in the production of the traits which ultimately distinguish the individual. There is no doubt that temperament, which plays so large
a part in the development of the personality, is largely an inborn affair. Infants
a week old, living in the same environment, present to trained observers differences of a temperamental kind; yet even as early as this the skilled nurse will also
detect the reaction of a child which is unwanted. Thus early does the psychological
environment play a part. The observation of twins gives some means of estimating
the relative importance of environment and inheritance. Identical twins, even if
reared apart, show a remarkable similarity in their traits of temperament, while
dissimilar twins, brought up together, show obvious divergences from the earliest
age.

The post-natal development of traits of temperament and character proceeds
as a result of friction arising from within and without, and whatever views may
be held with regard to the share of inheritance, there is no doubt of the modifi-
ability of this development by changes in the external factors.

Some characteristics are the more or less direct expression of innate qualities
—as, for example, energetic activity, impulsiveness, cheerfulness, persistence and
pugnacity. They naturally undergo a progressive socialization in the course of
time. Where the environment enters unusually early or forcibly the trait may be
regarded as either imitative of the environment, *e.g.* vanity in the child of a doting
mother (the mother dotes on the child and the child dotes on himself) or, as a
reaction against it, *e.g.* sullenness in response to a nagging parent. Some traits,
however, have a more complicated origin, of the same form as a neurotic symptom—they are reactions against certain inner tendencies and attitudes, which
may of course themselves be largely determined by environmental influences.
Such in many instances are shyness and over-conscientiousness.

In any case, an attempt should be made from the main facts to surmise at least
what may have been the exact cause of any trait so disadvantageous as to bring
the child for treatment.

Paranoid and schizoid personalities can be discerned occasionally among children, especially from about twelve years onwards. Their occurrence is of particular importance, of course, for the topic of predisposition to and prevention
of a psychosis in later life; and they deserve much more attention than they have
yet received, both as to cause and treatment.

The following example illustrates many such points. The patient had already
from the beginning of our observation been regarded as a psychopathic personality. He represents one of many possible varieties.

CASE No. 59

Solitariness, temper tantrums and a fanatical interest in religious ritual were the principal marks of a boy, age 12½. His mother added that he was 'difficult', slept badly and
was easily frightened. He went to bed at 9 p.m. but did not fall asleep till midnight,
and insisted on one of his parents remaining by his bedside the while. At meal-times he
frequently refused to stay at table, alleging as his reason for this that his mother 'did
not eat right' or 'was not dressed right'. He had 'church on the brain'—his main topics
of conversation were ecclesiastical, and his principal recreation out of school hours
was rehearsing church services. His knowledge of these matters was said by his mother

to be astonishingly detailed, and when he went to church he would find fault with the minutiae of the service.

He played ordinary boys' games very little. Football he only took part in when compelled to do so by other boys. He had no friends of his own age and said that he did not want any. If his parents invited another boy to the home he 'sat and talked quite nice to him', but he would not accept invitations in return.

From his mother it was discovered in addition that he swore, even in front of his father (who never punished him). He was not cleanly in his bodily habits. His mother bathed him, to the accompaniment of screaming and fighting. At night in his bedroom when his mother sat with him, he terrified her with his restlessness, throwing his arms about and talking incessantly. He had the habit of harping on one theme to the intense and frequently expressed annoyance of his parents—for example, he would talk for hours to his cat, saying 'nice boy' over and over again, *ad nauseam*.

He was in a private school, and the school report said:

'I have pleasure in stating that he has never given us the slightest trouble. The boy is obedient, quiet and inoffensive; in fact, the one thing that strikes us is that he is apathetic, dreamy and slow on the "up-take". In some subjects—English and drawing —he is in advance of his years; in others—arithmetic—he is slow and backward. When he first came here he kept somewhat aloof, but he is now mixing gradually with the other boys.

'Judging from his behaviour here I cannot understand the trouble over this boy. Here he is perfectly docile, without vice or troublesome tendencies.'

This divergence in the reports from school and home furnishes an example of the differentiation of behaviour which is so frequent in children, and is one of the evidences of environmental influences.

Family History. The father was quiet and retiring, sensitive and gentle in manner. He never cared to play with other boys when he was a child, and when he first went to work had a 'stiff' time, as he could not hold his own in the company of others. He neither smoked nor drank and had no hobbies. He took little interest in Peter, but took his part against the grandmother in a negative way—refusing to scold him at her demand.

The mother herself, who gave much of the above information when she came up to hospital and afterwards added considerably to it, was obviously greatly perturbed by her child's conduct. She confessed her entire helplessness to alter it. She admitted that she herself was of a worrying disposition. Since childhood she had thought worry the 'right thing to do'. She had been taken to a doctor at the age of 14 as she was 'all shaky'. Being afraid of her mother, who was ill-tempered and often thrashed her, she would wander about the streets at night afraid to go home.

The grandmother had now resided with the parents for the past three years, and entertained a violent dislike for the boy with whom she frequently quarrelled, while, on the other hand, she took his part against his mother on any question of discipline.

Home Conditions. The family occupied a good-sized house which they were buying by instalments. The situation was somewhat complicated, as they borrowed the capital for this venture from the maternal grandmother, and instead of paying her interest they kept her. They used four rooms—well-furnished parlour and kitchen, a bedroom for the old lady and one for themselves. The home gave the impression of real comfort and prosperity. There was a garden, and the neighbourhood was a good one. Part of the house was let.

Previous History. Birth was normal and the child appeared perfectly normal during his infancy. When he was one year old his father went into the Army and his mother went out to work. Peter was left to the care of his maternal grandmother until the age of 5, when his father returned. From 5 to 10 years of age Peter went to an elementary school. He did not get on well with the other boys, and his parents were anxious for him to mix with a good type of boy. Also, when he was about 10, he began to be difficult and moody, and the parents decided to make a great sacrifice to meet the expense of sending him to a private school.

Mental Status. In appearance he was a well-grown but thin and sallow-complexioned boy, who carried himself in slovenly fashion, with rather bent shoulders, and looked older than his years. He had a glum expression, and he did not talk spontaneously at the interview but only in answer to questions, and then rather briefly. He did not look his interlocutor in the eye, but usually looked at the ground instead. The general impression gained from his demeanour was of a rather surly reluctance.

He denied being unhappy and gave no evidence of realizing that his conduct and interests were abnormal, or of any desire to change them. In reply to questions, he admitted his interest in religious ritual. His reading, besides the Bible, consisted almost exclusively of Shakespeare and Mark Twain. He was not interested, he said, in comics or in tales of adventure.

A psychological rating a year later, at $13\frac{1}{2}$, gave him an I.Q. of only 77 on the Binet-Simon scale and of 87 on a scale of performance tests. Educational achievement tests gave him a mental age of $10\frac{1}{2}$ years for mechanical arithmetic, 8 years for problems, 10 years for mechanical reading, 9 for appreciation of material read and 12 years for spelling. The report on the tests in general was as follows:

'Peter's school work is probably up to the level of his power. He is quite unsuited to prolonged education of a school type or to advanced work.'

These tests did not corroborate the schoolmaster's report in several important points. Part of the explanation lay in the lower general standard of pupils in certain private schools; but, from the subsequent history, it seems probable that the results of the tests were vitiated by temperamental factors.

Summary. It is clear that in this boy symptoms in the ordinary sense played an insignificant part. He was slow in going to sleep at nights and he had certain compulsions, but the preponderating abnormalities were in his conduct and in his trend of interests. The latter were unusual at his age—the Church and Shakespeare—and would be unusually one-sided at any age. He was preoccupied, like so many children of his type, with the problems of the hardship of life and the unkindness of fate. His predilection for the ritualistic aspect of religion perhaps reflected his own shrinking attitude to life, which was shown also in his shunning companions and their boisterous games. If we considered only these more subjective aspects we would conclude that we were dealing with a temperamentally abnormal boy, shy, timorous and tender-minded, weltering in difficulties of inner origin, sometimes perhaps hereditary, in the light of his father's history. But the more objective aspects of his behaviour were equally striking, and although they were the more immediate cause of his being brought for advice, they were much more suggestive of possibilities of treatment than the subjective characteristics which we have just considered. Evidently the boy had some inventiveness; his interests may have been perverse but they were strong, according to his mother's account, and they did not seem to derive anything directly from the parental example except some of the strength that springs from rebellion.

It was clear that the father was a minor factor in every sense; he had done little positive harm, but had erred rather in what he had failed to do, in not exerting some discipline. The mother was of much greater importance. She had been badly brought up by her own mother, knew no discipline except that of fear, and no attitude to difficulties except anxiety. The son unwittingly copied her timidity, and at the same time, not so unwittingly perhaps, took advantage of it, and of his father's feeble attitude. Also it was apparent that the follies of the parents were visited on the offspring in more subtle ways. The boy made use of the antagonism of mother and grandmother to play them off against each other, while he went himself unpunished. He saw that to defy his mother gave the grandmother opportunities for homilies to her daughter, and for maliciously gloomy forebodings that he was a little maniac and would end in an asylum; while, when he called his grandmother 'old cat', he earned but a mild reproof from his mother, whose inmost feelings to her own mother he was expressing only too well.

From the school report and from the results of psychological testing it was clear that the parents' ambition had placed the boy in an atmosphere too rare for his intellectual capacity. Probably also, their delicacy about allowing him to mix with rougher companions at his elementary school had something to do with his withdrawal from all companions later.

Treatment. 1. In view of the mismanagement at home and his mother's emotional condition, it was decided to send him for a time to a holiday home at the seaside. He remained there only two days, as he cried the whole time and was sent home.

2. Change of school. He was removed from the private secondary school he was attending and placed in a public (rate-aided) elementary school. This was followed by an immediate improvement in his behaviour; and he approximated much more closely to the normal in school.

3. Instruction was given to the parents, accompanied by reassurance and explanation of the true nature of the boy's condition.

4. The boy himself was encouraged to join some social bodies like the Scouts and a Church Club.

Results. Besides the appearance of normal behaviour in school and the improvement of his work there, he gained in several ways. He was no longer morbidly interested in Church. He bathed himself. At home he was no longer omnipotent. Outside of school he remained solitary, however.

Twenty months later the mother reported that she had found him a post in making artificial teeth. He had proved efficient at it but 'did not like having to do clearing up', so he had left of his own accord. After being unemployed for about fourteen days he had found a good job for himself in a stockbroker's office, which he still held. He had entirely dropped his interest in Church, and now went every week to a theatre or music hall. He had made only one friend, who dropped him, 'as Peter was so rude'. He attended hospital again after nearly two years. He was then a grand young man in a bowler hat, and appeared to be happily settled in the stockbroker's office. He spoke with much feeling and bitterness against the grandmother, who, he said, was getting old and silly and was the cause of much friction at home. Peter had one friend, and was strongly advised to make more and if possible join a club. (It is an interesting and significant fact that this boy was at least three years retarded when given Intelligence Tests and had an I.Q. of 77, and yet apparently managed to pass muster as a clerk.)

The subsequent history of this youth, in spite of all the more that has been done with him, has not been encouraging. He is solitary, seldom goes out, except after dark, and has been back to Church again. In fact he appears to be heading for a schizophrenic psychosis.

Behaviour Disorders

These include such complicated actions as truancy from school, wandering, lying, stealing, refusal of food and refusal to speak, cruelty and temper outbursts.

These are positive acts, isolated or habitual, of the child as a whole, *i.e.* in relation to the society in which he finds himself. More uniformly and definitely than any of the previously described symptoms, they betoken a conflict of his urges with what his environment allows or requires. The point of outbreak, so to speak, of the abnormal behaviour does not necessarily represent the point of conflict. There is frequently a displacement from the real source of friction, and the large part of the psychiatric diagnosis and therapeutic task depends on detecting the true cause of the discontent.

It is important to realize that none of the disorders enumerated are themselves 'abnormal' in the strict sense. Ask any group of normal adults whether they have ever stolen anything in their lives and they will almost to a man answer 'yes'. Few people have not in their childhood secretly admired the boy who had the courage to play truant. Lying is a universal tendency. Cruelty, being less useful, is much more readily discarded and is a common enough trait in any child.

But when any of these reactions occur flagrantly or persistently, inquiry is indicated, lest the tendency become a habit and worse things befall.

Truancy may be a negative or avoidance phenomenon, as when a child funks going back to school in face of a threatened punishment or disgrace, or it may be a more primitive phenomenon, as the expression of the boy's urge for adventure and variety. Wandering is only a prolonged truancy, usually with a similar basis and in older children who have left school. Lying may be done for defence or prestige. Sometimes it depends on simple confusion of phantasy with fact. In the latter instance it is usually elaborate and based on egoistic phantasy. Stealing may be a simple matter of opportunity having presented itself, or it may also be done for prestige, as when a child spends the proceeds on gifts to his friends. It may, on the other hand, be a rebellion against discipline, directly as in deprivation of pocket-money, or indirectly against some other form of frustration. Rare instances have been described by Healy, where stealing represented a neurotic symptom, a compulsion being felt to steal because of the similarity of the guilty feeling aroused by the deed to that attaching to sexual curiosity which had been repressed. It has been suggested that some habitual stealing comes from the child's urge to compensate for what he feels to have been denied him, namely the love of his parents or their substitutes. Acts of cruelty express either an innate tendency, common to everyone but usually soon brought under discipline (except in places where it is tacitly encouraged, as it used to be in certain public schools), or as a response in kind to an unfriendly environment, as jealousy and revenge. Temper outbursts are either negativistic in origin or matters of egoistic self-display, or more usually composed of both, and refusal to eat or speak have similar origins.

Behaviour disorders are often of such a nature as to bring the child under the notice of the law; they then constitute the delinquencies which crowd the children's courts.

The following is an example, principally of temper tantrums:

CASE No. 60

Gavin T., age 13¾, was referred to hospital by the school authorities because the mother complained of the boy's tantrums, in which, for example, he threw the coal shovel at her. When asked by her to tidy the sitting-room and do some shopping for her, he refused and flew into a rage, and when she pleaded with him he threw a book at her. Headaches were also reported, for which no physical cause could be discovered at a school medical examination.

2 K

Family History and Home Environment. He was the third of a family of five children, the fourth being a girl while the other three were boys. The father, age 41, was a manager in a local shop. He had had to work very hard when he was young, and said that he had suffered headaches worse than Gavin's. He said that the boy would grow out of them. Towards his wife he was curt and unsympathetic in the presence of the social worker, and took sides with the children against the mother in any difference that arose.

The mother was the youngest of a large family whose father was comfortably off and died when she was young. At the time of her marriage at 21 she had furnished the house, 'bought a job' for her husband and given a sum of money to his mother, all from money which she had inherited. She had a 'nervous breakdown' the year before the boy came for advice. She had had fits (hysterical) since the birth of the daughter, then aged 10.

The father's mother had lived with the parents for a considerable time after they married. She adored her son and he reciprocated the attachment. She constantly made trouble between her son and his wife, insisting that he could not digest dishes made by the latter. If Mrs. T. (the younger) suggested that she and her husband should go anywhere, or buy anything, he always consulted his mother first and usually followed her advice. The grandmother also interfered with the discipline of the children, while at the same time disliking Gavin and pinching him when he was younger and making him cry. After the younger Mrs. T.'s return from hospital, she found the home so unbearable that she refused to have the grandmother live any longer with them. The grandmother now lived alone, her son making her an allowance.

As an example of the atmosphere which had been engendered, the following example may be quoted. The eldest boy refused to make the tea, told his mother to shut her —— mouth, jumped up, caught both her elbows and held them right back, breaking her brassière and causing her pain. When the father was informed in the evening he was merely abusive.

The house itself was physically comfortable—a six-roomed house, clean and well kept by the mother, who did all the work, including the washing. The father had refused to allow her any help, saying that when a woman married she must be prepared for hard work.

Personal History. The patient was born during an air raid. Nothing abnormal was noted in his early years, but for some years he had displayed fits of temper. Recently at school he had not been allowed to enter for a scholarship examination, as in the opinion of his teachers he could not apply himself to home work. His school report stated that he reached a fair average in a class where the average age was three months less than his, but in manual work and drawing he was reported 'very good'. He was not good at games, however, which were the touch-stone at this school, and was regarded as 'too much of a nincompoop to be a prefect'. There was no trouble with his behaviour.

Mental Examination. He exhibited nothing abnormal in his attitude. When his tantrums were mentioned he looked embarrassed and would not talk about them at the first interview. His I.Q. on the Binet-Simon scale was 93, but his performance with Porteus mazes was much better, and he attained the average for the sixteenth year. The examiner stated that 'he perfectly understood the problem, made no impulsive mistakes and planned the whole path before he began to work'. Physically he was sound.

Summary. It was clear that the boy's sole form of misdemeanour depended on his mother's feebleness of discipline, the subversive attitude of the grandmother and the father's failure to adjust to his wife on account of his own maternal attachment. As far as factors in the boy himself were concerned, the self-assertion, which had no outlet at school (he was far from scholarship standard, had little ability at games and had never had conferred on him any work of authority in any official way among the other boys), found distorted expression in his tantrums at home.

Treatment. The boy and his parents were all interviewed and advised in turn. The boy was encouraged to take an interest in his manual abilities, and led to understand that the criteria by which his school judged him were not the only ones possible. At the same time, a standard of behaviour at home more suited to his age was held up to him; and an attitude of protectiveness towards his mother was fostered. The mother was given a simple exposition of the reasons for the boy's outbursts, and was supported in a more courageous disciplinary attitude. At the same time, she herself was recommended convalescent home treatment, as she suffered not only from hysterical fits but complained of feeling weak and ill.

The father was at first aggressive and resentful of outside interference, but was ultimately persuaded to support his wife to some extent—at least in her attempt to keep control of the family, to the extent of corporal punishment, which he inflicted on one occasion on Gavin with a marked improvement in the latter's behaviour. Soon afterwards the mother went to a convalescent home for two months, and in the meantime Gavin was invaluable as cook and housekeeper. When she returned home there were no further complaints about his conduct. He left school six months later and went to work at a wholesale hosier's.

Aggressive sexual behaviour, self-ostentation, a hypochondriacal trend and disobedience were all exhibited by

CASE NO. 61

Gladys B., age 14, was referred to hospital by the school authorities for advice, principally on account of her behaviour towards the opposite sex. She showed much less than the normal reserve, and was particularly bent on making friends with men in uniform, especially policemen! She talked so readily to strangers that her parents were chary of allowing her out of the house. At home she was untidy, disrespectful and disobedient. She would not perform services for those at home but would perform them readily for strangers. She showed little perseverance and had not learned to sew or knit. When playing games, or at school, she always wanted the limelight and to be first. She would appear in school with her arm in a sling and make a great fuss over a small cut. From time to time she complained of various aches and pains, to the mother's alarm, so that the latter took her to hospital, where, however, nothing physical was discovered amiss. In school her achievement was poor. This had been attributed to her day-dreaming. It was considered by the school authorities that she would be capable of the average work of her class if she concentrated on it.

Family History. The patient was the youngest of four children, the others being capable and successful. The father, age 52, a tram driver, was a kindly, respectable, home-loving and sentimental man. He had been brought up strictly by his father and did not drink or smoke. He was apparently on the best of terms with his wife. The mother was an ailing woman with various minor physical complaints and inclined to lean on her second daughter. She had spoiled the patient constantly. The eldest daughter was married, capable and much more successful than the parents in managing Gladys. The second daughter, age 28, was superintendent of a Sunday School, hard-working, economical and self-sacrificing. The third member of the family was a young man, recently married, and capable at his work of motor mechanic. None of them were outstanding at school, but they made excellent citizens.

The patient's history showed that her mother had found her difficult to manage from her earliest years. There had been no serious illnesses. At school her record had always been indifferent. Her school report for the current year showed that she was much below the class average in achievement, though seven months older than the average age of her classmates. Spelling was 'poor', arithmetic 'very poor' and composition 'fair'. She did not mix well with other children and had no friends, and had a reputation for being untruthful. For example, she was heard telling her class-mates that the teacher had given her sole charge of her desk, which was untrue. She reacted to lessons in mothercraft by telling a policeman friend that she was about to enter a maternity home. The mothercraft lessons were swiftly discontinued by her scandalized parents.

Physically she was well developed and good-looking. She had a coquettish air and wore clothes of a showy type. Her pleasure at being taken notice of by being brought to the clinic seemed to outweigh any sense of social transgression she may have had when the doctor talked to her about the behaviour. She claimed to have friends, older than herself, including one who had recently had a baby.

Her *intelligence rating* gave her a mental age of $10\frac{1}{2}$ on the Binet-Simon scale. Scores on performance tests ranged from 7 to 11 years, the average value being $8\frac{1}{2}$. In the Porteus mazes she showed a power to plan only under the simplest conditions. She attempted the tests generally too rapidly and inaccurately. Her perception for form was poor. She tried to cover up her deficiencies by gossiping. It was shown that the school report, already quoted, erred in supposing that her difficulties depended on lack of concentration, and that she was actually subnormal.

Summary. The intelligence rating gave the clue to much of her behaviour. It definitely accounted for the backwardness in school and for some of her behaviour there and outside. In her pleasing appearance and address she had found her main asset, and her erotic drive was allowed fuller play than a child capable of more intelligent social adaptation would have allowed it. Her ill-discipline at home and her unpopularity with other girls probably depended more on the faults in her parents' management than upon her subnormality.

Treatment. The position was explained to the parents and a more consistent discipline enjoined, with allowances to be made for her lack of common sense, *i.e.* she was to be supervised in her activities much more closely than the average child of her age. The mother was advised to invite the child's young married friends to tea, so that they might undergo inspection, and, if considered desirable, they were to be invited to co-operate in managing Gladys.

A training in domestic service was arranged for, and it was decided that if by the time she reached 16 she still required social supervision, she would be notified as subnormal (mentally defective) to the local authority.

CASE NO. 62

Stealing as rebellion was well shown by a boy of 13 who was brought by his mother, who was in great distress. He was the eldest child and only boy in the family, and had been the apple of his parents' eye, but two years previously he had begun to steal anything of value that he could find lying about the house. He stole his mother's money, his father's cigars and his sister's sweets. He was incorrigible; no punishment was of any avail. This hardened young delinquent, when interviewed, rapidly dissolved into tears. It came out bit by bit that after day-school, which ended about 4 o'clock, he was expected by his mother to do two hours' lessons; thereafter to practise the violin (which he loathed) for half an hour, and after that to help his mother in the garden. If any leisure remained before bedtime he was allowed to play with his sister in the garden; the village boys were considered 'too rough'. Nominally he had ample pocket-money for one of his years—8d. a week—but 4d. of this he gave (under duress) to foreign missions, and the other 4d. he placed in his bank against the purchase of Christmas and birthday presents for the rest of the family. A reasonable rearrangement of pocket-money and of the other conditions of his life led to an immediate cessation of stealing.

The following boy's stealing was secondary to his truancy, which in turn was dependent on the reaction of a timidly evasive personality to scholastic difficulties.

CASE NO. 63

William C., aged 14, was referred to hospital by the Probation Officer on account of truancy and stealing, with the report: 'About four months ago he truanted success-fully for a whole fortnight. When found out he ran away from home and slept out. He has done this four or five times since, sometimes staying away for several nights at a time. He never goes far away, but sleeps in the blocks round where he lives. He has also stolen from his younger brother's and sister's money boxes and has borrowed money from the neighbours under false pretences. . . .'

Family History and Circumstances. The father was a boiler-coverer whose work took him much away from home. He was an intelligent man, much interested in his children's welfare, but, according to his wife, he had a bad temper. The stepmother was a pleasant woman who married Mr. C. when the second boy was a baby, and the boys had been brought up to believe that she was their mother. She had one child, a girl, age 9. Willie had also a younger brother, age 11. Both parents had become extremely worried over Willie. The father was very bitter about the effect of his delinquencies on the peace of the household and was very anxious that he should be 'sent away' (*i.e.* to an approved school). The house was in a rough district but clean and comfortable. The income was sufficient to prevent hardship. The children were mostly with their mother in their free time and were not given much opportunity of mixing with others. Willie had 1s. a week pocket-money, of which he spent 3d. and saved the rest for camp. He belonged to the Boys' Brigade, whose officers had often been out at night searching for him.

Personal History. Willie had had an uneventful career until the recent outburst of truancy. His stepmother, however, had always found him more difficult to manage than the other children. He was well-behaved when his father was at home, but inclined to torment the younger ones in his absence, while very resentful of any teasing himself. At the Boys' Brigade his reputation was that he 'could not say boo to a goose'.

His *school report* from a Central school (*i.e.* of scholarship boys) was that he was at the bottom of a class of 40, the average age of the class being 13, *i.e.* slightly younger than Willie. He was reported as below average capacity. His marks at the various examinations had been—Arithmetic, 0; Spelling, 0; Algebra, 0; French, 17 out of 75. Totals of 317 out of 1000, and 411 out of 1000 were some of his results at the end of term examinations.

Psychiatric Examination. The boy himself presented a reserved appearance at first; but he soon talked readily enough. He was very unhappy about himself, and especially about his position at school. He declared that he truanted because he hated lessons and was always being given lines. Having stayed away from school he was afraid to go home, and so in order to provide food while he lived out he took it from home just before truanting from school. On the second last occasion his father had thrashed him when he returned from his escapade. On the final occasion, which brought him ulti-mately to hospital, when he heard his father was coming, Willie took 2s. 6d. which his aunt had given him to do some shopping and stayed out all night. He was found next day, soaking wet, and his aunt undertook to charge him with stealing.

He was very anxious to leave school and go to work, but he did not want to leave home.

The impression was of a timid, likeable boy, who was over-dependent on his home, shy of friends and evasive of difficulties. An intelligence test showed that with an I.Q. of 90 he belonged to the low average group. In performance tests his results ranged from 10 (Dearborn and cube construction) to 14 years (substitution test and Healy, 2). Scholastic tests gave, for reading: comprehension, 10 years; speed, 11 years for three-letter words, and 9 years, continuous prose. In dictation he scored 11. 8/12 for separate words, and 11–12 years, running. These tests were made because an independent attempt had been proposed to apprentice him in the printing trade. They showed him to be unfit to be a compositor.

Physically he presented no signs of organic disease.

Treatment. As his delinquencies had occurred since he had been de-moted to a class below his previous one, evidently the easing of school work had little effect. It was accordingly recommended that he should leave school forthwith and go to work. The headmaster demurred, and advocated his entering the third year in six months' time, but with the intention of working on the technical side and having opportunities for hand-work instead of shorthand and other commercial subjects. The boy was much upset at this decision, and the stepmother removed him without further consultation with anyone. He started work in an office and went willingly to evening classes, but at Christmas failed to bring home his wages for the week. When his parents pressed him he disappeared, slept anywhere he could and when found by them was put to bed for several days. It transpired that a practical joke had been played on him at his work—he was told that he would be given handsome overtime for doing extra work before Christmas. He went to work an hour early every day for a week, and expected to get 4s. or 5s. extra on Christmas Eve, instead of which he received only his normal pay. He was dreadfully disappointed, and apparently tried to realize his hopes by giving his stepmother 4s., which he said was overtime, and pretending that he would not get his week's pay till after Christmas. This of course involved him in a tangle of lies, and when he could not escape from the tangle he ran away again. He was found five nights later by his stepmother.

On this occasion work was found for him as a page boy and he continued at evening classes. Three months later he was reported to have remained well.

Cruelty. There is another kind of dog which is apt to be given a bad name and hanged in consequence, and that is the child who is labelled spiteful and cruel, and whom the doctor is sometimes asked in consequence to exclude from school.

CASE NO. 64

A small child called Gladys, age 6, was reported to scratch, kick and bite other children, to be disobedient and unmanageable at home and to be beyond control at school.

Family Circumstances. The father was a labourer, age 40, and the mother about the same age. They got on well together and had five children, of whom Gladys was the youngest but one. The second oldest child, also a girl, was reported to have been disobedient and unruly at one time, but by 'severe discipline', that is, by whipping, she was said to have been made into a normal child. The whole family of seven people lived in two rooms and they all slept in one of these rooms. The other room was very clean and tidy, and was kept so in case anyone called. Gladys and the other children were not allowed to play in anything but the bedroom.

Personal History. Until she was about 4 years of age Gladys was a perfectly normal and very affectionate, attractive child. Until the same age she was never allowed to play with her older brothers and sisters, but was kept altogether with the mother. The reason alleged for this was that the grandmother, who lived downstairs, complained of the noise that the children made in the yard, and it was felt that Gladys would be the last straw which would break the grandmother's back, and so Gladys was sacrificed.

At 4 she went to school and the mother began to allow her out to play, but the elder children regarded her as a nuisance, and as a rule made her stay in a corner. If she emerged from this she was set on by the other children, and made to go back to what they considered was a place of safety for her. In the meantime, her restless liveliness in the confined precincts of the narrow space of the home became more than the mother could stand and she tried to repress it. If the child would not keep quiet she was smacked, and this happened often—so frequently in fact that ultimately it had no effect. Threats were tried, but Gladys screamed if deprived of her weekly penny, and found that by this means she could always get it back. Putting her to bed was of no use, as the mother did all the housework in the room where the child slept. Thus repressive discipline completely broke down with the triumph of Gladys, but at the expense of a feeling of defeat and exasperation on the part of the mother.

Furthermore, the child followed instinctively the rule of doing as she was done by, through lack of being taught the other rule, to love one's neighbour as oneself. For example, Gladys had begun by being fond of the baby, but, just before she came to hospital, there had been an occasion on which, after being punished by her mother, she went and stuck pins into the baby.

Psychiatric Examination. When Gladys was first seen by the doctor she screamed and wept. The mother explained that she was always being punished and so was afraid. Later after playing with toys, she came happily to the examination room and talked quite freely. It was interesting that her favourite toys were soldiers, and she loved shooting them, and when she played with a doll she confessed quite blithely that she enjoyed sticking pins into it. She asserted without any sign of rancour that everybody hit her, as though this were the normal order of things. Our impression was that she lacked no moral sense but simply moral teaching, and that her spitefulness and cruelty were direct reactions to her environment. They could hardly be innate tendencies, as until she was 4 she was regarded as a pleasant and affectionate child.

An *intelligence test* showed that she was one year backward. This was by no means sufficient to account for her behaviour.

Treatment consisted in stopping all physical punishment forthwith and removing her to a different environment. We do not like removing a child from its environment when it is giving difficulty, but prefer to adjust the environment, so that the child need no longer be ill-behaved in order to assert itself in some way. In this instance, however, the conditions were so cramped, and it seemed so difficult to make a complete alteration in the attitude of the family without at least a preliminary absence of the child from home, that we decided to place her in a foster home.

Soon after her arrival in the foster home we received the following report: 'This child is not at all difficult to manage here. She has at times attacked other children, but not often, and lately she has been perfectly good. She takes very little real interest in any occupation; she only wants to rush about and give vent to her enormous activity.'

Finally, after some months, she returned home, and the report was that she was a happy child at home and there was seldom any difficulty. The school report was that Gladys was less given to kicking and unruly behaviour and seemed to be forgetting to do nasty and unkind things.

Some months later it was said that she was no bother unless she was kept indoors too long. The school report said that kicking was not unknown but was comparatively rare.

A delinquent act may represent, according to Healty and Bronner (Healy, 1915; Healy and Bronner, 1936):

1. An attempt to avoid, even as a temporary measure, the unpleasant situation by escape or flight from it.

2. An attempt to achieve substitutive compensatory satisfactions through delinquent activities—by adventures or through notoriety.

3. An attempt to strengthen or bolster up the ego wounded by feelings of inadequacy or inferiority—by obtaining status with the delinquent crowd, or, in a solitary individual, by proving his courage and worth to himself.

4. A delinquency may also represent an attempt to get certain satisfactions through direct and conscious or even unconscious expression of revenge attitudes, perhaps through a hidden desire to punish parents or others by conduct that will make life difficult for them.

5. An attempt to gain a maximum of self-satisfaction, to inflate the ego, by generally aggressive, antisocial attitudes.
6. A response to instinctual urges felt to be thwarted—sometimes in the form of sexual misbehaviour, but more often of attempts at emancipation.
7. A wish for punishment which is always a response to a conscious or unconscious sense of guilt.

Habit Disorders

Habit disorders include thumb-sucking, nail-biting, head-rolling, masturbation, enuresis (nocturnal and diurnal), faecal incontinence, stammering (some cases) and other speech disorders. These, for the most part, are either primarily auto-erotic in basis or represent a regression to infantile sources of satisfaction in face of environmental frustration. They readily become associated secondarily with defiance (negativism).

Treatment again consists in analysing the situation in each case and making appropriate readjustments. Frustration in any direction, 'babying' by the parents, erotic stimulation by the parents (usually unrealized by them), jealousy of another child in the family and defiance of the parents from lack of their affection, or mismanagement in other ways, are the commonest causes.

It is particularly in this group that successes are obtained in young children with Thom's method of encouraging the child to keep a diary in which a star is marked on each successful day, and the dates of failure are left blank, and the child is mildly praised or rewarded in some small material way for successes.

CASE No. 65

Simon J., aged 5, was brought by his mother on account of a 'nervous habit' of a curious kind. On going to bed he would put his arm up to and round his head (without actually touching it) and rock his head and arm at increasing speed until he was 'hysterical', to use the mother's phrase. By this she meant that he seemed not to be able to hear when at the height of the habit, and could only be stopped by placing one's hand on him. The habit occurred every time he lay down and was also repeated if he woke up in the night.

Family History. The father was a professional man of an intelligent, stable type. The mother was a highly intelligent woman, and the married life was happy and marital relations normal. There was one younger child, a girl aged 2½, of whom the patient was very fond. He displayed little jealousy of her, and would himself place her on his mother's knee.

History of Patient. His birth was two months premature and the labour was induced for gynaecological reasons. His habit of head and arm rocking began at about 18 months, just after circumcision. He had an anaesthetic for the operation, but he screamed a good deal for three weeks after. He touched his penis so much that it was difficult to procure healing. Walking did not occur till 2 years of age, and he was still later in talking (3 years). The mother brought him up very strictly on Truby King methods. The régime was relaxed, however, when the baby sister arrived.

He had recently gone to school in the mornings from 9.30 till 12.30. He slept at midday and was in bed by 6.30. No food was given after 4.30. He now slept in the same room as his sister. Formerly he had talked a little about the 'dark coming in at the door', but less was heard of this after his sister had been put to sleep in the same room.

He bit his nails for a time, but his mother's old nurse succeeded in stopping this. During a visit to his grandmother, who thought she could cure his head-rocking, the latter became worse.

His mother declared that his pleasure in his habit was obvious.

Psychiatric Examination. The boy was a bright-looking, lively youngster, with intelligence above the average. He had a very definite ambivalent reaction to the habit, a look of pleasure passing over his face when it was mentioned, while at the same time he flatly denied indulging in it.

The inference was that his habit was an auto-erotic phenomenon. His mother had let him feel that it was 'naughty' on the basis that it was against her wishes. This, combined with the pleasure obtained, probably accounted for his abnormal attitude. The mother's opinion that she had been unduly severe in her discipline in the first three years of his life was of interest, especially in view of the fact that among his leading characteristics already were obstinacy and persistence.

Treatment. The mother was advised that the habit could not hurt him physically unless he banged himself against some hard object, and it was pointed out that the physical damage would be limited to that. An attempt was also made to reassure her on the whole subject, by explaining that while the form of the tic was unusual the motive behind it was not. The importance was stressed of trying to get rid of any guilt feeling he might have by getting him to co-operate with her in trying to remove it. She was advised to talk to him about it and to give him a small diary, asking him to keep it himself and to put a cross against the days when he managed not to do it, and to give him little rewards for slight improvement.

A light meal of easily assimilated carbohydrate about an hour before he went to sleep was recommended, such as toast with butter and a sugary drink or some simple sticks of barley sugar.

Three months later the habit was reported to have ceased.

Nocturnal Enuresis. This is probably the commonest habit disorder. By the age of three most children have attained control of the sphincter of the bladder both by night and day. The term nocturnal enuresis is applied to bed-wetting occurring after that stage. This is one of the commonest disorders of childhood. It is a problem both in the home and in the institution; although the degree to which it persists in the latter varies considerably and depends on a number of factors. Nocturnal enuresis is also much more prevalent in some families than in others— three out of four siblings may show it, and very often one or two in the previous generation as well. It appears to be more prevalent in boys. Commonly it ultimately ceases spontaneously, at various ages. Few people suffer from it after adolescence has been passed. In an individual case it may occur every night, or nearly every night, or with intervals of days or weeks or months. There is no morbid anatomy of the condition, although it has been associated at times with vesical calculus, spina bifida occulta and other local anomalies. Rarely in cases of spina bifida, improvement has been reported following the surgical division of the fibrous band that in such cases passes from the extremity of the conus medullaris. But, as a general rule, no gross physical disorder is to be found that has any relevance.

From the psychological aspect the possible causes are these:

1. Lack of training. According to Levy, this is the most important cause.
2. Lack of educability, from subnormality (mental defect).

3. Anxiety on the part of a timid child who has learned to fear his enuresis, or who fears other difficulties.
4. Regression to infancy, associated with too much maternal attachment.
5. Negativism.
6. Possibly a substituted erotic manifestation.

A familial incidence has been reported by various observers. The significance of this is as yet uncertain. We suspect on several grounds a constitutional factor not as yet further definable.

The first two factors are not frequent. The function of nocturnal control establishes itself even in the subnormal, except in those of the lowest grades. The timid, anxious, excitable, often very intelligent, child of asthenic habitus is the most frequent type. Apprehension is one of the principal factors here. It is this type principally which Cameron refers to when he emphasizes that nocturnal enuresis rarely occurs if a child is removed to hospital, where a child is, in a way, expected to wet the bed and so does not fear it any more. When bed-wetting occurs as a negativistic phenomenon, it is permissible to suspect that it is not always unconsciously performed. Direct suggestion itself is sometimes sufficient either in the waking state or under hypnosis.

The psychological treatment should, as a rule, be of the type fitted to the type of maladjustment that has been discovered, and should follow the general lines indicated in this chapter.

Faecal incontinence in any but the severely abnormal is so much more amenable to treatment than nocturnal enuresis that its origin must be very close to consciousness. Sheer unhappiness is often an important factor. Negativism is the basis in others: and in some the aspect of sensuous pleasure suggests itself, associated with anal-erotic phantasies. It usually clears up when the child is made to discover disadvantages associated with it—not of the repressive type, but such disadvantages as the deprivation of some treat that would otherwise have been shared with companions. The method works best in association with other children living in the same house and with a tradition of cleanliness.

Stalker and Band in an important paper on 'Persistent Enuresis' (1946) emphasized how under war-time conditions the frequency of nocturnal enuresis increases, and persists into adolescence and adult life. A group of 67 cases was examined, and some of the more significant features encountered were noted. For instance, abnormalities of the lumbosacral spine such as fusion defects and lumbarization and sacralization are so common in ordinary life that they probably have no special relation to enuresis. Enuresis may be described as an autonomic symptom complex assuming a variety of forms, *e.g.* nocturnal enuresis, rising at night, diurnal enuresis, diurnal frequency and urgency and encopresis. The majority of enuretic patients have cystometrograms of the uninhibited neurogenic type showing a lack of cerebral inhibition similar to that present in certain organic cerebral diseases.

Clinically, the anxious-minded states and the psychopathic personality types predominate; the physiological state of disordered function can be correlated with the emotional and social anomalies which are so frequent. Enuresis predominates in the male sex, it is accompanied by associated autonomic disorders, *e.g.* deep sleep, and not infrequently by a family history of psychosomatic disorders.

From the point of view of treatment, Stalker and Band had good results with ephedrine hydrochloride, B.P. In adults $1\frac{1}{2}$ gr. at night-time which may be increased by $\frac{1}{2}$ gr. every few nights, according to tolerance, to a maximum of 3 gr. The dosage in children is modified according to age. A varying degree of improvement occurred in 23 out of the 67 cases treated in the above way.

Sleep-walking. This is a fairly common phenomenon, which usually occurs only on a few occasions in the child and does not persist, except in rare instances, into adult life. It must depend on an extensive dissociation of cortical function, and, like similar dissociations in waking life, can result from either psychological or physiological factors. It is, very rarely, an epileptic symptom. Sometimes it is found in several members of the family, *e.g.* mother, son and daughter, and may then be a peculiar physiological anomaly. It occurs, however, principally in children of emotionally labile, excitable disposition, and in children with definite discoverable conflicts, where the somnambulism is the equivalent of an hysterical symptom. In the hysterical group the goal of the sleep-walking may in itself suggest the psychological interpretation. For example, a boy of 10, very much attached to his mother, who had until recently slept in the same room with her, walked frequently in his sleep to his mother's bedroom, saying, 'You know about it', 'What is it?' 'Tell me the secret'. Talk of this kind is rarely recorded, but the apparent setting of a definite objective, especially the parent's room, is not rare.

It is not unknown, although it is very unusual, for a somnambulist to injure himself and even another person.

Treatment consists in adjusting psychological difficulties and prescribing a sedative at night.

Stammering. There are broadly two types of stammering: that acquired for the first time in adolescent or adult life in relation to some emotional problem, and stammering originating in childhood.

The first, of recent origin, and commonly of short duration, is a form of speech disorder that is easily and obviously imitable by voluntary effort, and is, in effect, an hysterical symptom. The more usual type of stammering is not so susceptible of close imitation and can often attain considerable complication in the form of tonic or clonic spasm of the articulatory movements. The former is entirely psychogenic; the latter type is mainly due to physiological instability in the neuromuscular organization, although it may be provoked or increased by emotional causes. In many instances it induces a secondary shyness, but some stammerers of this type are remarkably unembarrassed by their disability.

The evidence for a physiological basis of some sort lies in a family history of stammering, which is fairly often elicited, or of some speech defect which may not always amount to stammering, but may consist in lisping, or of mere slowness in enunciation. The not infrequent discovery of a family history of left-handedness has given rise to the theory that the fundamental fact is an incomplete dominance of the leading hemisphere. E.E.G. records tend to confirm this view, the alpha waves of the two hemispheres being out of phase. The incidence of stammering in the population is thought to be about 1 per cent.

The treatment of the physiological type of stammering must obviously depend on re-education, in addition, of course, to removal of any emotional factors which may reinforce the stammering. There are many varieties of re-educational method, but they all depend on a mixture of suggestion and a mechanical trick of articulation. Attempts at a deeper psychotherapy of stammering of this type have usually been unsuccessful, but it is nevertheless possible that some stammers originating in the first few years of speech development may be mainly or preponderantly of psychological origin. It has been shown in some cases that stammering can originate around infantile conflicts even as early as the suckling phase (Despert, 1943). Any threat to the mouth area at a time when phantasies are apt to centre round it, especially those concerned with aggressive impulses and fears of retribution, is likely to elicit stammering as a neurotic symptom (Orton, 1937).

The prognosis for a stammer of early origin of the physiological type is usually of spontaneous disappearance in the course of later adolescence. Few seem to persist into middle age. Naturally, a previous habit of stammering may be re-aroused under emotional stress.

Night Terrors. Night terrors are distinct from nightmares. In the latter, a dreamer, who may be child or adult, wakes from the dream in fear, with recollection as a rule of part of the dream content. In night terrors, which are almost confined to childhood, the child sits up in bed in fright, but evidently unconscious of his surroundings. He does not wake spontaneously, and in the morning has rarely any recollection of the occurrence. Where recollection does occur it is of a terrifying but indescribable and unformed visual hallucination.

Night terrors are physiological disturbances on an emotional basis and are not susceptible to treatment by psychological symbolic interpretation. They are practically confined to the over-active, intelligent, anxious type of child, and they tend to be transient phenomena.

Neuroses

Hysteria. Hysterical symptoms in children appear to be determined largely by the influence of suggestion, coupled with the desire for self-assertion or sympathy, or for evasion. Gross hysterical symptoms of the type of paralysis of limbs are not a common reaction but may appear nevertheless early. Hysterical symptoms of the type of somatic complaints (headache, bodily aches and pains and nausea) are frequent enough.

The influence of environmental example in determining the nature of the symptoms, not only in the hysterical type of reactions but in the anxiety type as well, was demonstrated by E. Richards, who pointed out that 'their symptom-pictures of distress are strangely similar to those of the adult invalid types—palpitation; shaking in stomach; headaches; pain in chest, abdomen and legs; giddy spells; fullness in the epigastrium; 'I feel all played out'; 'Sometimes I vomit a lot, too'. Here we see children who expressed complaints that they had absorbed from an atmosphere charged with hypochondriacal utterance and fear of disease, objectively reinforced by numerous prescriptions, patent medicines and the medical folk-lore of neighbourhood gossip. With the pattern of these reactions well established through the daily contact of actual behaviour, it needed but the catalysing agent of some unusual circumstance or emotional strain to produce a symptom-picture quite baffling to the ordinary approaches of clinical procedure.'

Disregard of the symptom and care that nothing merely 'invalidish' is gained by the child in having it, coupled with the means already advocated for the treatment of the expression of psychological distress in children, are the necessary therapeutic methods in the hysteria of childhood.

In addition to hysterical symptoms it is possible to find in some children all the makings of a so-called hysterical personality. It is only necessary to encounter such a case to realize how wrong it is to regard the hysterical type of personality as 'child-like'. 'Childish' it is, but not 'child-like'.

Rose V. furnishes a crude example of a hysterical reaction.

CASE No. 66

Rose V., age 9½, was referred by the District Organizer of Children's Care (L.C.C.). The child was reported to have attacks in school, in which she called out that she was going blind and was going to die, and that people were after her. She had refused some of her meals and would baulk at certain kinds of food.

Family History. The father, age 41, of Cornish descent, had been a sign-writer, then a stable-man and had now been unemployed for two years. He felt he had come down in the world, but did not give the impression of being fit for much except labouring.

He had met his wife during the war, and after a few weeks' acquaintance married her, partly out of pity. She had been neglected by her parents, who were addicted to drink, and she was often without food or shelter. The mother was a very unstable person. During the previous year she had had attacks in which she would get up in the night, dress and go out, followed by her husband. About the same time she had attacks of trembling and said that she was dying. These episodes occurred intermittently over a period of six months. She made a great fuss over her child's behaviour, which was her stock subject of gossip. She called on the headmistress of Rose's school and was excessively voluble. She even called at the private address of Rose's class teacher. The mother was practically illiterate and the more apt in consequence to think she was being imposed upon. There was one other child, a boy, age 6, who was lively and pugnacious, but got on well with his sister with only occasional quarrels.

Home Conditions. The home consisted of two rooms in a tenement scantily furnished and not very clean. The children slept in the parent's bedroom.

History of the Child. During the mother's pregnancy the father lost his employment, and circumstances became so reduced that part of the home had to be sold to pay expenses. Food was inadequate in consequence, both before and after Rose's birth.

Rose first came under hospital care when the mother complained that she screamed at night. Impetigo and bad teeth were also noted and treated at that time. No further special difficulty was noted until she was referred for the complaints noted above. It was also reported from the school that Rose had had a peculiar 'fit' in school, in which she said she was going to die, and frightened the teachers considerably on her account. On her way to hospital she had an attack of shrieking. Subsequently the class teacher concluded that she was given to 'acting' to escape work. If the teacher paid special attention to her she would begin to pay unnecessary services to the teacher, showing her pictures and so on.

Psychiatric Examination. No abnormality emerged in conversation. She was willing enough to talk about impersonal topics, but her illness was touched on only in a general way.

Her *intelligence rating* was 92·8 on the Binet-Simon scale, but she succeeded in getting into the low-average group mainly on the basis of her memory. After the eighth year she succeeded in four tests. Two of them were in age 10 and were both memory tests. Of the other two in year nine, one was repetition of digits backwards. In performance tests there was a scatter from 0 (Healy form board) to 10 (Porteus).

Her school report regarded her as average for her age. She was bad at arithmetic, but improving.

Physically there was no evidence of organic disease.

Treatment. The mother was instructed to ignore the attacks and the difficulty about food. If the child refused some article of food, nothing was to be said and nothing was to be substituted in its place. The mother was also asked to conceal her own symptoms, as far as possible, in the child's presence, and was encouraged to come for treatment herself. At the same time, she was asked to understand that Rose's symptoms probably betokened a desire for some display of affection as well as for attention, and that she could let her have this in the ordinary course of events. A similar line had already been taken by the school. The child herself was simply told that she would soon be quite well. An attempt was made to deal with the mother's own symptoms, but she did not co-operate in that respect.

The course of action taken with Rose was rapidly followed by an improvement, and when last heard of she had been free from symptoms for the past four months.

Anxiety States. Neurotic anxiety states are frequently the result of conscious or unconscious imitation of an atmosphere of anxiety in the home. The anxious mother especially is apt to produce an anxious child, and later an anxious adult. But whereas the treatment of an adult of this kind is a long process of investigation and recapitulation of a life history, too frequently with a final result that is still unsatisfactory, in children the re-education of the parents, together with the provision of healthy contacts and outlets for the child, can result in a product that is robustly happy and promises well for future stability. If resort is made to the (in some ways feeble) expedient of removing the child from the home, the symptoms are apt to disappear with characteristic rapidity and finality. The symptoms are the same as in adults and the causes are in part identical. Parental over-solicitude, motivated not infrequently by dissatisfactions in the parents' own love-life, is by far the commonest cause. The exceptionally strong attachment of the child to the parent that usually results is not invariably to the parent of the opposite sex. Worrying fathers can produce anxious sons.

Some of these anxiety states may be dependent on an Oedipus situation in the Freudian sense. So far, such children's neuroses as we have treated have not suggested that the proportion so determined is high, and the effect of such treatment suggests that such an explanation is not by any means always the most far-reaching or practical. It might, of course, be assumed that in treatment of this kind the external readjustments, which are made automatically, bring about a redirection of libido within the patient, but we prefer to work with the ascertainable facts and to reserve possible interpretations of a Freudian kind for the rare cases that do not respond to our usual measures, and to wait until the play technique had been used repeatedly by persons with a sound psychiatric and scientific training.

Phobias are much more difficult to treat than the other symptoms of neurotic anxiety. The special origin of the more usual phobias, such as fear of the dark, often remains undetermined. Probably some will never be further analysable and may be regarded as primitive or instinctive fears. Others can probably be produced in the manner of conditioned reflexes, by some accidental association, after the pattern of Watson's experiments on the effect of noise on infants. Some are produced by parental example, like the other symptoms of neurotic anxiety, while a residuum have the symbolic value of a symptom in the Freudian sense.

CASE No. 67

Kenneth C. is an example of an anxiety state which illustrates the above remarks.

This boy, age 12, was brought to hospital by his mother. She said that he slept badly, had terrifying dreams and twitchings of the limbs. He was not going to school on account of these symptoms and spent his time moping at home. He complained also of pain behind the ears and of headache. He was afraid of being left alone; out of doors he was terrified of traffic.

From his mother it was learned that he did not play with other boys, that his only recreation was reading and that he was so scared of the dark that his mother had to allow him to sleep with her. She had felt obliged to make a fuss of him because of his 'nervousness', and to show preference for him over her younger son. She tried to arrange special conditions for him in school, and kept him away from it often for trifling ailments. He attended an elementary school and was in Standard 5, but his work was not up to that standard. He had of course been frequently absent on account of his symptoms.

Family History. His father was said to be 'nervous', *i.e.* anxious, unstable and impatient, sometimes striking the boy when he refused to go to school. His mother admitted that she also was 'nervous', *i.e.* apprehensive, but claimed that she could conquer this. The paternal grandfather died in a mental hospital. The mother, who married at 30, had had three pregnancies. The first resulted in a miscarriage, the patient was the second and the youngest boy, now 10 years of age, was reported healthy. The patient was born when his mother was 32. The boys slept together in their parents' room. When the latter proposed moving to a room downstairs, Kenneth refused to be parted from his mother at night.

Early History. His mother said that he had been a very quiet baby, that he was late in walking, but that he talked at about one year and cut his teeth at the normal age. His quietness and lack of spontaneity were the only abnormal signs in infancy. His only acute physical illnesses had been measles and rheumatic fever.

Mental Condition on Examination. He wept and shrank away when spoken to, and clung to his mother's skirts. At the first interview he would not answer at all. He looked terrified and altogether miserable. No information was to be obtained from him on this first occasion. Subsequently a Binet-Simon rating was done, and gave him an I.Q. of 97. The psychologist's report was as follows:

'No specific defects in elementary processes were detected except (*a*) a slight reduction in visual discrimination and retention of forms, which possibly influenced spelling ability; (*b*) some lowering of normal power in auditory retention (immediate and distant).

'Motor response was good, suggestions were resisted and association was good.

Reasoning showed badly on tests (mental age, 10 years) but was probably influenced by emotional factors.

'The main mental characteristics revealed in the boy's whole work and attitude were:
(1) a marked distrust of his own capacity;
(2) inability to make efforts in the face of difficulty or adverse criticism.

'The test results are probably not a true indication of his native intelligence, but show the operation of intelligence, in many ways above the average, hampered by emotional and temperamental factors. Failure in school work may be largely attributable to similar causes.'

Physical Status. There was no physical abnormality. He was fairly well grown and developed.

Treatment. In view of the exceptional difficulty of the boy's disposition, it was decided to give him the benefit of a period away from home among other boys. This was done and seemed to be meeting with a fair measure of success, when he became very depressed and threatened to take his own life if he were not allowed home. He was found in a dark pantry with an open penknife. He walked on one occasion in his sleep, and was reported to have narrowly escaped falling downstairs. His parents were instructed in the necessity of encouraging him to emancipate himself from them, especially from his mother. They were to encourage him to play football and to join the Scouts. It was arranged that he should sleep with his brother, in a bedroom of their own. His brother undertook to teach him to box.

On his return home he walked once in his sleep and frequently talked in it; he slept and ate better and expressed a desire to join a football club, which he had never done before. Also he played more readily with his brother.

Fifteen months after he was first seen, a letter was received from his mother, stating that he was much better, had been chosen to play for his school at football and was mixing well with other boys.

We might have preferred to consider this as an example principally of timidity, induced and fostered principally by the mother's attitude, rather than of an anxiety neurosis in a child, because the former hypothesis is simpler and covers all the facts without making the invocation of hypothetical factors necessary, and forms a successful basis for treatment.

As a result of child and mother being excessively dependent on one another, a child may suffer acutely from separation anxiety on going to school. This is perhaps the commonest basis of a 'school phobia', where the child at any stage in its school career may openly refuse to go to school and pose a considerable problem to the parents and to the family doctor. The condition has recently been discussed in a leading annotation in the *British Medical Journal* (1960). Timid, spoilt children, only children and those much younger than their siblings are said to be especially at risk: and mothers who are overprotective, insecure and inconsistent in the handling of their children's problems predispose them to fears of this and other kinds. The child may also be unhappy at school because of poor performance there or a disturbed relationship with other children and teachers. The sooner the child can be returned to school the better; but the acutely anxious child cannot be forced to return—it would often require physical violence to overcome his fearful holding back. The reaction is usually complexly determined and both child and mother need help. If the child is off school for more than a week or two, specialist advice should be sought. However inconvenient it may be administratively, it must be recognized that certain children cannot fit happily into the normal pattern of schooling and special, more flexible, arrangements may have to be made for their education.

OBSESSIVE-COMPULSIVE SYMPTOMS as they occur in children have been discussed briefly in the chapter on adult neuroses. It is only necessary to add here that in children they seldom by themselves constitute a condition that is brought for treatment.

Some delinquent acts are produced in a way precisely analogous with the mode of production of neurotic symptoms. They are the outcome of conflict, or a substitute or compromise between opposing tendencies, and are symbolic, while the delinquent is unaware of their real source and may suffer from neurotic symptoms in the ordinary sense at the same time.

Thus, reporting instances of incendiarism in children, Yarnell (1940) observed the following characteristics: 1. They set the fires with accompanying daydreams of burning some member of the family who had either withheld his affection from the child or become too serious a rival for the parental love; 2. the fires were made in or around their own homes, causing little damage and being usually put out by the child himself, a sign therefore, as Yarnell points out, that the act was chiefly symbolic; 3. the children showed anxiety and suffered from terrifying dreams at night and terrifying phantasies in the day-time; and 4. all the children had some recent mental conflict.

One of the most striking things about this study was the similarity of the children's thoughts to what is found in Biblical writings. Thus, they felt that anyone bad was doomed to destruction by fire, but in the end everything became new and perfect by the purifying effect of fire. They seemed to feel that killing by fire would render the object of their act good, and that he would then be restored to life or 'reborn'.

All the children had suffered from deprivation of love from parents or their substitutes, and many had lacked even food and economic security; in fact, what seemed to distinguish them from neurotic children and made them delinquent rather than neurotic in the ordinary sense was the intensity of their deprivation.

Psychoses

Psychoses in childhood are rare. Parents commonly fear that any oddity of behaviour in their children may be a sign of insanity, particularly if there is a family history of mental illness; but it is very unusual for the psychiatrist to have to confirm their fears. It is axiomatic that behaviour which would be considered psychotic in an adult may be normal in a child. This does not mean that certain trends of behaviour in childhood may not be factors, if left uncorrected, in the development of a psychosis in adult life.

Even if patients up to the age of 16 years are included, the numbers of psychotic illnesses remain small. Adding together the figures for several large series of admission to mental hospitals in various parts of the world, it was found that only 1 per cent. of 21,000 admissions were of children or young adolescents (Gillespie, 1939). Even this figure probably implies the use of the word psychotic in a wide sense.

2 L

Though the numbers involved are small, these illnesses are important, not only on account of the great suffering that they cause to the children themselves and to their parents, but because of the possibility that an understanding of the psychoses of childhood may throw light on the aetiology of the much more numerous psychoses of adult life. Clinical differentiation is still at an elementary stage. A great deal more research is required in this field: we need more detailed case reports, more intensive investigations of both the mental and physical aspects (using the most accurate biochemical and other laboratory techniques), and more long-term follow-up studies.

Schizophrenia. This is very uncommon in childhood, and by no means all children labelled schizophrenic are psychotic—some we have seen wrongly diagnosed have been severely subnormal (mentally defective) from birth. Understandably, the older the child the more nearly the clinical picture resembles that of adult schizophrenia, but differentiation into adult sub-types is very difficult. Kanner (1957) draws attention to the following features. The child's scholastic ability begins to deteriorate, concentration becomes impaired, interest in and contact with others begins to be lost. There is day-dreaming, seclusiveness, lack of rapport, irritability, and in some cases hypochondriasis. Speech and general behaviour become disordered, the latter in the direction either of great restlessness and impulsiveness, or immobility with katatonic features. Delusions tend to be simple and symbolization naïve.

Early Infantile Autism. Kanner first described this condition in 1943, and since then many other psychiatrists have confirmed his reports. In his textbook (1957) he includes early infantile autism in the chapter on schizophrenia: but it is by no means certain that the condition is allied to schizophrenia. The aetiology is unknown, and follow-up studies have not yet given us a clear picture of the outcome.

Children suffering from early infantile autism are commonly first suspected of being deaf or subnormal (mentally defective). But these children, though they are inaccessible to formal intelligence testing, do not look unintelligent. What is most characteristic is their 'extreme autistic aloneness', and this may be apparent from the first year of life, the child not stretching out its arms, for example, to be picked up. They are abnormally self-sufficient, interested in things (and able to manipulate them skilfully) but apparently not in people, with whom they seem quite unable to form normal emotional relationships. In their behaviour they show an obsessive need for the maintenance of the exact *status quo* in their environment. Speech is grossly disturbed: about one third are mute, the others have great difficulties in various ways—they cannot form sentences, or use personal pronouns easily, or understand the concept 'Yes', and they may exhibit echolalia: rote memory on the other hand is often excellent. It is a striking clinical syndrome.

Autistic children appear to come usually from notably intelligent stock: many of the parents are university or college graduates. Kanner (1954) described the majority of the parents as detached, humourless perfectionists, 'more at home in the world of abstractions than in the world of people. . . . They treat their children about as meticulously and impersonally as they treat their automobiles.

. . . It is possible to speak of them as successfully autistic adults.' Kanner thought that the autistic children of these parents had suffered 'emotional refrigeration'. Whether upbringing or inheritance is the more important is, however, still uncertain: and though physical and laboratory investigations have so far produced negative findings, the condition may be organically determined.

Manic-Depressive Psychosis. Both manic and depressive psychotic reactions can occur in childhood, but both are rare, the former especially so. States of depression of a transient kind with self-accusation are probably common enough in childhood, but they very infrequently attain psychotic form or intensity. Schilder and Bender (1937) in an investigation of 65 child patients with suicidal preoccupations do not appear to have encountered any who were suffering from a manic-depressive form of illness. These children either came from very unhappy homes, or were themselves psychopathic—reacting to frustration, real or imagined, of their affectionate impulses with intolerance and vengeful phantasies of suicide. The few attempted suicides in children that we have encountered have been in children from very unhappy homes. Of completed suicides in children below the age of 15 years, only one-fifth occur before 13 and four-fifths occur between 13 and 15 (that is, in early adolescence).

Occasionally in the history of a manic-depressive psychosis in an adult, one finds evidence of a depressive phase having occurred within the first ten years of life.

Dementia Infantilis. Heller (1908) described a condition, with onset usually in the third or fourth year, characterized by a specially rapid and profound disturbance of speech, leading to its almost complete loss, by extreme restlessness, and by a uniformly unfavourable outcome (only one case has been reported as improving) in a state of dementia, which is reached in a few months. Stereotyped and tic-like movements, episodes of anxiety, apparently hallucinatory experiences, and cruel and aggressive behaviour have also been described. The deterioration has been said to differ from a schizophrenic one in that there is retention of the emotional response to joy or shock, and of anxiety at an elementary level. The facial expression remains intelligent, the physical health is relatively well maintained, and there are no gross neurological signs or fits. Various quite different pathological changes in the brain have been reported, including inflammation and diffuse sclerosis.

This is probably not a clinical entity, and further research is required.

Hyperkinesia. Hyperkinesia is not uncommon in young children who are subnormal (mentally defective) and have suffered a brain injury. Hyperkinesia may or may not in these cases be associated with epilepsy, but there appears to be a connection between the two symptoms. It has been reported that about 8 per cent. of epileptic children may become hyperkinetic.

Ounsted (1955) has given a comprehensive account of a series of seventy children who suffered from fits and hyperkinesia. Some intellectual deficit is common but not invariable: intelligence ranged from high normal to severely subnormal. The hyperkinesia is global, the over-activity (which may continue for months or years) being at about double the speed and energy level of the normal child. Attention and concentration are poor. Brief intense outbursts of rage, aggression and destructive behaviour are common. The mood may be unstable, but is usually euphoric and often constantly so. Shyness and fear are absent and spontaneously affectionate behaviour tends to be lost. Sleep is profound. These children are extremely disturbing at home and intolerable in school.

Ounsted draws attention to these other features. Male children predominate among these cases, and he considers male sex a significant aetiological factor. The epilepsy, initiated usually by cerebral damage of a heterogeneous kind prenatally or perinatally, commences in most cases in the first five years of life and all types of epileptic seizures are found, except *petit mal*. In some cases status epilepticus appeared to have initiated or exacerbated the mental disorder. The left and right hemispheres were equally often affected as shown by hemiplegia, focal seizures, E.E.G. foci and dominant handedness. Primidone was found to be the most useful anticonvulsant, but it did not relieve the behaviour disorder. Dextro-amphetamine sulphate produced improvement in one-quarter of the cases, and a depressive reaction in two-thirds.

Subnormality (Mental Defect)

Subnormality has been described in another chapter. Reference may be made here to the large numbers of the dull and backward group—those who are intellectually below average but not sufficiently so to be regarded as subnormal (mentally defective). They furnish many of the problems seen at psychiatric clinics for children. It is often not until they begin to play truant or behave badly in some way as the result of their difficulty in school work that an opportunity is given for a precise assessment of their intelligence. The disturbances they exhibit are not, however, different in kind from those described elsewhere in this chapter.

It is important to distinguish intrinsic from accidental retardation. A child may be backward at school and also score badly on intelligence tests as the result of emotional difficulties, or of faulty attitudes on the part of his teachers, or from lack of stimulation such as occurs in the institutionalized child, or from a local deficit such as word blindness with which some children struggle through school undiagnosed. We have known a child's intelligence quotient rise considerably in a few months when such difficulties have been dealt with along the lines indicated by the diagnostic conclusions. Ingram and Reid (1956) have shown how educational retardation and difficulties due to developmental aphasia, may lead to behaviour disorders of many different kinds. They present a detailed account of 78 children of average intelligence referred to a department of child psychiatry, who were found to have specific dyslexia and dysgraphia due to developmental aphasia. Retarded speech development, expressive and receptive aphasia and speech defects were commonly also found in these children.

The relation between subnormality and psychosis in children is complicated. Some cases classed as subnormal are probably states of defect following a psychotic process such as schizophrenia. Differentiation is often difficult clinically and depends a great deal on the history. As in the adult, a psychosis may be superimposed on one who is already subnormal.

Disorders Associated with Physical Disease

Epidemic encephalitis in children has already been dealt with under the organic-reaction types, and the emotional instability associated with chorea is well known. Regarding trauma, it is difficult to assess the effects of head trauma on subsequent behaviour and the nervous disorders of children. Head trauma of some kind has almost invariably occurred, and great weight is laid upon it by the parents, so that of all incidents in the history it is likely to be singled out for special attention by them.

Our impression, however, in cases where there has been undoubted brain trauma, sometimes of a severe kind, is that the prolonged after-effects in children are surprisingly few and slight. There are rare cases in which injury has been so severe as to lead to permanent subnormality (mental defect). In one case in our experience the only prolonged residuum of a severe head trauma (which produced delirium in a girl of 9 for several weeks immediately following an accident) was a slight defect in immediate memory (retention). Epileptic fits and irritability can also occur.

Results like this are rare. More usually it is disorders of behaviour and neuroses which are attributed to head trauma. Investigation in these cases nearly always shows that the symptom existed before or otherwise independently of the head injury. It not infrequently happens that the extra consideration given to the child who has had a head injury, and the additional allowances made for it, lead to spoiling, and it is this spoiling and not the injury which is responsible for most of the after-effects of which the parents subsequently complain.

Nervousness is often associated with rheumatism but the association is, more often than is commonly supposed, an unreal one (Winnicott, 1939) since the diagnosis 'rheumatic' is often applied to vague aches and pains where no objective evidence of rheumatism is forthcoming, and the term 'chorea' when the movements are impulsive or, at most, fidgety. In such cases the 'neurosis' and the 'rheumatic' manifestations may alike be indicative of mental conflict associated with unconscious phantasies of the type alluded to under 'Play therapy'.

Endocrine Disease. This has influences that are mainly indirect. The more direct associations between endocrine disease and personality remain somewhat conjectural, just as in adults.

As regards indirect effects, precocity of physical development or immaturity or abnormality produce obvious difficulties of adjustment to other children, who in any case are not sufficiently developed in social sentiments to attempt to make life easier for those who are in any way conspicuously different from the rest.

The direct effects of endocrine disease are the physical urges, which, like the excessive appetite of some patients with pituitary disease, or the excessive sexual urge of those having a precocious development of the gonads, will tend to produce behaviour disorders rather than deviations of personality. It is important on the other hand not to jump to conclusions that just because a child is sluggish and indolent and has, say, a Fröhlich's syndrome, there is a necessary causal connection between the two, since we have encountered children with Fröhlich's syndrome in whom such characteristics were not well marked.

REFERENCES

British Medical Journal (1960) School Phobia, **2**, 848.
Despert, J. L. (1943) *Amer. J. Psychiat.*, **99**, 881.
Freud, A. (1928) *Introduction to the Technic of Child Analysis*, New York.
Healy, W. (1915) *The Individual Delinquent*, Boston.
Healy, W., and Bronner, A. F. (1936) *New Light on Delinquency and its Treatment*, London.
Heller, T. (1908) *Z. Erforsch. Jugendl. schwaehsinns*, **2**, 17.
Ingram, T. T. S., and Reid, J. F. (1956) *Arch. Dis. Childh.*, **31**, 161.
Kanner, L. (1954) *Res. Publ. Ass. nerv. ment. Dis.*, **33**, 378.
Kanner, L. (1957) *Child Psychiatry*, Illinois.
Klein, M. (1932) *The Psycho-analysis of Children*, London.
Orton, S. T. (1937) *Reading, Writing and Speech Problems in Children*, New York.
Ounsted, C. (1955) *Lancet*, ii, 303.
Rogerson, C. H. (1939) *Play Therapy in Childhood*, London.
Schilder, P., and Bender, L. (1937) *Amer. J. Orthopsychiat.*, **7**, 225.
Stalker, H., and Band, D. (1946) *J. ment. Sci.*, **92**, 324.
Winnicott, D. W. (1939) *A Survey of Child Psychiatry*, London.
Yarnell, H. Y. (1940) *Amer. J. Orthopsychiat.*, **10**, 272.

20

OCCUPATIONAL THERAPY

An active, well-organized department of occupational therapy is an essential, integral part of every hospital dealing with the physical or psychological rehabilitation of those who are in need of such specialized help. It enlists the co-operation of the patients so that they themselves can form an estimate of their own progress and be encouraged to make further efforts. It adds to their resources and hastens a satisfactory and healthy adaptation to their bodily and psychological needs. Furthermore the prescription of suitable occupation can attain its purpose: 1. through its own merit; 2. by being complementary to any other form of treatment; and 3. by its utilization not only during the course of the illness but even after recovery has been effected. Its scope has recently been defined by a Committee of the American Occupational Therapy Association (1960), and its success, in a general way, is considered likely to depend on the activity undertaken, the atmosphere in which it is performed, and the relationship established with the professional staff.

The principles embodied in the above statement are by no means new. The acolytes, priests and other attendants who formed the staff at the 'healing temples' of Aesculapius, where it was believed that even the dead could be restored to life, were well aware of them. They did everything possible to promote the right atmosphere, the proper state of mind, so that the person might be more susceptible of cure. An attractive site was chosen for the temple, its natural beauties were enhanced, and everything possible was done to exteriorize the patient by employing his leisure in a purposeful, constructive manner, rather than by allowing him to sink into a state of contemplation which could so easily lead to apathy and stagnation. Unfortunately, however, the above healing methods were not followed up and organized as they might have been, and it was not until the Humane Period of the treatment of the mentally disordered had been instituted that occupation as a form of therapy became recognized. The archives of many of our mental hospitals in Europe and Great Britain can verify these facts. The physician superintendents of those institutions in their annual reports invariably emphasized the value of suitable employment as a means of promoting efficiency, happiness, a sense of accomplishment. Life, even in a mental hospital, could be made constructive, the monotony of hospitalization could be alleviated, and the chance of improvement and recovery expedited. Congenial work was found to be an antidote to irritation, friction, gossip, boredom, introspection and bad habits. In a more positive way it bred interest, skill and orderly habits of mind and body. As an example reference may be made to the records of the Glasgow Royal Mental Hospital which date back to 1814. The evidence they provide is impressive. For instance in 1817 it is stated: 'Two looms and five spinning wheels are generally kept at work; clothes are made or mended, stockings and worsted gloves are knit, and occasionally a little muslin is flowered though, on the whole, this is the least profitable manufacture, because when any freak or wrangling occurs the figures are apt to rise on the wrong side. Every encouragement, however, is given to the exertions of industry, because nothing contributes so much to promote a cure, and prevent a relapse.'

Another excerpt from the enlightened report of 1820 is worthy of recording: 'Sociality has often been promoted, while the irksomeness of confinement has been alleviated by various occupations and amusements. Bowls and billiards have been favourite games, and reading, music and drawing have often served to arrest attention and to dispel illusion. Some write letters or poems, one solves mathematical problems, and another has been busily engaged in composing the history of a voyage round the world. . . . Some have laboured in the garden or shrubbery grounds; shoes have been made and cloth woven by various individuals, and one patient is at present very useful as a joiner. Some of the females have knitted and sewed diligently, and so many of them have been industriously employed in spinning that almost all the bed and table linen now used in the asylum is the product of their labour.'

A much wider aspect was also kept in mind because in 1821 we find the following: 'Our asylum, we believe, is the first establishment of the kind in which a sermon was ever preached. . . . We are not aware that divine service, as in Church, was ever performed in any lunatic establishment in this country until it was introduced into our asylum, and we are much gratified to find that our example in affording the benefit of religious instruction and consolation to the insane begins now to be generally followed.' The above innovation became so appreciated that one of the patients thanked the clergyman for his kind condescension and added that he was particularly gratified to be thought worthy of attending public worship.

The social side of hospital life was also developed. Weekly dances, ward parties, indoor games, e.g. billiards, cards, draughts, etc., outside activities such as cricket, hockey, curling, golf, tennis, all provided an opportunity for patients and staff to meet informally. Charitable organizations, by providing lectures, concerts, plays, did much to brighten the lives of all those patients whose illness might require continued treatment over many years. The so-called 'therapeutic communities', whose praises we sing to-day, were not unknown to our psychiatric forebears!

It must be admitted, however, that the institutional and economic needs of the hospital were probably given precedence over the more individual aspects which are the hall-mark of well organized occupational therapy. The criticism that good hard-working willing patients were exploited for the benefit of the institution would not be easy to refute. The patients were recommended, in a more or less haphazard way, to the laundry, kitchen, sewing-room, piggery, garden or artisan's department. They were sent where they were most needed, and they accepted hospital life uncomplainingly, so long as they received the extra privileges and perquisites which they were so well entitled to. But the withdrawn, listless, apathetic, depressed, delusional patients many of whom had never been accustomed to manual work were far too numerous, and came to be regarded as unemployable. It was only when it became more fully recognized that the success of an occupational therapy department could be measured by its ability to provide work for those who were thought to be unemployable that its organization was justified.

In Scotland (and perhaps in Great Britain) the earliest attempt to organize the employment of patients, on a specialized and systematic basis, was launched in 1880 when a far-sighted and charitably minded woman, Lady Brabazon, offered a grant of money to any workhouse or infirmary which developed a plan to employ their 'crippled and infirm inmates'. The challenge was taken up in 1895 by the managers of the Barnhill Poor House, Glasgow, and in 1898 Dr. Hamilton Marr at the Woodilee Mental Hospital, Glasgow, introduced a similar scheme. It was arranged that, once a week, a group of ladies interested in handicrafts should visit the hospital so as to teach certain forms of handicraft. That particular day, subsequently known as 'Brabazon Day', became eagerly anticipated. In official circles, however, occupational therapy did not receive a very warm reception; it was regarded as a well-intentioned fad. In 1899 an editorial in the *Journal of Mental Science* commented as follows: 'Provided the work be carried on with the sympathy and accord of the asylum officials, as doubtless it would be, we see no objection to the Brabazon scheme in these institutions; at any rate for our pauper asylums it appears to be well worthy of an extended trial'. We need not be too severe in our criticism of that somewhat niggardly snobbish comment because government financial help was at a minimum, there were no adequate facilities and many mental hospitals were dependent for their existence on bequests and voluntary contributions. The maintenance of the institution was regarded as the first priority, and no surplus funds were available for necessary amenities which were regarded as luxuries. It is only in very recent years that we have witnessed the shift from rough-and-ready group methods to individualization, to the intensive study of the needs of each person. The majority of those who suffer from nervous and mental illness resent it, their pride and sense of prestige is hurt, they would love to exhibit an objective lesion to justify their apparent failure. They feel that they have been lacking in faith and determination, that they should have striven harder, that they are not suffering from an illness at all but merely sheer lack of will power. The truth is that they have struggled on for far too long, and have become exhausted bodily and mentally. It is our immediate duty to help them at once, and to supply them as speedily as possible with those physical and spiritual vitamins which they are so much in need of. Psyche responds to companionship, friends, attention and interest, congenial work and occupation, suitable literature and all those other things which a well-organized occupational department can supply. The programme must always be of an elastic nature, and so geared as likely to obtain a quick response.

When thinking along the above lines we were reminded of an address delivered in 1903 by that great philosopher-physician, Sir William Osler, to the undergraduates of Toronto University. Its title was the 'Master-Word in Medicine'. He said: 'Though a little one the master-word looms large in meaning. It is the open sesame to every portal, the great equalizer in the world, the true philosopher's stone which transmutes all the base metal of humanity into gold. The stupid man among you it will make bright, the bright man brilliant, and the brilliant student steady. With the magic word in your heart all things are possible, and without it all study is vanity and vexation. The miracles of life are with it; the blind see by touch, the deaf hear with eyes, the dumb speak with fingers. . . . The master-word is "Work" . . . a little one, as I have said . . . directly responsible for all advances in medicine during the past twenty-five centuries.' While those words were addressed as a principle, precept and injunction to medical students yet they appear peculiarly appropriate to the topic which concerns us here, and are not too great a digression from our chronological account of work as a healing agent.

Adolf Meyer in a paper entitled 'The Philosophy of Occupational Therapy' described how in 1893 he began to realize that 'the proper use of time in some helpful and gratifying activity appeared to be fundamental in the treatment of any neuro-psychiatric patient'. At a later date his interest was stimulated by Dr. W. R. Dunton, Jr., one of the founder members of the American Occupational Therapy Association. In 1902 at the Psychiatric Institute, Wards Island, New York, with the valuable help of Mrs. Meyer, and the enthusiastic support of Dr. Dent and Dr. Mabon the successive medical superintendents of the Manhattan State Hospital, an occupational therapy department with associated recreational activities was established. One of the staff nurses of the Manhattan State Hospital was chosen to attend a course of training under Miss Lathrop at the Chicago School of Civics and Philanthropy, and afterwards returned to the Manhattan State Hospital to organize occupational work. In this humble way organized occupational therapy took its rise to become, in due course, welded into the World Federation of Occupational Therapy which exercises great influence, and sets a high standard.

It seems appropriate enough that the Glasgow Royal Mental Hospital, whose archives have already given up some of their secrets, should have earned the distinction of being the first mental hospital in Scotland to organize an occupational therapy department. The occupational work we had seen and been able to take part in, in the United States, had impressed us so much that we were impelled to follow the example which had been set. In consequence, in 1919 a scheme was submitted to Dr. L. R. Oswald, the Physician Superintendent, and to the Managers of the Glasgow Royal Mental Hospital for their approval. Their support was most cordial, and with the co-operation of Miss Darney, the matron, and selected members of the nursing staff, and the patients themselves, classes of an occupational and recreational nature were arranged. In 1922 Miss Dorothea Robertson, a resourceful, intelligent and charming woman was appointed to be in charge of the department. Pavilions were erected apart from the main hospital buildings, and an attempt was made to make them as attractive as possible; a great variety of crafts were made available. In 1924 the Scottish Division of the Royal Medico-Psychological Association met at the hospital to discuss the value and importance of occupational therapy; that meeting constituted the first meeting ever devoted to that topic in Great Britain. It was the forerunner for the development of organized occupational departments in the mental hospitals throughout the British Isles. But to make such departments really effective it was soon realized that the establishment of training schools, for those wishing to adopt such work as a career, was an imperative necessity. Thus it was that in 1933 an occupational therapy department was opened at the Astley Ainslie Hospital, Edinburgh. In the first instance it was staffed by senior Canadian therapists recommended by the Canadian Medical Association. In 1937 the Training Centre was opened so that students could be prepared for occupational work both in the physical and psychiatric fields. The comprehensive course of instruction extends over a period of three years.

We have always been strongly of the opinion that the person in charge of such a department in a mental hospital should have been specially trained for the post. It has been argued that a trained mental hospital nurse would be more appropriate. That, however, is not our experience. The fact that the occupational therapist provides a different social and educational standard, and is not so concerned with the disciplinary side of hospital life as the nurse constitutes a great advantage. We believe, however, that the trained occupational therapists should have the ability to transmit their knowledge to others, and possess the sympathetic understanding whereby they can gain the co-operation both of patients and nursing staff. Jealousy and rivalry between hospital staff merely retards the improvement or recovery of the patients. There is much to be done to enable them to overcome their difficulties. While every effort must be made to produce work of a satisfying standard yet the work *per se* is not the main thing. The essential thing is to stimulate the patient to produce something, no matter how simple, so as to create a sense of accomplishment. A word or two of praise, a pat on the back, the individual touch can work wonders. Frequent discussions between the therapists and the medical and nursing staff regarding the progress of the patient are essential. Sometimes the doctor seems to think he has fulfilled his function by referring the patient to the occupational department, and may take no further interest in that part of the treatment. But occupational treatment should be prescribed with as much care and consideration as a drug, and should be altered or changed according to the progress, or lack of it, which is taking place. Those in charge of the occupational department can often make valuable contributions at the medical staff meetings when individual cases come up for discussion.

The accommodation provided for an occupational division should be quite simple, but it should be made attractive, well lit, with plenty of window-space, modern tools and appliances, and sufficient rooms so that, if necessary, certain crafts requiring quiet surroundings and special skill can be practised separately. It is of great advantage to provide a display room for completed articles. In addition to the work centre it is most advantageous to provide a play centre where games, physical exercises and dancing can be indulged in.

For the smooth and efficient working of the department it has seemed to us to be important to grade the patients into classes so that the less skilled do not feel over-awed by their more expert neighbours, and so that more individual attention can be given to those most in need of help. Some patients like to spend all their available time in the occupational department, but as a general rule the classes should not be longer than 1–2 hours, depending upon the patient's ability to maintain his interest and concentration. The work should never be allowed to become too monotonous and fatiguing.

Frequently we have been asked whether one type of work is more applicable to a particular form of mental or nervous disorder than to another. We have never found it to be so. The potential talent of each patient has to be considered anew apart altogether from the mental disorder from which he may be suffering. 'Familiarity breeds contempt' would seem to be the order of the day in an occupational department for there it is not uncommon to see depressed patients who, if unoccupied, might be suicidal, using sharp tools and other lethal instruments with impunity. It is, however, important that such instruments should be carefully accounted for before the patient returns to his ward unit. When the patient goes to the department for the first time the work given should be able to yield quick results; the use of bright colours is preferred to something drab. Some patients adapt themselves easily to raffia and cane work, basket- and chair-making, weaving, joinery, toy making; others of a more aesthetic and artistic type may prefer china painting, drawing, embroidery, leather work, pottery, brass hammering, or a host of other crafts all of which may create a feeling of something well done. It should always be possible to cater for every taste. Nor must the scope of employment be limited to the department alone. Our hospitals are usually situated in pleasant surroundings which provide ample opportunity for outside games, pleasant exercise, gardening and other out-door work. The house-keeping departments are always in need of good workers who prefer such employment to more exotic tasks.

THE PURPOSES OF THE DEPARTMENT

1. It affords an additional outlet for a variety of interests and offers facilities for constructive work not only during the period of hospital treatment but also after the patient has returned home. For instance, a single man, 40 years old, who resented his admission to hospital, stated that he was unlawfully detained, that it was a 'frame-up'. He paced the floor continuously, was influenced by hallucinations of hearing, taste and smell, and resented being questioned. He thought the other patients were laughing at him, slept poorly, and looked ill both physically and mentally. He was persuaded, eventually, to visit the occupational division where he was amazed by the activity and happiness. He said that he would like to learn rug-making. He proved a diligent, capable worker who found great pleasure in working out his own designs. He became co-operative, his symptoms abated, and he made a satisfactory recovery. On returning to his own home he added considerably to his income by continuing his work at the craft which he had learned.

Another striking example of the curative value of an occupational department was instanced, in the case of a young man, 20 years old, who was sullen, perverse and antagonistic. He was determined to make things unpleasant for all who had to care for him. He refused to wash or shave, or dress himself. After much persuasion he was induced to visit the occupational department. There, fortunately, he soon found he was able to sublimate his feelings of antagonism and resentment. China painting proved an attraction, he expressed a wish to try it. He was given a bowl on which he drew his own design, and became so successful and talented that at a crafts exhibition, held in the city, he was awarded a first prize. The occupational department made his temporary hospital residence much more bearable, and indirectly helped him to tackle his problems in a better balanced frame of mind.

2. An occupational department creates a new series of contacts.

The trained teachers whose task it is to appeal to the patient's practical interests—irrespective of the disorder from which they may be suffering—establish a relationship which is different from that of doctor or nurse. Patients who are antagonistic to the medical and nursing staff may, and often do, establish a most harmonious relationship with the occupational therapist. As an example we can report the case of a male schizophrenic patient who had been a 'wallflower' for over forty years. When it was suggested that he might be tried in the occupational department the nurses who were in charge of him shook their heads in wonder. They said that many attempts had been made to employ him but they had been useless. The result, however, which followed exceeded all expectations. He responded to the therapist and to the general activity of the department. He learned the art of cane-weaving so as to make seats for stools and chairs, and soon became a rug-maker as well. He acquired an interest which he never had had previously, life became pleasanter, and the monotony of his hospital residence was alleviated. He was weaned back into a constructive occupation.

3. An occupational department creates a work-atmosphere where there is a spirit of competition so that a healthy rivalry comes into play. The desire to be occupied becomes infectious.

All the above-mentioned factors work together to create a spirit of hope, faith and accomplishment. And these objects can be attained in every type of case from the subnormal child to the geriatric patient. It is only a matter of modifying techniques and of having the capacity to form a good personal relationship or rapport with the particular patient. Every occupational therapist is not suited for psychiatric work any more than every doctor is. It requires patience, understanding and a natural flair or aptitude for being able to get in touch with the nervous and mentally affected. The aim in view is to substitute good habits and thinking in place of bad ones, to establish a philosophy of life and work in place of fantasy thinking in terms of the unattainable. Through suitable work we can help the spark of light in the subnormal to burn a little brighter, the depressed anxious-minded patient can be made to feel that life has still something in store, the manic can direct his energy aright, the paranoid can be side-tracked from his supposed wrongs, and even those with organic brain disease and dwindling intellectual powers may be prevented from sinking into a profound dementia.

OCCUPATIONAL THERAPY AT HOME

Occupational therapy does not necessarily begin and end in hospital. What has been learned in hospital can often be continued at home, there is no reason why occupational therapists should not provide a home service analogous to that of the psychiatric social worker. There are many subnormal and geriatric patients who do not require hospital treatment but who would benefit from the imaginative advice of a skilled occupational therapist. The fascination of acquiring new knowledge, the recognition of a talent which had lain dormant, the ability to transform a hobby into a profitable vocation can all create intense satisfaction. The biggest incentive lies in the possibility of preserving one's general health, but if even a small financial reward is forthcoming it adds to one's enthusiasm and persistence of effort.

OCCUPATION AS A METHOD OF PREVENTION

As the teaching of psychiatry becomes more firmly welded into the medical curriculum the doctor of the future, whether general practitioner or specialist, will become more appreciative of its medico-social importance. As a result he will become a better informed doctor because he will have learned not to confine his interest to the disease or problem *per se*, but to the person who is suffering from it. This widens the scope of treatment enormously, because with his intimate knowledge of the family, their illnesses, circumstances and resources, the general practitioner will be in a good position to advise not only in relation to the use of medicinal remedies, but also to the mental hygiene of childhood, and of how a successful adaptation to education (school, university, workshop), marriage and other social and business responsibilities can be best effected. The whole-hearted application and acceptance of the above principles is likely to place the general practitioner in the forefront of preventive medicine; he will become something of a social scientist.

Many large business and industrial organizations have been gravely concerned with the problem of wastage turn-over caused by discontented and inefficient workmen who are often the cause of friction arising between employer and employee. Works doctors and personnel managers have been appointed to deal with those situations. They recognize very clearly that complaints of irritability, restless impatience, indigestion, headache, palpitation, fatigue, etc., stem—not always from some physical lesion—but from underlying emotional factors which require to be thoroughly investigated. Tonics and tranquillizers are not enough. They need to be replaced, or at least complemented by, social measures and a study of the personality. Organizations such as The National Institute of Industrial Psychology and the Industrial Fatigue Research Board have constantly emphasized the above matters, and stressed how, both in peace and war, every effort should be expended to fit the man for his job so as to minimize the chance of a nervous or mental break-down.

We do not, therefore, regard occupational therapy in a narrow sense as merely providing an agreeable craft for an idle moment while a patient is in hospital. Our horizon is infinitely wider so that we regard habit formation and work therapy as the most important agents in preventing boredom and monotony, and in building up constructive useful lives which can be lived at a level of efficiency and consequent happiness.

Dr. Clarence B. Farrar, has recorded that William James in his discussion on 'Habit' summed it up in the following epigram: 'Sow an action, and you reap a habit; sow a habit, and you reap a character; sow a character, and you reap a destiny'. The following extract by the same distinguished author from the chapter on 'Habit' may also be quoted: 'Nothing we ever do is, in strict scientific literalness, wiped out. Of course this has its good side as well as its bad one. As we become permanent drunkards by so many separate drinks, so we become saints in the moral, and authorities and experts in the practical and scientific spheres, by so many acts and hours of work. Let no youth have any anxiety about the upshot of his education, whatever the line of it may be. If he keep faithfully busy each hour of the working day, he may safely leave the final result to itself. He can with perfect certainty count on waking up some fine morning, to find himself one of the competent ones of his generation, in whatever pursuit he may have singled out.'

We would suggest that the above-stated philosophy of work forms the core of healthy living.

REFERENCES

American Occupational Therapy Association (1960) *Occupational Therapy Reference Manual for Physicians*, Dubuque, Iowa.

Dunton, William R., Jn., and Licht, Sidney, eds. (1957) *Occupational Therapy: Principles and Practice*, 2nd ed., Springfield, Ill.

Farrar, Clarence B. (1958) *Portraits*, American Psychiatric Association, printed privately.

Henderson, D. K., and Thompson, A. G. W. (1925) Occupational Therapy, *J. ment. Sci.* **71**, 59.

James, William (1890) *Psychology*, New York Co.

Le Vesconte, H. P. (1961) Pioneer in Rehabilitation Medicine—William R. Dunton, Jn., *Amer. J. Psychiat.*, **117**, 751.

Meyer, Adolf (1952) The Philosophy of Occupational Therapy, in *Collected Papers*, Vol. IV, Baltimore.

Osler, Sir William (1910) *Aequanimitas*, Philadelphia.

21

RELATIONS OF PSYCHIATRY AND LAW

England and Wales, and Scotland

A Royal Commission was appointed in 1954, to inquire into the law in relation to mental illness and defect. The new Mental Health Acts (1959–1960) which have resulted are applicable both to England and Wales, and Scotland. They reflect the progressive trends which have been taking place, not only in the general administration of our hospitals, but also in regard to the admission of patients and to their care and treatment. The English Act differs from the Scottish one in certain minor particulars, which will be noted later, but they are in complete agreement on the broad principles on which the reforms have been based. These are:

1. To give the maximum encouragement to patients suffering from any form of mental illness or disability to seek treatment promptly and informally.

2. To ensure adequate restraint and safeguards where patients, in the interests of safety, must be compulsorily treated and detained.

It should be noted that the National Health Service Acts (1947) make the necessary provision for mental and nursing care and treatment whether carried out in hospital or at home. Every effort is being made to extend and improve the community services whereby the mental patient or mental defective can be successfully cared for without recourse to hospital treatment, or if that becomes necessary, then the period of residence should be of as short duration as possible. The purpose and policy of the Mental Health Acts and of the National Health Service Act is to effect an integration so that harmonious working relationships can be established between them. The local health authority, in the case of mentally disordered persons, may—and, if so directed, should—carry out certain functions for the prevention of illness, and after-care:

1. the provision of residential accommodation, and the care of persons resident therein;

2. the exercise of functions in respect of persons under guardianship, and the supervision of mental defectives not in hospital or subject to guardianship;

3. the ascertainment of mental deficiency in persons not of school age (education authorities have already a statutory duty in respect of children of school age);

4. the appointment of mental health officers to carry out duties relating to compulsory detention and guardianship; and

5. ancillary and supplementary services.

In addition to the above, it is the duty of the local authority to provide suitable training and occupation for children under sixteen years of age who are unsuitable for education or training in a special school, and for mental defectives over

16 years of age. Provisions are also incorporated whereby the local authority can arrange for visits to mentally disordered persons while in hospital. It is also laid down that there should be complete co-operation between education authorities and the local health authority. Such an arrangement is particularly necessary in the development of occupation centres some of which might be made residential.

The Mental Health Act (England and Wales), 1959, repeals the Lunacy and Mental Treatment Acts, 1890 to 1930, and the Mental Deficiency Acts, 1913 to 1938. It effects a completely new orientation in relation to the classification and care and treatment of mentally disordered persons. For instance the statutory designation of mental, and mental deficiency hospitals is abolished, and any suitable hospital can admit mentally disordered patients. This, of course, does not mean that specialized psychiatric clinics and hospitals can be dispensed with, but it may lead to the quicker and more general development of psychiatric wards and clinics as part of general hospitals. Such informal admission of patients has already been in action in mental deficiency hospitals, and already 27,000 of the 60,000 in residence are on the same basis as any other hospital patients; about 70 per cent. of the new patients admitted in 1958 entered informally (Maclay, 1960).

The English Act recognizes 4 groups of mentally disordered patients: 1. Mentally ill; 2. Severely subnormal; 3. Subnormal; 4. Psychopathic.

These categories have been defined as follows:

1. 'Mental disorder' means mental illness, arrested or incomplete development of mind, psychopathic disorder, and any other disorder or disability of mind; and 'mentally disordered' shall be construed accordingly.
2. 'Severe subnormality' means a state of arrested or incomplete development of mind which includes subnormality of intelligence and is of such a nature or degree that the patient is incapable of living an independent life, or will be so incapable when of an age to do so.
3. 'Subnormality' means a state of arrested or incomplete development of mind (not amounting to severe subnormality) which includes subnormality of intelligence and is of a nature or degree which requires or is susceptible to medical treatment or other special care or training of the patient.
4. 'Psychopathic disorder' means a persistent disorder of mind (whether or not accompanied by subnormality of intelligence) which results in abnormally aggressive or seriously irresponsible conduct on the part of the patient, and requires, or is susceptible to, medical treatment.

It is further laid down by the Act that subnormal and psychopathic patients should not be compulsorily admitted to hospital over the age of 21 years except for a short period of observation or after conviction in the courts. They are, however, liable to compulsory admission under the age of 21 years, but unless admitted through the courts or considered dangerous they should not be detained beyond the age of 25 years.

The above regulations may prove most difficult to implement. There seems to be no particular point in attempting to differentiate closely between subnormality

2 M

and severe subnormality—the one shades into the other, it is a matter of degree which, for administrative purposes, could safely be left to the decision of the medical specialist.

The definition of the term 'psychopathic disorder' might have been phrased much more in keeping with its clinical symptoms. We would suggest that it is not necessarily 'a persistent disorder of mind'. If it were so, then the last part of the definition suggesting that such a person 'requires or is susceptible to medical treatment' becomes superfluous. We have no accurate knowledge of how or why a psychopathic personality is determined, or how much is due to innate constitutional factors as compared with acquired characteristics of a multiple nature derived from a variety of personal, social and economic causes. In the absence of such knowledge it is perhaps a little presumptuous to speak in terms of 'persistence' or lack of it. From our own personal experience we can remember a considerable number of psychopathic persons who have made reasonably good readjustments. The definition also makes use of qualifying terms, e.g. 'abnormally aggressive' or 'seriously irresponsible'. Such qualifications are open to much argument and are likely to lead to endless difficulty, especially in the law courts. We prefer to think of psychopathic states as inclusive of persons who conform to a certain intellectual standard, sometimes high, sometimes approaching intellectual subnormality, but yet not amounting to it, who throughout their lives have exhibited disorders of conduct of an antisocial or asocial nature, usually of a recurrent or episodic type, which, in many instances, have proved difficult to influence by social, personal or medical measures.

Furthermore, the introduction of an age basis during which the compulsory treatment of the subnormal and the psychopath must be carried out—under 21 years and not beyond 25 years—is an assumption of knowledge and an attempt at certainty which is hardly justifiable.

The Board of Control of England and Wales which formerly was the responsible supervisory body concerned with mental illness and deficiency has been dissolved, and its duties have become merged in the work of the Ministry of Health, and in Mental Health Review Tribunals consisting of legal, medical and other members who will consider applications from patients or their relatives, for release from hospital. There will be one Tribunal for each of the fifteen Hospital Regions. The members in each region will be drawn from three panels, one of legal members, one of medical members, and one of other members of relevant experience. The extent to which those Tribunals will be used, and their exact procedure remains to be seen (Maclay). We are inclined to think that the term 'Tribunal' is unfortunate—it smacks more of a court-martial or of criminal proceedings than of the beneficent purpose for which it has been introduced.

The Mental Health (Scotland) Act, 1960, appears to have had the skill to evade some of the unnecessary complications of the English Act which we have drawn attention to. It repeals the Lunacy (Scotland) Acts 1857 to 1914 and the Mental Deficiency (Scotland) Acts 1913 to 1940. It provides that patients may, in future, be treated in hospitals or nursing homes for mental disorder without any formality, and makes new provision for those cases in which use of compulsory powers may be necessary, specifying the circumstances in which mentally disordered persons (including those involved in criminal proceedings) may be detained in hospital or placed under guardianship. It sets up a Mental Welfare Commission (in place of the General Board of Control) for Scotland to exercise protective functions in respect of mentally disordered persons who may be unable to protect themselves or their interests, and makes other provision for the protection of patients and their property. The Board will include, at least, two medical practitioners amongs its members of whom there are to be not fewer than five, and not more than seven. The Act makes minor amendments to the National Health Service (Scotland) Act, 1947, and other Acts relating to care and treatment and services that may be provided by local authorities for persons suffering from mental disorder. It provides for the registration of private hospitals and residential homes for persons suffering from mental disorder. For instance 'State Hospitals' replace the provision in the Mental Deficiency and Lunacy (Scotland) Act, 1913, for State institutions, and in the Criminal Justice (Scotland) Act, 1949, for State Mental Hospitals. The 'State Hospitals' are for patients requiring treatment under conditions of special security on account of their dangerous, violent or criminal propensities.

Mental disorder is used in the Act as a general term to cover mental illness and mental deficiency however caused or manifested. These are the only categories referred to, and thus the questionable differentiations detailed in the English Act are avoided.

In those cases in which compulsion may be required for admission to hospital the application must receive the approval of the Sheriff as has heretofore been the case. In England the judicial authority has now been abrogated. The application must be supported by two medical recommendations—one by a doctor approved by the Regional Hospital Board who has had special experience in the diagnosis and treatment of mental disorder, the other by the patient's general practitioner, or by another doctor with previous acquaintance of the patient. Apart from the above-mentioned differences the regulations governing the care of patients and their interests follow an almost identical pattern to those in England. When compulsion is required, the application and medical recommendations must state the form of the patient's disorder which warrants the detention of the patient in a hospital, and that the interests of the patient's health and safety or the protection of other persons cannot be secured otherwise than by such detention. The application may be made by the nearest relative of the patient or by a mental welfare officer; in the latter case, the nearest relative should have been consulted, previously, by the mental welfare officer except in cases involving unreasonable delay in making arrangements. The patient should have been seen within the period of fourteen days ending with the date of the application; the medical recommendations require to be given by practitioners who have personally seen the patient either together or at an interval of not more than seven days. The application shall be addressed to the managers of the hospital to which admission is sought, and shall specify the qualification of the applicant. In this respect certain *statutory prohibitions* must be complied with. For instance, a medical recommendation cannot be given by: 1. the applicant; 2. a partner of the applicant or of a practitioner by whom another medical recommendation is given for the purposes of the same application; 3. a person employed as an assistant by the applicant or by any such practitioner aforesaid; 4. a person who receives or has an interest in the receipt of any payments made on account of the maintenance of the patient; or 5. in the case of a private patient, by a practitioner on the staff of the hospital to which the patient is to be admitted.[1]

In cases of *emergency* the application may be made either by a mental welfare officer or by any relative of the patient. The patient can be detained for seven days in Scotland, and three days in England so as to provide time for the normal procedure to be effected.

Similar provision is made for application, founded on two medical recommendations, for reception of a patient into guardianship. The guardian may be a person or a local health authority. It is, however, specified that two classes of patient are not to be liable to admission to hospital or into guardianship under compulsion if they are over the age of 21 years. These are:

1. persons who, though mentally defective, are not so defective as to be unable to lead an independent life or to guard themselves against serious exploitation; and

2. mentally ill persons with a persistent disorder manifested only by abnormally aggressive or seriously irresponsible conduct. Such patients are to be discharged on reaching the age of 25 years, unless likely to act dangerously.

While, therefore, the Scottish Act does not mention psychopathic persons it subscribes to and adopts the definition given in the English Act which we have already criticized.

According to the English Act a patient who is compulsorily detained may apply to a Mental Health Review Tribunal within the period of six months since admission, or when he attains the age of 16 years, to have his case reconsidered. In Scotland the appeal may be made to the Sheriff of the County in which the patient resides, or to the Mental Welfare Commission which has a right to discharge a patient at any time, and a duty to do so in certain circumstances. The Commission will also be constantly available to hear and investigate any complaint of wrongful detention or improper treatment.

The foregoing is merely a general summary of the main changes which have been effected by the new Acts which now operate in Great Britain. For the detailed changes the respective Acts should be consulted.

In all cases in which a patient is advised to seek admission to a hospital or clinic either informally or under compulsion, the doctor has a highly important and serious responsibility. It is almost too easy to advise hospital care and treatment, and we strongly support the view that every other avenue should be explored before such a course is taken. No deception should ever be utilized: when admission to hospital is considered necessary the patient and his relatives should be fully informed regarding all the legal implications which may be involved. And it is advisable in cases of mental illness of whatsoever kind that

---

[1] Here the provisions of the Mental Health Act, 1959, have been quoted.

the doctor should keep detailed notes of the circumstances which led him to the opinion that hospital treatment was necessary. There are a number of cases who may prove to be unco-operative, and for whom compulsion might seem to be the only practicable method of providing adequate care and treatment, but social or economic or business circumstances may be such that attempts at compromise should be persevered with. There should, however, so as to avoid a disastrous occurrence, be no undue delay. The particular aims in employing compulsion are: 1. to protect the public from injury; 2. to protect the patient from self-injury; 3. to give treatment with a view to care or amelioration which cannot otherwise be given; and/or 4. to protect the patient from injury due to want of care. The prescribed forms require to be filled in with meticulous care, and with sufficient detail to satisfy the officials of the Ministry of Health (England and Wales) and the Sheriff of the County (Scotland) that all the regulations have been complied with, and that the patient's condition is such that hospital care is imperative.

A good general plan to follow is to describe the appearance of the patient, whether depressed, elated, excited, suspicious, antagonistic. Any abnormality of conduct should be noted, whether unduly talkative, restless, destructive, liable to self-injury; or mute, inactive, stereotyped in speech and action. It is important to describe any hallucinatory or delusional symptoms which may be present, and if possible to give a short verbatim statement of abnormal remarks uttered by the patient. If the patient's intellectual functions are involved, then attention should be drawn to memory impairment, facility, lack of insight and judgement, and the obvious necessity for hospital treatment. It is wiser to avoid a definite diagnosis; it may be wrong, or at least arguable, and is more an inference than a fact.

The reason for exercising so much care is because, at a later date, a person who has been compelled to accept hospital treatment may demand an examination by two independent medical men, and may seek compensation by an action of damages for unnecessary and wrongful treatment. The doctors, therefore, who have made the recommendation must be able to produce proof that they have acted in good faith, and with reasonable care.

The above-mentioned beneficial changes and improvements which have now been introduced into Great Britain were anticipated or forestalled by the Irish Acts, which deserve special consideration.

The Republic of Ireland

The Mental Treatment Act, 1945, may be said to have ushered in a new era in the care and treatment of mentally ill persons. It abolished judicial certification, and transferred complete responsibility for the care and treatment of mentally ill persons to the Minister of Health. That arrangement has proved eminently successful. The main provisions of the Act are as follows:

Reception Orders. An application for the reception and detention of a patient is made to an authorized medical practitioner. The applicant must be over the age of 21 years, and must have seen the patient within a period of fourteen days. The authorized medical practitioner shall, within twenty-four hours: 1. visit and examine the person to whom the application relates; and 2. shall either accept or reject the recommendation. If the patient is accepted for care and treatment then (*a*) the recommendation shall be dated and signed on the same day; (*b*) the recommendation shall contain a certificate stating that the person concerned is of unsound mind, is a proper person to be taken charge of and detained under care and treatment, and is unlikely to recover within six months from the date of such examination; (*c*) the facts as determined by the examiner, and as obtained from others require to be stated. The certificate should be acted on within fourteen days. When the resident medical superintendent or his deputy examines the patient at the local mental hospital he must decide whether the patient is suitable for care and treatment. If not suitable then a statement to that effect, with reasons for refusal, must be transmitted to the Minister of Health.

Temporary Reception Orders. A *temporary reception order* may be utilized in those cases in which the patient is likely to recover within six months or if he is an addict to drugs or intoxicants, and will require at least six months preventive and curative treatment. Temporary orders may be extended for a period not exceeding 18 months.

Voluntary Patients. The application for admission is directed to the medical officer in charge of the mental hospital, and must be supported by a recommendation from an authorized doctor.

Northern Ireland

The Mental Health Act (N.I.), 1948, has also effected many improvements, and has simplified and expedited the admission of mentally ill patients to hospital.

Judicial certification has been abolished and all admissions to a mental hospital are arranged on a voluntary or temporary basis.

Temporary Patients. In the case of *temporary patients* a written application is made to the medical superintendent of the mental hospital by a relative of the patient, or, when a relative is not available, by a welfare officer. The application requires the recommendation of one medical practitioner stating reasons why such treatment is considered necessary. The initial period of temporary treatment extends for not longer than twelve months. This period may be extended by application to the Northern Ireland Ministry of Health and Local Government by two further periods not exceeding six months each. In exceptional circumstances an additional extension may be obtained. When a person alleged to be suffering from mental illness is brought to a place of safety, or is not under proper control, or cruelly treated, a judicial order is required for his removal to a mental hospital, but the order requires the patient to be dealt with on a temporary basis. If the temporary patient is considered unlikely to recover, and if further care in the mental hospital is required, then a judicial order becomes necessary. But certification is effected while the patient is still in the mental hospital.

Addicts. Addicts can be dealt with on a temporary basis. They are defined as persons who: 1. by reason of their addiction to drugs or intoxicants are dangerous to themselves or others, or incapable of managing themselves, or their affairs, or of ordinary proper conduct; or 2. by reason of their addiction are in serious danger of mental disorder. The net appears to have been spread very wide; almost anyone might be caught in it.

Mentally Infirm. Elderly persons who are mentally unable to care for themselves or their affairs are specially provided for.

Mental Defectives. These patients are defined as persons requiring special care on account of arrested or incomplete development of mind whether arising from inherent causes or induced by disease or injury which renders them socially inefficient to such an extent that they require supervision, training or control in their own or the public interest. The responsibility for the ascertainment and community care of the mentally subnormal is vested in the Northern Ireland Hospital Authority.

LEGAL RESPONSIBILITY

Evidence

Mental disorder is usually a bar to the ability to give evidence. There are, however, occasions on which a mentally disordered person has been adjudged able to do so. It is a matter for the Judge to determine whether the individual in question understands the nature and obligations of an oath. Before he is sworn he may be examined, and evidence given of the state of his mind. If he is admitted as a witness it is for the jury to determine how much weight or importance should be given to his evidence. Before an affidavit (written evidence) is sworn there is a similar inquiry.

Contract

The general theory of contract is that there must be free and full consent of each of the contracting parties, and the consent must be an act of reason accompanied by due deliberation. A contract made by a person during a state of mental disorder is regarded as void. With the object, however, of preventing the mentally disordered person from benefiting from his act, he is required to make restitution to the other party if the latter has suffered. A contract made during a 'lucid' interval is as binding as if made by a person of sound mind. Patients compulsorily detained as a result of mental disorder are permitted to execute deeds and similar documents provided the responsible medical officer of the hospital in which they are certifies that the nature of the act is understood by the patient.

In the case of 'necessaries' there is an exception to the above general rule. 'Necessaries' are such articles as clothing, and whatever other articles the Court may decide in a particular case. They include, for instance, all expenses necessarily incurred in caring for the patient. An obligation rests upon the patient whether compulsorily detained or not to repay a person who has supplied necessaries to him, if such necessaries are suitable to his position in life. The same rule holds in the case of a contract made by a person under the influence of alcohol.

Marriage. Marriage is a type of contract. Marriage with a person who is mentally disordered is null and void, when it is proved in a court of law that either contracting party was unable to comprehend the nature, or to fulfil the physical conditions of the marriage contract. The incapacity must be such that the party was, at the time of the marriage, incapable either of understanding the nature of the contract, and the duties and responsibilities it creates, or of taking care of his own person or property. Only a modest degree of understanding is necessary to comprehend the marriage contract. Hence impairment or weakness of mind, as distinguished from mental illness, does not invalidate a marriage unless fraud by the other party is proved. A person who marries during his mental disorder may sue for divorce on his recovery; while he is mentally disordered he may not sue, but his friends may do so on his behalf.

Contract of Insurance and Suicide. The Suicide Act, 1961, abrogates in England and Wales the law whereby it was a crime for a person to commit suicide. If a person who has insured his life while sane, commits suicide as a result of becoming mentally ill or disordered, a contract of life insurance will stand, unless the policy contained a special clause designed to meet the contingency of suicide.

Supervention of Mental Disorder. Mental disorder supervening after a contract has been made does not release either party from his obligations under the contract, unless the nature of the mental disorder makes fulfilment impossible. For instance, mental disorder supervening after marriage does not *per se* entitle either party to a divorce or to a judicial separation. On the other hand, it is not a sufficient defence to proceedings for divorce or separation by the partner of the marriage on the ground of cruelty or misconduct, unless it can be shown that the mental disorder was such as to render the mentally disordered person incapable of appreciating the character and consequences of the acts which led the partner to seek divorce or separation, and unless it can be shown that the mental disorder is persistent, and not merely transitory or intermittent.

Torts. Torts consist of wrongs done to the person, reputation or estate of an individual, and render the offender liable under the civil but not under the criminal law. The chief forms are trespass, libel, slander, fraud, nuisance and negligence. A mentally disordered person is considered as incapable of committing a tort unless it can be shown, to the satisfaction of the court, that the mental disorder did not preclude the person from understanding the nature and probable consequence of the act complained of.

Receiver (England), Judicial Factor or Curator Bonis (Scotland)

A patient who has been compulsorily admitted to a mental hospital is deprived of his civil rights, and in consequence it is often of considerable importance to safeguard the management of his affairs. In England a 'receiver' may be appointed by a Judge in Lunacy upon application being made by the petitioner. In Scotland a *curator bonis* or judicial factor is appointed by petition to the Junior Lord Ordinary of the Court of Session. When the estate in question does not exceed £100 per annum the application may be made in the Sheriff Court. If the patient is not ill enough or is not so circumstanced as to require compulsory treatment and yet cannot or will not grant a Power of Attorney then the above procedure may be carried out by a statement to the effect that by reason of mental infirmity arising from disease or age the patient is incapable of managing his affairs. The petition may be presented by:

1. The nearest relative, failing whom, any party having an interest.
2. In Scotland there is also a duty on the local health authority to petition the Court for such an appointment wherever it seems to them that it ought to be made, and no other person (a relative or creditor) is taking the necessary action.
3. The patient himself, if capable of understanding the effect of his doing so.

In the latter case the patient usually prefers to grant a Power of Attorney. Two medical certificates are required to support the application. The certificate is given on Soul and Conscience, and in Scotland it is sufficient to state that the patient's mental state is such as to render him incapable of managing his affairs or of giving instructions to others for their management. This petition must be served on the patient unless it is considered injurious to his interests to do so. In addition the petition is intimated on the walls and in the Minute Book of the Court, and any person wishing to oppose it must do so within a statutory period of eight days. The Curator makes an inventory of the estate, and renders annual accounts to the Accountant of Court under whose supervision he acts.

In England and Wales the medical certificates are much more detailed and explanations must be given as to why such a course is necessary.

Certificate of Sanity

A certificate of sanity may be required in a variety of cases; for instance, a patient who has been compulsorily admitted may believe that there is no justification for his detention in a mental hospital, and may demand an examination by two independent medical men, whom he is at liberty to name. If, after examination, medical certificates are granted stating that the patient has recovered and the Ministry of Health or Mental Health Review Tribunal (England) or the Mental Welfare Commission or Sheriff (Scotland) approves then the patient may be discharged. If the Tribunal or Mental Welfare Commission are satisfied by their own examination that the patient is recovered, then his discharge can be effected. Eight days' notice in writing is given to the person at whose instance the patient is detained, or failing such, to the nearest relative.

When a patient who has been compulsorily detained has been discharged either as relieved or recovered, a certificate of sanity may be required as presumptive evidence of his capacity to make a will, or sign a legal document. Furthermore, certificates of sanity are required to rescind a curatory, or receivership. The patient may require to be seen on several occasions before such a certificate is granted.

Testamentary Capacity

The point in this matter is to determine, not whether the testator is sane or mentally disordered, but whether his mental capacity is adequate to the testamentary act. This matter was put very clearly by Lord Chief Justice

Cockburn in Banks *v.* Goodfellow, 1870, when he said:

'It is essential to the exercise of the powers of making a will that the testator shall understand the nature of the act and its effects; shall understand the extent of the property of which he is disposing; shall be able to comprehend and appreciate the claims to which he ought to give effect; and, with a view to the latter object, that no disorder of the mind shall poison the affections, pervert his sense of right, or prevent the exercise of his natural faculties; that no insane delusion shall influence his will in disposing of his property and bring about a disposal of it which, if the mind had been sound, would not have been made.'

He said further: 'No doubt when the fact that a testator has been subject to any insane delusion is established, a will should be regarded with great distrust, and every presumption should in the first instance be made against it. When an insane delusion has ever been shown to have existed it may be difficult to say whether the mental disorder may not possibly have extended beyond the particular form or instance in which it has manifested itself. It may be equally difficult to say how far the delusion may not have influenced the testator in the particular disposal of his property, and the presumption against a will made under such circumstances becomes additionally strong when the will is an inofficious one, that is to say, one in which natural affection and the claims of near relationship have been disregarded.'

It may be seen then that testamentary capacity can be interpreted within very wide limits, and that it may be consistent with mental disorder. Each case has to be decided on its merits, but there are certain points which the testator should be thoroughly cognizant of. He must be able at the time when he makes his will to recall and to keep clearly before his mind:

1. the nature and extent of his property;
2. the persons who will have claims upon his bounty; and
3. his judgement and will must be so unclouded and free as to enable him to determine the relative strength of these claims.

Furthermore, it is essential that a will, to maintain its validity, should be made by 'a person of full age and sound disposing mind, executed in due form'. 'A sound disposing mind' is not necessarily synonymous with perfect sanity, as there are persons who are mentally ill, who are compulsorily detained in a hospital, and yet are capable of making a satisfactory will. The most usual types of mental illness in which testamentary capacity may be questioned are those associated with the mental enfeeblement of old age, delusional states, delirium and other conditions in which the mind of the testator may be easily influenced, *e.g.* subnormality. In addition to any information and opinion we may have regarding the testator's appreciation of his act, the extent of his property, and the nature and effect of his act, it is advisable to inquire regarding the behaviour and conversation of the testator as known to his friends, relatives and business associates. His entire life history should be passed under review and especially his ability to transact business. The case of Thoms and Others *v.* Thoms' Trustee and Others (reported by Glaister) contains many instructive points; it shows how gross eccentricity may be combined with business acumen. The actual writing in the case of a holograph will, both from the point of view of expression and writing, may prove important. Spelling, tremors, ambiguous and involved statements have all to be taken into account. It should also be remembered that a person may be capable of making a simple will but not an involved one; it is only the actual will, however, which can be taken into account. In a case of physical disease it requires to be shown that there is a correlation between the physical and mental health leading to mental impairment. If the will can be proved not to be capricious or frivolous or venomous, even though it may appear so, but is really the expression of the person's real mind and intention, it should stand.

The same principles which govern the making of a will also hold good to enable it to be revoked.

It should be noted that in the judgment in Banks v. Goodfellow, quoted above, it has been held that the clauses must be read conjunctively and not disjunctively, *i.e.* 'no disorder of the mind shall poison the affections (and) that no insane delusion shall influence his will' (Mr. Justice Langton in Bohrman v. Bohrman).

The Matrimonial Causes Act, 1937 (England)

The Act applies equally to Scotland with one important exception in relation to voluntary patients, which will be noted in the appropriate place.

1. No petition for divorce shall be presented to the High Court unless at the date of the presentation of the petition three years have passed since the date of the marriage:

A judge of the High Court, however, may allow a petition to be presented before three years have passed on the ground that the case is one of exceptional hardship suffered by the petitioner, or of exceptional depravity on the part of the respondent.

2. A petition for divorce may be presented to the Court either by the husband or the wife on the ground that the respondent—

   (*a*) has since the celebration of the marriage committed adultery; or
   (*b*) has deserted the petitioner without cause for a period of at least three years immediately preceding the presentation of the petition; or
   (*c*) has since the celebration of the marriage treated the petitioner with cruelty; or
   (*d*) is incurably of unsound mind, and has been continually under care and treatment for a period of at least five years immediately preceding the presentation of the petition; and by the wife on the ground that her husband has since the celebration of the marriage, been guilty of rape, sodomy or bestiality.

3. It should be noted, however, that a patient who has been admitted, informally, to a mental hospital in Scotland cannot be divorced because of his insanity.

4. The following section shall be substituted for Section 178 of the principal Act:

   (*a*) On a petition for divorce it shall be the duty of the Court to inquire, so far as it reasonably can, into the facts alleged and whether there has

been any connivance or condonation on the part of the petitioner and
whether any collusion exists between the parties and also to inquire
into any countercharge which is made against the petitioner.

(*b*) If the Court is satisfied on the evidence that—

    (i) the case for the petition has been proved; and

    (ii) when the ground of the petition is adultery, the petitioner has not
in any manner been accessory to, or connived at, or condoned
the adultery, or where the ground of the petition is cruelty the
petitioner has not in any manner condoned the cruelty; and

    (iii) the petition is not presented or prosecuted in collusion with the
respondent or either of the respondents;

the Court shall pronounce a decree of divorce, but if the Court is not satisfied
with respect to any of the aforesaid matters, it shall dismiss the petition.

Provided that the Court shall not be bound to pronounce a decree of divorce it
may dismiss the petition if it finds that the petitioner has during the marriage been
guilty of adultery or if, in the opinion of the Court, the petitioner has been guilty—

    (*a*) of unreasonable delay in presenting or prosecuting the petition; or

    (*b*) of cruelty towards the other party to the marriage; or

    (*c*) where the ground of the petition is adultery or cruelty, of having without
reasonable excuse deserted, or having without reasonable excuse wilfully separated himself or herself from the other party before the
adultery or cruelty complained of; or

    (*d*) where the ground of the petition is adultery or mental disorder or
desertion, or such wilful neglect or misconduct as has condoned to
the adultery or mental disorder or desertion.

5. In addition to any other grounds on which a marriage is by law void or
voidable, a marriage shall be voidable on the ground—

    (*a*) that the marriage has not been consummated owing to the wilful refusal
of the respondent to consummate the marriage; or

    (*b*) that either party to the marriage was at the time of the marriage suffering
from mental disorder; or

    (*c*) that the respondent was at the time of the marriage suffering from
venereal disease in a communicable form; or

    (*d*) that the respondent was at the time of the marriage pregnant by some
other person other than the petitioner.

Provided that, in the cases specified in paragraphs (*b*), (*c*) and (*d*) of this sub-
section, the Court shall not grant a decree unless it is satisfied—

    (i) that the petitioner was at the time of the marriage ignorant of the facts
alleged;

    (ii) that proceedings were instituted within a year from the date of the
marriage; and

    (iii) that marital intercourse with the consent of the petitioner has not taken
place since the discovery by the petitioner of the existence of the
grounds for a decree.

One of the first legal points that arose was the meaning of 'incurably of unsound mind'. The interpretation proved quite simple. It means irrecoverable by any means whatever—whether in the course of nature, or in consequence of mental treatment.

'Recoverable' means that degree of recovery which would enable the patient (respondent) to undertake again the ordinary responsibilities of marriage. It does not mean capable of improvement to the extent merely of being able to live outside of a mental hospital, or of being released from certificate while still being under some kind of supervision.

A very important point for the medical witness is what degree of certainty must attach to the statement that a patient is irrecoverable; must he be absolutely irrecoverable, as in the case of some of the organic dementias, or must recovery be only extremely improbable? Rulings in these cases show that the latter is the legal view. There must be a reasonable certainty that the patient will not recover, but it is not necessary to be able to say that recovery is utterly inconceivable. Thus where the case was one of chronic schizophrenic type of reaction and the chances were stated to be at least 30 to 1 against recovery, a decree was granted.

The medical problem of the prognosis after five years' continuous mental illness is an interesting one, and one of which few statistical studies appear to have been made. In organic dementias, once the diagnosis is definitely established, the problem is, of course, simple. A patient with an alcoholic or syphilitic or arteriosclerotic dementia, who has been detained in hospital for that reason for five years or more, may safely be regarded as incurable. A very rare case of recovery from long-standing epileptic type of dementia has been recorded, but this is so rare that for the purposes of this Act the knowledge of its occurrence could not influence the Judge.

The problem is more difficult with the chronic forms of manic depressive and schizophrenic illness, especially the former. Of the 'late recoveries' that have been recorded in the literature, most cases have been designated 'chronic mania'. The medical witness should therefore beware of emphasizing too greatly the impossibility of recovery in a case of this sort. Examples of recovery in chronic mania have been recorded after five or seven or even more years; but they are, of course, very rare, the aggregate of such cases being small anyhow.

Recovery from chronic depression, whether manic depressive or involutional in type, can be said to be very exceptional after five years; and this statement applies even more to the chronic schizophrenic reactions.

The introduction of leucotomy has produced an additional possibility of recovery even after many years of illness. The implications of this procedure with regard to the present Act have not yet been resolved.

The other matters connected with these Acts are mainly of a legal kind. 'Continuous detention' means that he must be uninterruptedly under care and control. Thus, if the patient be allowed home on leave for a few days this will invalidate subsequent proceedings. But if the sojourn outside of the mental hospital occurs under certain conditions of supervision, e.g. in a home run specially for mental invalids, as those conducted by the Mental After-Care

Committee, then this ranks as part of the continuous detention—provided at least that it is only for a short period.

CRIMINAL RESPONSIBILITY

The criminal responsibility of those offenders who are suffering from some degree of mental disorder has always been far from easy to assess, and has constituted a controversial problem which has led to much argument between doctors and lawyers. But the introduction of the Criminal Justice Act, 1949, the Homicide Act, 1957, and the Mental Health Act, 1959, have been instrumental in clarifying certain issues, and have led to greater unanimity of opinion. The result attained has been the development of a greater sense of social justice whereby more imaginativeness is being practised in relation to the rehabilitation and social adjustment of the individual; the reformatory aspect rather than the deterrent is in the ascendant. It is important that it should be so because prison and police statistics show that a significant increase of criminal conduct is occurring throughout every epoch of life, and every grade of society. We know that behaviour disorders may stem from a vast variety of sources, and when they involve the young—as they so frequently do—are a matter of grave concern to parents, teachers, doctors, social workers and to organizations such as special schools, approved schools, Borstals and occupational centres. The aim of everyone dealing with such matters is to organize specific methods of treatment so as to counteract, or at least minimize, those faulty and unhygienic reactions which so often lead to frustration, defeatism and dangerous antisocial over-compensation mechanisms. We suggest that in dealing with all such matters the same tactics should be employed as in all other branches of medical and social work—to prevent criminal conduct, and any accompanying mental disorder from developing, rather than to attempt the somewhat futile task of remedying it after it has become fully established. If we are to be successful it is important that the laws which govern us should keep in step with our ever-increasing knowledge of medical, legal and social practice. We have made considerable progress towards that goal, and the conformity of opinion between doctor and lawyer is ever so much closer than it used to be. The pioneer work of Dr. Edward Glover at the Institute for the Scientific Treatment of Delinquency has done much to bridge the gap between the professions; we may also hope, with confidence, that the recently established chair of Criminology at Cambridge University will provide a real stimulus to the study and understanding of the science of man whereby we may become more fully acquainted with the working of the psychobiological forces which so often influence human nature. It may be that with such advances it will soon become unnecessary to stress the different attitudes between doctors and lawyers which previously existed. It was suggested that the doctor's interest was centred in the individual, the lawyer's in the criminal act; the doctor thinks in terms of illness and disease, the lawyer is concerned with the protection of the public; the medical concept is of functions actuated by emotion, and determined by intrinsic factors operating at a subconscious level, the legal concept is of mind dominated by reason and free-will operating at a conscious level. The above differences are not nearly so irreconciliable as they might appear. It is generally agreed that there is no sharp dividing line between sanity and insanity, or perhaps better expressed between normality and abnormality or some degree of unsoundness of mind—the two shade into one another by imperceptible gradations. The degree of individual responsibility varies equally widely; no clear boundary can be drawn between responsibility and irresponsibility.

A considerable number of those who exhibit criminal conduct may suffer from some degree of mental disorder or defect, but the clinical form of the disorder differs in no way from that which may involve an ordinary member of the community. Sometimes the development of the disorder has been so insidious that warning signs of an approaching crisis have not been seriously considered and the criminal act itself may be the first tragic indication of abnormal brain functioning. In any case, however, in which the least suspicion of mental disorder has been aroused, it has become the almost routine practice to ask for a psychiatric examination and report; that refers not only to cases of serious crime, *e.g.* murder and dangerous assault, but also to minor crime, *e.g.* theft, housebreaking, fraud, sexual offences. This procedure has constituted a great advance, has stimulated research into causation and motivation, has led to greater differentiation in relation to treatment and punishment, and has shown the importance of effecting a correlation between the criminal act and the setting or background in which it occurs. If that is not done then the issue becomes prejudiced and the judgement both of the Court and the public may become distorted so that injustice may result. Sometimes it may seem that the criminal act was motiveless but there is always some reason—trivial though it may appear—which has set it in motion. Criminal behaviour is not a haphazard affair any more than mental disorder is; it is the expression of facets in the individual's personality which are more prominent or more easily provoked than in other people. Criminal behaviour, therefore, is much more than a mere symptom, it is a psychobiological reaction dependent on a person's particular make-up or constitution however that may have been determined. The criminal is not simply a wicked person who with purpose and malice attempts to injure others, but, like everyone else, he may be the victim of emotional storms and distorted ideas which dominate his behaviour so that he may act, temporarily, in an uncontrollable manner. It may be months or years before he comes to a full realization of his conduct. Dostoevsky has described in *Crime and Punishment* how nearly every criminal, at the moment of the crime, is subject to a collapse of reason and will power, exchanging them for an extraordinary childish heedlessness when judgement and caution are most indispensable. 'That eclipse of reason and failure of will attacked a man like an illness, developed gradually and reached its height shortly before the commission of the crime.' Wertham in his account (*Dark Legend*) of the Italian boy who committed matricide emphasizes the same aspect in the form of a katathymic crisis—an emotionally determined situation which may have developed gradually then crystallizes out in action, and may not be followed by insight for a long time afterwards.

In those cases in which a person on account of his disordered mental state is unable to understand the charge against him or instruct his defence, he cannot be tried. He is found insane 'in bar of trial'. Similarly, if the jury find that an accused person did the act charged but was insane at the time he may be 'acquitted because insane'. Under such circumstances he will be ordered to be detained in a State Hospital or such other hospital as, exceptionally, the Court may specify; the sanction of the Secretary of State will be necessary to effect transfer to another hospital, leave of absence, or discharge.

The plea of insanity in bar of trial has been extended to summary proceedings in the Sheriff Court. If the accused person is found to be insane, the sheriff may order his detention in a hospital without hearing evidence as to whether or not he committed the crime charged. It should be noted, however, that the Court does not accept mental deficiency as a plea in bar of trial or acquittal. If a person so affected is convicted, and if it is proved that he is a mental defective, the Court is empowered (but not required) to place him in a hospital for defectives.

The above-mentioned matters are of immense medico-legal importance and must be most scrupulously dealt with. It is the duty of the medical witness to assist the court to come to a fair judgement. He must be non-partisan, be able to speak as to the medical facts disclosed by his examination, and to avoid hypothesis unless in answer to the Judge. It may be necessary to examine the prisoner on several occasions, and to interview relatives or those likely to be able to supply pertinent information. The medical report should be phrased in non-technical language, or when technical terms are used they should be defined in a manner that both judge and jury can fully understand. It is always most important to explain to the accused who you are, why you have come to see him, and who has instructed you. In the first place, you must attempt to determine whether the prisoner's mental state is such that he is likely to understand the evidence, instruct counsel, and follow the court procedure. He should be asked to tell his story with as little interruption as possible, leading questions are best avoided, and to make your account as telling as possible examples of the prisoner's spontaneous statements should be incorporated. In the second place, as the result of your examination, you should be able to group together the salient features, and correlate them with the hereditary, constitutional and environmental factors which may have played a part in determining his action. If you have discovered reasons which appear to justify a mitigation of sentence, you should not hesitate to suggest to Counsel that a plea of diminished responsibility might be considered. Other general points which may be helpful to keep in mind are the following:

1. The criminal act is rarely the first indication of a disordered mental state. If the person has managed his life satisfactorily, up until the time of the criminal act, the presumption is that he is of sound mind.
2. Those prisoners who state that they have no memory of the criminal act of which they are accused should always be viewed with considerable suspicion especially when there is no previous history of amnesia; under such circumstances the excuse may be more an evasion than a reality.
3. The probability is that the accused may be suffering from some degree of

mental disorder if he (*a*) reports the matter to the police and gives himself up, (*b*) attempts suicide after the homicidal act, (*c*) commits the deed during daylight when he is sober, (*d*) attacks a person to whom he has been deeply devoted.

The current law in relation to cases of capital crime was formulated in 1843 and centred round the trial of a Glasgow man, McNaghten, a paranoiac who was tried in London for the wilful murder of Mr. Edward Drummond, the private secretary to Sir Robert Peel. McNaghten's history showed that, for many years, he had suffered from delusions of persecution as a result of which he had visited various countries in an attempt to escape from his persecutors. His complaints to his parents, and to public authorities, were unavailing, he became embittered, and so with the object of drawing attention to his case and of righting his supposed wrongs he devised a plan to kill Sir Robert Peel. He kept a watch on his house, and when he saw a man come out he shot Mr. Drummond under the mistaken belief that he was shooting Sir Robert Peel. At his trial McNaghten was most ably defended by Mr. Cockburn (afterwards Lord Chief Justice), who concluded his speech in the following terms: he did not bring forward this as a case of complete, but of partial insanity; of what a great French authority had denominated homicidal monomania. He trusted he had satisfied the jury, by the authorities he had quoted, that there existed such a disease as partial insanity, or homicidal monomania, in which the unhappy patient, acting under the influence of instinct, was led on by delusion to commit crime for which morally he could not be held responsible. Cockburn's plea was upheld and McNaghten was certified as of unsound mind and detained in a lunatic asylum.

The verdict in the above case created a great sensation and much controversy ensued. A few days after the trial the case was debated in the House of Lords by a number of distinguished law lords, *e.g.* the Lord Chancellor (Lyndhurst), Lord Brougham, Lord Cottenham and Lord Campbell. The opposing viewpoints were expressed by Lord Brougham and Lord Cottenham in the following extracts: Lord Brougham said: 'If the perpetrator knew what he was doing, if he had taken precautions to accomplish his purpose, if he knew at the time of doing the desperate act that it was forbidden by the law, that was his test of sanity; he cared not what judge gave another test, he should go to his grave in the belief that it was the real, sound and consistent test.'

On the other hand Lord Cottenham, with whose opinion the other judges concurred, 'thought it was impossible to listen to any doctrine which proposed to punish persons labouring under insane delusions. Their lordships could not mean to say that the man who was incapable of judging between right and wrong, of knowing whether an act were good or bad, ought to be made accountable for his actions. Such a man had not that within him which formed the foundation of accountability either from a moral or legal point of view. It appeared very strange that any persons should be labouring under a delusion and yet be aware that it was a delusion; in fact if they were aware of their state there could be no delusion.'

As a result of the difference of opinion which was expressed, the House of

2 N

Lords put certain specific questions to the judges in the hope that the position might be clarified. These questions were as follows:

1. What is the law respecting alleged crimes committed by persons afflicted with insane delusions in respect of one or more particular subjects or persons; as, for instance, where at the time of the commission of the alleged crime the accused knew he was acting contrary to law, but did the act complained of, with a view, under the influence of insane delusion, of redressing or revenging some supposed grievance or injury or of producing some supposed public benefit?

2. What are the proper questions to be submitted to a jury when a person afflicted with insane delusions respecting one or more particular subjects or persons is charged with the commission of a crime (murder, for instance) and insanity is set up as a defence?

3. In what terms ought the question to be left to the jury as to the prisoner's state of mind at the time when the act was committed?

4. If a person under an insane delusion as to existing facts commits an offence in consequence thereof, is he thereby excused?

There was also a fifth question, but it was essentially of a hypothetical nature and does not require to be discussed here.

The answers given, of which we shall state the gist, became known as the *McNaghten Rules* and are still operative in our courts of law. They are as follows:

1. If the accused person did the act complained of under the influence of an insane delusion, but with a view to redress or revenge some supposed grievance or injury, or to produce some public benefit, he was nevertheless punishable according to the nature of the crime committed, if he knew at the time of committing such a crime that he was acting contrary to law.

2. and 3. These two questions are the crux of the matter and were answered in in this way:

> Jurors ought to be told, in all cases, that every man is presumed to be sane, and to possess a sufficient degree of reason to be responsible for his crimes, until the contrary be proved to their satisfaction; and that to establish a defence on the ground of insanity *it must be clearly proved that at the time of the committing of the act the accused party was labouring under such a defect of reason from disease of the mind as not to know the nature and quality of the act he was doing; or if he did know it, that he did not know that he was doing what was wrong.*

4. The judges considered that if the delusion was only a partial delusion, and if otherwise the individual was not insane that he should be considered responsible for his act. They stated that if, under the influence of his delusion, he supposed another man to be attempting to take his life, and he killed that man, as he supposed in self-defence, he would be exempt from punishment. If, however, his delusion was that the deceased had inflicted a serious injury to his character and fortune, and he killed him in revenge, he would be liable to punishment.

According to that type of reasoning it would appear that one person can kill another with impunity, if he believes he is doing it in self-defence, but he can be sent to the gallows if he commit homicide in the belief that the victim was reading his thoughts, tampering with his genitals or spreading slanderous stories about him.

It is not surprising that medical and legal controversy should still persist in reference to the applicability of the McNaghten Rules to present-day psychiatric practice. A few opinions expressed by distinguished legal authorities are illuminating. Lord Brougham stated : 'Nobody is hardly ever really mad enough to be within the definition of madness laid down in the judges' answers.' Lord Coleridge, the Lord Chief Justice of England, in 1888 said: 'the judicial decisions on questions of insanity are bound by an old authority which, by the light of modern science, is altogether unsound and wrong'. At a later date he added: 'It was said by a legal authority, when he was a young man, that if a person was found guilty of murder he should be hanged whether he was insane or not, for if he was sane he deserved it, and if he was mad it was to him no harm.' That seemed to him to be a horrible doctrine, and he was glad that it was no longer held. Lord Blackburn stated that he had never been able to find an accurate definition of responsibility. 'You must take it that in every individual case you must look at the circumstances, and do the best you can to say whether it was the disease of the mind which was the cause of the crime or the party's criminal will.'

Another high legal authority, Sir James Fitzjames Stephen, although not concerned in the above controversy, expressed a view which is probably entirely consistent with present-day opinion. He said that 'the man's power of controlling his actions should be the test. The proposition which I have to maintain and explain is that if it is not it ought to be the law of England that no act is a crime if the person who does it is, at the time when it is done, prevented either by defective mental power, or by any disease affecting his mind from controlling his own conduct, unless the absence of the power to control has been produced by his own default.' For an even more succinct statement we would refer to the charge to the jury made by Lord Justice Clerk Inglis in 1863 when he said that if they were satisfied that the murderer was suffering from insane delusions at the time of the offence they did not need to inquire whether he knew right from wrong, or whether he knew what was murder in the eyes of the law, or what was a punishable act. In a strictly legal sense there is no insane criminal. The act of the insane, which in the sane would be criminal, lacks every element of crime.

As we review the matter anew we recognize that the McNaghten Rules smack of the ancient and medically out-of-date doctrine of the mental faculties, the mind being regarded as divided up into a series of independent compartments, the cognitive faculty being one of the large subdivisions. With this doctrine there flourished almost inevitably the belief in the existence of partial insanities in which one mental compartment and faculty was affected, and not any other; monomania, for instance, was freely translated as 'being insane on only one subject'. Medicine has now come to recognize that the mind is a whole, one and indivisible. There is no mental disorder, however partial, that does not have its reverberations throughout the rest of the affected mind. Consequently the purely intellectual criterion of responsibility falls to the ground, for the intellect as intellect may be unimpaired, but an emotional disturbance will alter, or impede, or nullify its effect on conduct. Conversely, intellectual defect means deficient emotional control. Allowance is now being made for all such well-known phenomena as the disordered ideation of the schizophrenic, post-hypnotic and epileptic automatisms, and the overwhelming influence of affective disorder, which may, for example, cause a depressed person to murder his children whom he loves, and whom he knows full well it is morally wrong to kill.

The practical issue is this, that whereas it is nominally required in the trial of a person pleading insanity in extenuation of the crime that evidence be taken bearing both on his general state of mind at the time of the commission of the crime, and on his particular knowledge of the moral nature of the act, it is to the latter—the knowledge of the criminal act—that attention is particularly or entirely devoted by the Court. Consequently it may happen that a person who, from a general survey of his mental state, was undoubtedly insane at the time of examination, is found sane in respect of the commission of the criminal act. It follows that a man can legally be hanged for murder, and yet be regarded by the same court as unfit to take care of himself or his property. It is, however, important to point out that in the application of the McNaghten Rules certain statutory medical inquiries can be utilized 'to bridge the gap . . . between the criteria of irresponsibility according to law and the medical criteria of insanity', so that insane persons, though they may sometimes be sentenced to death, are never executed. Such inquiries are held under Section 2 (4) of the Criminal Lunatics Act, 1884, which provides that when the Secretary of State is informed, by any means, that there is reason to believe that a person under sentence of death is insane, he shall appoint two or more legally qualified practitioners to examine such prisoner, and to inquire as to his insanity. If the medical men, or a majority of them, find he is insane, the Secretary of State may, if he thinks fit, direct the prisoner's removal to Broadmoor (the hospital for criminals suffering from mental disorder).

The prisoner, therefore, may be judged at his trial 'insane but worthy of punishment', only to be exempted while awaiting execution of his sentence. A case in point was that of Ronald True, who was tried at the Old Bailey, London, in May 1922. Justice McCardie, in his summing up, stated that all the doctors who had examined True considered that he was certifiably insane now and when the crime was committed, but the jury had to consider whether he was insane at the time of committing the offence within the meaning of the Criminal Law. Insanity, he said, from the medical point of view was one thing, and from the point of view of the Criminal Law was another. The jury found the prisoner guilty of 'wilful murder' and he was sentenced to death; the verdict was upheld by the Court of Criminal Appeal. It was then represented to the Home Secretary that True was insane, whereupon he called upon three experienced medical men to examine True, and to report. Their report was that he was an insane person who required care and treatment in Broadmoor on the ground of non-responsibility.

In England and Wales, the practice of holding an inquiry whenever there is anything to suggest that the prisoner may have been insane or mentally abnormal at the time of the crime or have become insane since his conviction has been used more frequently. For instance, 'if a plea of insanity is raised at the trial and rejected by the jury an inquiry is almost invariably held'. Furthermore, in cases where some mental abnormality is suspected, but not amounting to insanity, an inquiry can be instituted informally. The inquiry, whether statutory or extra-statutory, is normally held by three specialists. The panel usually includes the Medical Superintendent of Broadmoor and the Medical Commissioner of Prisons, the Director of Prison Medical Services or a person who has previously held one of these posts; the other person may be an independent consultant. They have access to all reports of the case, they are not bound by the McNaghten Rules but are free to consider all the medical aspects. In cases of minor abnormality it is their duty to report whether in their opinion the abnormality was associated with the crime. (Capital Punishment Report, 1949–1953.)

In Scotland there is no statutory obligation to hold a medical inquiry, but if there is any doubt about the prisoner's mental condition the Secretary of State appoints two Medical Commissioners with special psychiatric qualifications and experience to hold an inquiry.

Subnormality (Mental Deficiency)

In its relationship to criminal responsibility subnormality also poses many important and difficult questions which have never been adequately answered. It has been described as 'a condition of arrested or incomplete development of mind existing before the age of eighteen years whether arising from inherent causes or induced by disease or injury'. It therefore would appear to be the most serious catastrophe that can afflict one of God's creatures. It is something which is inherited or acquired through no fault of the person, it is much more incapacitating than any physical involvement, or even any mental illness which may develop from causes which are remediable. And yet the law has always been chary of making sufficient allowance for the disordered conduct of anyone so affected unless the condition is of so gross a nature that reason and judgement are in complete abeyance. The law presumes that a child under the age of 8 years cannot be guilty of any offence. A child between 8 and 14 is presumed to be incapable of criminal intent, although the presumption may be rebutted. But no statutory provision exists in relation to the criminal responsibility of adult subnormal persons of the feeble-minded class. Indeed many members of the medical and legal professions and of the public still believe that in such cases punishment might produce a salutary effect. Nothing could be further from the truth; a prison sentence, long or short, in such cases has no deterrent or remedial effect, it merely adds insult to injury, and is apt to create an increased hostility to society, and result in recidivism. We have knowledge of many tragic cases in which we have testified that the prisoner was a subnormal person but have been informed by counsel that such a plea was not a sufficient defence in bar of trial or sentence, and that the accused must be tried in a public court just like any other person accused of a criminal offence. In Scotland, fortunately, the usual practice, in murder cases, has been to reduce the charge from murder to culpable homicide, but in England and Wales it still remains possible that a death sentence may be passed; it is in such cases that the Home Secretary may recommend the exercise of the Prerogative of Mercy. Such procedure seems a travesty of human justice whereby mentally incapacitated persons, so affected from birth or early age, should be considered, legally, as capable of pleading to the charge against them, of instructing their defence, and of following the evidence in Court. As a concrete instance of what may happen we report the case of an unmarried woman, 24 years of age, who murdered her newly born child by inserting scissors or other sharp instrument into the mouth and throat of the child. The accused, when 7 years old, had been certified as a mentally defective person. At the time of her trial one of us (D. K. H.) found her to be a feeble-minded person with considerable intellectual and emotional impairment. As, however, she was regarded as 'merely feeble-minded' she was allowed to plead and was tried with all the awe-inspiring ceremony of the Criminal Court. It was in this case that the Lord Justice Clerk (Aitchison) made the scathing comment: 'If the law had kept pace with medical practice this prosecution would never have arisen. On the medical evidence this woman should never have been brought to trial.' That opinion may not have conformed to the letter of the law but it showed humanity and understanding.

It is on the basis of the above facts that we believe that a recasting of the criminal law in regard to the legal responsibility of subnormal persons is long overdue. We are glad to note that the Royal Commission on Capital Punishment (1949–1953) was of the same opinion and stated: 'We have no doubt that the law requires amendment.' It added, however, 'that mental deficiency, which is a failure of development of the intellectual faculties, is not necessarily a disease of the mind in the ordinary sense of the word, and is not therefore within the ambit of the McNaghten Rules'. In practice, however, the Commission admitted that the McNaghten Rules were often interpreted to include mental deficiency, but when that plea was rejected it was usually because the jury were not satisfied that the accused did not know the nature and quality of the act or did not know that it was wrong. The notorious Straffen case is cited as one in which a medical witness expressed the somewhat illogical opinion that the accused was labouring under a defect of reason but that it was 'not due to a disease of the mind'. We do not know of any more seriously affected mind than the one which has not developed, and never will develop, and that is why we are of the opinion that mentally defective persons who have committed serious criminal offences might well receive the benefit of the plea of diminished responsibility and after a period of observation in prison be transferred to the State Hospital, Rampton, in England, Carstairs in Scotland. When the sentence has been one of life imprisonment or for a fixed term of years, discharge should be effected with the consent of the Secretary of State. We would venture to suggest that persons who are so seriously affected are always, potentially, most dangerous, and in consequence approval of a return to social and family life should not be considered advisable until a sense of social responsibility has been consolidated.

Diminished Responsibility

The doctrine of diminished responsibility in cases of capital crime has for many years been the accepted practice of the Scottish Courts. When such a plea is introduced the charge may be reduced from murder to manslaughter or (in Scotland) to culpable homicide. That provision suggests a return to the concept of 'partial' responsibility, which is not, however, equated with a particular form of mental disorder, but with the presence of mitigating circumstances. The Report of the Royal Commission on Capital Punishment (1949–1953) refers to a memorandum submitted by the Crown Agent and Faculty of Advocates in which in 1867 in the case of *Dingwall* Lord Deas directed the jury to take note of the fact that the mental state of the prisoner might constitute an extenuating circumstance and that it was not beyond their province to find a verdict of culpable homicide. In 1923 the matter was formulated more fully in the case of *Rex v. Savage* by Lord Alness as follows: 'Formerly there were only two classes of prisoner, those who were completely responsible, and those who were completely irresponsible. Our law has now come to recognize in murder cases a third class, those who, while they may not merit the description of being insane, are nevertheless in such a condition as to reduce the quality of their act from murder to culpable homicide . . . there must be aberration or weakness of mind; there must be some form of mental unsoundness; there must be a state of mind bordering on, though not amounting to insanity; there must be a mind so affected that responsibility is diminished from full responsibility to partial responsibility; the prisoner in question must be only partially responsible for his action.' The above doctrine is now accepted by the High Court of Justiciary as part of the Common Law of Scotland: '. . . in the view of the Criminal Authorities it has worked satisfactorily and has the effect of preventing convictions of murder in the technical sense and consequent sentences of death where the prisoners are abnormal from a mental aspect, and tends greatly to the side of mercy'.

It is possible that the success of our Scottish practice has been instrumental in effecting its applicability to England by its inclusion into the Homicide Act, 1957. According to that Act it is stated: 'Where a person kills or is a party to the killing of another, he shall not be convicted of murder if he was suffering from such abnormality of mind (whether arising from a condition of arrested or retarded development of mind or any inherent causes or induced by disease or injury) as substantially impaired his mental responsibility for his acts and omissions in doing or being a party to the killing.' Under the above circumstances the verdict will be one of manslaughter and not of murder.

The interpretation of the type of case which should be included under the category of diminished responsibility is still a matter of considerable controversy. Many years may require to elapse before we can come to an absolute decision, and in the meantime we can only advise that each case must be determined on its individual merits irrespective of whether the predominating state is one of subnormality (mental deficiency), psychopathic personality, epilepsy, neurosis or other state in which a degree of abnormality of mind can be demonstrated. We would like to see the concept extended so that it might be made applicable, or at least be taken into careful consideration, not only in murder cases, but also where the offences have been of a minor nature, *e.g.* theft, sexual offences, assault, fire-raising and so on. The enlargement of our outlook in such directions might lead to much greater research into the causation and motivation of criminal conduct, and in that way foster a closer alliance between lawyer and doctor whose mutual aim, as has been stated previously, is to do everything possible to rehabilitate the individual compatible with the safety of the lieges.

Criminal Justice (Scotland) Act, 1949

The introduction of this Act, which is similar to the Criminal Justice Act (England and Wales), 1948, has resulted in many beneficial changes in dealing with offenders of all kinds and classes. The Act requires to be studied in detail by those interested in its application, but it is important to mention here those special parts concerned with offenders whose mental condition merits consideration.

Probation Orders requiring Treatment for Mental Condition. Where the Court is satisfied on the evidence of a medical practitioner who has knowledge and experience of mental disorders that the offender requires or is likely to benefit from treatment, it may make a probation order for a period not exceeding twelve months. The probationer may receive treatment as an in-patient or out-patient at an appropriate hospital, or under the direction of a registered medical practitioner.

The necessary arrangements for the reception and treatment of the patient should be made before the probation order is sanctioned. The medical practitioner under whose direction the probationer is being treated is allowed considerable discretion if special circumstances arise, *e.g.* if a surgical operation should become necessary. A probationer retains his right to refuse surgical, electrical or other treatment if the Court, in view of all the circumstances, is satisfied that the refusal is reasonable.

Orders for the Detention of Persons who are suffering from Mental Disorder. When a person is charged, summarily, in the Sheriff Court with an offence punishable with imprisonment and the Court is satisfied that he is mentally disordered he may be removed to an appropriate mental hospital. If he is regarded as a dangerous person, he may be removed to a State Mental Hospital.

Mental Defectives. Similar procedures to the above can be utilized in the case of those persons who are affected with mental deficiency (subnormality.) In those circumstances in which a mental defective is detained in a prison, remand home or other suitable place, he may be transferred to a hospital for defectives, or be placed under guardianship. Another possibility is that a person who may be liable to a term of imprisonment can be remanded in custody or placed on bail pending a medical examination and report.

Establishment of State Mental Hospitals. The Secretary of State may arrange that mentally disordered persons, who for precautionary reasons require strict custody, should be accommodated in a State Mental Hospital during Her Majesty's pleasure; those other mentally disordered persons who cannot be suitably cared for in a mental hospital can be transferred to a State Hospital.

The terms 'criminal lunatic' and 'criminal lunatic asylum' have been discarded, and replaced by 'state mental patient' and 'State Mental Hospital'. In Scotland the State Mental Hospital is under the aegis of the Mental Welfare Commission. If it is necessary, for judicial or medical reasons, mentally disordered persons in a State Hospital can be taken, under custody, to the appropriate place. Furthermore, a state mental patient may be transferred from Scotland to England and vice versa. Similar arrangements are in force in relation to mentally defective (subnormal) patients.

From what has been said it is obvious that the Criminal Justice Act has greatly facilitated the treatment of those offenders who, by reason of their mental state, are not considered suitable for prison treatment, and yet are not so seriously disordered as to be detained compulsorily. It is now possible for them to be admitted, informally, to a hospital for a period of twelve months. Some may discharge themselves in a lesser time, but others who realize the benefit they are receiving often remain for much longer.

Previous to the introduction of the Act a considerable number of dangerous, aggressive patients were cared for in the ordinary mental hospitals. This caused considerable anxiety both to the medical and nursing staff, and, there is no doubt, it is easier both for the patient and the staff of the hospital, that such cases be transferred to a more secure place.

Infanticide Act, 1938

The Courts have invariably dealt with a woman who has been convicted of the murder of her child under one year old with the greatest kindness and consideration. 'No woman has been executed for such an offence since 1849.' In all such cases allowance is made for all the mitigating circumstances which may be present. The statute states that, when a woman causes the death of her child under the age of 12 months, but that at the time of her act the balance of her mind was disturbed by reason of her not having fully recovered from the effect of giving birth, or by reason of the effect of lactation consequent upon the birth of her child, the verdict will be one of infanticide in lieu of murder.

The Infanticide Act does not apply to Scotland. In Scotland, under similar circumstances, the woman would be tried on a charge of culpable homicide.

As an indication of the leniency with which such cases are regarded the Royal Commission in its Report states that during the years 1923 to 1948, 602 women were tried for infanticide of whom 512 were convicted. 'Of these five were sentenced to penal servitude, 167 were sentenced to imprisonment or Borstal detention, 161 were bound over with a probation order, 165 were bound over on their own recognizances, and 14 were dealt with under the Mental Deficiency Acts.'

Homicide Act, 1957

This Act, which is applicable to the United Kingdom, introduces a new concept in regard to the trial and punishment of those persons who are accused of murder. It defines five categories of murder which alone carry the fixed penalty of death, subject to a possible reprieve on the recommendation of the Secretary of State. The categories are:

1. Murder committed in the course or furtherance of theft.
2. Murder by shooting or causing an explosion.
3. Murder in the course or for the purpose of resisting arrest.
4. Murder of a policeman in the course of duty or anyone assisting a policeman; and murder of a prison officer by a prisoner.
5. Two murders 'done on a different occasion'.

The Royal Commission on Capital Punishment had had this matter of defining degrees of murder very much in mind, and in order to get first-hand information they visited the United States where, in certain States, 'degrees of murder are an established institution'. The Commission, however, after a most exhaustive and penetrating inquiry, came to the conclusion that they could not recommend that such a system of categorization and delimitation of murder should be introduced into the United Kingdom.

The limitations of effecting such a differentiation of murder are at once evident when we note that murder by poisoning—a most deliberate and cruel form of causing death—and murder committed in the course of a sexual crime are not included in those offences which carry the death penalty.

But it has also been pointed out (*The Observer*, March 20, 1960) that the most odious types of murder are those connected with the strangulation of small children; but under the new Act these are no longer capital murders unless accompanied by theft or are double murders. Crimes of passion have, also, usually been deliberately planned and carried out. The case of the young college lecturer, Bernard Walden, who had been rejected by a 21-year-old student may be instanced. A week later he shot the girl and her male friend. The defence advanced the opinion that this was a case of diminished responsibility but the plea was unsuccessful.

These brief notes indicate some of the difficulties which may be experienced in carrying out the statutory obligations of the Homicide Act. A good many years may have to elapse before we can come to a proper and fair estimate of its advantages and disadvantages.

A further point of considerable importance is that a person under the age of 18 years at the time the offence was committed can neither be sentenced to death nor to life imprisonment. He will be sentenced to be detained during Her Majesty's pleasure under such conditions as the Secretary of State may direct.

Summary and Conclusions

We trust that the foregoing account of some of the mental aspects of criminal responsibility indicates clearly the steady development towards a more humanitarian outlook. Much has been accomplished: 1. to make the law more consistent with medical knowledge; 2. to train doctors in forensic psychiatry; 3. to balance more accurately the welfare of the individual with the safety of society; and 4. to educate the public so that crude, revengeful, primitive reactions may be replaced by more tolerant ones. Such an alteration in professional and lay opinion is, to a considerable extent, dependent on the greater realization that the germ of criminal conduct is deeply implanted in a person's constitution, develops insidiously and may exhibit malignant characteristics which cannot easily be eradicated. Retributory methods of punishment of a drastic, deterrent nature such as flogging, solitary confinement, penal servitude and the death penalty are, for the most part, out-moded. In their stead we are hoping that rehabilitation techniques based on a knowledge of the character and personality of the individual will provide more successful results. We must, however, consider all such matters realistically—there is no place for false sentiment or naïve optimism. Our common sense should tell us that the human material with which we are dealing is often loaded with imperfection and that we must be thankful for small mercies; for certain types of mentally abnormal persons, e.g. those of psychopathic disposition, who have been convicted of criminal conduct may remain as potentially dangerous persons all the days of their life. They may require to be safeguarded to a far greater extent than those frankly psychotic persons who are suffering from temporary disabilities from which they may make a good recovery. Indeed our experience has taught us to exercise the greatest care in forming a prognosis in relation to all those persons who have been diagnosed as belonging to the diminished responsibility category. A sentence of life imprisonment, in such cases, should mean what it says, unless a state of emotional stability and social responsibility has been reached so that mitigation of sentence and discharge can be recommended with confidence. It is quite impossible to predict how long such a process of readjustment may take. That is why we believe that in all such cases a strong argument can be advanced for the introduction into the statute books of an indeterminate sentence. Arbitrary time-limits of short or long duration are pure guess-work. A right of appeal, at a prescribed period, by or on behalf of the prisoner, would constitute a sufficient safeguard to prevent a sense of injustice. The above procedure would be in harmony with the practice we employ for those mentally incapacitated persons who are, compulsorily, detained in mental hospitals; discharge is not regarded as advisable unless they can fend adequately for themselves, or be looked after with safety by relatives or friends. Such a plan is really the application of the concept that individualization is the dominant truth of modern medical science whether applied to disease or crime; it is the realization of that fact which allows us to look forward to the future with greater optimism. Research into the science of man will become intensified and more specifically directed towards the possibility of creating states of psychobiological integration. Success in doing so will depend on our ability to see more deeply into the person's mind, to understand the instinctive and emotional forces which dominate conduct and on learning more about the action of those ancillary forms of treatment of a pharmacological and physical nature which have been proving so helpful. Mental disorder and criminal conduct have many things in common. They may stem from the same sources, start early in life, are susceptible to similar methods of investigation and are dealt with most successfully at a preventive rather than a curative level.

So far as the McNaghten Rules are concerned we believe that, in their day, they marked a great advance over the rough-and-ready legal procedure of earlier times. They stimulated discussion and argument which led to an elucidation of the many important principles involved. But now they have outlived their usefulness, and they no longer keep in step with medical knowledge, or even with well-informed legal or lay opinion. It has become evident that abnormal mental states—of which there are so many varieties—do not fit into rigid categories, and cannot be defined in terms of degrees of mental unsoundness. One person is not necessarily more mad than another. It follows, therefore, that to exonerate a person from a criminal act the issue must be widened so that something more than mere consciousness of the physical act, of knowing its 'nature and quality', or whether it was 'right or wrong' requires consideration. We believe that medically and legally in order to assess the matter fairly we should attempt to gauge as accurately as possible the circumstances under which the criminal act took place, the subjective, emotional and instinctive forces which seemed to blind the person to the suffering of the victim and the ensuing consequences to himself. If it can be conclusively shown that the accused is so mentally unsound, or so defective, or so abnormal that his criminal act has been determined by his diseased state, then we suggest that he should have the benefit of any doubt and be regarded as a sick man rather than a person who has acted with malice aforethought. Rules and formulae in determining culpability are both too easy and too unfair; the issue of life or death is much too serious to be settled by a formula or yardstick. We have always therefore been insistent in suggesting that the McNaghten Rules should be abrogated. In place of them we believe that a judge well versed and experienced in criminal procedure is eminently suited to sum up the salient features in the case so that the jury will be able to base their verdict on all the various aspects of the evidence, lay or medical, which has been put before them. The use of a formula may easily prevent a comprehensive summing up because the judge, witnesses and jury may become sidetracked in ethical and moral questions which are impossible to answer.

The Report of the Royal Commission on Capital Punishment supports our point of view. The Report states, categorically, that the test of responsibility laid down in England by the McNaghten Rules 'is so defective that the law on the subject ought to be changed'. As a possible alternative the Commission thought that, if the Rules were retained, they should be extended by the addition of the words: 'or was unable to prevent himself from committing it' (the criminal act). We can see no particular value in the suggested addendum—it might prove to be an added complication rather than a help. Neither recommendation, however, has been written into the Homicide Act, 1957, and we continue to accommodate ourselves to the McNaghten Rules as they were first formulated. We can only trust that the Courts will continue to interpret them in a liberal spirit.

The acceptance by the Court of the plea of diminished responsibility in cases of capital crime cuts into the McNaghten Rules to a significant extent. It has now been laid down by the Homicide Act, 1957, that no one shall be convicted of murder if he is suffering from such abnormality of mind as has substantially impaired his mental responsibility. Furthermore no person under the age of 18 years can be sentenced to death.

As a result of our experience with all such cases we venture to make the following recommendations:

1. More adequately trained psychiatrists should be encouraged to enter the prison medical service.

2. In addition to the State Hospitals such as Broadmoor (England), Carstairs (Scotland) we favour the establishment of psychiatric departments integrated within the prison system. Such departments might prove particularly valuable in the rehabilitation of those psychopathic and other abnormal persons who require much more security than the ordinary hospital provides; as an indication of what may be expected the Home Secretary on July 1, 1960, laid the foundation stone of Grendon Psychiatric Prison designed for the psychological treatment of crime.

3. The plea of diminished responsibility should be extended so that cases of a less serious character than that of murder would be included, *e.g.* assault, sexual offences.

4. The transfer of patients from State Hospitals to civil hospitals and vice versa should be simplified.

5. There should be no embargo on any forms of medical or surgical treatment which might prove helpful.

6. More liberal arrangements for the employment of prisoners in up-to-date workshops should be introduced.

7. The Probation Service should be greatly extended not only in preference to imprisonment, but also to facilitate parole and after-care in the case of the discharged prisoner.

8. Discharge of the mentally abnormal prisoner should be determined on the basis of social stability. An elastic scale of sentence might be devised, with minimum and maximum periods, but we believe that the introduction of an indeterminate sentence would be of immense value.

In previous editions of this textbook we attempted to give a survey of the laws governing the care and treatment of the mentally disordered in many other countries. Owing, however, to the many rapid and varied changes which are being effected throughout the civilized world, that task has now become impossible. The World Health Organization, Palais des Nations, Geneva, published, in 1955, a booklet entitled *Hospitalization of Mental Patients* which gives a comprehensive survey of the most recent enactments both in the United States of America and in Europe. Anyone desirous of detailed information should apply to the World Health Organization.

REFERENCES

Criminal Justice (Scotland) Act (1949) London, H.M.S.O.

East, W. Norwood (1936) *Medical Aspects of Crime*, London.

East, W. Norwood, and Hubert, W. H. de B. (1939) *The Psychological Treatment of Crime*, London, H.M.S.O.

Gibbens, T. C. N. (1956) Psychiatry and the Abnormal Offender, *Med.-leg. J. (Camb.)*, **24,** 142.

Henderson, David K. (1955) *Society and Criminal Conduct*, Edinburgh, Royal College of Physicians.

Homicide Act (1957) 5 & 6 Eliz. 2. Ch. 11, London, H.M.S.O.

Maclay, W. S. (1960) *Amer. J. Psychiat.*, **116,** 777.

Mental Health Act (1959) 7 & 8 Eliz. 2. Ch. 72, London, H.M.S.O.

Mental Health (Scotland) Act (1960) London, H.M.S.O.

Mercier, Charles (1905) *Criminal Responsibility*, Oxford.

Radzinowicz, L., and Turner, J. W. C., eds. (1944) *Mental Abnormality and Crime*, London.

Royal Commission on Capital Punishment, 1949–1953, London, H.M.S.O.

Tuke, D. H. (1892) *A Dictionary of Psychological Medicine*, London.

A SHORT BIBLIOGRAPHY

General Psychiatry

ARIETI, S. (Ed.) *American Handbook of Psychiatry*, 1959.
BLEULER, E. *Textbook of Psychiatry*, 1924.
BRAIN, W. R., and STRAUSS, E. B. *Recent Advances in Neurology and Neuropsychiatry*, 6th ed., 1955.
BUMKE, O. *Handbuch der Geisteskrankheiten*, 1928.
CAMERON, N. *The Psychology of Behavior Disorders*, 1947.
CLOUSTON, T. S. *Mental Diseases*, 6th ed., 1904.
CURRAN, D., and PARTRIDGE, M. *Psychological Medicine*, 4th ed., 1955.
JOURNAL OF MENTAL SCIENCE, *Recent Progress in Psychiatry*, Vol. I, 1944; Vol. II. 1950; Vol. III, 1959.
KRAEPELIN, E. *Psychiatrie*, 8th ed., 1913.
LIEF, A. (Ed.) *The Commonsense Psychiatry of Dr. Adolf Meyer*, 1948.
MAYER-GROSS, W., SLATER, E., and ROTH, M. *Clinical Psychiatry*, 2nd ed., 1960.
MEYER, ADOLF. *Collected Papers*, 1950.
NOYES, A. P., and KOLB, L. C. *Modern Clinical Psychiatry*, 5th ed., 1958.
TANNER, J. M. (Ed.) *Prospects in Psychiatric Research*, 1953.

History

ACKERKNECHT, E. H. *A Short History of Psychiatry*, 1959.
JONES, E. *Sigmund Freud: Life and Work*, 1953–1957.
TIFFANY, *Life of Dorothea Lynde Dix*, 1890.
TUKE, D. H. *A History of the Insane in the British Isles*, 1882.
TUKE, D. H. *A Dictionary of Psychological Medicine*, 1892.
ZILBOORG, G., and HENRY, G. W. *A History of Medical Psychology*, 1941.

Heredity

HARRIS, H. *Human Biochemical Genetics*, 1959.
KALLMANN, F. J. *Heredity in Health and Mental Disorder*, 1953.
LANGE, J. *Crime as Destiny*, 1931.
PENROSE, L. S. *The Biology of Mental Defect*, 1949.
SLATER, E., and SHIELDS, J. *Psychotic and Neurotic Illnesses in Twins*, 1953.

Constitution

EYSENCK, H. J. *Handbook of Abnormal Psychology*, 1960.
KRETSCHMER, E. *Physique and Character*, 2nd ed., 1936.
PARNELL, R. W. *Behaviour and Physique*, 1958.
SHELDON, W. H. *The Varieties of Human Physique*, 1940.

Physiology and Biochemistry

COBB, S. *Foundations of Neuropsychiatry*, 6th ed., 1958.
CUMINGS, J. N., and KREMER, M. (Eds.) *Biochemical Aspects of Neurological Disorders*, 1959.
ECCLES, J. C. *The Neurophysiological Basis of Mind*, 1953.
GELLHORN, E. *Physiological Foundations of Neurology and Psychiatry*, 1953.
MCILWAIN, H. *Biochemistry and the Central Nervous System*, 2nd ed., 1959.

Sexual Behaviour

ALLEN, C. *The Sexual Perversions and Abnormalities*, 2nd ed., 1949.
FORD, C. S., and BEACH, F. A. *Patterns of Sexual Behaviour*, 1951.

MEAD, M. *Male and Female*, 1949.
RADZINOWICZ, L. *Sexual Offences* (English Studies in Criminal Science), 1957.

Social Aspects

BROWN, J. A. C. *Social Psychology of Industry*, 1954.
EATON, J. W., and WEIL, R. J. *Culture and Mental Disorders*, 1955.
FARIS, R. E. L., and DUNHAM, H. W. *Mental Disorders in Urban Areas*, 1939.
HALLIDAY, J. L. *Psychosocial Medicine*, 1948.
HOLLINGSHEAD, A. B., and REDLICH, F. C. *Social Class and Mental Illness*, 1958.
JONES, K. *Lunacy, Law and Conscience, 1744-1845*, 1955.
LEMERT, E. M. *Social Pathology*, 1951.
MALZBERG, B., and LEE, E. S. *Migration and Mental Disease*, 1956.
STANTON, A. H., and SCHWARTZ, M. S. *The Mental Hospital*, 1954.
WOOTON, B. *Social Science and Social Pathology*, 1959.

Psychosomatic Medicine

ALEXANDER, F. *Psychosomatic Medicine*, 1952.
DUNBAR, F. *Emotions and Bodily Changes*, 4th ed., 1954.
TANNER, J. M. (Ed.). *Stress and Psychiatric Disorder*, 1960.
WOLFF, H. G. *Stress and Disease*, 1953.

Neuroses Examination

BELL, J. E. *Projective Techniques*, 1948.
BURT, C. *Mental and Scholastic Tests*, 2nd ed., 1947.
CRONBACH, L. J. *Essentials of Psychological Testing*, 1949.
WECHSLER, D. *Measurement of Adult Intelligence*, 3rd ed., 1944.

Psychoneuroses and Psychopathology

ABRAHAM, K. *Selected Papers on Psycho-analysis*, 1927.
ADLER, A. *Problems of Neurosis*, 1929.
DAVIS, D. R. *An Introduction to Psychopathology*, 1957.
DEJERINE, and GAUCKLER, *Les Psychonévroses*, 1911.
DEUTSCH, H. *The Psychology of Women*, 1946.
DUBOIS, P. *The Psychic Treatment of Nervous Disorders*, 1906.
FENICHEL, O. *The Psychoanalytic Theory of Neurosis*, 1945.
FREUD, S. The Standard Edition of the Complete Psychological Works, 1953.
HART, B. *Psychopathology*, 2nd ed., 1929.
HART, B. *The Psychology of Insanity*, 5th ed., 1957.
JANET, P. *The Major Symptoms of Hysteria*, 2nd ed., 1920.
JANET, P. *Psychological Healing*, 1925.
JONES, E. *Papers on Psycho-analysis*, 5th ed., 1948.
JONES, E. *Essays in Applied Psycho-analysis*, 1951.
JUNG, C. G. *Psychological Types*, 1923.
JUNG, C. G. *Two Essays on Analytical Psychology*, 1928.
KRETSCHMER, E. *A Textbook of Medical Psychology*, 2nd English ed., 1952.
MACCURDY, J. T. *The Psychology of Emotion*, 1925.
ROSS, T. A. *The Common Neuroses*, 2nd ed., 1937.
SUTTIE, I. D. *The Origins of Love and Hate*, 1935.

Manic-Depressive Psychoses

BELLAK, L. *Manic-Depressive Psychosis*, 1952.
HOCH, A. *Benign Stupors*, 1921.

HOCH, P. H., and ZUBIN, J. (Eds.) *Depression*, 1954.
KRAEPELIN, E. *Manic-Depressive Insanity and Paranoia*, 1921.

Schizophrenia
BELLAK, L. *Schizophrenia*, 1958.
BLEULER, E. *Dementia Praecox or the Group of Schizophrenias*, 1950.
JUNG, C. G. *The Psychology of Dementia Praecox*, 1936.
MEYER, A. *Collected Papers*, Vol. II, 1950.
RICHTER, D. (Ed.) *Schizophrenia—Somatic Aspects*, 1957.

Paranoid Psychoses
BLEULER, E. *Affektivität, Suggestibilität, Paranoia*, 1936.
MEYER, A. *Collected Papers*, Vol. II, 1950.

Alcoholism
JELLINEK, E. M. (Ed.) *Alcohol Addiction and Chronic Alcoholism*, 1958.
JELLINEK, E. M. *The Disease Concept of Alcoholism*, 1960.

Infection-Exhaustion States
BONHOEFFER, K. *Die Psychosen im Gefolge von akuten Infektionen*, 1910.

Epidemic Encephalitis
ECONOMO, C. VON. *Encephalitis Lethargica*, 1931.

Old Age
ANDERSON, W. F. *Care of the Elderly Sick in General Practice*, 1957.
CIBA FOUNDATION, *Colloquia on Ageing*, Vol. I, 1955.
KAPLAN, O. J. (Ed.) *Mental Disorders in Later Life*, 1945.

Epilepsy
HILL, D., and PARR, G. (Eds.) *Electroencephalography*, 1950.
HUGHLINGS JACKSON, J. *Selected Writings*, Vol. I, 1931.
PENFIELD W., and JASPER, H. *Epilepsy and the Functional Anatomy of the Human Brain*, 1954.

Psychopathic States
HENDERSON, D. K. *Psychopathic States*, 1939.
SCHNEIDER, K. *Psychopathic Personalities*, 1958.

Mental Deficiency
HILLIARD, L. T., and KIRMAN, B. H. *Mental Deficiency*, 1957.
O'CONNOR, N., and TIZARD, J. *The Social Problem of Mental Deficiency*, 1956.
TREDGOLD, R. F., and SODDY, K. *A Textbook of Mental Deficiency*, 9th ed., 1956.

War Neuroses
GILLESPIE, R. D. *Psychological Effects of War on Citizen and Soldier*, 1942.
GRINKER, R. R., and SPIEGEL, J. P. *Men under Stress*, 1945.

Psychiatry of Childhood
ALLEN, F. H. *Psychotherapy with Children*, 1942.
BOWLBY, J. *Maternal Care and Mental Health*, 2nd ed., 1952.
BURT, C. *The Young Delinquent*, 4th ed., 1957.
CAMERON, H. C. *The Nervous Child*, 5th ed., 1946.

2 o

FREUD, A. *The Psychoanalytic Treatment of Children*, 1946.
HEALY, W., and BRONNER, A. F. *New Light on Delinquency*, 1936.
KANNER, L. *Child Psychiatry*, 3rd ed., 1957.
KLEIN, M. *The Psychoanalysis of Children*, 3rd ed., 1949.
LEWIS, H. *Deprived Children*, 1954.
STOTT, D. H. *Delinquency and Human Nature*, 1950.

Treatment. (See also under Psychoneuroses)
BALINT, M. *The Doctor, His Patient, and the Illness*, 1957.
DIETHELM, O. *Treatment in Psychiatry*, 3rd ed., 1955.
FREEMAN, W., and WATTS, J. W. *Psychosurgery*, 2nd ed., 1950.
JONES, M. *Social Psychiatry*, 1952.
POWDERMAKER, F. B., and FRANK, J. D. *Group Psychotherapy*, 1953.
SARGANT, W., and SLATER, E. *Physical Methods of Treatment in Psychiatry*, 3rd ed., 1954.

Crime and Legal Aspects
EAST, N. *Society and the Criminal*, 1949.
EAST, N. (Ed.) *The Roots of Crime*, 1954.
GLOVER, E. *The Roots of Crime*, 1960.
MENTAL ABNORMALITY AND CRIME: English Studies in Criminal Science, Vol. II, 1944.

INDEX

PRINTED IN GREAT BRITAIN BY R. & R. CLARK, LTD., EDINBURGH